Lung Transplantation

This book provides a detailed account of the principles and practice of contemporary lung transplantation. An accomplished international team of contributing authors has provided the latest scientific developments and clinical knowledge based on their experience. The book covers the pulmonary vascular and parenchymal lung diseases that necessitate transplantation, together with all aspects of the multidisciplinary management of lung transplant patients. The volume concludes by looking at future developments in the treatment of advanced respiratory failure. The book is suitable for physicians, surgeons and nurses working in the field of lung transplantation. The interdisciplinary approach makes the publication of value to other specialists who contribute to lung transplantation, including those in haematology, radiology and psychology, as well as to pulmonary physicians who refer patients for transplantation. It will serve as a valuable source of reference and practical information for all those working in thoracic organ transplant units.

Nicholas Banner is a consultant physician at the Royal Brompton and Harefield NHS Trust, Harefield Hospital, and also an honorary senior lecturer at Imperial College London. He is the senior transplant physician at Harefield and has extensive experience in the care of patients both before and after heart or lung transplantation. His research interests include the medical aspects of transplantation. He is a Fellow of the Royal College of Physicians, London and of the European Society of Cardiology.

Julia Polak is Professor of Endocrine Pathology at Imperial College London and Director of the Imperial College Tissue Engineering and Regenerative Medicine Centre. In 1995 Julia underwent a heart and lung transplant at Harefield because of severe primary pulmonary hypertension. After her transplant she was able to return to full time research and changed the focus of her work to address the twin problems of lung transplantation: the lack of donor organs and the risk of organ rejection. In collaboration with Professor Larry Hench, she now leads a team of researchers investigating tissue repair and regeneration. She is a member of the Council of the Academy of Medical Sciences, a founder governor of the Tissue Engineering Society International and European Editor of *Tissue Engineering*.

Magdi Yacoub is British Heart Foundation Professor of Cardiothoracic Surgery and the Director of Research for the Harefield Heart Science Centre and Harefield Research Foundation. He founded the heart and lung transplant programs at Harefield Hospital and was Clinical Director for Transplantation at the Royal Brompton and Harefield NHS Trust for many years. His research interests include clinical transplantation, pulmonary hypertension, the scientific basis of organ transplantation and alternative ways of treating cardiac and respiratory failure including gene therapy and cell transplantation. He is a Fellow of the American College of Cardiology and of the Royal Society.

Lung Transplantation

Edited by

Nicholas R. Banner

Royal Brompton and Harefield NHS Trust and
National Heart and Lung Institute, Imperial College London

Julia M. Polak

Imperial College London

and

Magdi H. Yacoub

Harefield Research Foundation and Imperial College London

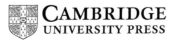

CAMBRIDGE
UNIVERSITY PRESS

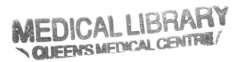

PUBLISHED BY THE PRESS SYNDICATE OF THE UNIVERSITY OF CAMBRIDGE
The Pitt Building, Trumpington Street, Cambridge, United Kingdom

CAMBRIDGE UNIVERSITY PRESS
The Edinburgh Building, Cambridge CB2 2RU, UK
40 West 20th Street, New York, NY 10011-4211, USA
477 Williamstown Road, Port Melbourne, VIC 3207, Australia
Ruiz de Alarcón 13, 28014 Madrid, Spain
Dock House, The Waterfront, Cape Town 8001, South Africa

http://www.cambridge.org

First published 2003

Printed in the United Kingdom at the University Press, Cambridge

Typefaces Utopia 8.5/12 pt and Dax   *System* LaTeX 2$_\varepsilon$ [TB]

A catalogue record for this book is available from the British Library

ISBN 0 521 65111 5 hardback

Every effort has been made in preparing this book to provide accurate and up-to-date information which is in accord with accepted standards and practice at the time of publication. Nevertheless, the authors, editors and publisher can make no warranties that the information contained herein is totally free from error, not least because clinical standards are constantly changing through research and regulation. The authors, editors and publisher therefore disclaim all liability for direct or consequential damages resulting from the use of material contained in this book. Readers are strongly advised to pay careful attention to information provided by the manufacturer of any drugs or equipment that they plan to use.

Contents

Contributors

Agnes M. Azimzadeh
Research Assistant
Department of Cardiothoracic Surgery
Vanderbilt University Medical Center
2986 The Vanderbilt Clinic
Nashville
TN 37323-5734
USA
Present address
   Assistant Professor of Surgery
   University of Maryland
   Cardiac Surgery N4W94
   22 South Greene St.
   Baltimore MD 21201-1595
   USA
   aazimadeh@smail.umaryland.edu

Nicholas R. Banner
Consultant in Cardiology and Transplant Medicine
Royal Brompton and Harefield NHS Trust
Harefield Hospital
Harefield
Middlesex
UB9 6JH
UK
n.banner@rbh.nthames.nhs.uk

Emma J. Birks
Specialist Registrar in Cardiology
Harefield Research Foundation
Harefield Hospital
Harefield
Middlesex
UBP 6JH
UK
ebirks@ic.ac.uk

Anne E. Bishop
Senior Lecturer
 Tissue Engineering and Regenerative Medicine Centre
Imperial College Faculty of Medicine
Chelsea and Westminster Hospital
369 Fulham Road
London
SW10 9NH
a.e.bishop@ic.ac.uk

Michael J. Boscoe
Consultant Anaesthetist
Harefield Hospital
Harefield
Middlesex
UB9 6JH
UK
m.boscoe@rbh.nthames.nhs.uk or boscoemj@aol.com

Michael Bristow
Professor of Medicine
Division of Cardiology
University of Colorado Health Sciences Center
University of Colorado
Health Science Center
4200 East 9th Avenue #C310
Denver
CO 80220–3706
USA

Margaret M. Burke
Consultant Histopathologist
Harefield Hospital
Harefield
Middlesex
UB9 6JH
UK
m.burke@rbh.nthames.nhs.uk

R. Jane Chambers
Consultant Radiologist
Harefield Hospital
Harefield
Middlesex
UB9 6JH
UK
jane.chambers@rbh.nthames.nhs.uk

Carlyne Cool
Assistant Professor
Department of Pathology
University of Colorado Health Sciences Center
University of Colorado
Health Science Center
4200 East 9th Avenue #C310
Denver
CO 80220–3706
USA

Paul A. Corris
Professor of Thoracic Medicine
The Freeman Hospital
High Heaton
Newcastle upon Tyne
NE7 7DN
UK
paul.corris@ncl.ac.uk

David Cummins
Consultant Haematologist
Harefield Hospital
Harefield
Middlesex
UB9 6JH
UK
d.cummins@rbh.nthames.nhs.uk

John Dark
Professor of Cardiothoracic Surgery
Regional Cardiothoracic Centre
The Freeman Hospital
Newcastle upon Tyne
NE7 7DN
UK
j.h.dark@ncl.ac.uk

R. M. du Bois
Professor of Respiratory Medicine
Royal Brompton Hospital
Sydney Street
London
SW3 6NP
UK
r.dubois@rbh.nthames.nhs.uk

William J. Federspiel
Department of Chemical Engineering, Departments of
    Surgery and Bioengineering
McGowan Institute of Regenerative Medicine
University of Pittsburgh
Pittsburgh PA 15219
USA
federspielwj@msx.upmc.edu

Juliet Foweraker
Consultant Microbiologist
Microbiology Laboratory
Papworth Hospital
Papworth Everard
Cambridgeshire
CB3 8RE
UK
juliet.foweraker@papworth-tr.anglox.nhs.uk

Shane J. George
Consultant in Anaesthesia and Intensive Care
Harefield Hospital
Harefield
Middlesex
UB9 6JH
UK
s.george@rbh.nthames.nhs.uk

Mark Geraci
Associate Professor
Division of Pulmonary Sciences and Critical Care
    Medicine
University of Colorado Health Sciences Center
University of Colarado
Health Science Center
4200 East 9th Avenue #C310
Denver
CO 80220–3706
USA

Allan R. Glanville
Associate Professor of Medicine
St Vincent's Hospital
Xavier 4
Victoria Street
Darlinghurst
Sydney
NSW 2010
Australia
aglanville@stvincents.com.au

Claire N. Hallas
Health Psychologist
Harefield Hospital
Harefield
Middlesex
UB9 6JH
UK
c.hallas@rbh.nthames.nhs.uk

Rachel Harrison
Research Fellow
Division of Medical Genetics
Adrian Building
University of Leicester
University Road
Leicester
LE1 7RH
reh17@le.ac.uk

Brack G. Hattler
Professor of Surgery
Artificial Lung Program
University of Pittsburgh
200 Lothrop Street
C-700
Pittsburgh
PA 15213
USA
Hattlerbg@msx.upmc.edu

Larry L. Hench
Professor of Materials
Centre for Tissue Regeneration and Repair
Imperial College of Science Technology and Medicine
Prince Consort Road
London
SW7 2BP
UK
l.hench@ic.ac.uk

Marshall I. Hertz
Professor of Pulmonary/Critical Care Medicine
Pulmonary Medicine/Lung Transplant Program
University of Minnesota
420 Delaware Street SE
276 Mayo Mail Room
Minneapolis
MN 55455
USA
hertz001@umn.edu

Margaret Hodson
Professor of Respiratory Medicine
Department of Cystic Fibrosis
Royal Brompton Hospital
Sydney Street
London
SW3 6NP
UK
s.hockley@ic.ac.uk

Duncan C. S. Hutchison
Consultant in Respiratory Medicine
King's College Hospital
Denmark Hill
London
SE5 9RS
UK
dhutchison@arlingtonave.demon.co.uk

Ian V. Hutchinson
Professor of Immunology
Manchester University
Oxford Road
Manchester
M13 9PL
UK
ian.hutchinson@man.ac.uk

Julian R. Jones
Research Associate
Department of Materials
Imperial College of Science Technology and Medicine
Prince Consort Road
London
SW7 2BP
UK

Mary T. Keogan
Consultant Immunologist
Papworth Hospital
Papworth Everard
Cambridge
CB3 8RE
UK
Present address
  Consultant Immunologist
  Beaumont Hospital
  Department of Immunology
  Beaumont Road
  Dublin 9
  Ireland
  mary.keogan@beaumont.ie

A. Khaghani
Clinical Director of Transplantation
Harefield Hospital
Harefield
Middlesex
UB9 6JH
UK
a.khaghani@rbh.nthames.nhs.uk

Rubia F. S. Lenza
Research Associate
Federal University of Minas Gerais
Department of Metallurgical and Materials Engineering
Rua Espirito Santo, 35–200 Andar
30160–030 Belo Horizonte
MG
Brazil

Haifa Lyster
Transplant Pharmacist
Harefield Hospital
Harefield
Middlesex
UB9 6JH
UK
h.lyster@rbh.nthames.nhs.uk

Janet R. Maurer
Medical Director
LIFESOURCE Transplant Network
CIGNA HealthCare
900 Cottage Grove Road
Bloomfield
CT
USA
Janet.Maurer@CIGNA.com

Keith McNeil
Consultant Physician
Papworth Hospital
Papworth Everard
Cambridge
CB3 8RE
UK
Present address
  Department of Thoracic Medicine
  Prince Charles Hospital
  Rode Road
  Chermside
  Brisbane
  Queensland 4032
  Australia
  keith_mcneil@health.qld.gov.au

Richard N. Pierson III
Associate Professor of Surgery
Department of Cardiothoracic Surgery
Vanderbilt University Medical Centre
2986 The Vanderbilt Clinic
Nashville
TN 37232–5734
USA
Present address
    Associate Professor of Surgery
    University of Maryland
    Cardiac Surgery N4 W94
    22 South Greene St.
    Baltimore
    MD 21201-1595
    USA
    rpierson@smail.umaryland.edu

Julia M. Polak
Professor of Endocrine Pathology
Tissue Engineering and Regenerative
    Medicine Centre
Imperial College Faculty of Medicine
Chelsea and Westminster Hospital
369 Fulham Road
London
SW10 9NH
UK
julia.polak@ic.ac.uk or s.lock@ic.ac.uk

Robert Quaife
Assistant Professor
Division of Cardiology
University of Colorado Health Sciences Center
University of Colorado
Health Science Center
4200 East 9th Avenue #C310
Denver
CO 80220–3706
USA

Rosemary Radley-Smith
Consultant Paediatric Cardiologist
Harefield Hospital
Harefield
Middlesex
UB9 6JH
UK
j.henning@rbh.nthames.nhs.uk

Stuart Rich
Professor of Medicine and Director
Center for Pulmonary Heart Disease
Rush Presbyterian St Luke's Medical Center
1725 West Harrison Street
Suite 020
Chicago
IL 60612
USA
PPH@rush.edu

Marlene Rose
Professor of Immunology
Harefield Hospital
Harefield
Middlesex
UB9 6JH
UK
marlene.rose@ic.ac.uk

Carsten Schroeder
Research Fellow
Department of Cardiothoracic Surgery
Vanderbilt University Medical Center
2986 The Vanderbilt Clinic
Nashville
TN 37232–5734
USA
Present address
    University of Maryland
    Cardiac Surgery
    22 South Greene St.
    Baltimore
    MD 21201-1595
    cshroeder@smail.umaryland.edu

Gordon L. Snider
Professor of Medicine
Boston University School of Medicine
VA Boston Healthcare System (111RmB9–74)
150 South Huntington Avenue
Boston
MA 02130
USA
Gordon.Snider@med.va.gov

Susan Stewart
Consultant Histopathologist
Department of Histopathology
Papworth Hospital
Papworth Everard
Cambridge
CB3 8RE
UK
susan.stewart@papworth-tr.anglox.nhs.uk

Richard C. Trembath
Professor of Medical Genetics
Division of Medical Genetics
Departments of Medicine and Genetics
Adrian Building
University of Leicester
University Road
Leicester
LE1 7RH
UK
rtrembath@hgmp.mrc.ac.uk

Rubin M. Tuder
Associate Professor of Pathology and Director of
    Cardiopulmonary Pathology
Department of Pathology
Johns Hopkins Medical School
Ross Research Building, Room 519B
Baltimore
Maryland 21205
USA

Wander L. V. Vasconcelos
Professor
Federal University of Minas Gerais
Department of Metallurgical and Materials Engineering
Rua Espirito Santo, 35–200 Andar
30160–030 Belo Horizonte
MG
Brazil

Norbert F. Voelkel
Professor of Emphysema Research and Director of the
    Pulmonary Hypertension Center
Pulmonary Sciences and Critical Care Medicine
University of Colorado
Health Sciences Centre
4200 East 9th Avenue
Box C272
Denver
Colorado 80262
USA
norbert.voelkel@uchsc.edu

Jo Wray
Health Psychologist
Harefield Hospital
Harefield
Middlesex
UB9 6JH
UK
j.wray@rbh.ivthames.nhs.uk

Tim Wreghitt
Consultant Virologist and Director
Addenbrookes Hospital
Clinical Microbiology and Public Health Laboratory
Box 236 Hills Road
Cambridge
CB2 2QW
UK
tim.wreghitt@msexc.addenbrookes.anglox.nhs.uk

Magdi H. Yacoub
Professor and Director of the Harefield
    Research Foundation
Heart Science Centre
Harefield Hospital
Harefield
Middlesex
UB9 6JH
UK
m.yacoub@ic.ac.uk

Preface

Organ transplantation has been one of the major medical achievements of the twentieth century. Transplants have saved the lives of countless patients with failure of one, or more, of their vital organs and have returned most to a happy and productive existence. The lung proved to be one of the most difficult organs to transplant and clinically successful lung transplantation was first achieved two decades after the first renal allografts were performed. The results of lung transplantation have steadily improved and the procedure is now accepted as a standard therapy for patients with advanced parenchymal or vascular pulmonary disease. This success has produced a growing population of lung transplant recipients but has also highlighted the problems and limitations of lung transplantation that now represent challenges for the twenty-first century.

Currently, the potential long-term benefits of lung transplantation are reduced by the frequent occurrence of bronchiolitis obliterans, which leads to progressive dysfunction of the pulmonary allograft and eventually to respiratory failure. Our understanding of the pathogenesis of this condition remains limited but there is some hope that newer approaches to pharmacological immunosuppression, including the use of drugs with antiproliferative properties, together with more effective prophylaxis against infection may reduce the impact of this condition. The burden of long-term pharmacological immunosuppression (infection and malignancy), as well as side effects of individual immunosuppressive drugs, are other important problems faced by transplant recipients. Progress has been made in this area through the more effective use of drug combinations to minimize the side effects of individual agents, the introduction of agents with better side effect profiles, and prophylaxis against some specific complications, such as infection with *Pneumocystis* or cytomegalovirus and against corticosteroid-related osteoporosis. In the longer term, however, it is to be hoped that our growing understanding of transplant immunology will provide methods of producing immunosuppression that are specific for the allograft without the need for continuing drug therapy.

The number of lung transplant operations that can be performed is now limited by availability of donor lungs that are suitable for transplantation; there is an urgent need for effective alternative medical and surgical treatments for the conditions that currently require transplantation. Recently, significant progress has been made both in our understanding of the pathogenesis of pulmonary hypertension and in its medical treatment. It is to be hoped that scientific progress in other areas of pulmonary disease will lead to new therapeutic approaches for these conditions as well. Nevertheless, there is likely to be a continuing need for 'pulmonary replacement' therapy for the foreseeable future. New approaches such as the development of an artifical lung to bridge patients to transplantation may lead to technology that will become a long-term alternative to transplantation. In the future, growth of replacement organs using the techniques of molecular and developmental biology together with tissue engineering may provide alternative sources of lungs for transplantation. The use of genetically modified xenotransplants may provide another route to this goal if the concerns about safety can be addressed adequately.

Lung transplantation is a complex endeavour that requires the cooperation of physicians, surgeons and scientists working in many different fields. The care and assessment of the patient before surgery can have a profound effect on the outcome of transplantation and a successful programme must integrate all stages and aspects of the patient's care. In this book, we have gathered contributions from specialists working in many of the fields that contribute to a lung transplant programme; they have produced a comprehensive account of contemporary lung transplantation. The first section addresses specific aspects of the medical conditions that commonly necessitate transplantation; this highlights some recent advances and issues that are of particular importance from the transplant perspective. The second section provides a detailed and systematic account of the various aspects of transplantation. The final section looks at some of the directions that 'pulmonary replacement' therapy may take in the future.

The contributors come from Europe, North America and Australia and they have provided a 'state of the art' description of this rapidly developing field. Evidence to determine the optimum practice in some aspects of lung transplantation is lacking or equivocal. Consequently, there are significant variations in clinical practice between institutions; whenever possible, these have been highlighted by individual authors or by differing perspectives between authors. We believe that this book will be of value to those working in all aspects of lung transplantation as well as to pulmonary specialists and family physicians who either refer patients as potential candidates for transplantation or who cooperate with a transplant centre in providing long-term care for transplant recipients.

We offer our heartfelt thanks to the friends and colleagues who have contributed to this book. In addition we would like to acknowledge Peter Silver, Athena Horsten, Sandi Irvine and Lucille Murby at Cambridge University Press for their excellent support and guidance throughout the project. We thank Joan Green and Sandra Lock for their help with the management of the manuscripts and the authors as well as of the editors! Finally, we must thank our families who have supported and encouraged us throughout this project and in our many other professional endeavours.

Nicholas R. Banner
Julia M. Polak
Magdi H. Yacoub

Harefield and London

Editorial note

For consistency, the recommended international nonproprietary names of drugs have been used. These some times differ from those that have been used in many countries e.g. ciclosporin is used here rather than cyclosporin or cyclosporine.

Part 1

Pulmonary disease

Primary pulmonary hypertension: pathophysiology and therapy

Stuart Rich

Rush Medical College, Chicago, Illinois, USA

Introduction

Primary pulmonary hypertension (PPH) is a progressive and fatal disease, whose pathobiology has been elusive. It is clear, however, that the initial explanations that this was a disease of vasoconstriction of the pulmonary vasculature was a gross oversimplification of the biological mechanisms that are involved [1]. With our better understanding of vascular biology and the various mediators involved in the regulation of vascular tone and growth, we now realize that a number of pathways may be involved in what we call PPH, and that many different cell types within the arteries may be implicated in the aetiology. For example, some have suggested that an abnormality in the endothelium can account for the changes that are noted in both the intima and media [2]. However, it is also possible that a primary abnormality of the pulmonary artery smooth muscle cell or the extracellular matrix may be causative in this disease. Given the heterogeneous nature of the pathological changes that have been described in patients with primary and secondary forms of pulmonary arterial hypertension, it is likely that more than one abnormality is playing a key role [3,4]. Nonetheless, over recent years in treating patients with PPH there has been considerable progress that has arisen from our attempts to understand the pathogenesis of the disease.

The genetic basis of primary pulmonary hypertension

A familial pattern of disease transmission for PPH has been well characterized. Recently, the gene for familial PPH, known as *PPH-1*, has been described [5]. It is autosomal dominant with markedly reduced penetrance, and is located on chromosome 2q33 (Chapter 2). Using a positional candidate approach it has been shown that a mutation in the gene for bone morphogenic protein receptor 2 (*BMPR2*) is responsible. BMPs fall within the super family of transforming growth factor beta (TGF-β) receptors, and have been shown to regulate a diverse number of biological processes including cell differentiation, proliferation, apoptosis and morphogenesis [6]. The precise way that this defect causes PPH remains unclear, and it may be that the presence of either an exogenous risk factor (such as the fenfluramines) or a second genetic abnormality is necessary to induce the disease. Of particular interest is that these genetic mutations have also recently been described in 25% of patients with 'sporadic' PPH [7].

The rationale behind vasodilator therapy

In nearly all pathological series on PPH, varying degrees of medial hypertrophy exist that have been interpreted to be an expression of underlying vasoconstriction [3,4,8]. Indeed, some of the earliest physiological studies in patients with PPH have shown that the administration of a vasodilator such as a acetylcholine can cause immediate and pronounced vasodilatation [9,10]. Since the vessels are characterized by marked thickening of the media, it was originally postulated that this represented uncontrolled growth and constriction of the smooth muscle cells in the pulmonary vascular bed. The fact that a wide spectrum of responsiveness has been noted in patients with PPH has been interpreted as a reflection of the chronicity as well as the severity of the underlying disease [1,11]. It has been suggested that patients who present earlier appear to be more likely to respond to an acute vasodilator challenge, and those that are more advanced are less likely to be responsive [2,12].

Nonetheless there remains considerable uncertainty regarding the role of vasoconstriction in PPH and the favourable effects of vasodilators. Although vasoconstriction can be demonstrated in some patients with PPH, it is uncommon to demonstrate any pulmonary vasodilator response to any agent in patients who present with advanced disease, suggesting that vasoconstriction is not a feature of the disease in the late stages. A close look at the histopathology of PPH, however, would suggest that this clinical observation should be of no surprise. Patients with PPH will typically have severe concentric laminar intimal fibrosis, often with obliteration of the vessels representative of an angioproliferative vasculopathy. This suggests that a dominant problem in PPH may be uncontrolled myointimal growth, consistent with the recent genetic observations.

It has been reported that patients with PPH may also possess an abnormality in the function of the potassium channels in pulmonary artery smooth muscle cells that causes membrane depolarization and increased cytoplasmic calcium, which was not apparent in patients with secondary pulmonary hypertension [13]. This could promote pulmonary vasoconstriction, as well as pulmonary arterial smooth muscle cell proliferation and raises the possibility that some patients with PPH may have a unique mechanism for their pulmonary hypertension arising in the pulmonary smooth muscle cells. This may also explain why calcium channel blockers seem to be effective predominantly in patients with PPH, and only rarely with secondary pulmonary hypertension.

Calcium channel blockers were the first oral vasodilators that were demonstrated to have sustained, pronounced benefits in patients with PPH [14]. Published data, however, illustrated that only a minority of patients (approximately 20%) will respond to calcium channel blockers at the time that they initially present with the diagnosis of PPH [14,15]. Given the complexity, as well as reported hazards of high doses of calcium channel blockers in patients with PPH, it is widely advocated that patients be tested acutely with a short acting vasodilator to select those patients that would be most likely to respond to calcium channel blockers chronically [16–19].

It is important to note that calcium channel blockers may in some cases have no effect, and more importantly may have an adverse affect [20]. Concerns over calcium blockers being associated with increased cardiovascular mortality in patients with coronary disease are based on factors that may also play a role in PPH. If there is no demonstrable vasoconstriction as an underlying abnormality in a patient presenting with pulmonary hypertension, there would be

no justification for the use of chronic vasodilators. In addition, a patient who presents at an advanced stage may no longer have the ability to respond to a vasodilator, given the extensive nature of the vascular changes. More importantly, however, calcium channel blockers can cause neurohormonal activation that could be very problematic in these patients [21], and many possess negative inotropic properties that could worsen underlying right ventricular dysfunction [22].

On the basis of the published data, our group makes the following recommendations regarding the use of vasodilators in PPH. First, because these drugs have the potential for serious deleterious effects, acute testing of short acting vasodilators should be done in all patients before chronic calcium channel blocker therapy is used. At the present time it does not appear that there is any superiority over using intravenous adenosine, intravenous epoprostenol (prostacyclin), or inhaled nitric oxide as the testing agent. The decision to initiate chronic therapy should be based on the demonstration of a pronounced acute pulmonary vasodilator effect. Although there is no agreement on this definition, we believe that there should be at least a reduction in the mean pulmonary artery pressure to under 30 mmHg (4 kpa) associated with an increase in cardiac output. Patients who deteriorate while on calcium channel blocker therapy should have it withdrawn, and not have it increased, as it may worsen underlying cardiac function.

The rationale behind anticoagulation

One of the most common findings in patients with PPH is the presence of eccentric intimal pads that are presumed to be caused by thrombosis in situ, as well as recanalized thrombotic lesions that are randomly scattered throughout the pulmonary vascular bed. The assumption that this represents recurrent microembolization has been abandoned, as several studies have characterized the presence of a procoagulant state in patients with PPH that would logically predispose to the development of thrombosis in situ [23]. Studies on the value of anticoagulation in these patients support the notion that ongoing thrombosis might either be causative or serve to perpetuate PPH in some patients (Figure 1.1). A retrospective study of patients with PPH followed at the Mayo Clinic, Rochester, Minnesota, demonstrated improved survival of those who received warfarin anticoagulation versus those who did not [24]. Similarly, patients who developed PPH from exposure to the diet pill aminorex fumarate seemed to have improved survival when treated with warfarin anticoagulation [25]. In the only

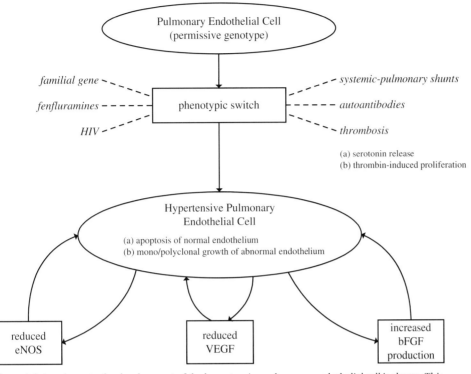

Figure 1.1 A pathway to the development of the hypertensive pulmonary endothelial cell is shown. This cell is characterized by reduced levels of endothelial nitric oxide synthase (eNOS) and increased production of basic fibroblast growth factor (bFGF). Reduced vascular endothelial growth factor (VEGF) from normal endothelial cells is also likely. HIV, human immunodeficiency virus.

prospective study to date, patients who were unresponsive to calcium channel blockers also had improved survival when treated with warfarin anticoagulation versus those who did not [15].

Whether the development of arterial thrombosis in PPH is a result of localized endothelial cell injury, circulating procoagulant factors, or platelet activation has not been fully elucidated. It is possible that any or all of these may be playing a role in these patients. Recently there have been newer antithrombotic agents that work via platelet-mediated mechanisms [26]. Whether these agents would be effective in PPH is completely unknown at this time.

On the basis of the published data, we recommend that chronic warfarin anticoagulation be used in the treatment of all patients with PPH unless there is an underlying contraindication. Although the intensity of the anticoagulant therapy has never been addressed, the common practice currently is to use a target international normalized ratio (INR) of 2.0–3.0 times control. Because of the similarities that exist, at least histologically, in patients with primary and secondary forms of pulmonary hypertension, we use warfarin anticoagulation in all patients who present with pulmonary arterial hypertension.

The rationale behind prostacyclin therapy

A wide spectrum of endothelial cell proliferation and fibrosis is extremely common in patients with PPH, as is the development of plexogenic lesions in advanced cases presumed to be derived from the endothelial cell line [27]. Whether this represents primary endothelial cell injury, endothelial cell dysfunction secondary to an extrinsic trigger, or some other process remains unknown. A multitude of factors that could adversely affect endothelial cell function and proliferation have been described. These include a reduction in circulating prostacyclin metabolites [28], which are presumably derived from the pulmonary vascular endothelium, as well as an increase in thromboxane metabolites, presumably derived from platelet activation (Figure 1.2) [27]. Marked elevations in circulating endothelin have been noted [29], which at a minimum could perpetuate endothelial cell proliferation and dysfunction. Similarly, increased expression of angiotensin converting enzyme activity in the pulmonary vascular endothelium of patients with pulmonary hypertension has now been described [30], as have reduced levels of endothelial nitric oxide synthase, implicating inadequate nitric

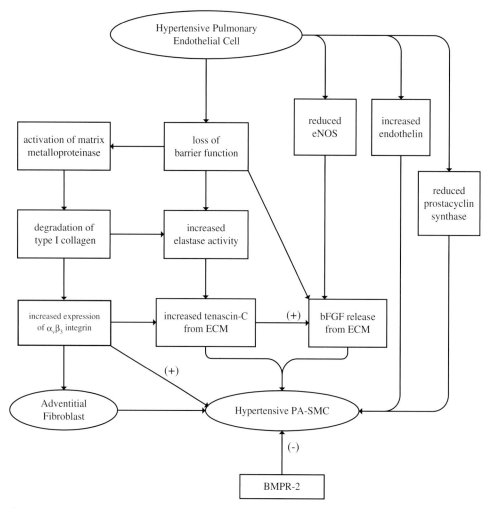

Figure 1.2 Multiple pathways to the development of the hypertensive pulmonary artery smooth muscle cell (PA-SMC) are shown. Pathways on the left have been elucidated from animal models, whereas pathways on the right are from human studies. BMPR-2, bone morphogenic protein receptor 2; ECM, extracellular matrix; eNOS, endothelial nitric oxide synthase; bFGF, basic fibroblast growth factor; +, increase; −, decrease.

oxide production [31]. All of these observations make for exciting possibilities of selected therapies targeted at reversing these abnormalities.

To date, the only long-term studies of a therapy that has the potential to correct these abnormalities have focused on the use of chronic intravenous epoprostenol (prostacyclin). Prostacyclin has a number of biochemical properties, which include vasodilatation, platelet inactivation, and antiproliferative effects [32]. Several studies on the acute and chronic effectiveness of epoprostenol in PPH have all shown that it is associated with increased exercise tolerance, improved haemodynamics, and improved survival [33,34]. A recent study, demonstrating that chronic haemodynamic changes attributed to epoprostenol appear to go beyond acute vasodilatation suggests that the compound

may also initiate reversal of the vascular remodelling that is part of PPH [35].

On the basis of the published data, our group believes that intravenous epoprostenol is indicated for all patients with advanced PPH that remain symptomatic in spite of conventional therapy. Indeed, this would be the ideal drug to use in all patients with PPH were it not that its current availability is very limited because of its expense, and because of the requirement for a chronic indwelling central venous catheter, which carries substantial associated morbidity. Clearly, analogues of prostacyclin that may be given through subcutaneous, inhaled, or oral routes need to be evaluated [36,37]. In addition, the mechanisms by which epoprostenol produces favourable effects in these patients need to be better understood.

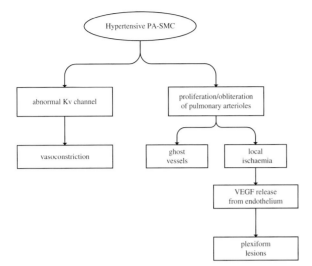

Figure 1.3 Pathways illustrating the pathobiological expression of the hypertensive pulmonary artery smooth muscle cell (PA-SMC) are shown. Vasoconstriction is an early phenomenon, whereas plexiform lesions represent chronic severe disease. VEGF, vascular endothelial growth factor.

Growth inhibitors: a new approach

From advances made in our understanding of the molecular basis of vascular growth and the response to stimuli one can assemble a molecular pathway that may explain the pathobiology of primary pulmonary hypertension (Figures 1.1 to 1.3). Most of these pathways have been derived from the hypoxic- and monocrotaline-induced pulmonary hypertensive rat, and from immunohistochemical studies of human lung tissue. What becomes apparent is that PPH appears to represent an angiogenic-obliterative pulmonary vasculopathy as a result of abnormal or uncontrolled pulmonary vascular arterial growth. It is likely that there are multiple and redundant pathways responsible for this disease.

Recent observations provide evidence that the pulmonary hypertension initiates a positive feedback loop that serves to sustain the clinical disease entity. In an interesting study using the monocrotaline rat model, it was shown that, when a pulmonary hypertensive lung is removed and transplanted into a normal rat, the lung will reverse its disease [38]. This has been attributed to the reduction in mean pulmonary pressure that exists in the animal receiving the transplant, and subsequent absence of growth factors necessary to sustain the disease process. Interestingly, a case report of a patient who underwent single lung transplantation for PPH provides a look at the reverse experiment [39]. In this instance, a diseased patient received one normal lung, which not only resulted in a reduction in the pulmonary artery pressure but, over the ensuing years, reversed the severity of the disease process on the native lung. Taken together these observations suggest that the body may be able to produce growth inhibitors to reverse the vascular changes of advanced pulmonary hypertension. Two types of inhibitor currently being evaluated clinically are the endothelin receptor blockers and nitric oxide.

Endothelin (ET) is a constrictor of human pulmonary arteries through its action on smooth muscle ETA receptors, but can also induce vasodilatation through endothelial ETB receptors [40]. In addition to its vasomotor actions, it has been implicated in vascular remodelling in a number of animal models. ET, for example, is overexpressed in rats developing hypoxic pulmonary hypertension; this can be prevented and reversed using an ET receptor antagonist [41]. A central role for endothelin in the pathogenesis of PPH has been proposed because plasma levels are increased and there is evidence of local production in the lung [42]. Thus, if effective, endothelin receptor antagonists could produce favourable short-term haemodynamic changes by virtue of their vasodilator properties, and perhaps longer-term favourable changes by growth inhibition and potentially reversal of the chronic myointimal proliferation that exists with the disease.

Chronic elevations in endothelin levels in patients with PPH have been described by several investigators [42]. Although the exact role that endothelin is playing in this disease remains undefined, it is appealing to believe that inhibiting this potent mitogen might have beneficial effects in arresting the disease process, reversing the disease, or improving cardiac function. Two pilot clinical trials have been conducted, with favourable results of endothelin receptor blockers in patients with PPH. Their role in the spectrum of treatments for chronic pulmonary arterial hypertension remains to be defined.

Endothelial-derived nitric oxide is a mediator that controls vascular remodelling by acting as a negative regulator of vascular smooth muscle proliferation in response to a remodelling stimulus [43]. In the absence of nitric oxide, luminal remodelling is impaired and vessel wall thickness increases due to the proliferation of vascular smooth muscle cells. The mechanism by which nitric oxide works is under investigation. It may, for example, stimulate an inhibitor of vascular smooth muscle proliferation such as TGF-β or counteract the actions of known smooth muscle mitogens such as fibroblast growth factor [44]. In experimental models, high levels of nitric oxide can be both cytotoxic and apoptosis promoting.

Several strategies are under study to increase nitric oxide in patients. For example, nitric oxide can be inhaled and has been reported to be clinically effective in treating PPH [45].

Table 1.1. Possible futuristic therapy of pulmonary hypertension

	Target	Treatment
Phase I	Increase nitric oxide levels	Phosphodiesterase inhibitor
	Reverse local prostacyclin/thromboxane imbalance	Epoprostenol (prostacyclin)
Phase II	Maintain local nitric oxide production	L-arginine
	Reverse vasoconstriction	Calcium channel blockers
	or	
Phase I	Reversal of intimal proliferation	Epoprostenol (prostacyclin)
	Blockade of neurohormonal activation	Angiotensin converting enzyme inhibitor
Phase II	Increase endogenous nitric oxide production	Nitric oxide synthase gene transfer
	Reduce vascular smooth muscle cell hypertrophy	Endothelin receptor blocker

The use of nitric oxide precursors, such as L-arginine, has been employed to increase nitric oxide production by the endothelial cell [46]. The cholesterol-lowering statin drugs can increase levels of endothelial nitric oxide synthase in vessels with impaired endothelium [47]. The use of phosphodiesterase inhibitors, which prolong the activity of nitric oxide, is currently being studied in a response to case reports of patients with PPH responding to oral sildenafil [48]. Finally, cell-based gene transfer of endothelial nitric oxide synthase has been effective in inhibiting monocrotaline-induced pulmonary hypertension and may provide another strategy worthy of clinical pursuit [49].

Future treatment strategies

Because it is not clear whether PPH is a result of an abnormality of a single cell type or a pathophysiological abnormality, we should begin looking at combination therapies designed to correct as many of the abnormalities associated with PPH as possible (see Table 1.1). Indeed, the combined use of warfarin anticoagulation with calcium channel blockers has been the first step in this approach. One lesson that has been learned in treating PPH, similar to the treatment of congestive heart failure, is that acute haemodynamic changes need not occur for drugs to produce chronic effectiveness. Finally, we should also learn from our oncology colleagues that staged therapy should also be considered. If, in fact, epoprostenol has the ability to reverse vascular remodelling of PPH, then it may be possible to administer it over the short term for patients with PPH, as part of initial therapy, in order to allow the pulmonary vascular bed to recover so that medication may be replaced with another therapy, such as oral calcium channel blockers, which might not otherwise have been effective.

Although the basis of primary pulmonary hypertension still remains unclear, the advances that have been made in our understanding of the basis of the disease have already led to exciting improvements in patient responsiveness and survival. Indeed, we anticipate that the next 10 years will continue to hold promise for the rapid development of new, effective therapies.

REFERENCES

1 Wood P. Pulmonary hypertension with special reference to the vasoconstrictive factor. *Br Heart J* 1958; **20**: 557–570.

2 Rich S. Clinical insights into the pathogenesis of primary pulmonary hypertension. *Chest* 1998; **114**: 237S–241S.

3 Wagenvoort CA, Wagenvoort N. Primary pulmonary hypertension: a pathologic study of the lung vessels in 156 clinically diagnosed cases. *Circulation* 1970; **42**: 1163–1184.

4 Pietra GG, Edwards WD, Kay JM, et al. Histopathology of primary pulmonary hypertension: a qualitative and quantitative study of pulmonary blood vessels from 58 patients in the National Heart, Lung, and Blood Institute Primary Pulmonary Hypertension Registry. *Circulation* 1989; **80**: 1198–1206.

5 Newman JH, Wheeler L, Lane KB, et al. Mutation in the gene for bone morphogenetic protein receptor II as a cause of primary pulmonary hypertension in a large kindred. *N Engl J Med* 2001; **345**: 319–324.

6 Loscalzo J. Genetic clues to the cause of primary pulmonary hypertension. *N Engl J Med* 2001; **345**: 367–371.

7 Thomson JR, Machado RD, Pauciulo MW, et al. Sporadic primary pulmonary hypertension is associated with germline mutations of the gene encoding BMPR-II, a receptor member of the TGF-beta family. *J Med Genet* 2000; **37**: 741–745.

8 Wagenvoort CA. Vasoconstriction and medial hypertrophy in pulmonary hypertension. *Circulation* 1960; **22**: 535–556.

9 Dresdale DT, Schultz M, Michtom RJ. Primary pulmonary hypertension. 1. Clinical and hemodynamic study. *Am J Med* 1957; **11**: 686–705.

10 Samet P, Bernstein WH, Widrich J. Intracardiac infusion of acetylcholine in primary pulmonary hypertension. *Am Heart J* 1960; **60**: 433–439.

11 Samet P, Bernstein WH. Loss of reactivity of the pulmonary vascular bed in primary pulmonary hypertension. *Am Heart J* 1963; **66**: 197–199.

12 Celermajer DS, Cullen S, Deanfield JE. Impairment of endothelium dependent pulmonary artery relaxation in children with congenital heart disease and abnormal pulmonary hemodynamics. *Circulation* 1993; **87**: 440–446.

13 Yuan JXJ, Aldinger AM, Juhaszova M, et al. Dysfunctional voltage-gated K^+ channels in pulmonary artery smooth muscle cells of patients with primary pulmonary hypertension. *Circulation* 1998; **98**: 1400–1406.

14 Rich S, Brundage BH. High-dose calcium channel blocking therapy for primary pulmonary hypertension: evidence for long-term reduction in pulmonary arterial pressure and regression of right ventricular hypertrophy. *Circulation* 1997; **76**: 135–141.

15 Rich S, Kaufmann E, Levy PS. The effect of high doses of calcium-channel blockers on survival in primary pulmonary hypertension. *N Engl J Med* 1992; **327**: 76–81.

16 Rubin LJ, Barst RJ, Kaiser LR, et al. Primary pulmonary hypertension. *Chest* 1993; **104**: 236–250.

17 Groves BM, Badesch DB, Turkevitch D, et al. Correlation of acute prostacyclin response in primary (unexplained) pulmonary hypertension with efficacy of treatment with calcium channel blockers and survival. In: Hume JR, Reeves JT, Weir EK, eds. *Ion flux in pulmonary vascular control.* Plenum Press, New York, 1993: 317–330.

18 Schrader BJ, Inbar S, Kaufmann L, et al. Comparison of the effects of adenosine and nifedipine in pulmonary hypertension. *J Am Coll Cardiol* 1992; **19**: 1060–1064.

19 Ricciardi MJ, Knight BP, Martinez FJ, et al. Inhaled nitric oxide in primary pulmonary hypertension: a safe and effective agent for predicting response to nifedipine. *J Am Coll Cardiol* 1998; **32**: 1068–1073.

20 Packer M, Medina N, Yushak M. Adverse hemodynamic and clinical effects of calcium channel blockade in pulmonary hypertension secondary to obliterative vascular disease. *J Am Coll Cardiol* 1984; **4**: 890–896.

21 Epstein M. The calcium antagonist controversy: the emerging importance of drug formulation as a determinant of risk. *Am J Cardiol* 1997; **79**(10A): 9–19.

22 Michalewicz L, Messerli FH. Cardiac effects of calcium antagonists in systemic hypertension. *Am J Cardiol* 1997; **79**(10A): 39–46.

23 Eisenberg PR, Lucore C, Kaufmann E, et al. Fibrinopeptide A levels indicative of pulmonary vascular thrombosis in patients with primary pulmonary hypertension. *Circulation* 1990; **82**: 841–847.

24 Fuster V, Steele PM, Edwards WD, et al. Primary pulmonary hypertension: natural history and the importance of thrombosis. *Circulation* 1984; **70**: 580–587.

25 Mlczoch FH, Huber K, Schuster E, et al. The effect of anticoagulant therapy in primary and anorectic drug-induced pulmonary hypertension. *Chest* 1997; **112**: 3, 714–721.

26 Lefkovits J, Plow EF, Topol EJ. Platelet glycoprotein IIb/IIIa receptors in cardiovascular medicine. *N Engl J Med* 1995; **332**: 1553–1559.

27 Tuder RM, Groves B, Badesch DB, et al. Exuberant endothelial cell growth and elements of inflammation are present in plexiform lesions of pulmonary hypertension. *Am J Pathol* 1994; **144**: 275–285.

28 Christman BW, McPherson CD, Newman JH, et al. An imbalance between the excretion of thromboxane and prostacyclin metabolites in pulmonary hypertension. *N Engl J Med* 1992: **327**: 70–75.

29 Yoshibayashi M, Nishioka K, Nakao K, et al. Plasma endothelin concentration in patients with pulmonary hypertension associated with congenital heart defects: evidence for increased production of endothelin in the pulmonary circulation. *Circulation* 1991; **84**: 2280–2285.

30 Schuster DP, Crouch EC, Parks WC, et al. Angiotensin converting enzyme expression in primary pulmonary hypertension. *Am J Respir Crit Care Med* 1996; **154**: 1087–1091.

31 Giaid A, Saleh D. Reduced expression of endothelial nitric oxide synthase in the lungs of patients with pulmonary hypertension. *N Engl J Med* 1995; **333**: 214–221.

32 Moncada S, Korbut R, Bunting S, et al. Prostacyclin is a circulating hormone. *Nature* 1978; **273**: 767–768.

33 Barst RJ, Rubin LJ, Long WA, et al. A comparison of continuous intravenous prostacyclin versus conventional therapy in primary pulmonary hypertension. *N Engl J Med* 1996; **334**: 296–301.

34 Shapiro SM, Oudiz RJ, Cao T, et al. Primary pulmonary hypertension: improved long-term effects and survival with continuous intravenous epoprostenol infusion. *J Am Coll Cardiol* 1997; **30**: 343–349.

35 McLaughlin VV, Genthner DE, Panella MM, et al. Reduction in pulmonary vascular resistance with long-term prostacyclin therapy in primary pulmonary hypertension. *N Engl J Med* 1998; **338**: 273–277.

36 Olschewski H, Walmrath D, Schermuly R, et al. Aerosolized prostacyclin and iloprost in severe pulmonary hypertension. *Ann Intern Med* 1996; **124**: 820–824.

37 Saji T, Ozawa Y, Ishikita T, et al. Short-term hemodynamic effect of a new oral PGI_2 analogue, beraprost, in primary and secondary pulmonary hypertension. *Am J Cardiol* 1996; **78**: 244–247.

38 O'Blenes SB, Fischer S, McIntyre B, et al. Hemodynamic unloading leads to regression of pulmonary vascular disease in rats. *J Thorac Cardiovasc Surg* 2001; **121**: 279–289.

39 Levy NT, Liapis H, Eisenberg PR, et al. Pathologic regression of primary pulmonary hypertension in left native lung following right single-lung transplantation. *J Heart Lung Transpl* 2001; **20**: 381–384.

40 Dupuis J, Jasmin JF, Prie S, Cernacek P. Importance of local production of endothelin-1 and of the ET_B receptor in the regulation of pulmonary vascular tone. *Pulm Pharmacol Ther* 2000; **13**: 135–140.

41 McCulloch KM, MacLean MR. Endothelin_B receptor-mediated contraction of human and rat pulmonary resistance arteries and the effect of pulmonary hypertension on endothelin responses in the rat. *J Cardiovasc Pharm* 1995; **26**: S169–S176.

42 Chen YF, Oparil S. Endothelin and pulmonary hypertension. *J Cardiovasc Pharm* 2000; **35**: S49-S53.

43 Rudic RD, Shesely EG, Maeda N, et al. Direct evidence for the importance of endothelin-derived nitric oxide in vascular remodeling. *J Clin Invest* 1998; **101**: 731–736.

44 Norrby K. Nitric oxide suppresses bFGF- and IL-1-alpha-mediated but not VEGF$_{165}$-mediated angiogenesis in natively vascularized mammalian tissue. *APMIS* 1998; **106**: 1142–48.

45 Perez-Penate G, Julia-Serda G, Pulido-Duque JM, et al. One-year continuous inhaled nitric oxide for primary pulmonary hypertension. *Chest* 2001; **119**: 970–973.

46 Nagaya N, Uematsu M, Oya H, et al. Short-term oral administration of L-arginine improves hemodynamics and exercise capacity in patients with precapillary pulmonary hypertension. *Am J Respir Crit Care Med* 2001; **163**: 887–891.

47 Laufs U, LaFata V, Plutzky J, Liao JK. Upregulation of endothelial nitric oxide synthase by HMG CoA reductase inhibitors. *Circulation* 1998; **97**: 1129–1135.

48 Prasad S, Wilkinson J, Gatzoulis MA. Sildenafil in primary pulmonary hypertension. *N Engl J Med* 2000; **343**: 1342.

49 Campbell AIM, Kuliszewski MA, Stewart DJ. Cell-based gene transfer to the pulmonary vasculature: endothelial nitric oxide synthase overexpression inhibits monocrotaline-induced pulmonary hypertension. *Am J Respir Cell Mol Biol* 1999; **21**: 567–575.

2

Genetics of primary pulmonary hypertension

Richard C. Trembath and Rachel Harrison

University of Leicester, Leicester, UK

Introduction

Primary pulmonary hypertension (PPH) is typically de-scribed as a sporadic disorder. However, patients with at least one affected relative have been increasingly recognized since early reports of the disorder over 50 years ago [1]. Interestingly, the natural history of PPH appears similar in both familial and sporadic forms of the disease. Recent advances in understanding the genetic basis of familial PPH are therefore likely to shed light on the pathogenic processes common to all forms of the disease.

Molecular genetic studies have identified that mutations within the gene *BMPR2* on the long arm of chromosome 2 underlie familial PPH [2,3]. This chapter describes the studies that led to these discoveries, explores the prospects for future research into the molecular mechanisms involved in the disease process and emphasizes the immediate implications for assessment and management of patients and their relatives, as a consequence of the identification of the gene associated with PPH.

Patterns of inheritance

Figures from the American National Institute of Health Registry demonstrate that at least 6% of patients with PPH have a family history of the disease [4]. However, familial cases may be difficult to detect due to delayed or missed diagnosis, inadequate case finding or the markedly reduced penetrance by which the disease gene acts. Hence, PPH individuals in families may inherit and transmit the disease gene without developing overt clinical features of the disease. This observation may explain the recognition of remote common ancestry occasionally observed in patients with apparently sporadic PPH [5].

Families with PPH demonstrate an autosomal dominant mode of inheritance, yet because the disease gene acts with reduced penetrance [6] any individual harbouring a PPH gene defect is estimated to have no greater than 10–20% chance of developing the disease [7]. This suggests that, although the gene confers a susceptibility to develop PPH, additional genetic and/or environmental factors are required for the initiation or progression of the disease. Women are twice as likely as men to develop the disease, suggesting hormonal factors may be particularly important. Of interest, a similar sex ratio is observed for cases with or without a family history of the disease. The age of onset of clinical disease is highly variable both within and between PPH families. Anticipation, a phenomenon by which successive generations are affected at an earlier age [8], has been observed.

Approach to finding the gene – positional cloning
(Figure 2.1)

By 1997, two groups working independently had performed genome wide searches for the location of putative PPH genes. Linkage was established on the long arm of chromosome 2, within a broad interval of 25 cM [9,10]. Of interest, in linkage studies performed on over 40 independently ascertained kindreds, all appear to share the same chromosomal region [3,11], suggesting this to be the location of the major genetic determinant for inherited PPH. By analysis of cross-over (recombination) events, the critical interval for the PPH gene was reduced to a 4.8 cM region, flanked by polymorphic *D2S115* (centromeric) and *D2S1384* (telomeric) [12].

The region at 2q31–33 included a large number of genes, each a potential candidate for the putative PPH gene by virtue of its position. These included the apoptosis related

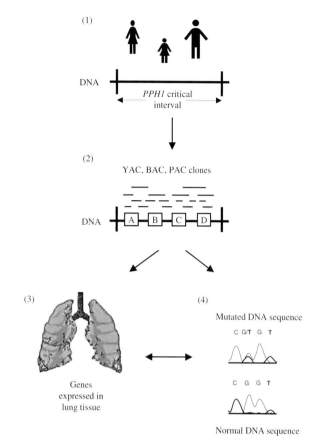

Figure 2.1 Idealized positional cloning strategy. (1) The critical interval for the PPH gene was reduced by detection of recombinant events. In brief, segments of chromosome 2q33 shared by affected individuals within a family were identified. (2) Data from the human genome project were used to identify genes and expressed sequence tags (partially sequenced genes or ESTs) located within the critical interval for the PPH gene (e.g. genes *A*, *B*, *C* and *D*). To place these genes, ESTs and other DNA markers in the correct order, a series of overlapping DNA clones inserted into yeast, bacteria or plasmid artificial chromosomes (YACs, BACs and PACs, respectively) were created; a process known as physical mapping. (3) Studies were performed to identify genes expressed in lung tissue that were potential candidates for the PPH gene. (4) Finally, direct analysis of genes to detect a mutation or DNA sequence variant was performed in affected individuals and compared with normal controls. (After Thomson JR, Trembath RC. Primary pulmonary hypertension: the pressure rises for a gene. *J Clin Path* 2000; **53**: 899–903, reproduced with permission.)

genes (caspases 10 and 8, CASP8 and FADD-like apoptosis regulator, and usurpin), genes related to immune modulation (T-cell membrane glycoprotein CD28, cytotoxic T-lymphocyte-associated protein 4, and activation-inducible lymphocyte immunomediatory molecule) and

BMPR2 (the gene for bone morphogenetic protein receptor II) – the gene for a receptor in the transforming growth factor beta (TGF-β) superfamily [12]. Bone morphogenetic proteins (BMPs) have multifunctional cytokine activity, regulating cell differentiation, growth and apoptosis. The *BMPR2* product (BMPR-II) is a receptor member of the TGF-β signalling pathway and TGF-β expression has been shown to be upregulated in remodelling pulmonary vasculature in PPH [13].

When detailed genetic analysis of the coding sequences of *BMPR2* was performed, a range of mutations was identified, each segregating with the disease, providing compelling evidence that *BMPR2* represents a PPH-causing gene.

Mutations found in familial PPH

Over 40 unique *BMPR2* mutations have now been identified in patients with a known family history of PPH [2,3,11]. These are all heterozygous mutations, occurring in only one copy of the gene. It is also important to note that these represent germline mutations transmitted from parents at the point of conception, which are therefore represented in all cell types. From these studies, a number of conclusions can be reached. Mutations are widely dispersed throughout the gene, each family appearing to have its own private or unique defect (Figure 2.2). Hence, no mutational 'hot spot' has been identified in *BMPR2*. This will certainly confound attempts to design simple molecular diagnostic genetic tests for the disease (Figure 2.3). None of the identified mutations was found in over 200 independent samples taken from a healthy population, suggesting that they are unlikely to represent more common susceptibility alleles of pulmonary hypertension, and adding weight to the argument that they are truly pathogenic.

The range and type of mutations is also of interest as these observations can provide initial clues as to the important functional domains of the *BMPR2* gene in PPH (see Figure 2.2). Missense mutations occur when one nucleotide is substituted for another, altering a triplet codon so that it specifies a different amino acid. Disease causing missense mutations affect highly conserved and functionally important sites of the BMPR-II protein [12]. For example, missense mutations present in the extracellular domain would be predicted to disturb ligand binding, and those within the kinase domain to inhibit phosphorylation and prevent normal receptor complex function [2]. Nonsense mutations occur when a nucleotide substitution changes a codon from one that previously specified an amino acid, to

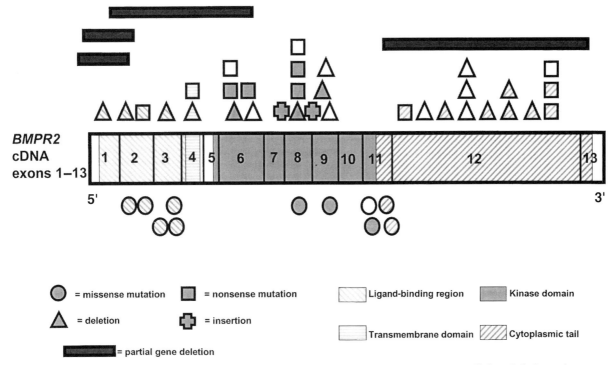

Figure 2.2 Position of *BMPR2* mutations. Structure of *BMPR2* indicating position of identified mutations. Filled symbols denote known familial cases of PPH; open symbols denote sporadic cases.

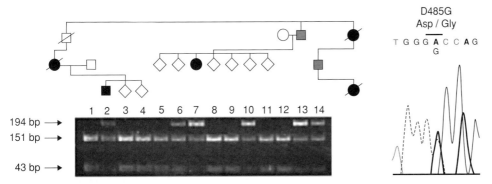

Figure 2.3 Cosegregation of mutations of *BMPR2*. Symbol shading is as follows: Filled symbol, affected; open symbol, unaffected; shaded symbol obligate disease gene carriers. An open diamond has been used to anonymize 'at risk' family members. Arrows indicate the sizes of the observed fragments for the restriction endonuclease. The DNA sequence change associated with the D485G amino acid substitution leads to loss of the normal restriction site. Heterozygotes can therefore be identified by the detection of the remaining 194 bp fragment as well as the two digestion fragments of 151 and 43 bp. (After The International PPH Consortium, Lane KB, Machado RD, Pauciulo MW, et al. Heterozygous germline mutations in *BMPR2*, encoding a TGF-β receptor, cause familial primary pulmonary hypertension. *Nature Genet* 2000; **26**: 81–84, reproduced with permission.)

a stop codon that terminates transcription of the gene. This can lead to a shortened, dysfunctional form of the protein, or RNA transcripts that are rapidly degraded within the endoplasmic reticulum, a process known as RNA-mediated decay. Frameshift mutations occur when nucleotides are inserted or deleted, so that they alter the translational reading frame of the gene. This will also lead to a premature termination codon, causing loss of gene expression.

Taken together, assessment of published *BMPR2* mutations in PPH suggests that the likely mechanism for the inherited basis of the disease is an overall reduction in the amount of the protein present at the cell surface, or haploinsufficiency [11]. However, the molecular impact of these mutations will require further detailed analysis.

Sporadic disease and mutations of *BMPR2*

Whilst only a minority of patients with PPH have a declared family history of the disease, misdiagnosis or incomplete family details may lead to underassessment of the extent of familial disease. In a study of 50 PPH patients with no identified family history of PPH, germline mutations in *BMPR2* were identified in almost one third [14]. The range of mutations paralleled that seen in recognized familial cases, with detection of inherited as well as de novo or spontaneous defects (see Figure 2.2).

Why have *BMPR2* mutations not been found in all subjects with PPH?

Mutations have now been described for 55% (40 of 73) of families with familial PPH [2,3]. A number of explanations may account for the failure to detect mutations in the remaining 45%. Direct DNA sequencing methods have to date been confined to the coding sequence of *BMPR2*, yet deleterious mutations may occur in other gene regions, including regulatory or intronic sequences. Direct sequencing will also miss large-scale gene rearrangements. Additionally, it remains possible that other genes, yet to be identified, contribute to the genetic basis of PPH. PPH is likely to be aetiologically heterogeneous. In support of this, detailed molecular genetic analysis of plexiform lesions from sporadic cases of PPH have identified the accumulation of a range of somatic or acquired mutations, including defects in genes known to play an important role in cell growth [15].

Anticipation revisited

Some families with a history of PPH show anticipation, in which successive generations are affected at an earlier age [8]. The underlying defect of genetic anticipation as observed in several neurodegenerative disorders may in part be explained by unstable expansion of trinucleotide repeat sequences of DNA. However, polymerase chain reaction (PCR) analysis of a GCC repeat close to the initiation codon of *BMPR2* showed no evidence of expansion in a cohort of patients with PPH [3,11]. The appearance of anticipation may be explained by associated environmental factors, whilst bias in ascertainment of such data is difficult to eliminate entirely.

BMPR-II and the role of the TGF-β superfamily

BMPs were originally identified as proteins regulating growth and differentiation of bone and cartilage. More recent studies have shown BMPs to be members of the TGF-β family of growth factors, behaving as multifunctional cytokines responsible for the regulation of growth, differentiation and apoptosis of various cell types [16].

The TGF-β superfamily regulates the proliferation and differentiation of most cell types including endothelial, epithelial, neuronal and connective tissue cells, but also plays a critical role in embryonic development, angiogenesis, and wound healing [17]. Altered TGF-β function has been implicated in a wide range of disease states, including fibrotic disease of the kidney, liver and lung, and atherosclerosis. Mutations in the genes for TGF-β, its receptors or the associated intracellular signalling molecules, have also been shown to contribute to the pathogenesis of cancer, together with the inherited vascular disorder hereditary haemorrhagic telangiectasia [17].

The mechanism of TGF-β signalling requires activation by ligand of at least two receptor types (I and II), together with a family of intracellular signalling proteins (the Smad proteins) (see Figure 2.4). TGF-β or BMPs bind to type II receptors, including BMPR-II, stimulating formation of a receptor complex with type I receptors. Complex formation activates the protein kinase domain of the type I receptor, resulting in phosphorylation and activation of Smad proteins. The resulting Smad complex moves into the nucleus, leading to cell-specific transcriptional regulation. More recently TGF-β receptors have been shown to act as a mitogen and to act through stress-activated protein kinase pathways [17].

Role of TGF-β cell signalling in human disease

Role of TGF-β in cancer

Defects in the TGF-β pathway are associated with the development of cancer. In most endothelial, epithelial and haematopoietic cells, TGF-β is a potent inhibitor of cell proliferation [17]. Inhibition of cellular proliferation,

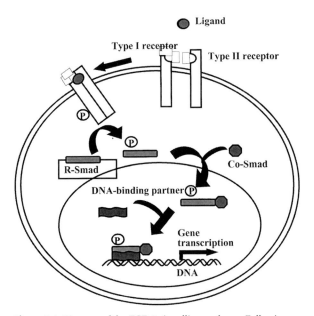

Figure 2.4 Diagram of the TGF-β signalling pathway. Following ligand binding, BMPR-II, a type II receptor, forms a heteromeric complex with a type I receptor, resulting in kinase domain activation. This initiates phosphorylation of cytoplasmic signalling proteins named Smads, leading to signal transduction. Co-Smad, common partner Smad; R-Smad, receptor-regulated Smad. (After Thomson JR, Machado RD, Pauciulo MW, et al. Sporadic primary pulmonary hypertension is associated with germline mutations of the gene encoding BMPR-II, a receptor member of the TGF-β family. *J Med Genet* 2000; **37**: 741–745, reproduced with permission.)

or promotion of either apoptosis or cellular differentiation, results in a tumour suppressor effect. If somatic cells acquire mutations causing loss of expression of the genes for components of the TGF-β pathway, loss of TGF-β-mediated growth inhibition allows uncontrolled proliferation of cells. For example, 100% of pancreatic cancers and 83% of colon cancers have a somatic mutation affecting at least one component of the TGF-β pathway [18,19].

Role of TGF-β in hereditary haemorrhagic telangiectasia and blood vessel formation

Hereditary haemorrhagic telangiectasia (HHT) is an autosomal dominant disorder characterized by a vascular dysplasia. Mutations underlying HHT have been reported in two genes encoding TGF-β receptors, the endoglin gene (*ENG*) on chromosome 9, and the gene for activin-receptor-like kinase 1 (*ALK1*) on chromosome 12 [20,21]. Mice lacking endoglin or ALK-1 die early in embryonic life from defects in angiogenesis. Primary defects in the endothelial and smooth muscle cells of the developing blood

vessels confirm that the TGF-β pathway has a vital role in angiogenesis [22,23].

TGF-β signalling and pulmonary hypertension

HHT is associated with abnormalities in vessel wall development leading to mucocutaneous telangiectases. Clinically patients present with recurrent epistaxis or gastrointestinal blood loss, and arteriovenous malformations may develop within the pulmonary, hepatic and cerebral circulations. Patients with HHT may develop pulmonary hypertension that is clinically and pathologically identical with PPH [24,25]. Recent clinical and molecular studies in HHT families have produced further evidence for a critical role of the TGF-β cell signalling pathway in the pathogenesis of the pulmonary lesions characteristic of pulmonary hypertension.

Five kindreds and one individual were identified with a family history of HHT and cases of pulmonary hypertension [26]. In each family, novel defects of *ALK1* were identified (see Figure 2.5). The apparent diversity of impact of *ALK1* mutations on vessel wall integrity is not necessarily surprising given the recognized role TGF-β signalling has in regulating many intracellular pathways. For example, overexpression of TGF-β simultaneously promotes intimal growth and apoptosis of vascular endothelium [27]. Dysfunction of receptors such as ALK-1, BMPR-II, or endoglin can result in varying effects, depending on local vascular interactions or other environmental or genetic effects. Elucidating these cell-specific interactions will be crucial to gaining a detailed molecular understanding of the pathogenesis of PPH.

Why do defects in *BMPR2* lead to defects of the pulmonary vasculature?

BMPR2 is expressed throughout developing and adult tissues and has a high level of expression in lung tissue [28]. With such wide patterns of expression it remains unclear why mutations in *BMPR2* lead to specific or predominant lung pathology. However, the effect of BMP signalling is determined by numerous intracellular regulatory molecules, which vary in different tissues. Stimulation of *BMPR2* will therefore lead to radically different responses, depending on the cell type. Immunohistochemical analysis has shown expression of ALK-1 to be predominantly in the vascular endothelium of normal and diseased lungs (see Figure 2.6). It has also been observed in the endothelium of occlusive and plexiform lesions [26]. These observations directly

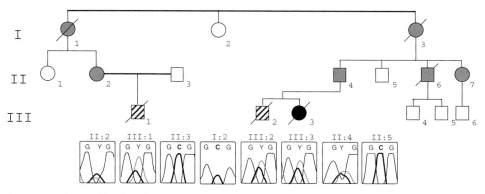

Figure 2.5 Pedigree of family with members affected by hereditary haemorrhagic telangiectasia and pulmonary hypertension, showing segregation of the cytosine-to-thymine mutation at position 1450 in *ALK1*. Black symbols denote family members with both pulmonary hypertension and hereditary haemorrhagic telangiectasia; grey symbols members with hereditary haemorrhagic telangiectasia only; hatched symbols members with pulmonary hypertension only; and open symbols members unaffected by either condition.

The DNA sequence chromatograms for the subjects tested are shown below the pedigree. Unaffected family members (II:3, I:2, and II:5) have two normal alleles (cytosine, C) at position 1450 of *ALK1*. Family members with pulmonary hypertension, hereditary haemorrhagic telangiectasia or both (II:2, III:1, III:2, III:3, and II:4) have one normal allele and one mutant allele at position 1450, indicated by the letter Y. (After Trembath RC, Thomson JR, Machado RD, et al. Clinical and molecular genetic features of pulmonary hypertension in patients with hereditary haemorrhagic telangiectasia. *N Engl J Med* 2001; **345**: 325–334, reproduced with permission. Copyright © 2001 Massachusetts Medical Society. All rights reserved.)

implicate the pulmonary endothelial cell in the aetiology of PPH but provide little insight into the apparent tissue specificity of the disease.

Implications of research

Molecular pathogenesis

All identified *BMPR2* mutations are heterozygous defects of the gene. This immediately raises questions regarding the mechanism of action and the impact of such genetic alterations. In autosomal dominant disorders the presence of an altered form of the protein is typically expected to impair the activity of the product of the normal gene – a so-called dominant negative effect. Evidence of the cellular impact of PPH causing *BMPR2* mutations is now eagerly awaited. However, it is clear that heterozygous mutations of *BMPR2* are not sufficient to lead to the clinical disorder of PPH. It will therefore be important to identify other factors, either genetic or environmental, that contribute to the onset of disease.

Clinical implications

The recent findings of germline mutations have immediate implications for counselling and family management in PPH. In those families and individuals in whom a germline mutation in *BMPR2* or *ALK1* has been identified, it is now possible to offer presymptomatic genetic testing to other family members. Those who have inherited a disease-related mutation can be offered clinical screening to identify disease early, as early treatment may potentially improve outcome. They will also be aware of the potential benefits of avoiding exposures known to worsen PPH, including pregnancy or hypoxic environments. Families must be offered comprehensive counselling regarding the implications of the findings, and there is a clear need for additional research before interventions and care plans for life style management can be developed on the basis of objective evidence.

Summary

Investigative strategies that combine clinical observations with detailed molecular genetic analyses are beginning to yield important insights into the pathogenesis of PPH. Whilst ultimately these findings will necessarily lead to a revised classification of PPH, it is already apparent that a significant proportion of patients who develop this intriguing yet devastating disorder, do so because of an inherited defect in receptor members of the TGF-β cell signalling system. These observations provide a target for the development of focused research in the field of pulmonary

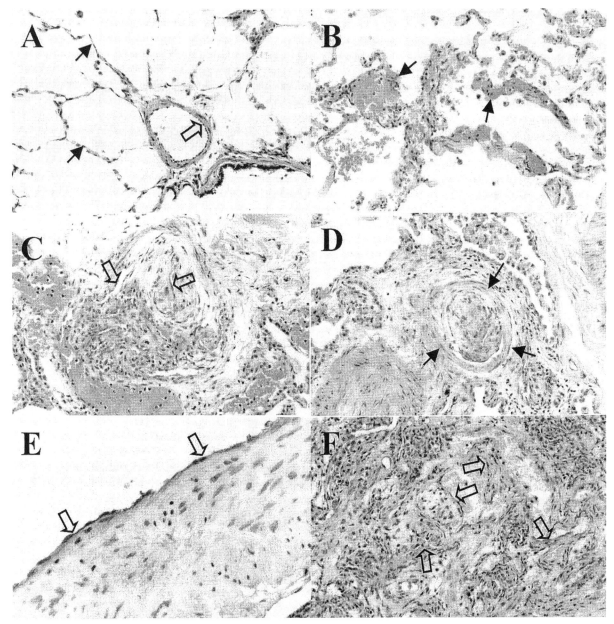

Figure 2.6 Photomicrographs of paraffin-embedded lung sections from a control subject (A) and subjects with plexogenic pulmonary hypertension and mutations in *ALK1* (B, C, D, E and F). Histological analysis of normal lung shows thin-walled peripheral pulmonary arteries (open arrow in A) and normal alveolar capillaries (solid arrows in A). In contrast, regions of the alveolar capillary bed in subjects with pulmonary hypertension show capillary dilatation (arrows in B), the presence of plexiform lesions composed of thin-walled capillary channels (open arrows in C), and thick-walled peripheral pulmonary arteries occluded by a cellular intimal proliferation (arrows in D). Immunohistochemical analysis performed with a polyclonal antibody against activin-receptor-like kinase 1 demonstrated cellular localization of activin-receptor-like kinase 1 to the pulmonary vascular endothelium in normal arteries and in arteries of patients with pulmonary hypertension (open arrows in E), including the capillary channels containing occlusive and plexiform lesions (open arrows in F). (After Trembath RC, Thomson JR, Machado RD, et al. Clinical and molecular genetic features of pulmonary hypertension in patients with hereditary haemorrhagic telangiectasia. *N Engl J Med* 2001; **345**: 325–334, reproduced with permission.)

hypertension, but also have pressing consequences for the management of the individuals and relatives in whom such genetic mutations are identified.

Acknowledgement

Much of the work described in this chapter has been funded by the British Heart Foundation, who continue to support research into the genetics of PPH. Rachel Harrison is a British Heart Foundation Clinical Research Fellow.

REFERENCES

1 Dresdale DT, Schultz M, Michton RJ. Primary pulmonary hypertension: clinical and hemodynamic study. *Am J Med* 1951; **11**: 686–705.

2 The International PPH Consortium, Lane KB, Machado RD, et al. Heterozygous germline mutations in *BMPR2*, encoding a TGF-β receptor, cause familial primary pulmonary hypertension. *Nature Genet* 2000; **26**: 81–84.

3 Deng Z, Morse JH, Slager SL, et al. Familial primary pulmonary hypertension (gene *PPH1*) is caused by mutations in the bone morphogenetic protein receptor-II gene. *Am J Hum Genet* 2000; **67**: 737–744.

4 Rich S, Dantzker DR, Ayres SM, et al. Primary pulmonary hypertension. A national prospective study. *Ann Intern Med* 1987; **107**: 216–223.

5 Elliott G, Alexander G, Leppert M, Yeates S, Kerber R. Coancestry in apparently sporadic primary pulmonary hypertension. *Chest* 1995; **108**: 973–977.

6 Loyd JE, Primm RK, Newman JH. Familial primary pulmonary hypertension: clinical patterns. *Am Rev Respir Dis* 1984; **129**: 194–197.

7 Rich S. Executive summary from the world symposium on primary pulmonary hypertension (Evian, France, 1998). Website: www.who.int/ncd/cvd/pph.htm

8 Loyd JE, Butler MG, Foroud TM, Conneally M, Phillips JA III, Newman JH. Genetic anticipation and abnormal gender ratio at birth in familial primary pulmonary hypertension. *Am J Respir Crit Care Med* 1995; **152**: 93–97.

9 Nichols WC, Koller DL, Slovis B, et al. Localization of the gene for familial primary pulmonary hypertension to chromosome 2q31–32. *Nature Genet* 1997; **15**: 277–280.

10 Morse JH, Jones AC, Barst RJ, Hodge SE, Wilhelmsen KC, Nygaard TG. Mapping of familial primary pulmonary hypertension locus (*PPH1*) to chromosome 2q31–q32. *Circulation* 1997; **95**: 2603–2606.

11 Machado RD, Pauciulo MW, Thomson JR, et al. *BMPR2* haploinsufficiency as the inherited molecular mechanism for primary pulmonary hypertension. *Am J Hum Genet* 2001; **68**: 92–102.

12 Machado RD, Pauciulo MW, Fretwell N, et al. A physical and transcript map based upon refinement of the critical interval for *PPH1*, a gene for familial primary pulmonary hypertension. *Genomics* 2000; **68**: 220–228.

13 Botney MD, Bahadori L, Gold LI. Vascular remodeling in primary pulmonary hypertension. Potential role for transforming growth factor-beta. *Am J Pathol* 1994; **144**: 286–295.

14 Thomson JR, Machado RD, Pauciulo MW, et al. Sporadic primary pulmonary hypertension is associated with germline mutations of the gene encoding BMPR-II, a receptor member of the TGF-β family. *J Med Genet* 2000; **37**: 741–745.

15 Yeager ME, Halley GR, Golpon HA, Voelkel NF, Tuder RM. Microsatellite instability of endothelial cell growth and apoptosis genes within plexiform lesions in primary pulmonary hypertension. *Circ Res* 2001; **88**: e2–e11.

16 Massague J, Wotton D. Transcriptional control by the TGF-β/Smad signaling system. *EMBO J* 2000; **19**: 1745–1754.

17 Blobe GC, Schiemann WP, Lodish HF. Role of transforming growth factor β in human disease. *N Engl J Med* 2000; **342**: 1350–1358.

18 Villanueva A, García C, Paules AB, et al. Disruption of the antiproliferative TGF-β signalling pathways in human pancreatic cancer cells. *Oncogene* 1998; **17**: 1969–1978.

19 Grady WM, Myeroff LL, Swinler SE, et al. Mutational inactivation of TGF-β receptor type II in microsatellite stable colon cancers. *Cancer Res* 1999; **59**: 320–324.

20 McAllister KA, Grogg KM, Johnson DW, et al. Endoglin, a TGF-β binding protein of endothelial cells is the gene for hereditary haemorrhagic telangiectasia type I. *Nature Genet* 1994; **8**: 345–351.

21 Johnson DW, Berg JN, Baldwin MA, et al. Mutations in the activin receptor-like kinase 1 gene in hereditary haemorrhagic telangiectasia type 2. *Nature Genet* 1996; **13**: 189–195.

22 Li DY, Sorenson LK, Brooke BS, et al. Defective angiogenesis in mice lacking endoglin. *Science* 1999; **284**: 1534–1537.

23 Oh SP, Seki T, Goss KA, et al. Activin receptor-like kinase 1 modulates transforming growth factor-β1 signalling in the regulation of angiogenesis. *Proc Natl Acad Sci USA* 2000; **97**: 2626–2631.

24 Sapru RP, Hutchinson DC, Hall JI. Pulmonary hypertension in patients with pulmonary arteriovenous fistulae. *Br Heart J* 1969; **31**: 559–569.

25 Trell E, Johansson BW, Linell F, Ripa J. Familial pulmonary hypertension and multiple abnormalities of large systemic arteries in Osler's disease. *Am J Med* 1972; **53**: 50–63.

26 Trembath RC, Thomson JR, Machado RD, et al. Clinical and molecular genetic features of pulmonary hypertension in hereditary hemorrhagic telangiectasia. *N Engl J Med* 2001; **345**: 325–334.

27 Schulick AH, Taylor AJ, Zuo W, et al. Overexpression of TGF-β1 in arterial endothelium causes hyperplasia, apoptosis, and cartilaginous metaplasia. *Proc Natl Acad Sci USA* 1998; **95**: 6983–6988.

28 Rosenweig BL, Imamura T, Okadome T, et al. Cloning and characterization of a human type II receptor for bone morphogenetic proteins. *Proc Natl Acad Sci USA* 1995; **92**: 7632–7636.

3

Pathology of pulmonary hypertension

Anne E. Bishop and Julia M. Polak

Imperial College London, UK

Introduction

The pulmonary circulation receives the entire cardiac output and its vessels are uniquely structured to provide a low resistance system to accommodate the high flow. Thus the vessels are thin walled, comparatively wide, and acutely sensitive to raised pressure. The pulmonary arterial pressure for a normal resting adult at sea level is 14 ± 3 mmHg (1 mmHg $\approx$ 133.3 Pa) (mean $\pm$ standard error of the mean) and so pulmonary hypertension is defined as a level that would be expected to occur in fewer than 1% of a normal population; 25 mmHg or above at rest [1,2]. This allows a clinical diagnosis to be made. At present, in line with the National Institutes of Health (NIH) Registry, exclusion of possible causative conditions, such as cardiac, respiratory, thromboembolic or connective tissue diseases, allows a diagnosis of idiopathic (or primary) rather than secondary pulmonary hypertension. For secondary disease, the predisposing condition is usually evident and patients can be monitored for possible hypertensive changes. The idiopathic form is insidious and, when it does finally present clinically, it is with nonspecific symptoms of dyspnoea and fatigue, so diagnosis is delayed, on average by two years [2]. The principal pathological feature of chronic pulmonary hypertension is pulmonary vascular remodelling, where both the cellular and extracellular components of the arteries undergo dramatic reorganization.

Our knowledge of the pathogenesis of pulmonary hypertension is limited and, consequently, despite major advances in recent years, pharmacological therapy is not always successful. For primary disease in particular, there is no real cure and lung or heart–lung transplantation is often the only option for survival [3]. Why has this disease remained such an enigma? A major factor has been the comparative lack of interest in the pulmonary circulation shown by the medical fraternity. It is only 45 years since the importance of the pulmonary circulation was finally acknowledged, with the first ever conference devoted entirely to it being held in 1958 [4]. In the same year, the first detailed study of the morphological abnormalities that occur in the hypertensive lung was published [5]. The progress made in the clinical and surgical management of pulmonary hypertension is described in other chapters in this volume. On the histopathology side, the Heath and Edwards system of grading has been updated over the years [6–8] but, in essence, remains in present-day use despite criticisms, for example, that the variability of the pathological changes seen restricts its usefulness [9]. Recent work, notably by the Denver collaboration of Rubin Tuder and Norbert Voelkel and by Marlene Rabinovitch's group in Ontario, has argued for a re-evaluation of the classification of the pathological features of the hypertensive lung not just for diagnostic purposes but also to further our understanding of the pathogenesis of the disease. In studying the hypertensive lung, the perspective of the pathologist has largely been one of viewing the structural consequences of raised blood pressure; most of the original observations were made on lungs taken at cardiac surgery. This view has been confounded by the detailed documentation of the histological changes that occur in animal models of pulmonary hypertension created, for example, by systemic to pulmonary artery shunt [7,10,11]. No satisfactory model of primary pulmonary hypertension exists to provide the means to study its genesis from the early stages.

These days, the histopathologist is no longer confined to describing morphology alone. In-depth analysis is possible through the application of modern technology, including immunocytochemistry, molecular biology and selective tissue culture. In this chapter, the authors review both the histological features that can be seen in chronic pulmonary hypertension and the progress that has been made towards gaining insight into the pathobiology of the disease through the application of histological analysis of the diseased lung.

Histopathology

Vascular disease in the lung is usually associated with pulmonary hypertension and so the histopathology covers a variety of clinical conditions. The histopathological description that follows is restricted to plexogenic arteriopathy [1,12], a term adopted for the characteristic morphological pattern seen in chronic pulmonary hypertension that encompasses the entire range of pathological alterations that the pulmonary vessels can undergo. Plexogenic pulmonary arteriopathy is seen in primary pulmonary hypertension and in association with certain conditions including congenital cardiac shunts [13,14], portal vein thrombosis/portal hypertension [15–17] and, most recently recognized, human immunodeficiency virus (HIV) infection [18,19]. Conventional histopathological assessment shows no morphological features that can allow a distinction to be made between primary and secondary forms of plexogenic pulmonary arteriopathy [20].

Medial hypertrophy

Thickening of the media of the pulmonary arteries, through hypertrophy/hyperplasia of smooth muscle cells in muscularized arteries and formation or extension of muscle into normally nonmuscularized arteries, is the most frequent lesion in the hypertensive lung. It is, therefore, not specific to plexogenic arteriopathy and can be seen, albeit in a milder form, even in lungs from subjects without pulmonary hypertension. In the undistended normal postmortem lung, the muscular component of the pulmonary arteries forms around 5% of the external diameter of the vessel [21,22] and, for medium to large arteries, this rises to about one quarter of the diameter in severe pulmonary hypertension [22,23]. It has been reported, on the basis of ultrastructural studies, that there are two types of vascular smooth muscle within muscular arteries in plexogenic arteriopathy [24]. The cytoplasm of most of the muscle cells was found to be light but some showed relatively dark cytoplasm. These dark muscle cells were seen to migrate towards the inner media of the vessels and into the intima (see below). However, apart from this ultrastructural analysis and measurements of medial thickness, little has been done to establish the phenotypic and functional alterations that the medial muscle undergoes during the pathogenesis of plexiform arteriopathy.

Intimal cellular hyperplasia

Proliferation of the intima, the formation of a layer of cells between the endothelium and the internal elastic lamina, is not specific to pulmonary hypertension and can be a feature of the ageing lung as well as being associated with certain diseases [5]. It is usually seen first in small muscular arteries and arterioles and causes vessel occlusion. Migration of smooth muscle cells from the inner half of the media, as mentioned above, has long been thought to be the basis of the intimal expansion [24–26]. It has been reported that the endothelium does not contribute directly to the cellular intimal proliferation [27], although it may affect the activity and proliferation of smooth muscle cells [28]. However, the endothelium is thickened in individuals with congenital heart defects [29] and shows ultrastructural evidence of increased metabolic activity [8]. In addition, it has recently been suggested [30] to contribute through transdifferentiation to smooth muscle cells [31,32]. When the muscle cells have reached the intima, significant numbers appear to dedifferentiate to myofibrobasts [24] and there is a gradual build up of collagen and elastic fibres. This intimal fibrosis has a characteristic, concentric laminar pattern, also known as onion skin configuration. At later stages, concentric elastic fibrils are deposited. The fibrosis often leads to total obliteration of the vessel lumen and represents an irreversible stage in the pathogenesis of plexogenic arteriopathy.

Arterial dilatation

Dilatation of muscular arteries and arterioles, both generalized and localized, is present in plexogenic arteriopathy and is thought to be due to the incapacity of a segment of vessel wall to cope with excessive intraluminal pressure. Local dilatations, such as thin-walled, dilated branches of hypertrophied muscular arteries, have been termed dilatation lesions [5]. In extreme, so-called angiomatoid lesions form. These are clusters of dilated vessels usually arising from a muscular artery proximal to a fibrotic occlusion.

Fibrinoid necrosis and arteritis

The term fibrinoid necrosis refers to the infiltration of the vascular wall by fibrin, with consequent breakdown of the media and elastic laminae. These lesions, which typically occur just after the ramification of a branch from its parent artery, have been suggested to give rise to plexiform lesions [7,27]. Although there is not always an inflammatory response to the fibrinoid necrosis, an acute reaction can occur, particularly in patients with congenital cardiac

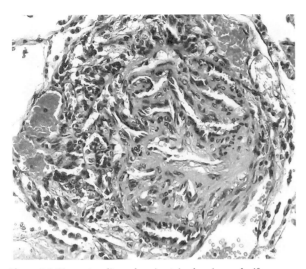

Figure 3.1 Haematoxylin and eosin stain showing a plexiform lesion in the lung of a patient with primary pulmonary hypertension (285×).

shunts. The entire arterial wall is infiltrated by neutrophils and the exudate often spills over into the surrounding lung. Affected arteries frequently show thrombosis.

Plexiform lesions

These lesions often occur distal to a site of arterial ramification and are dilated segments of artery filled by a compact bundle of tortuous vascular channels (Figure 3.1). Plexiform lesions have been suggested to be pathways for communication between the pulmonary arterial and venous systems [33–36] but serial sectioning [37–39] and, more recently, three-dimensional reconstruction [40,41] have shown that they are entirely arterial in nature. As mentioned above, they were previously supposed to arise at sites of fibrinoid necrosis [7,27] or post-thrombotic scarring [42] and be a proliferative response to injury rather than neo-angiogenesis. Recent evidence suggests, however, that they are produced by endothelial cell growth in a process of local angiogenesis [43,44].

The presence of fibrinoid necrosis and plexiform lesions in the lung is associated with poor prognosis as, although irreversibility of the arteriopathy occurs earlier, their formation seems to represent a stage of enhanced disease progression.

Molecular mechanisms

The composition and structure of the vascular wall is clearly under the control of a delicately balanced system of soluble mediators, principally growth factors and cytokines. These mediators are released not only from cells normally present in the wall but also from other cell types including, for example, platelets containing the potent mitogen platelet-derived growth factor (PDGF) [45], mast cells that can affect matrix production [46] and macrophages that produce several potentially contributing bioactive substances, including transforming growth factor β (TGF-β) [45]. Changes within the pulmonary vascular system, hypoxia, haemodynamic alterations and/or inflammation, precipitate a cascade of events in the wall that lead to structural remodelling of the vasculature. This can be compensatory and reversible during an adapative physiological response or pathological, as in pulmonary hypertension. Although in recent years considerable advances have been made in unravelling the complexities of the molecular basis of vascular remodelling, the whole process still remains largely enigmatic. The following is an account of some of the most recent advances made in this area and concentrates on the possible contributions of major vasodilator and vasoconstrictor substances to vascular remodelling.

Nitric oxide

It has been recognized comparatively recently that the endothelium may be a mediator of pulmonary hypertension as it produces a number of vasoactive factors including the free radical gas nitric oxide (NO). As its original name of endothelium-derived relaxing factor indicates, NO is a potent vasodilator with profound effects on blood flow [47]. Nitric oxide is produced from L-arginine by the action of NO synthase (NOS), an enzyme that exists in three isoforms; one that is calcium independent and inducible (type II or iNOS) and two that are calcium dependent and mainly expressed constitutively in neurons (type I or nNOS) and endothelium (type II or eNOS) [47].

In view of its vasodilatory action, inhalation of NO was an obvious choice for the treatment of pulmonary hypertension and it has been shown to reduce pulmonary vascular resistance in the disease [48]. An advantage of the clinical use of NO is that it is relatively specific to the pulmonary bed as its binding to haemoglobin in lung capillaries reduces its activity in the systemic circulation. In view of this compensatory effect of exogenous NO, functional studies of hypoxic animal models [49,50] and humans [51,52] were made. The results indicated impairment of the eNOS system in pulmonary hypertension. In addition, deletion of the eNOS gene results in systemic hypertension [53] and pulmonary vasoconstriction [54]. Subsequent morphological studies confirmed this by showing abnormal levels of eNOS expression in the hypertensive human lung. In general, a reduction was seen in the endothelium of pulmonary

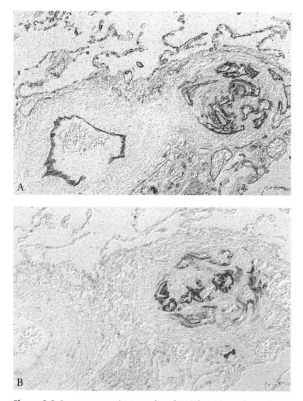

Figure 3.2 Low power micrographs of serial sections through an artery and a plexiform lesion. (A) Immunostaining for CD31 to demonstrate endothelium and in (B) immunostaining for endothelial nitric oxide synthase shows dense immunoreactivity in cells lining the plexiform lesion but not in the artery.

arterial vessels [55,56] (Figure 3.2). Considerable evidence exists to show that NO derived from the endothelium has a negative effect on vascular smooth muscle growth [57–60]. Therefore, the lack of endothelial NO production, in addition to reducing the intrinsic mechanism controlling the relaxation of the vessel wall, may also underlie the extensive remodelling that characterizes pulmonary hypertension, particularly in its chronic form. It was also shown that the expression of eNOS is increased in the endothelium of plexiform lesions [56] (Figure 3.2). An additional effect of eNOS is to mediate the actions of the potent endothelial mitogen vascular endothelial growth factor [61–63] (see below). Thus the increase of eNOS in these lesions gives support to the suggestion that these are sites of active endothelial proliferation rather than passive scarring [43].

Vascular endothelial growth factor

The highly specific endothelial mitogen vascular endothelial growth factor (VEGF) [64–66] is found in a range of cell types, including the vascular smooth muscle [67–69]. The importance of its role in vasculogenesis and angiogenesis [70–72] is underlined by the lethality of targeted disruption of the VEGF gene [73,74]. VEGF stimulates endothelial cells by binding to tyrosine kinase receptors on the cell surface known as Flt-1 (or VEGFR-1) and Flk-1/KDR (or VEGFR-2) [75–77], with eNOS acting as a downstream mediator, as mentioned above. Upregulation of VEGF has been demonstrated in a variety of conditions where there is pathological angiogenesis, apparently in reponse to tissue hypoxia [78]. There is some evidence for upregulation in pulmonary hypertension. In experimental animals, chronic hypoxic pulmonary hypertension is associated with increased expression of VEGF gene and receptors [79]. More recently, increased levels of VEGF have been reported in the lungs [68,69] and plasma/serum [80,81] of patients with primary pulmonary hypertension. A recent study using northern blotting and in situ hybridization demonstrated the upregulation of the RNA for Flt-1, as well as the angiopoietin receptor Tek (or Tie-2), in peripheral lung from patients with end-stage primary pulmonary hypertension as compared with normal controls [82] (Figure 3.3). Gene expression of the KDR receptor was found to be unaltered. Similar selective upregulation of the transcription of Flt-1 has been shown to occur in hypoxia [83,84].

Prostacyclin

Another vasodilator that has given substantial success in the treatment of pulmonary hypertension, particularly the primary form, is prostacyclin (epoprostenol) [85–87], although it has been observed that the dosage needed to maintain its effects has to be increased with time [87]. This may be the result of desensitization and/or vascular remodelling, as was suggested some time ago [88]. Like NO, prostacyclin suppresses the growth of smooth muscle cells [89–93]. Prostacyclin is formed from the precursor prostaglandin H_2 in an isomerization reaction catalyzed by prostacyclin synthase [92,94,95]. It is found in endothelial cells from which it is released to act locally and maintain the low vascular resistance normally found in the lung [96]. A study of the expression of prostacyclin synthase in the hypertensive lung showed that the protein is present in endothelium of vessels that have undergone relatively little remodelling but lacking from those that have altered their structure significantly [97]. The biological actions of prostacyclin are expressed through binding to membrane-associated receptors and consequent increase in intracellular cyclic AMP concentrations via direct stimulation of adenylyl cyclase [98]. Investigation of the distribution of the prostacyclin receptor protein in end-stage pulmonary

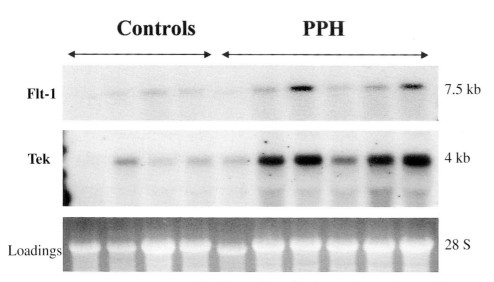

Figure 3.3 Northern blots of RNA extracts of lung from patients with primary pulmonary hypertension (PPH, $n = 6$) and unused donor lungs ($n = 4$). Clear upregulation of RNA for the VEGF receptor Flt-1 can be seen, as well as for the angiopoietin receptor Tek.

hypertension revealed that there is significantly less in lung from patients with primary disease, irrespective of whether they received epoprostenol treatment, compared with patients with secondary disease and normal controls [99] (Figure 3.4). In addition, work on animal models supports a role for prostacyclin in the pulmonary vascular response to chronic hypoxia. Transgenic mice that overexpress the prostacyclin gene are protected against the development of hypoxic pulmonary hypertension while prostacyclin receptor knockout mice are reported to develop more severe pulmonary hypertension and vascular remodelling than their wild-type counterparts in response to chronic hypoxia [100,101].

The loss of both prostacyclin synthase and prostacyclin receptors indicates a major defect in this intrinsic vasodilatory pathway in pulmonary hypertension. The significantly greater loss of receptor protein in primary disease may help to explain why the condition is more severe and bears a worse prognosis than the secondary form, as well as providing a basis for a possible differential diagnostic tool.

Endothelin

In direct contrast to nitric oxide and prostacyclin, another endothelial factor, endothelin, is not only the most potent vasoconstrictor known [102], but also a mitogen for smooth muscle cells [103,104]. Increased production and activity of endothelin would thus be expected in pulmonary hypertension and there is considerable evidence that this is indeed the case. Circulating levels of endothelin have been

reported to be elevated in primary pulmonary hypertension [105,106] and appear to correlate with the severity of the disease [107]. Morphological analysis has revealed increased expression of endothelin-1, its mRNA and its synthetic enzyme, endothelin-converting enzyme (ECE-1), in the vascular endothelium of lung from patients with pulmonary hypertension as compared with normal controls [28,108]. These findings have led to suggestions that specific blockade of endothelin A receptors, present on smooth muscle cells, may be used to treat pulmonary hypertension.

Renin–angiotensin system

The effector molecule of the homeostatic renin–angiotensin system, angiotensin II, is not only a vasoconstrictor like endothelin but also a potent stimulator of vascular smooth muscle proliferation and hypertrophy [109–111], although some variability in the growth response has been reported [112–113]. Angiotensin II is formed from angiotensin I by the hydrolytic action of angiotensin-converting enzyme (ACE), which is thought to determine the local concentrations of angiotensin II at the tissue level. ACE is attached to the luminal surface of the vascular endothelium by a carboxyl residue. Chronic hypoxia increases the expression of ACE in experimental animals [114] and long-term inhibition of the enzyme's activity reduces vascular remodelling in the animals [115,116]. ACE inhibitors have also been tested in humans with primary pulmonary hypertension and, although they do not appear to cause acute pulmonary vasodilatation

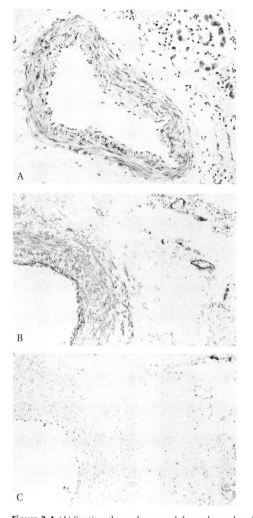

Figure 3.4 (A) Section through unused donor lung showing immunoreactivity for prostacyclin receptor protein on the wall of an arterial vessel. (B) and (C) show serial sections through lung taken from a patient with primary pulmonary hypertension immunostained for alpha smooth muscle actin (B), to show the vascular muscle, and for prostacyclin receptor protein (C) where, unlike the normal lung, little receptor protein can be seen on the vessel wall.

[117], long-term administration is associated with reduced pulmonary vascular resistance (118,119). A role for angiotensin II in human pulmonary vascular remodelling is supported by the finding of increased immunoreactivity for ACE in the endothelium of pulmonary arteries in primary pulmonary hypertension as compared with normal controls [120] and the presence of angiotensin II type 1 (AT_1) receptors on human pulmonary artery smooth muscle cells in vivo and in vitro that are coupled to activation of DNA and protein synthesis (121).

BMPR2

A major step forward in unravelling the pathobiology of primary pulmonary hypertension was made recently with the discovery of heterozygous germline mutations of the bone morphogenetic protein receptor II (*BMPR2*) gene in familial primary pulmonary hypertension [122]. These mutations have also been reported in 32% of sporadic cases of the disease [123]. BMPR II is a member of the transforming growth factor beta (TGF-β) cell signalling superfamily and thus these defects could contribute in various ways to the pathogenesis of pulmonary hypertension as TGF-β ligands modulate a large range of cellular functions, including vasculogenesis, angiogenesis and wound healing [124]. Little is known about the distribution of BMPR II in the lung. An initial report suggests that, in normal lung, it occurs on endothelium, with minimal expression on airway or vascular smooth muscle, and in primary pulmonary hypertension, in addition to endothelial expression, it is present on myofibroblasts of concentric laminar and obliterative lesions in small arteries [125] (see Chapter 2).

Conclusions

Major progress has been made in the past decade in the management of pulmonary hypertension, leading to significant improvements in both patient survival and quality of life. However, despite the considerable advances made in our understanding of the mechanisms controlling vascular activity and growth, pulmonary hypertension remains a life-threatening condition. It is hoped that, through the discovery of further potential regulators and the in-depth understanding of how they all work, the momentum gained in recent years will be maintained and new diagnostic approaches and more effective treatments will soon be available.

Acknowledgements

The authors wish to thank the Wellcome Trust, the Jonathan Sparkes Memorial Fund and United Therapeutics for support.

REFERENCES

1 Hatano S, Strasser T. Primary pulmonary hypertension. *WHO Reg Publ Eur Ser* 1975; 7–45.
2 Rich S, Dantzker DR, Ayres SM, et al. Primary pulmonary hypertension. A national prospective study. *Ann Intern Med* 1987; **107**: 216–223.

3 Higenbottam TW, Spiegelhalter D, Scott JP, et al. Prostacyclin (epoprostenol) and heart–lung transplantation as treatments for severe pulmonary hypertension. *Br Heart J* 1993; **70**: 366–370.

4 Adams W, Veith I. *Pulmonary circulation.* Grune & Stratton, New York. 1959.

5 Heath D, Edwards, JE. The pathology of pulmonary hypertensive disease. A description of six grades of structural changes in pulmonary arteries with special reference to congenital cardiac septal changes. *Circulation* 1958; **18**: 533–547.

6 Wagenvoort CA, Wagenvoort N. Primary pulmonary hypertension. A histopathologic study of the lung vessels in 156 clinically diagnosed cases. *Circulation* 1970; **42**: 1163–1184.

7 Wagenvoort CA, Wagenvoort N. *Pathology of pulmonary hypertension.* John Wiley, New York, 1977.

8 Rabinovitch M, Keane JF, Fellows KE, Castaneda AR, Reid L. Quantitative analysis of the pulmonary wedge angiogram in congenital heart defects. *Circulation* 1981; **63**: 152–154.

9 Edward WD. Pathology of pulmonary hypertension. *Cardiovasc Clin* 1988; **18**: 321–359.

10 Ferguson DJ, Varco RL. The relation of blood pressure and flow to the development and regression of experimentally induced pulmonary arteriosclerosis. *Circ Res* 1955; **3**: 152–158.

11 Blank RH, Muller WH, Damman JF. Experimental pulmonary hypertension. *Am J Surg* 1961; **101**: 143–153.

12 Wagenvoort CA, Mooi WJ. Vascular diseases. In: Dial DH and Hammar SP, eds. *Pulmonary pathology*, 2nd edn. Springer-Verlag, New York, 1994: 985–1026.

13 Wagenvoort CA. Open lung biopsies in congenital heart disease for evaluation of hypertensive pulmonary vascular disease. Predictive value with regard to corrective operability. *Histopathology* 1985; **9**: 417–436.

14 Haworth SG. Pulmonary vascular diseases in ventricular septal defect: structural and functional correlations in lung biopsies from 85 patients, with outcome of intra-cardiac repair. *J Pathol* 1987; **152**: 157–168.

15 Saunders JB, Constable TJ, Heath D, Smith P, Paton A. Pulmonary hypertension complicating portal vein thrombosis. *Thorax* 1978; **34**: 281–283.

16 Edwards BS, Weir EK, Edwards WD, Ludwig J, Dykoski RK, Edwards JE. Coexistent pulmonary and portal hypertension: morphological and clinical features. *J Am Coll Cardiol* 1987; **10**: 1233–1238.

17 Robalino BD, Moodie DS. Association between primary pulmonary hypertension and portal hypertension: analysis of its pathophysiology and clinical laboratory and hemodynamic manifestations. *J Am Coll Cardiol* 1991; **17**: 492–498.

18 Speich R, Jenni R, Opravil M, Pfab M, Russi EW. Primary pulmonary hypertension in HIV infection. *Chest* 1991; **100**: 1268–1271.

19 Petitpretz P, Brenot F, Azarian R, et al. Pulmonary hypertension in patients with human immunodeficiency virus infection: comparison with primary pulmonary hypertension. *Circulation* 1994; **89**: 2722–2727.

20 Caslin AW, Heath D, Madden B, Yacoub M, Gosney JR, Smith P. The histopathology of 36 cases of plexogenic pulmonary arteriopathy. *Histopathology* 1990; **16**: 9–19.

21 Heath D, Best PV. The tunica media of the arteries of the lung in pulmonary hypertension. *J Pathol Bacteriol* 1958; **76**: 165–174.

22 Wagenvoort CA, Mooi WJ. *Biopsy pathology of the pulmonary vasculature.* Chapman & Hall, London, 1989.

23 Chazova I, Loyd JE, Zhdanov VS, Newman JH, Belenkov Y, Meyrick B. Pulmonary artery adventitial changes and venous involvement in primary pulmonary hypertension. *Am J Pathol* 1995; **146**: 389–397.

24 Heath D, Smith P, Gosney J. Ultrastructure of early plexogenic pulmonary arteriopathy. *Histopathology* 1988; **12**: 41–52.

25 Esterly JA, Glagov S, Ferguson DJ. Morphogenesis of intimal obliterative hyperplasia of small arteries in experimental pulmonary hypertension. An ultrastructural study of the role of smooth muscle cells. *Am J Pathol* 1968; **52**: 325–327.

26 Smith P, Heath D, Yacoub M, Madden B, Caslin A, Gosney J. The ultrastructure of plexogenic pulmonary arteriopathy. *J Pathol* 1990; **160**: 111–121.

27 Harris P, Heath D. *The human pulmonary circulation.* Churchill Livingstone, Edinburgh, 1986.

28 Giaid A, Yanagisawa M, Langleben D, et al. Expression of endothelin-1 in the lungs of patients with pulmonary hypertension. *N Engl J Med* 1993; **328**: 1732–1739.

29 Hall SM, Haworth SG. Onset and evolution of pulmonary vascular disease in young children: abnormal postnatal remodelling studied in lung biopsies. *J Pathol* 1992; **166**: 183–193.

30 Voelkel NF, Tuder RM. Cellular and molecular biology of vascular smooth muscle cells in pulmonary hypertension. *Pulmon Pharmacol Ther* 1997; **10**: 231–241.

31 Arciniegas E, Sutton AB, Alled TD, Schor AM. Transforming growth factor-beta-1 promoted the differentiation of endothelial cells into smooth muscle-like cells in vitro. *J Cell Sci* 1992; **103**: 521–529.

32 DeRuiter MC, Poelmann RE, Van Munsteren JC, Mironov V, Markwald RR, Gittenberger-deGroot AC. Embryonic endothelial cells transdifferentiate into mesenchymal cells expressing smooth muscle actins in vivo and in vitro. *Circ Res* 1997; **80**: 444–451.

33 Rutishauser E, Blanc W. Anastomoses arterioveineuses glomiques du poumon avec syndrome d'insuffrance droite et cyanose. *Schweiz Z Allg Pathol Bakteriol* 1950; **13**: 61–65.

34 Spencer H. Primary pulmonary hypertension and related vascular changes in the lungs. *J Pathol Bacteriol* 1950; **62**: 489–493.

35 Jewett JF, Ober WB. Primary pulmonary hypertension as a cause of maternal death. *Am J Obstet Gynecol* 1956; **71**: 1335–1341.

36 Jamison BM, Michel RP. Different distribution of plexiform lesions in primary and secondary pulmonary hypertension. *Hum Pathol* 1995; **26**: 987–993.

37 Brewer DB. Fibrous occlusion and anastomosis of the pulmonary vessels in a case of pulmonary hypertension associated with patent ductus arteriosus. *J Pathol Bacteriol* 1955; **70**: 299–309.

38 Wagenvoort CA. The morphology of certain vascular lesions in pulmonary hypertension. *J Pathol Bacteriol* 1959; **78**: 503–510.

39 Naeye RL, Vennart GP. The structure and significance of pulmonary plexiform structures. *Am J Pathol* 1960; **36**: 593–597.

40 Ogata T, Iijima T. Structure and pathogenesis of plexiform lesion in pulmonary hypertension. *Chin Med J Engl* 1993; **106**: 45–48.

41 Tuder RM, Lee SD, Cool CD. Histopathology of pulmonary hypertension. *Chest* 1998; **114**(1 Suppl): 1S–6S.

42 Fuster V, Steele PM, Edwards WD, Gersh BJ, McGoon MD, Frye RL. Primary pulmonary hypertension: natural history and the importance of thrombosis. *Circulation* 1984; **70**: 580–587.

43 Tuder RM, Groves BM, Badesch DB, Voelkel NF. Exuberant endothelial cell growth and elements of inflammation are present in plexiform lesions of pulmonary hypertension. *Am J Pathol* 1994; **144**: 275–285.

44 Cool CD, Kennedy D, Voelkel NF, Tuder RM. Pathogenesis and evolution of plexiform lesions in pulmonary hypertension associated with scleroderma and human immunodeficiency virus infection. *Hum Pathol* 1997; **28**: 434–442.

45 Kaplan DR, Chao FC, Stiles CD, Antoniades HN, Scher CD. Platelet alpha granules contain a growth factor for fibroblasts. *Blood* 1979; **53**: 1043–1052.

46 Tozzi CA, Thakker-Varia S, Yu SY, et al. Mast cell collagenase correlates with regression of pulmonary vascular remodelling in the rat. *Am J Respir Cell Mol Biol* 1998; **18**: 497–510.

47 Moncada S, Palmer RMJ, Higgs EA. Nitric oxide: physiology, pathophysiology and pharmacology. *Pharm Rev* 1991; **43**: 109–142.

48 Pepke-Zaba J, Higenbottam TW, Dinh-Xuan AT, Stone D, Wallwork J. Inhaled nitric oxide as a cause of selective pulmonary vasodilatation in pulmonary hypertension. *Lancet* 1991; **338**: 1173–1174.

49 Adnot S, Raffestin B, Eddahibi S, Braquet P, Chabrier PE. Loss of endothelium-dependent relaxant activity in the pulmonary circulation of rats exposed to chronic hypoxia. *J Clin Invest* 1991; **87**: 155–162.

50 McQuillan LP, Leung GK, Marsden PA, Kostyk SK, Kourembanas S. Hypoxia inhibits expression of eNOS via transcriptional and post-transcriptional mechanisms. *Am J Physiol* 1994; **267**: H1921–H1927.

51 Dinh-Xuan AT, Higenbottam TW, Clelland CA, et al. Impairment of endothelium-dependent pulmonary-artery relaxation in chronic obstructive lung disease. *N Engl J Med* 1991; **324**: 1539–1547.

52 Brett SJ, Bibbs SR, Pepper JR, Evans TW. Impairment of endothelium-dependent pulmonary vasodilation in patients with primary pulmonary hypertension. *Thorax* 1996; **51**: 89–91.

53 Huang PL, Huang Z, Mashimo H, et al. Hypertension in mice lacking the gene for endothelial nitric oxide synthase. *Nature* 1995; **377**: 239–242.

54 Steudel W, Ichinose F, Huang PL, et al. Pulmonary vasoconstriction and hypertension in mice with targeted disruption of the endothelial nitric oxide synthase (*NOS 3*) gene. *Circ Res* 1997; **81**: 34–41.

55 Giaid A, Saleh D. Reduced expression of endothelial nitric oxide synthase in the lungs of patients with pulmonary hypertension. *N Engl J Med* 1995; **333**: 214–221.

56 Mason NA, Springall DR, Burke M, et al. High expression of endothelial nitric oxide synthase in plexiform lesions of pulmonary hypertension. *J Pathol* 1998; **185**: 313–318.

57 Garg UC, Hassid A. Nitric oxide-generating vasodilators and 8-bromo-cyclic guanosine monophosphate inhibit mitogenesis and proliferation of cultured rat vascular smooth muscle cells. *J Clin Invest* 1989; **83**: 1774–1777.

58 Sarkar R, Gordon D, Stanley JC, Webb RC. Cell cycle effects of nitric oxide on vascular smooth muscle cells. *Am J Physiol* 1997; **272**: H1810–H1818.

59 Rudic RD, Shesely EG, Maeda N, Smithies O, Segal SS, Sessa WC. Direct evidence for the importance of endothelium-derived nitric oxide in vascular remodeling. *J Clin Invest* 1998; **101**: 731–736.

60 Steudel W, Scherrer-Crosbie M, Bloch KD, et al. Sustained pulmonary hypertension and right ventricular hypertrophy after chronic hypoxia in mice with congenital deficiency of nitric oxide synthase 3. *J Clin Invest* 1998; **101**: 2468–2477.

61 Papapetropoulos A, García-Cardena G, Madri JA, Sessa WC. Nitric oxide production contributes to the angiogenic properties of vascular endothelial growth factor in human endothelial cells. *J Clin Invest* 1997; **100**: 3131–3139.

62 Ziche M, Morbidelli L, Choudhuri R, et al. Nitric oxide synthase lies downstream from vascular endothelial growth factor-induced but not basic fibroblast growth factor-induced angiogenesis. *J Clin Invest* 1997; **99**: 2625–2634.

63 Murohara T, Asahara T, Silver M, et al. Nitric oxide synthase modulates angiogenesis in response to tissue ischemia. *J Clin Invest* 1998; **101**: 2567–2578.

64 Gospodarowicz D, Abrakam JA, Schilling J. Isolation and characterization of a vascular endothelial cell mitogen produced by pituitary-derived folliculo-stellate cells. *Proc Natl Acad Sci USA* 1989; **86**: 7311–7315.

65 Ferrara N, Henzel WJ. Pituitary folliculo-stellate cells secrete a novel heparin-binding growth factor specific for vascular endothelial cells. *Biochem Biophys Res Commun* 1989; **161**: 851–858.

66 Neufeld G, Cohen T, Gengrinovitch S, Polotorak Z. Vascular endothelial growth factor (VEGF) and its receptors. *FASEB J* 1999; **13**: 9–22.

67 Shifren JL, Doldi N, Ferrara N, Mesiano S, Jaffe RB. In the human fetus, vascular endothelial growth factor is expressed in epithelial cells and myocytes, but not vascular endothelium: implication for mode of action. *J Clin Endocrinol Metab* 1994; **79**: 316–322.

68 Tuder RM, Wang J, Lee SD, Voelkel NF. Vascular endothelial growth factor (VEGF) expression in normal and remodelled pulmonary arteries in severe pulmonary hypertension. *Am J Respir Crit Care Med* 1997; **1555**: A627.

69 Shehata SMK, Mooi WJ, Okazaki T, El-Banna I, Sharma HS, Tibboel D. Enhanced expression of vascular endothelial growth factor in lungs of newborn infants with congenital diaphragmatic hernia and pulmonary hypertension. *Thorax* 1999; **54**: 427–431.

70 Tischer E, Mitchell R, Hartman T, et al. The human gene for vascular endothelial growth factor. Multiple protein forms are encoded through alternative exon splicing. *J Biol Chem* 1991; **266**: 11947–12154.

71 Shweiki D, Itin A, Neufeld G, Gitay-Goren H, Keshet E. Patterns of expression of vascular endothelial growth factor (VEGF) and VEGF receptors in mice suggest a role in hormonally regulated angiogenesis. *J Clin Invest* 1993; **91**: 2235–2243.

72 Jakeman LB, Armanini M, Phillips HS, Ferrara N. Developmental expression of binding sites and messenger ribonucleic acid for vascular endothelial growth factor suggests a role for this protein in vasculogenesis and angiogenesis. *Endocrinology* 1993; **133**: 848–859.

73 Ferrara N, Carvermoore K, Chen H, et al. Heterozygous embryonic lethality induced by targeted inactivation of the VEGF gene. *Nature* 1996; **380**: 439–442.

74 Carmeliet P, Ferreira V, Breier G, et al. Abnormal blood vessel development and lethality in embryos lacking a single VEGF allele. *Nature* 1996; **380**: 435–439.

75 Terman BI, Dougher-Vermazen M, Carrion ME, et al. Identification of the KDR tyrosine kinase as a receptor for vascular endothelial growth factor. *Biochem Biophys Res Commun* 1992; **187**: 1579–1586.

76 DeVries C, Escobedo JA, Ueno H, Houck K, Ferrara N, Williams LT. The fms-like tyrosine kinase, a receptor for vascular endothelial growth factor. *Science* 1992; **255**: 989–991.

77 Quinn TP, Peters KG, DeVries C, Ferrara N, Williams LT. Fetal liver kinase 1 is a receptor for vascular endothelial growth factor and is selectively expressed in vascular endothelium. *Proc Natl Acad Sci USA* 1993; **90**: 7533–7537.

78 Breier G, Damert A, Plate KH, Risau W. Angiogenesis in embryos and ischemic diseases. *Thromb Haemost* 1997; **78**: 678–683.

79 Tuder RM, Flook BE, Voelkel NF. Increased gene expression for VEGF and the VEGF receptors KDR/Flk and Flt in lungs exposed to acute or to chronic hypoxia. Modulation of gene expression by nitric oxide. *J Clin Invest* 1995; **95**: 1798–1807.

80 Maloney J, Voelkel NF. Plasma levels of vascular endothelial growth factor are increased in primary pulmonary hypertension. *Am J Respir Crit Care Med* 1999; **159**: A164.

81 Sediame S, Humbert M, Chouaid C, et al. Serum and platelet VEGF concentrations in patients with COLD or primary pulmonary hypertension. *Am J Respir Crit Care Med* 1999; **159**: A697.

82 Tuder RM, Chacon MR, Alger L., et al. Expression of angiogenesis-related molecules in plexiform lesions in severe pulmonary hypertension: evidence for a process of disordered angiogenesis. *J Pathol* 2001; **195**: 367–374.

83 Gerber HP, Condorelli F, Park J, Ferrara N. Differential transcriptional regulation of the two vascular endothelial growth factor receptor genes. Flt-1 but not flk-1/kdr, is upregulated by hypoxia. *J Biol Chem* 1997; **272**: 23659–23677.

84 Marti HH, Risau W. Systemic hypoxia changes the organ-specific distribution of vascular endothelial growth factor and its receptors. *Proc Natl Acad Sci USA* 1998; **95**: 15809–15814.

85 Rubin LJ, Groves BM, Reeves JT, Frosolono M, Handel F, Cato AE. Prostacyclin-induced pulmonary vasodilation in primary pulmonary hypertension. *Circulation* 1982; **66**: 334–338.

86 Rubin LJ, Mendoza J, Hood M, et al. Treatment of primary pulmonary hypertension with continuous intravenous prostacyclin (epoprostenol). Results of a randomized trial. *Ann Intern Med* 1990; **112**: 485–491.

87 Barst RJ, Rubin LJ, McGoon MD, Caldwell EJ, Long WA, Levy PS. Survival in primary pulmonary hypertension with long-term continuous intravenous prostacyclin. *Ann Intern Med* 1994; **121**: 409–415.

88 Badesch DB, Orton EC, Zapp LM, et al. Decreased arterial wall prostaglandin production in neonatal calves with severe chronic pulmonary hypertension. *Am J Respir Cell Mol Biol* 1989; **1**: 489–498.

89 Uehara Y, Ishimitsu T, Kimura K, Ishii M, Ikeda T, Sugimoto T. Regulatory effects of eicosanoids on thymidine uptake by vascular smooth muscle cells of rats. *Prostaglandins* 198; **36**: 847–857.

90 Shirotani M, Yui Y, Hattori R, Kawai C. U-61, 431F, a stable prostacyclin analogue, inhibits the proliferation of bovine vascular smooth muscle cells with little antiproliferative effect on endothelial cells. *Prostaglandins* 1991; **41**: 97–110.

91 Asada Y, Kisanuki A, Hatakeyama K, et al. Inhibitory effects of prostacyclin analogue TFC-132 on aortic neointimal thickening in vivo and smooth muscle cell proliferation in vitro. *Prostaglandins Leukot Essent Fatty Acids* 1994; **51**: 245–258.

92 Hara S, Miyata A, Yokoyama C, et al. Molecular cloning and expression of prostacyclin synthase from endothelial cells. *Adv Prostaglandin Thromboxane Leukotriene Res* 1995; **23**: 121–123.

93 Peiro C, Redondo J, Rodriguez-Martínez MA, et al. Influence of endothelium on cultured vascular smooth muscle cell proliferation. *Hypertension* 1995; **25**: 748–751.

94 Miyata A, Hara S, Yokoyama C, Inoue H, Ullrich V, Tanabe T. Molecular cloning and expression of human prostacyclin synthase. *Biochem Biophys Res Commun* 1994; **200**: 1728–1742.

95 Yokoyama C, Yabuki T, Inoue H, et al. Human gene encoding prostacyclin synthase (PTGIS): genomic organisation, chromosomal localisation and promoter activity. *Genomics* 1996; **6**: 296–304.

96 Gryglewski RJ, Korbut R, Ocetkiewicz A. Generation of prostacyclin by lungs in vivo and its release into the arterial circulation. *Nature* 1978; **273**: 765–767.

97 Tuder RM, Wang J, Cool CD, et al. Prostacyclin synthase expression is decreased in lungs with severe pulmonary hypertension. *Am J Respir Crit Care Med* 1999; **159**: 1925–1932.

98 Halushka PV, Mais DE, Morinelli TA. Thromboxane and prostacyclin receptors. *Progr Clin Biol Res* 1989; **301**: 21–28.

99 Mason NA, Bishop AE, Yacoub MH, Tuder RM, Voelkel NF, Polak JM. Reduced expression of prostacyclin receptor protein on remodelled vessels in pulmonary hypertension. *Am J Respir Crit Care Med* 1999; **159**; A166.

100 Geraci MW, Gao B, Shepherd DC, et al. Pulmonary prostacyclin synthase overexpression in transgenic mice protects against development of hypoxic pulmonary hypertension. *J Clin Invest* 1999; **103**: 1509–1515.

101 Hoshikawa Y, Voelkel NF, Gesell TL, et al. Prostacyclin receptor-dependent modulation of pulmonary vascular remodelling. *Am J Respir Crit Care Med* 2001; **164**: 314–318.

102 Yanagisawa M, Kurihara H, Kimura S, et al. A novel potent vasoconstrictor peptide produced by vascular endothelial cells. *Nature* 1988; **332**: 411–415.

103 Dubin D, Pratt RE, Kooke JP, Dzau VJ. Endothelin, a potent vasoconstrictor, is a vascular smooth muscle mitogen. *J Vasc Biol Med* 1989; **1**: 150–154.

104 Hirata Y, Takagi Y, Fukuda Y, Marumo F. Endothelin is a potent mitogen for rat vascular smooth muscle cells. *Atherosclerosis* 1989; **78**: 225–228.

105 Stewart DJ, Levy RD, Cernacek P, Langleben D. Increased plasma endothelin-1 in pulmonary hypertension: marker or mediator of disease? *Ann Intern Med* 1991; **114**: 464–469.

106 Yoshibayashi M, Nishioka K, Nakao K, et al. Plasma endothelin concentrations in patients with pulmonary hypertension associated with congenital heart defects. Evidence for increased production of endothelin in pulmonary circulation. *Circulation* 1991; **84**: 2280–2285.

107 Nootens M, Kaufmann E, Rector T, et al. Neurohormonal activation in patients with right ventricular failure from pulmonary hypertension: relation to hemodynamic variables and endothelin levels. *J Am Coll Cardiol* 1995; **26**: 1581–1585.

108 Giaid A. Nitric oxide and endothelin-1 in pulmonary hypertension. *Chest* 1998; **114**: 208S–212S.

109 Campbell-Boswell M, Robertson AL. Effects of angiotensin II and vasopressin on human smooth muscle cells in vitro. *Exp Mol Pathol* 1981; **35**: 265–276.

110 Gibbons GH, Pratt RE, Dzau VJ. Vascular smooth muscle cell hypertrophy vs. hyperplasia. Autocrine transforming growth factor beta-1 expression determines growth response to angiotensin II. *J Clin Invest* 1992; **90**: 456–461.

111 Naftilan AJ, Gilliland GK, Eldridge CS, Kraft AS. Induction of the proto-oncogene c-*jun* by angiotensin II. *Mol Cell Biol* 1990; **10**: 5536–5540.

112 Jackson CL, Schwartz SM. Pharmacology of smooth muscle cell replication. *Hypertension* 1992; **20**: 713–736.

113 Sachinidis A, Ko Y, Nettekoven W, Wieczorek AJ, Dusing R, Vetter H. The effect of angiotensin II on DNA synthesis varies considerably in vascular smooth muscle cells from different Wistar–Kyoto rats. *J Hypertens* 1992; **10**: 1159–1164.

114 Morrell NW, Atochina EN, Morris KG, Danilov SG, Stenmark KR. Angiotensin converting enzyme expression is increased in small pulmonary arteries of rats with hypoxia-induced pulmonary hypertension. *J Clin Invest* 1995; **96**: 1823–1833.

115 Morrell NW, Morris KG, Stenmark KR. Role of angiotensin converting enzyme and angiotensin II in development of hypoxic pulmonary hypertension. *Am J Physiol* 1995; **269**: H1186–H1194.

116 Zhao L, Al-Tubuly R, Sebkhi A, Owji AA, Nuñez DJR, Wilkins MR. Angiotensin II receptor expression and inhibition in the chronically hypoxic rat lung. *Br J Pharmacol* 1996; **119**: 1217–1222.

117 Leier CV, Bambach D, Nelson S, et al. Captopril in primary pulmonary hypertension. *Circulation* 1983; **67**: 155–161.

118 Stumpe KO, Schmengler K, Bette L, Overlack A, Kolloch R. Persistent hemodynamic and clinical improvement after captopril in patients with pulmonary hypertension. *Herz* 1986; **11**: 217–225.

119 Alpert MA, Pressly TA, Mukerji V, Lambert CR, Mukerji B. Short- and long-term hemodynamic effects of captopril in patients with pulmonary hypertension and selected connective tissue disease. *Chest* 1992; **102**: 1407–1412.

120 Schuster DP, Crouch EC, Parks WC, Johnson T, Botney MD. Angiotensin converting enzyme expression in primary pulmonary hypertension. *Am J Respir Crit Care Med* 1996; **154**: 1087–1091.

121 Morrell NW, Upton PD, Kotecha S, et al. Angiotensin II activates MAPK and stimulates growth of human pulmonary artery smooth muscle cells via AT$_1$ receptors. *Am J Physiol* 1999; **277**: L440–L448.

122 International PPH Consortium, Lane KB, Machado RD, Pauciulo MW, et al. Heterozygous germline mutations in *BMPR2*, encoding a TGF-β receptor, cause familial primary pulmonary hypertension. *Nature Genet* 2000; **26**; 81–84.

123 Thomson J, Machado R., Pauciulo M., et al. Familial and sporadic primary pulmonary hypertension is caused by BMPR2 gene mutations resulting in haploinsufficiency of the bone morphogenetic protein type II receptor. *J Heart Lung Transplant* 2001; **20**: 149.

124 Massague J, Chen YG. Controlling TGF-β signalling. *Genes Dev* 2000; **14**: 627–644.

125 Atkinson C, Stewart S, Imamura T, Trembath RC, Morrell NW. Immunolocalization of BMPR-II and TGF-β type I and type II receptors in primary plexogenic pulmonary hypertension. *J Heart Lung Transplant* 2001; **20**: 149.

4

Pulmonary hypertension and the right ventricle

Norbert F. Voelkel[1], Rubin M. Tuder[2], Carlyne Cool[1], Mark Geraci[1],
Robert Quaife[1] and Michael Bristow[1]

[1]University of Colorado Health Services Center, Denver, Colorado, USA
[2]Johns Hopkins Medical School, Baltimore, Maryland, USA

Introduction

Severe chronic pulmonary hypertension develops in patients with congenital cardiovascular abnormalities, patients with thromboembolism, interstitial lung diseases, collagen-vascular disorders, patients with sickle cell disease and in a group of diseases summarized under the rubric of primary pulmonary hypertension [1–3]. Although the prevalence of severe pulmonary hypertension in the population is not known, there are estimates that the prevalence of primary pulmonary hypertension (PPH) is 1–2 per million people. The use of the term 'primary pulmonary hypertension' continues to produce confusion among patients, physicians and insurance providers. Attempts should be made to change the nomenclature. Recently, our group has made such an attempt [4]. One of the many vexing aspects of PPH and other forms of plexogenic pulmonary arteriopathy is the multifactorial aetiology of such diseases.

Figure 4.1 demonstrates that a familial genetic disposition to high blood flow, elevated shear stress, collagen-vascular diseases, liver cirrhosis and portal hypertension, viral infections and appetite suppressant drugs [5–13] can all lead to the same histopathological pattern. How is this possible? Is there a common pathomechanism that can explain such a multifaceted aetiology? In search of a 'unifying' hypothesis, we arrived at the concept of 'misguided angiogenesis'.

Pathobiology

Vasoconstriction or increased blood flow, and therefore increased shear stress, causes vascular injury, and either this vascular injury carries inflammatory features [14] or there is endothelial cell proliferation, autonomously triggered in the pulmonary precapillary arteries, that causes obliteration of most of the precapillary arterioles and severe pulmonary hypertension (Figure 4.2). We recently found that patients with sporadic severe pulmonary hypertension [15] and patients with anorexigen-induced pulmonary hypertension [12] have monoclonal endothelial cell expansion, whereas the plexiform lesions in patients with pulmonary hypertension associated with collagen vascular disease or cardiovascular abnormalities are strictly polyclonal (Figure 4.2).

Regardless of whether the lesions are monoclonal or polyclonal, pulmonary vascular remodelling [16] always occurs, i.e. altered pulmonary vascular structures are predictably detected in the lungs of patients with pulmonary hypertension. Great emphasis has been put, in the past, on vasoconstriction as an important, perhaps the most important, mechanism leading to vascular remodelling. This notion is based to a large measure on observations derived from animal models, because of a lack of knowledge of the natural history of these diseases in humans. The information gathered from animal experiments has been transposed to the human condition.

It is not known whether vasoconstriction is very important or the most important pathogenetic factor leading to pulmonary vascular remodelling in human pulmonary hypertension. In fact, 75% of the patients at the time of their first right heart catheterization have a pulmonary vascular bed that is practically unresponsive to acute vasodilator treatment, indicating that significant structural vascular alterations are present. The commonly stated explanation for this finding is that the patients are being diagnosed late in their disease at a time when structural alterations are quite advanced and that the investigators are notoriously missing the early disease states. An alternative explanation, however, is that vasoconstriction may not be as important in the pathogenesis of pulmonary hypertension and

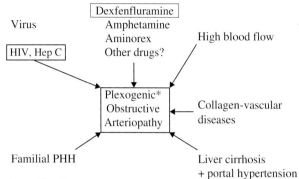

*Endothelial cell proliferation

Figure 4.1 The multiple causes of plexogenic pulmonary arteriopathy. PPH, primary pulmonary hypertension; HIV, human immunodeficiency virus; Hep C, hepatitis C.

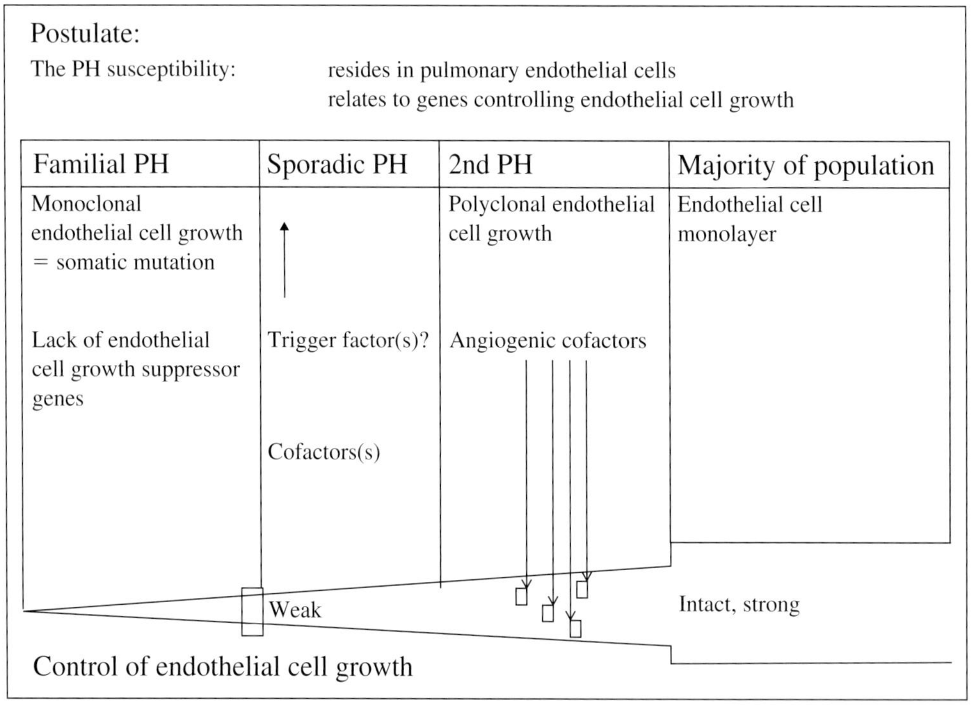

Postulate:

The PH susceptibility:　resides in pulmonary endothelial cells
relates to genes controlling endothelial cell growth

Familial PH	Sporadic PH	2nd PH	Majority of population
Monoclonal endothelial cell growth = somatic mutation		Polyclonal endothelial cell growth	Endothelial cell monolayer
Lack of endothelial cell growth suppressor genes	Trigger factor(s)?	Angiogenic cofactors	
	Cofactors(s)		
	Weak		Intact, strong

Control of endothelial cell growth

Figure 4.2 Comparison of monoclonal and polyclonal endothelial cell growth of plexiform lesions. Familial and sporadic forms of primary pulmonary hypertension (PH) show monoclonal endothelial cell growth in plexiform lesions, probably caused by somatic mutations of endothelial cells. In contrast, in severe pulmonary hypertension associated with liver disease or due to congenital cardiac malformation, the plexiform lesions show polyclonal endothelial cell growth. Angiogenic cofactors can change the endothelial cell phenotype and switch the endothelial cells towards proliferation. The usual state of the pulmonary vasculature is characterized by the fact that endothelial cells line up as a monolayer and it can be postulated that the control mechanisms preventing endothelial cells from piling up and proliferating are multigeneic and strong.

in the development of vascular remodelling as previously assumed in many of the patients with severe, progressive pulmonary hypertension.

For clarity, we can describe pulmonary vascular remodelling as a combination of alterations of the vascular smooth muscle layer and alterations that relate to endothelial cell structure and function. In pulmonary hypertension, the vascular smooth muscle cells extend further into the periphery of the vascular tree (longitudinal extension of the vascular smooth muscle cells). In addition, vascular smooth muscle cells (VSMCs) undergo hypertrophy, but little, if any, proliferation. The pulmonary hypertensive VSMC phenotype is likely to be noncontractile, i.e. the smooth muscle cell machinery that regulates contraction and relaxation is abnormal.

Endothelial cells are functionally and structurally abnormal, as evidenced by intimal thickening, altered gene and protein expression and by proliferation of endothelial cells that leads, via a process of 'misguided angiogenesis', to the formation of plexiform lesions (Figures 4.3–4.5).

Given that the pulmonary vascular remodelling includes both VSMC and endothelial cell abnormalities, we believe that what is fundamentally altered in vascular remodelling is the VSMC–endothelial interaction. Although separated by the internal elastic lamina, VSMCs and endothelial cells form essentially a syncytium. It makes 'sense' for the haemodynamically stressed pulmonary vessel to fortify its wall. This response, as already stated, is characterized by longitudinal extension of the VSMCs and by their hypertrophy. How increase of pressure, vessel wall tension and shear stress are sensed by the endothelial cells and translated into this vascular response is not understood. We can surmise that VSMC migration and perhaps pericyte differentiation occur in response to a combination of haemodynamic stress, hypoxia and inflammatory stimuli. In addition it can be speculated that endothelial cells may be able to 'help out' and quickly differentiate into VSMCs [17–18].

In order to comprehend the unusual intimal response, the nature of the normal adaptive response of the pulmonary vessels must be understood first. Or, to put it differently: why does the pulmonary vascular tree under conditions of chronic hypoxia with or without haemodynamic stress, respond with muscularization of the resistance vessels that is by and large completely reversible? Is it because the endothelial cells direct this process? Do plexiform lesions arise in regions of the lung vasculature where endothelial cell control of muscularization has become faulty?

Is it possible that neonatal pulmonary hypertension resembles more the muscularization response of the arteries and is more readily reversible when treated with epoprostenol (prostacyclin) than the adult plexiform presentation? Is the neonatal severe pulmonary hypertension of the muscular type due to something going wrong during the development of the lung or the lung vasculature? As stated above, we know very little about the full spectrum of endothelial cell–VSMC interactions. Known examples are control of VSMCs by endothelial cell-derived nitric oxide and prostacyclin together with effects on VSMCs by the interaction between vascular endothelial growth factor (VEGF) and its KDR receptors on endothelial cells.

We postulate that there are several principal mechanisms whereby the normal endothelial cell–VSMC interaction can be disrupted leading to vascular remodelling. First,

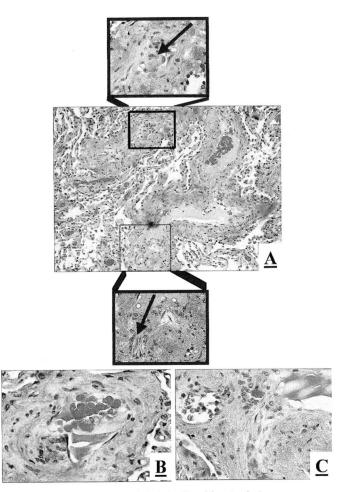

Figure 4.3 Example of early endothelial cell proliferation lesions. A low power photomicrograph of a medium-sized pulmonary artery is shown in (A). The insets of boxed areas show, at a higher magnification, the formation of conglomerates of round cells (arrow), heaping up from the intima towards the blood vessel lumen. A similar pattern is seen in a different vessel in (B). In (C), the endothelial cells appear to stream along the blood vessel branch, and already assume a somewhat spindle pattern, suggestive of progression to concentric proliferation and an abnormal phenotype.

there may be congenital or acquired endothelial cell gene mutations. Second, there may be a general genetic disposition facilitating the development of pulmonary hypertension because of a mutation in the transforming growth factor (TGF) beta 2 (TGF-β2) receptor or a mutation of the prostacyclin receptor (these are only two examples). Third, there may be mutations in the VSMC itself. Fourth, there are likely to be acquired VSMC alterations that go hand in hand with alterations in membrane ion channel expression [19–20] and alterations in the status of contractile proteins.

With this, a scenario emerges where the endothelial cell controls vascular remodelling and the disturbed

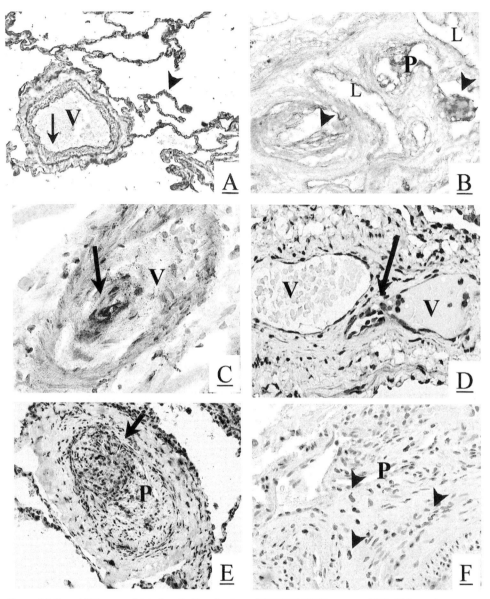

Figure 4.4 (A and B) Immunohistochemical localization of VEGF (D) VEGF receptor KDR, (E) hypoxia inducible factor-1 and (F) aryl hydrocarbon nuclear translocator (ARNT or HIF-1α) and (C) in situ hybridization for KDR mRNA in severe pulmonary hypertension with endothelial cell proliferation. (A) VEGF protein (V) is expressed along the basement membrane in alveolar septa (arrowhead) and internal and external elastic lamina in normal lung (165×). (B) VEGF protein is expressed within the endothelial cells (arrowheads) in a plexiform lesion (P) of a PPH patient. The remaining vascular lumen is marked (L) (150×). (C) KDR mRNA expression in endothelial cells present in the concentrically thickened intima in a pulmonary vessel (V) in a patient with PPH (300×). (D) KDR protein expression by a cluster of endothelial cells (arrow) in a pulmonary artery (V) of a patient with lupus-associated pulmonary hypertension. Note the weaker staining in the remainder of the endothelial cell lining of the same vessel. This cluster might represent an early stage of a plexiform lesion, such as shown in (B) and (E) (300×). (E) Intense expression of HIF-1α, one of the components of the HIF, in endothelial cells (arrow) of a plexiform lesion (P) (150×). (F) Expression of ARNT or HIF-1β, the second component of HIF, in the nuclei of the cells (arrowheads) in a plexiform lesion (P) (300×).

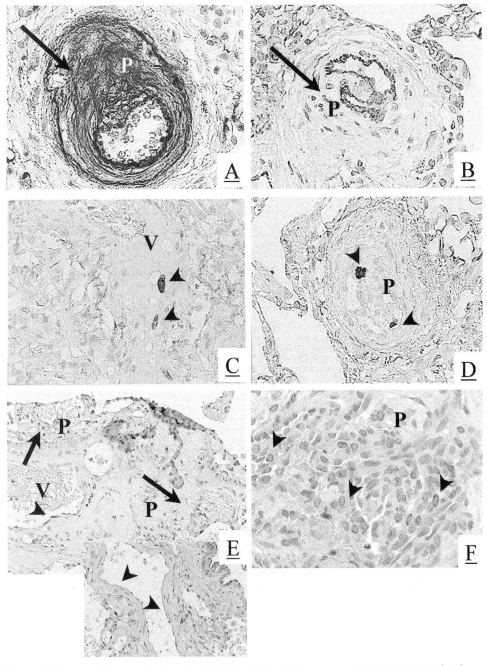

Figure 4.5 Phenotypic characterization of endothelial cells in plexiform lesions (P). (A) Factor VIII-related antigen (400×) reactivity of endothelial cells (arrow). (B) Platelet endothelial cell adhesion molecule (PECAM or CD31) immunostaining, which highlights exclusively the cells lining the slit-like vascular lumina of a serial section of the plexiform lesion shown in A (arrow) (280×). (E) Lack of prostacyclin synthase expression in a plexiform lesion (arrows), whereas there is preserved prostacyclin synthase expression in endothelial cells of the parent vessel (V) (arrowheads) (140×). (F) Expression of the anti-apoptotic molecule BCL-2 in the endothelial cells (arrowheads) of a plexiform lesion in a patient with severe pulmonary hypertension secondary to cardiac right to left shunting (280×).

VSMC–endothelial cell interaction is critical. Further, without (acquired?) endothelial cell mutations and/or without a pulmonary hypertensive genetic disposition, the pulmonary vasculature undergoes the usual muscularization.

In contrast to the morphological process involving VSMCs described above, which lack specificity and do not correlate closely with the degree of the haemodynamic alterations in severe pulmonary artery pressures, plexiform lesions occur in patients who have severe pulmonary hypertension with associated conditions or in an idiopathic form (PPH). This is one of the vascular lesions present in malignant forms of the pulmonary hypertension. Heath and Edwards included plexiform lesions in their grades 3 to 6, most characteristically as grade 4 [16].

It has been widely accepted that endothelial cells participate in the pathogenesis of PPH [21]. The elucidation of the role of endothelial cells in the disease process has relied on the detection of markers of altered cell pheonotypes, which can be assessed at the morphological level with a handful of cell markers [22–26]. As part of an overall endothelial cell dysfunction in PPH, we propose that deregulated endothelial cell growth (as present during angiogenesis) plays a role in the progression of PPH [14]. It follows that markers of angiogenesis such as VEGF and its KDR receptor can be used to define the abnormal pulmonary endothelial cells [27].

The use of endothelial cell markers allows us to identify correctly plexiform lesions and to include the concentric lesions as part of the spectrum of pulmonary endothelial cell proliferation in severe pulmonary hypertension. This approach may also help to define the so-called early lesions, which in the past would have been missed, thus explaining the diagnosis of pulmonary hypertension with medial hypertrophy (without plexiform lesions) described in a few patients in the PPH Registry [28]. We present an example of severe (pulmonary artery pressures = 50 mmHg (6.7 kPa)) pulmonary hypertension associated with liver cirrhosis and an undefined collagen vascular disease with lung tissue obtained by video-assisted thorascopic sampling. Note the clusters of endothelial cells, highlighted by Factor VIII-related antigen immunostaining, which represent the so-called 'early-lesion', prior to development of classical plexiform lesions (Figure 4.5A). The present case exhibited also medial hypertrophy, muscularization of arterioles and eccentric intimal thickening.

It is not known at what stage (i.e. early versus late, during the natural course of PPH) the endothelial cell proliferation occurs. If it occurs early in the disease process, the endothelial cell proliferation is related to both the initiation and maintenance of PPH. Alternatively, it has been proposed that classical plexiform lesions occur in the later stages of the disease, since most of the lung tissue is available only when the patient dies or when lung tissue is surgically obtained during transplantation and the disease is clinically end-stage. The different interpretations may originate from the fact that endothelial cell proliferation occurs as small clusters of cells, which, by the time of tissue sampling, have already developed into fully mature plexiform lesions.

We propose that endothelial cell proliferation in PPH occurs in progressive stages, which ultimately result in the formation of the classic plexiform lesion. The concept of lesion progression is best illustrated with studies concerning cancer formation. Several studies have demonstrated that cancer is a biological process with multiple genetic events (deletions, mutations, gene amplifications and silencing), that occur during the evolution of premalignant lesions prior to resulting in a malignant neoplasm [29]. By means of defining the genetic alterations of the cancer cell, it is possible to delineate the multiple stages required for the transformation of normal epithelial cells. Accordingly, the study of the pulmonary endothelial cell phenotype in biopsy or autopsy specimens can give us clues to the progressive cellular alterations that develop in the course of PPH.

It is possible to employ markers of altered pulmonary endothelial cell phenotypes such as increases in the expression in endothelin [22] or 5-lipoxygenase [26–30], and decreases in the expression of eNOS in advanced vascular lesions [23,24,31] and prostacyclin synthase [25], in the aid of the pathological approach to PPH.

The close association of vascular dilatation (lesion grade 4 of Heath and Edwards [16]) and plexiform lesions suggests that both lesions are the result of a complex process of 'misguided angiogenesis' in the lung, where endothelial cells are induced to form poorly organized blood vessels; a similar process occurs in angiopoietin-1 knockout mice [32].

The focus on angiogenesis is justified by the finding of clumps of endothelial cells in the plexiform lesions (Figures 4.3–4.5), the identification by immunohistochemistry of different phenotypes of endothelial cells in these lesions (Figure 4.6) and the localization of several factors involved in angiogenesis to these lesions. Angiogenesis in the adult has been associated both with cancer and with inflammation. There is clear evidence for inflammation in patients with PPH [14], whereas the monoclonal expansion of endothelial cells in PPH and plexiform lesions makes one consider a model that has components of the cancer paradigm [15]. We believe, on the basis of the concept of the genetic susceptibility requirement, that a two hit genetic hypothesis, as has been postulated for several cancers, can be considered. The chronic inflammation that is manifested in the lung tissue and the chronic vascular lesions by the presence of macrophage clusters, lymphocytes and the mast cells may initiate or modify the angiogenesis process.

PPH Vascular Lesions

VEGF mRNA	Present
KDR	Present
Tie 2	Present
PGI_2-S mRNA	Absent
PGI_2-S	Absent
5-LO	Present
Endothelin[a]	Increased
eNOS[b]	Decreased
eNOS[c]	Increased
TM	Decreased

Figure 4.6 Expression pattern of genes and proteins in plexiform lesions of patients with primary pulmonary hypertension. VEGF, vascular endothelial growth factor; KDR, vascular endothelial growth factor receptor; Tie 2, endothelial cell tyrosine kinase 2, PGI_2-S, prostacyclin synthase; 5-LO, lipoxygenase, eNOS, endothelial nitric oxide synthase; TM, thrombomodulin. (a) ref. 22, (b) ref. 23, (c) ref. 24.

A three-dimensional reconstruction of pulmonary arteries in plexiform pulmonary hypertension has shown that the plexiform lesions occur distal to branch points, that they express the VEGF receptor KDR intensely and that the endothelial cells in these lesions segregate into P27-negative cells in the central core of the lesions and into P27-positive cells in the periphery of the lesions. The latter findings indicate that the cells in the central core are proliferating [27].

The pressure-overloaded right ventricle

Patients with severe pulmonary hypertension die from right heart failure. Figures 4.7 and 4.8 show the enormously dilated right ventricle (RV) of a patient with PPH. The mean right atrial pressure elevation and the reduction in cardiac output are the best indicators of patient survival [33]. We have demonstrated in a retrospective study a correlation between elevated plasma uric acid levels in patients with PPH and elevated right atrial pressures [34].

Right ventricular reserve

The RV is one of the relatively unexplored 'white spots' on the landscape of human pathophysiology. Much more is known about mechanisms of acute right heart failure (from animal studies) than about the pressure-overloaded RV in severe chronic pulmonary hypertension. This lack of information is particularly remarkable in view of the fact that RV

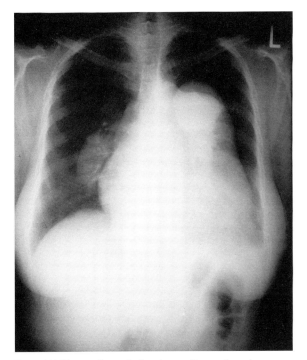

Figure 4.7 Chest radiograph showing cardiomegaly and very large, central pulmonary arteries.

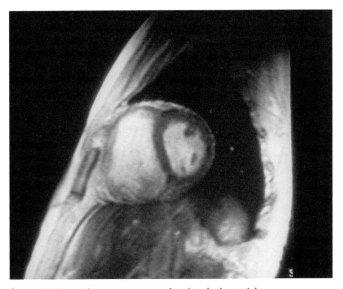

Figure 4.8 Magnetic resonance scan showing the large right ventricle of a patient with primary pulmonary hypertension.

performance is the most important predictor of outcome in severe, chronic pulmonary hypertension (i.e. New York Heart Association (NYHA) classification and mean right atrial pressure). Figure 4.9 shows the breakdown of a cohort of 99 patients with PPH according to the mean right atrial pressure at the time of the diagnosis. Prior to lung

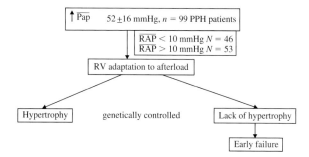

Figure 4.9 Of 99 patients with primary pulmonary hypertension, 46 had a mean right atrial pressure less than 10 mmHg (1.33 kPa) and 53 patients had a mean right atrial pressure greater than 10 mmHg at the time of the diagnosis. Apparently, the adaptation of the right ventricle (RV) to the same degree of afterload is variable in some patients, leading to hypertrophy of the muscle, and in others there is an inadequate hypertrophic response.

transplantation the consensus opinion was that the end-stage, pressure-overloaded RV was irreversibly damaged – now we know that, following transplantation, the RV does quickly and fully recover. It follows that the reversible structural and functional changes and the RV failure programme are in need of investigation – in particular at the level of gene expression [35–36]. Clinically, patients with severe pulmonary hypertension present *at the time of their first diagnosis* either with or without signs of RV failure – yet the mean pulmonary arterial pressure (the RV afterload) is identical for both groups [36].

One hypothesis that attempts to explain this difference in the presentation of patients with severe pulmonary hypertension (PPH) relates to molecular genetic variations (different genotypes of patients with PPH). One such genotypic variation is the the angiotensin converting enzyme (ACE) gene polymorphism, a form of which (the DD genotype) is associated with increased circulating and cardiac tissue ACE activity. This genotype may be related to preservation of RV function in PPH. Of 32 patients with PPH, 12 had the ACE DD phenotype (cardiac output higher than 5.9 ± 0.3 L/min) when compared with the non-DD phenotype (3.3 ± 0.3 L/min). Perhaps angiotensin has an RV inotropic action or affects RV myocyte hypertrophy resulting in development (and perhaps persistence) of the more advantageous *concentric* RV hypertrophy.

On the basis of gated cardiac magnetic resonance imaging studies [38] we classified RV phenotypes (Tables 4.1 and 4.2). Our group of severe pulmonary hypertensive patients had moderate to severe RV dysfunction and a spectrum of increased RV mass and wall thickness. Two of our PPH patients showed marked concentric hypertrophy

Severe Pulmonary Hypertension

Challenges

Endothelial cell mutations
Familial PPH genes
How does prostacyclin work?
Replacement of continuous prostacyclin infusion
How can we stabilize the RV?

Figure 4.10 The challenges to the investigators by the patients with severe pulmonary hypertension. RV, right ventricle.

with an RV wall thickness greater than 1.0 cm, which was associated with preserved or near-normal RV systolic function. In these subjects, an exaggerated increase in wall thickness may have normalized wall stress, leading to preservation of RV systolic function. The ability to identify mulitple phenotypes of ventricles subjected to a uniform insult, such as chronic pressure overload in PPH, sets the stage for the determination of the different patterns of gene expression (Table 4.3) and perhaps differential activation of specific signalling pathways [36–38] that account for these phenotypic differences. In this regard, in the RV, the molecular phenotype can be readily determined by quantitative reverse transcriptase/polymerase chain reaction (RT-PCR) performed on RNA extracted from endomyocardial biopsy material [36].

Summary and conclusion

Conceptual progress has been made in recent years that may lead towards a better understanding of the pathobiology of severe pulmonary hypertensive diseases. Endothelial cell proliferation is clearly an important mechanism in that it leads to occlusion of the precapillary arteries. In this process the 'law of the monolayer' is violated; this is probably determined by inherited and somatic mutations that result in a VEGF/KDR driven programme of angiogenesis. We continue to be impressed by the fact that the incidence of severe pulmonary hypertension is low in any of the known conditions. As patients do not die because of chronic pulmonary hypertension, but from RV failure, and as we observe how different individuals handle the pressure differently, we feel the need to explore the 'right ventricular reserve' at cellular, molecular and genetic levels. Figure 4.10 lists the challenges provided by the patients with severe pulmonary hypertension and the issues the investigators need to address in the immediate future. These issues include the question of the mechanisms by which long-term prostacyclin improves the survival of patients with PPH [38–40].

Table 4.1. Parameters by clinical/disease subject group

Group	EDV (mL)	EDV_1 (mL/m^2)	EF (%)	TH (cm)	Mass (g)	Mass index (g/m^2)
RV						
Normal values	111 ± 22	68 ± 13	60 ± 10	0.44 ± 0.09	42 ± 7	23 ± 5
PPH ($n = 10$)	122 ± 34	67 ± 13	$34 \pm 10^*$	$0.91 \pm 0.31^*$	$86 \pm 39^*$	$49 \pm 26^*$
LV						
Normal values	100 ± 20	69 ± 13	68 ± 6	0.66 ± 0.22	164 ± 21	92 ± 10
PPH ($n = 10$)	$71 \pm 24^*$	$40 \pm 14^*$	58 ± 17	$1.10 \pm 0.32^*$	$109 \pm 29^*$	$61 \pm 17^*$

Note: RV, right ventricle; LV, left ventricle; EDV, end-diastolic volume; EDV_1, end-diastolic volume index; EF, ejection fraction; TH, end-diastolic thickness; PPH, primary pulmonary hypertension; values expressed as mean $\pm$ standard deviation; $^*p < 0.05$ versus normal values.

Table 4.2. Parameters by RV phenotype

Category (no.)	PPH no.	RVEDV (mL)	RVEF (%)	RVTH (cm)	RV mass (g)
ConCmpHty (2)	2	122 ± 14	47 ± 1	$1.20 \pm 0.40^*$	132
ConFailHty (4)	4	124 ± 16	$28 \pm 5^*$	$0.95 \pm -0.10^*$	85
Failing, no Hty (2)	2	98 ± 19	$34 \pm 1^*$	0.85 ± 0.15	50

Note: RV, right ventricle; RVEDV, right ventricular end-diastolic volume; failing concentric hypertrophy; RVEF, RV ejection fraction; RVTH, RV free wall thickness at end diastole; RV mass, RV myocardial mass; ConCmpHty, compensated concentric hypertrophy; Failing no Hty, RV failure without hypertrophy; PPH, primary pulmonary hypertension; values expressed as mean $\pm$ standard error; $^*p < 0.05$ versus normal values.

Table 4.3. The known alterations in gene expression in the pressure-overloaded failing right ventricle (of PPH patients)

The increase in the β_2-adrenergic receptor gene expression may be unique to the pressure-overloaded RV. Whether any of these alterations in RV gene expression renders a survival benefit is unknown.

Gene (protein or mRNA)	Directional change	In failing RV but not in nonfailing LV
β_1-Adrenergic receptor	↓	Yes
β_2-Adrenergic receptor	↑	Yes
Angiotensin AT1 receptor	↓	Yes
Adenylyl cyclase	↓	Yes
ANP	↑	Yes
α-Myosin heavy chain	↓	Yes
β-Myosin heavy chain	↑	Yes

Note: RV, right ventricle; LV, left ventricle; ANP, atrionatriuretic protein.

REFERENCES

1 Voelkel NF, Tuder RM. Cellular and molecular mechanisms in the pathogenesis of severe pulmonary hypertension. *Eur Resp J* 1995; **8**: 2129–2138.

2 Tuder RM, Lee SD, Cool CD. Histopathology of pulmonary hypertension. *Chest* 1998; **114**: 1S–4S.

3 Voelkel NF, Cool C, Lee SD, Wright L, Geraci MW, Tuder RM. Primary pulmonary hypertension between inflammation and cancer. *Chest* 1998; **114**: 225S–230S.

4 Voelkel NF, Tuder RM. Severe pulmonary hypertensive diseases – a perspective. *Eur Resp J* 1999; **14**: 1246–1250.

5 Cool CD, Kennedy D, Voelkel NF, Tuder RM. Pathogenesis and evolution of plexiform lesions in pulmonary hypertension associated with scleroderma and human immunodeficiency virus infection. *Hum Pathol* 1997; **28**, 434–442.

6 Morse JH, Jones AC, Barst RJ, Hodge SE, Wilhelmsen KC, Nygaard TG. Mapping of familial primary pulmonary hypertension locus (PPH) to chromosome 2q31–q32. *Circulation* 1997; **95**: 2603–2606.

7 Nichols WC, Koller DL, Slovis B, et al. Localization of the gene for familial primary pulmonary hypertension to chromosome 2q31–32. *Nature Genet* 1994; **15**: 277–280.

8 Herve P, Lebrec D, Brenot F, et al. Pulmonary vascular disorders in portal hypertension. *Eur Resp J* 1998; **11**: 1153–1166.

9 Abenhaim L, Moride Y, Brenot F, et al. Appetite-suppressant drugs and the risk of primary pulmonary hypertension. *N Engl J Med* 1996; **335**: 609–616.

10 Voelkel NF, Clark WR, Higenbottam T. Obesity, dexfenfluramine and pulmonary hypertension. *Am J Resp Crit Care Med* 1997; **155**: 786–788.

11 Voelkel NF. Appetite suppressants and pulmonary hypertension. *Thorax* 1997; **52**: 563–567.

12 Tuder RM, Radisavljevic Z, Shroyer KR, Polak JM, Voelkel NF. Monoclonal endothelial cells in appetite suppressant-associated pulmonary hypertension. *Am J Resp Crit Care Med* 1998; **158**: 1999–2001.

13 Mark EJ, Patalas EC, Change HT, et al. Fatal pulmonary hypertension associated with short term use of fenfluramine and phentermine. *N Engl J Med* 1997; **337**: 602–605.

14 Tuder RM, Groves B, Badesch DB, Voelkel NF. Exuberant endothelial cell growth and elements of inflammation are present in plexiform lesions of pulmonary hypertension. *Am J Pathol* 1994; **144**: 275–285.

15 Lee SD, Shroyer KR, Markham NE, Cool CD, Voelkel NF, Tuder RM. Monoclonal endothelial cell proliferation is present in primary but not secondary pulmonary hypertension. *J Clin Invest* 1998; **101**: 927–934.

16 Heath D, Edwards JE. The pathology of pulmonary hypertensive disease. A description of six grades of structural changes in the pulmonary arteries with special reference to congenital cardiac septal changes. *Circulation* 1958; **18**: 533–547.

17 DeRuiter MC, Poelmann RE, VanMunsteren JC, Mironov V, Markwald RR, Gittenberger-deGroot AC. Embryonic endothelial cells transdifferentiate into mesenchymal cells expressing smooth muscle actins in vivo and in vitro. *Circ Res* 1997; **80**: 444–451.

18 Arciniegas E, Sutton AB, Alled TD, Schor AM. Transforming growth factor beta promoted the differentiation of endothelial cells into smooth muscle-like cells in vitro. *J Cell Sci* 1992; **103**: 521–529.

19 Weir KE, Reeve HL, Peterson DA, Michelakis ED, Nelson DP, Archer SL (1998) Pulmonary vasoconstriction, oxygen sensing and the role of ion channels. *Chest* 1998; **114**: 17S–22S.

20 Yuan XJ, Wang J, Juhaszova M, Gaine SP, Rubin LJ. Attenuated K+ channel gene transcription in primary pulmonary hypertension. *Lancet* 1998; **351**: 726–727.

21 Loscalzo J. Endothelial dysfunction in pulmonary hypertension. *N Engl J Med* 1992; **327**: 117–119.

22 Giaid A, Yanagisawa M, Langleben D, et al. Expression of endothelin-1 in the lungs of patients with pulmonary hypertension. *N Engl J Med* 1993; **328**: 1732–1739.

23 Giaid A, Saleh D. Reduced expression of endothelial nitric oxide synthase in the lungs of patients with pulmonary hypertension. *N Engl J Med* 1995; **333**: 214–221.

24 Mason NA, Springall DR, Burke M, et al. High expression of endothelial nitric oxide synthase in plexiform lesions of pulmonary hypertension. *J Pathol* 1998; **185**: 313–318.

25 Tuder R, Geraci MW, Wang J, et al. Prostacyclin synthase expression is decreased in lungs from patients with severe pulmonary hypertension. *Am J Resp Crit Care Med* 1999; **159**: 1925–1932.

26 Wright L, Tuder RM, Wang J, Cool CD, Lepley RA, Voelkel NF. 5-Lipoxygenase and 5-lipoxygenase activating protein (FLAP) immunoreactivity in lungs from patients with primary pulmonary hypertension. *Am J Resp Crit Care Med* 1993; **157**: 219–229.

27 Cool CD, Stewart JS, Werahera P, et al. Three-dimensional reconstruction of pulmonary arteries in plexiform pulmonary hypertension using cell-specific markers: evidence for a dynamic and heterogeneous process of pulmonary endothelial cell growth. *Am J Pathol* 1999; **155**: 411–419.

28 Pietra GG, Edwards WE, Kay JM, et al. Histopathology of primary hypertension. *Circulation* 1989; **80**: 1198–1206.

29 Kinzler KW, Volgestein B. Oncogenesis – landscaping the cancer terrain. *Science* 1998; **280**: 1036.

30 Voelkel NF, Tuder, RM, Wade K, et al. Inhibition of 5-lipoxygenase-activating protein (FLAP) reduces pulmonary vascular reactivity and pulmonary hypertension in hypoxic rats. *J Clin Invest* 1996; **97**: 2491–2498.

31 Xue C, John RA. Endothelial nitric oxide synthase in the lungs of patients with pulmonary hypertension. *N Engl J Med* 1995; **333**: 1642–1644.

32 Suri C, Jones PF, Patan S, Bartunkova S, et al. Requisite role of angiopoietin-1, a ligand for the TIE2 receptor, during embryonic angiogenesis. *Cell* 1996; **87**: 1171–1180.

33 Bristow MR, Zisman LS, Lowes BD, et al. The pressure-overloaded right ventricle in pulmonary hypertension. *Chest* 1998; **114**: 101S–106S.

34 Voelkel MA, Wynne KM, Badesch DB, Groves BM, Voelkel NF. Hyperuricemia in severe pulmonary hypertension. *Chest* 2000; **117**: 19–24.

35 Abraham WT, Raynolds MV, Gottschall B, et al. Importance of angiotensin-converting enzyme in pulmonary hypertension. *Cardiology Suppl* 1995; **1**: 9–15.

36 Lowes BD, Minobe W, Abraham WT, et al. Changes in gene expression in the intact human heart: downregulation of alpha-myosin heavy chain in hypertrophied, failing ventricular myocardium. *J Clin Invest* 1997; **100**: 2315–2324.

37 Quaife RA, Lynch D, Groves BE, et al. Elevated right ventricular circumferential wall stress inversely correlates with right ventricular systolic function in primary pulmonary hypertension. *Circulation* 1996; **94**(Suppl): 1–67.

38 Quaife RA, Lynch D, Badesch DB, et al. Right ventricular phenotypic characteristics in subjects with primary pulmonary hypertension or idiopathic dilated cardiomyopathy. *J Card Fail* 1999; **5**: 46–54.

39 Shapiro SM, Oudiz RJ, Cao T, et al. Primary pulmonary hypertension: improved long term effects and survival with continuous intravenous epoprostenol infusion. *J Am Coll Cardiol* 1999; **30**: 343–349.

40 McLaughlin VV, Genthner DE, Panella MM, Rich S. Reduction in pulmonary vascular resistance with long-term epoprostenol (prostacyclin) therapy in primary pulmonary hypertension. *N Engl J Med* 1998; **338**: 273–277.

5

Emphysema

Gordon L. Snider

Boston University School of Medicine, Boston, Massachusetts, USA

Introduction

Emphysema and chronic obstructive pulmonary disease (COPD), of which emphysema is a part, are major causes of disability and death in the developed world. After a brief discussion of definitions and pathophysiology, the epidemiology of COPD will be reviewed to highlight the magnitude and causes of the problem. The clinical aspects of usual and alpha-1-antitrypsin (AAT) deficiency COPD will be reviewed (see also Chapter 6). The history and worldwide experience with lung transplantation will be summarized and the outcome of transplantation for COPD and other lung conditions will be compared. The limited cost-effectiveness information that is available for lung, liver and heart transplantation will be summarized. Finally, some health care policy implications of lung transplantation as a therapeutic initiative for relieving the suffering and prolonging the life of patients with end-stage emphysema will be discussed.

Definitions and pathophysiology

Emphysema is defined as abnormal permanent enlargement of the air spaces distal to the terminal bronchioles accompanied by destruction of their walls and without obvious fibrosis. COPD is defined as the presence of emphysema or chronic bronchitis associated with chronic airflow obstruction. Emphysema occurs most commonly in association with chronic bronchitis [1].

The major cause of impaired blood gas exchange, dyspnoea, disability and death in COPD is chronic airflow obstruction. Airflow obstruction occurs in emphysema because of loss of elastic recoil of the lung and rupture of alveolar attachments to airways of < 2 mm diameter or bronchioles. As a result of these changes, the small, poorly

supported airways collapse and narrow at much larger lung volumes than normal, thus causing structural and irreversible airflow obstruction.

Chronic bronchiolitis is an important feature of chronic bronchitis and is a second mechanism of airflow obstruction in COPD. The bronchiolitis is manifest pathologically by cellular infiltration, fibrosis, goblet cell metaplasia, smooth muscle hypertrophy and secretory luminal obstruction. Bronchiolar inflammation, smooth muscle contraction and luminal secretion are potentially reversible causes of airflow obstruction and account for the limited amount of reversible airflow obstruction in COPD.

Epidemiology

Morbidity and mortality

In 1996 an estimated 16 million persons in the USA suffered from COPD, 2 million with emphysema and 14 million with chronic bronchitis, representing an increase in prevalence of 59% since 1982. In 1998, 107 146 deaths were attributed to COPD in the USA, constituting the most frequent cause of death. The age-adjusted death rate increased from 14.0 per 100 000 population in 1979 to 19.9 per 100 000 in 1998, a 42.1% increase; during this time the all-cause age-adjusted death rate decreased by 18% and the death rate for cardiovascular disease declined. The increase in mortality due to COPD has occurred despite the sharp decrease in smoking frequency among adults in the USA in recent decades – from about 41% in 1964 to 25.5% in 1990. The smoking prevalence among adults of 24.7% in 1997 was similar to that in 1990. Cessation of smoking stops the progression of COPD but lung inflammation and other aspects of the disease process are not reversed nor is lung function improved. There is a long lag between decrease

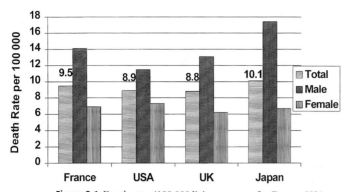

Figure 5.1 Death rates/100 000 living persons, for France, USA, UK and Japan, age standardized for Europe: bronchitis, chronic and unspecified, emphysema and asthma, 1992–1994 [3]. Total values are in a similar range for the four developed countries shown; in all, mortality for males is higher than for females.

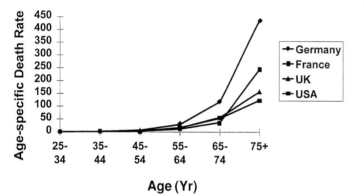

Figure 5.2 Age-specific death rates/100 000 living males, for Germany, France, UK and USA, age standardized for Europe: bronchitis, chronic and unspecified, emphysema and asthma, 1992–1994 [3]. Note the sharp increase in mortality after age 65 years.

in smoking frequency and decrease in COPD mortality rates [2].

Figure 5.1 shows mortality data (1992–1994) age-standardized for European age distribution, compiled by the World Health Organization, for France, the USA, the UK and Japan [3]. The value of the annual mortality rate due to COPD in the USA is lower than in the foregoing paragraph because deaths coded for COPD are not included, since the diagnosis of COPD as a cause of death is not widely used in Europe. Also, asthma, which causes few deaths in comparison to COPD, is included in these data. Mortality rates are similar in the four countries, and, in all, mortality is higher for males than for females. Figure 5.2, shows age-specific mortality for males for four countries (1992–1994). Note the sharp rise in mortality after age 65 years, which reflects the long time-course of usual COPD; disabling disease does not

usually develop until the seventh decade of life after many years of smoking.

Risk factors

Tobacco smoking and age account for more than 85% of the risk of developing COPD in the USA. Only severe AAT deficiency presents a comparable risk, but this factor accounts for only 1–2% of patients with COPD. Data from longitudinal, cross-sectional, and case control studies show that, as compared with nonsmokers, cigarette smokers have higher COPD mortality. They also have higher prevalence and incidence of productive cough, other respiratory symptoms, and airflow obstruction, as shown by a decrease in forced expiratory volume in 1 s (FEV$_1$) and a decrease in the ratio of FEV$_1$ to forced vital capacity (FVC) to < 0.75. A dose–response relationship exists between the severity of airflow obstruction and intensity of tobacco smoking; differences between smokers and nonsmokers increase as daily cigarette consumption and number of years of smoking increase. Pipe and cigar smokers have higher COPD mortality and morbidity than nonsmokers, although their rates are lower than those of cigarette smokers. For reasons not known, only about 15–20% of cigarette smokers develop clinically significant COPD. Familial aggregation of COPD has been established and genetic factors may account for increased susceptibility of a segment of the population [4].

Passive, or involuntary, smoking also known as 'second-hand smoke' is the exposure of nonsmokers to cigarette smoke indoors. Cigarette smoke in indoor air can produce eye irritation and may incite wheezing in asthmatic persons. An increased prevalence of respiratory symptoms and disease, and small but measurable decreases in lung function, have been shown in the children of smoking as compared with nonsmoking parents. Although the significance of these findings for the future development of COPD is unknown, children should be protected from environmental tobacco smoke [4].

Figure 5.3 shows the number of grams of tobacco sold annually per adult in four countries from 1964 to 1990. Per capita tobacco sales have a downwards trend in the USA and the UK. Sales have an upwards trend in France but a slight downwards trend in Japan since 1980. Since tobacco smoking is the major risk factor for COPD in developed countries, these data suggest that COPD will be a major public health problem in developed countries for the foreseeable future.

It is established that high levels of urban air pollution are harmful to persons with chronic heart or lung disease; peaks of urban air pollution are strongly associated with increases in morbidity and mortality due to COPD.

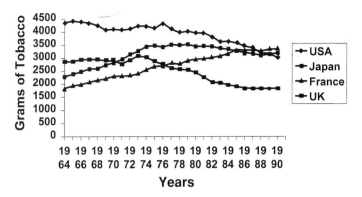

Figure 5.3 Annual grams of tobacco sold per adult, 1964 to 1990, in the USA, Japan, France and the UK [68]. Tobacco use has a trend downwards over time in the USA and the UK, but up in Japan and France.

Although the exact role of air pollution in producing COPD is unclear, its role is small compared with that of cigarette smoking [4].

Prevalence and mortality rates are higher in whites than in nonwhites. Incidence and mortality are generally higher in blue collar workers than white collar workers and in those with fewer years of formal education. Prevalence as well as mortality of COPD is higher for men than for women, presumably because of the lower frequency of smoking in women until recent years.

Working in an occupation in which the air is polluted with chemical fumes or a biologically inactive dust leads to increased prevalence of chronic airflow obstruction. There are increased rates of decline in FEV_1 and increased mortality from COPD. Interaction between cigarette smoking and exposure to hazardous dust such as silica or coal dust results in increased rates of COPD. In all these studies, however, smoking effects are much greater than occupational effects. Except for coal and gold dust exposure, which can alone cause COPD, the effects of occupational pollution and smoking appear to be additive [4].

It has been proposed but not proved that the atopic state or nonspecific airways hyperresponsiveness (usually measured as responsiveness to methacholine inhalation) predisposes smokers to the development of airways obstruction. In the absence of asthma, studies have failed to show a relation of manifestations of COPD in smokers to standardized levels of immunoglobulin (Ig) E, eosinophilia or skin test reactivity to allergens. Airways hyperreactivity in COPD is inversely related to FEV_1 and is predictive of an increasing rate of decline of FEV_1 in smokers. However, it is not clear whether airways hyperreactivity is a cause of development of airflow obstruction or results from the airway inflammation that occurs in smoking-related airflow obstruction [5]. Nonspecific airway hyperreactivity occurs in a significantly higher proportion of women than men [6].

Childhood respiratory infection may predispose to COPD. Chronic inflammation, which persists for years after smoking cessation, is the major cause of slow progression of the disease. There is increasing evidence that acute exacerbations of COPD, which are known to be associated with worsening inflammation, are also important in accelerating the rate of pulmonary function decline in persons with COPD [7,8].

Alpha-1-antitrypsin deficiency

The modern era of understanding of the pathogenesis of emphysema began with the discovery of severe AAT deficiency in 1963. Briefly, AAT is a glycoprotein composed of 394 amino acid residues, coded by a single gene on chromosome 14. The serum protease inhibitor phenotype (PI type) is determined by the independent expression of the two parental alleles. More than 75 polymorphisms are known, and they have been classified into normal (associated with normal serum levels of normally functioning AAT), deficient (associated with serum AAT levels lower than normal), null (associated with undetectable AAT in the serum), and dysfunctional (AAT is present in normal amount but does not function normally).

AAT is a member of the serpin superfamily, which has a reactive centre loop that acts as a pseudosubstrate for a proteinase. When AAT is exposed to a proteinase such as neutrophil elastase, the centre loop is cleaved and is inserted into the A-beta-sheet of the AAT molecule. The inhibitor becomes more stable and the proteinase is irreversibly locked into the altered AAT molecule.

Most variants of AAT occur because of point mutations that result in a single amino acid substitution. The Z variant results from the substitution of a lysine for a glutamic acid residue in the M protein. The substitution changes the conformation of the molecule allowing an interaction between the reactive centre loop of one molecule and the A-beta-sheet of a second molecule, resulting in polymerization of the molecule. The polymerized AAT molecules are too large to be excreted from the liver cells, which make most of the AAT in the body. The granules accumulate in the liver cells, may be seen with the periodic acid–Schiff–diastase reaction and are related in a poorly understood way to the liver disease of AAT deficiency. It is now clear that AAT deficiency is one of a growing number of molecular conformational diseases, which also includes Alzheimer's disease, Parkinson's disease and cystic fibrosis. One of the important aspects of this discovery is that chaperone molecules may be developed which can prevent the intracellular polymerization of the Z and similar molecules, thus permitting their secretion from the cell.

The normal M alleles occur in about 90% of persons of European descent with normal serum AAT levels; their phenotype is designated PI∗M. Normal values of serum AAT are 150 to 350 mg/dL or 20 to 48 μmol. More than 95% of persons in the severely deficient category are homozygous for the Z allele, designated PI∗Z, and will have serum AAT levels of 2.5 to 7 μmol (mean, 16% normal). Almost all of these persons are Caucasians of northern European descent; the Z allele is rare in Asians and African-Americans. Rarely observed phenotypes that are associated with these low levels of serum AAT include the following: PI∗SZ and persons with nonexpressing alleles, PI∗null, occurring in homozygous form, PI∗null-null; and PI∗Znull, occurring in heterozygous form with a deficient allele. Persons with phenotype PI∗S have AAT values ranging from 15 to 33 μmol (mean, 52% of normal). The threshold protective level of 11 μmol or 80 mg/dL (35% of normal) is based on the knowledge that PI∗SZ heterozygotes, with serum AAT values of 8 to 19 μmol (mean, 37% of normal), rarely develop emphysema. PI∗MZ heterozygotes have serum AAT levels that are intermediate between PI∗MM normals and PI∗ZZ homozygotes (12 to 35 μmol; mean, 57% of normal) who are index cases at increased risk for COPD [9].

Lung disease in severe AAT deficiency

The premature development of severe emphysema is the hallmark of homozygous AAT deficiency. The onset of dyspnoea occurs at a median age of 40 years in PI∗Z smokers, compared with 53 years in PI∗Z nonsmokers and about age 65 in PI∗M persons (usual COPD). Chronic bronchitis is present in about half of the symptomatic persons. Bronchiectasis, diagnosed by computed tomography, occurs in about 40% of persons with severe AAT deficiency. More than half of persons who are type PI∗Z die from pulmonary disease.

Symptoms or signs of pulmonary disease rarely develop before age 25 years. Tobacco smoking and the development of pulmonary disease are strongly associated; PI∗Z smokers have a significantly lower life expectancy than PI∗Z nonsmokers, although male and female nonsmokers also have a reduced life expectancy. Annual decline of FEV_1 is greater than normal in nonsmokers who are type PI∗Z, but is much greater in smokers who are type PI∗Z.

Severity of lung disease varies markedly; lung function is well preserved in some smokers who are type PI∗Z and severely impaired in some nonsmokers. Nonindex cases tend to have better lung function, whether they smoke or not, than do index cases (discovered because they have lung disease). The annual decline of FEV_1 in nonindex cases tends to be only moderately greater than normal. PI∗Z persons who are nonsmokers may live into their eighth or ninth decade; however, they usually develop some airflow obstruction as they age. In addition to cigarette smoking, asthma, recurrent respiratory infections, environmental dust and fume exposure and unidentified familial factors are identified as possible risk factors for chronic airflow limitation. There may well be other as yet undiscovered genetic factors that play a role in the phenotypic manifestations of AAT-COPD [9–11].

Radiographically, AAT-deficient patients characteristically have more definite evidence of emphysema than patients with usual COPD. The finding of basilar emphysema, denoting the presence of panacinar emphysema, while not constant in the plain chest X-ray film in PI∗Z patients, is strongly suggestive of the diagnosis.

Liver disease in AAT deficiency

Homozygous AAT deficiency is often associated in infancy with hepatomegaly or hepatosplenomegaly and evidence of cholestasis and elevation of hepatocellular enzymes. About 10% of infants with this abnormality go on to develop cirrhosis. Hepatic failure due to AAT deficiency can be treated with liver transplantation. Since the transplanted liver produces normal AAT, this effectively cures the disorder [12]. Cirrhosis, often with hepatoma, is the second most frequent cause of death in adults [13]. It occurs most often in nonsmokers, since they live longer than smokers, who die of lung disease before they develop cirrhosis.

Diagnosis of AAT deficiency

Estimates of the frequency of the PI∗ZZ phenotype in North America and Europe range from about 1 in 1600 to 1 in 4000, a prevalence approximating to that of cystic fibrosis and suggesting that severe AAT deficiency is among the most common potentially serious genetic conditions. Nevertheless, in large studies in both Sweden and Great Britain, rigorous attempts to collect all available cases have at most garnered 10% of estimated cases. This suggests that either most subjects who are type PI*Z are asymptomatic or they are masquerading under other diagnoses such as asthma.

The diagnosis of AAT deficiency is made by measuring serum AAT level, followed by PI typing for confirmation [9]. These tests should be performed in patients with premature onset of COPD, COPD occurring in nonsmokers or with a predominance of basilar emphysema, in bronchiectasis of uncertain origin and in patients with severe asthma. A screening test should also be done in persons with hepatic cirrhosis of uncertain origin. A strong argument can be made for screening all persons with COPD. Since they are already ill, the social and economic risks of genetic discrimination are less. Family studies in homozygotes might well keep children from starting to smoke or might increase the possibility of smokers stopping the habit. General population screening is controversial [10].

AAT augmentation therapy

Augmentation therapy with purified human AAT for patients with severe AAT deficiency is based on the concept that a deficient protein is being restored to protective levels in the body. Recent studies have shown elevation of desmosine, a biological marker of elastin degradation, in the urine of persons with AAT-COPD. The levels did not fall in 8–52 weeks of AAT augmentation therapy. However, there is suggestive evidence that: mortality is lower in AAT-deficient persons on augmentation therapy than those who are not [14]; augmentation therapy may decrease the rate of decline of FEV_1 [15,16]; and augmentation therapy may decrease the rate of progression of emphysema as shown by computed tomography of the lungs [17]. A survey of AAT subjects receiving and not receiving AAT augmentation therapy suggests that acute exacerbations of COPD are less frequent in those receiving augmentation therapy [18]. Augmentation therapy should be reserved for patients whose serum concentration of AAT is less than 11 μmol. It is not indicated for patients with usual COPD or persons with AAT-deficiency-associated liver disease, unless they also have lung disease.

Persons with normal lung function should have their lung function monitored regularly; augmentation therapy should be considered when serial studies show deterioration. There have been shortages of AAT for augmentation therapy in the USA and a number of countries do not have the agent available. Aerosol therapy using three different preparations (human AAT, human AAT made from the milk of transgenic sheep, and recombinant AAT made by yeast)

is currently under development by the pharamaceutical industry.

Other genetic influences in COPD

AAT deficiency comprises 1–2% of all COPD. However, only about 15% of smokers develop COPD. Accordingly it has long been suspected that there must be other genes that control the development of emphysema in smokers, and research in this area is active. Several reports have suggested that DNA polymorphisms in the flanking regions of the AAT gene may be associated with an increased frequency of development of emphysema in persons with normal serum protein. This polymorphism does not appear to be associated with altered baseline levels of AAT. However, the mutation appears to be located in a region that may serve as an interleukin (IL) 6 regulatory sequence. This raises the possibility that the polymorphism may be associated with a defective upregulation of AAT during stress. This could result in a relative AAT deficiency and increased risk for emphysema in the face of environmental or infectious exposures [11,19].

Pathogenesis of COPD

There is widespread agreement that inflammation with neutrophils, macrophages and lymphocytes, predominantly of CD8 type, is a constant association of COPD. Although cigarette smoke is the main cause of this inflammation, host factors, probably under genetic control, are also considered highly probable. Increased apoptosis is observed in human emphysema and in some animal models of the disease.

The main function in the body of AAT appears to be its ability to permanently inactivate neutrophil elastase and protease-3. The elastase–antielastase hypothesis of pathogenesis of emphysema in AAT deficiency suggests that lung destruction is due to inadequate neutralization of neutrophil elastase by the greatly decreased amount of AAT. The hypothesis has also been invoked for the emphysema of usual COPD. Since neutrophils are increased in the lungs of smokers, elastase–antielastase imbalance is postulated to occur as a result of increased neutrophil elastase and other enzymes. Inactivation of AAT by oxidation of the methionine residues in the molecule has also been posited. It has been suggested that the much slower course of usual COPD than AAT-COPD is because only the elastase portion of the ratio is affected rather than both the elastase and antielastase portions.

Macrophages produce metalloelastases that are inactivated by tissue inhibitors of metalloproteases (TIMPs) but not by AAT. These elastases appear to work in microenvironments where macrophages are in contact with elastic fibres rather than being excreted into the intercellular space. Mice with knocked out metalloprotease genes do not develop emphysema when exposed to cigarette smoke. These mice have decreased lung macrophages, but restoring these cells to normal levels by treating the mice with macrophage chemoattractant protein does not result in emphysema. The exact role of lymphocytes in causing emphysema is unclear, although these cells are prominent in emphysematous alveolar walls and may well have cytotoxic properties.

It seems highly likely that centriacinar emphysema (CAE) and panacinar emphysema (PAE), the two commonest forms, have different pathogeneses. Their different anatomical distributions in the lungs and different associations with elastic recoil and bronchiolar disease were noted earlier. Biochemical studies have shown that elastin concentration is decreased but collagen concentration is unchanged in lung tissue affected by PAE. In CAE, collagen concentration is increased even in mild disease but elastin concentration is not affected until the disease is severe. It has been suggested that PAE is caused primarily by elastase–antielastase imbalance. CAE is probably due to inflammation and fibrosis with collapse of alveoli, their incorporation into the interstitium and the enlargement of less involved respiratory airspaces by local distending forces [7,20,21].

Therapy of COPD

Therapy of COPD may be divided into four broad categories [4]:
1 Specific or preventive.
2 Symptomatic.
3 Secondary – therapy that improves the functioning of the whole person but does not affect lung function or structure.
4 Surgical therapy that is designed to improve lung function. Management of pneumothorax complicating emphysema will not be discussed.

Specific therapy

1 Smoking cessation is the cornerstone of specific therapy. COPD would be a much smaller public health problem than it is if smoking prevalence declined – by young people not starting and those who smoke giving up the habit. For those with diagnosed COPD, regardless of their age,

stopping smoking is important. On the other hand, tobacco smoking is highly addictive, even with the best professional help. Those who cannot stop smoking should never be sanctioned.
2 Vaccination against influenza and pneumococcal infection are useful.
3 Those exposed to dust or fumes in their work should be counselled to change jobs, something often easier said than done.

Symptomatic therapy

1 Bronchodilator drugs are the major element of symptomatic therapy. These drugs have generally been studied in COPD after they have been shown to be effective in asthma. The apparent superiority of inhaled ipratropium bromide in COPD, as compared to beta agonists, may be a result of the doses used for comparison. Studies have shown that there is no further bronchodilation when either ipratropium or a beta agonist is given after maximal bronchodilation produced with the other agent. There is no doubt that ipratropium has less toxicity than beta agonists. The combination of ipratropium and albuterol in a single metered dose inhaler (MDI) has the advantage of a rapid bronchodilator response because of the albuterol and less toxicity from the sustained response due to ipratropium. The combined MDI should be used for both timed-dose therapy and rescue therapy. Salmeterol given by MDI every 12 hours has the advantage of a sustained effect; the drug may also be given in combination with fluticasone in varying doses from a dry-powder inhaler.
2 Corticosteroids given systemically shorten the course of COPD exacerbations. Corticosteroids given by MDI do not delay the rate of decline of FEV_1 over time but they do decrease the frequency of exacerbations and improve disease-related quality of life.
3 Antibiotics have no effect on the roughly 25% of exacerbations that are due to viral infection. Neither do they affect exacerbations related to exposure to high levels of urban air pollution. However, when sputum has become purulent, often with evidence of an increased bacterial load in the lower respiratory tract, they appear to shorten the duration and severity of the exacerbation.
4 Cooperative self management enhances the chance of success in symptomatic therapy. Patients are educated to understand their disease and its therapy within the limits of their ability and are provided with a range of options for adjusting intensity of therapy to the varying severity of their disease [1,22].

Secondary therapy

1 Long-term oxygen therapy has a major impact on correcting the pathophysiology of hypoxaemia and tissue hypoxia. It prolongs life without improving lung function.
2 Another major component of secondary therapy is rehabilitation therapy, a multidisciplinary programme whose goals are to improve exercise capacity, independence, health status and quality of life. Exercise and educational programmes are the foundation of rehabilitation programmes.
3 Nocturnal mechanical ventilation using either intermittent negative pressure body respirators or intermittent positive pressure nasal mask respirators have been advocated for resting respiratory muscles with the expectation of improving daytime functioning. The literature on this topic is controversial but the largest randomized control trials suggest that the treatment is not effective [23–27].

Surgical therapy other than lung transplantation

Resection of giant bullae has been used for many years to restore lung function in occasional patients. Surgery is most effective when bullae are larger than one third of a hemithorax, there is evidence of lung compression (best judged by computed tomography), the compressed lung is believed to be normal or only minimally emphysematous and the FEV$_1$ is < 50% of the predicted value. In appropriate cases the results are often dramatic. Unfortunately only rare patients among the large numbers of patients with usual COPD meet these criteria. Giant bullous disease is most often a part of generalized emphysema and simple bullectomy is not indicated. In these cases, the criteria of lung volume reduction surgery should be applied [28].

Lung volume reduction surgery (LVRS) entails resection of 20–30% of the most diseased portion of each lung. Introduced by Brantigan [29] in the late 1950s, the operation was based on the theory that reducing lung size restores elastic recoil and circumferential pull on bronchioles, leading to improved pulmonary function, chest wall mechanics and exercise tolerance. The operation was abandoned because of the high operative mortality (18%) and failure to document subjective improvements with objective measurements. In the spring of 1994, Cooper reported his experience with a revival of LVRS [30]. Patients were highly selected; only about 15% of referred patients were accepted for surgery. All operated patients first underwent a rigorous rehabilitation programme. The operative mortality was approximately 5%. Objective assessment

showed improved pulmonary function, exercise tolerance and quality of life indices.

Large numbers of patients were operated upon in both academic and community medical centres. However, in the autumn of 1995, the Health Care Financing Administration (HCFA) announced that the agency considered LVRS to be investigational and discontinued reimbursement for the operation effective from 1 January 1996. Many other health insurers adopted a nonpayment policy and the number of lung volume reduction operations performed fell precipitously. In May of 1996 HCFA and the National Institutes of Health (NIH) announced joint sponsorship of the National Emphysema Treatment Trial (NETT) on LVRS. The study was designed to randomize 4700 Medicare patients between LVRS and the best available medical treatment, for five years, at 18 clinical sites throughout the USA. Patient eligibility criteria for NETT resembled the characteristics of the population in which the short-term efficacy of LVRS had already been established.

Subsequently, Blue Cross Blue Shield of Massachusetts (BCBSMA) in conjunction with 11 community and academic hospitals, affiliated with the four medical schools in the Commonwealth of Massachusetts, organized the Overholt Blue Cross Emphysema Surgery Trial (OBEST). This second multicentre randomized controlled trial (RCT) on LVRS in the USA randomizes patients between LVRS and the best available medical treatment for six months, followed by a cross-over option to surgery by those in the medical arm. The eligibility criteria adopted by OBEST are similar to those of NETT. The cross-over option allows access to LVRS by all qualified candidates but postpones the operation in the medical arm by six months. Comparison of the results in the medical and surgical groups at six months is expected to provide credible information about the long-term, palliative effect of LVRS; OBEST cannot provide information on long-term mortality. Fewer than one third of the anticipated number of patients have entered NETT and OBEST. NETT has cut back its original goal of enrollment from 4700 to 2500 patients. OBEST has joined forces with the Canadian Lung Volume Reduction Trial in an attempt to obtain statistically meaningful six month outcome data [31].

Two randomized controlled trials from the USA (37 and 49 patients), and one each from the UK (48 patients), Sweden (38 patients), and Italy (60 patients) compared LVRS with the best available medical treatment. All five studies reported better subjective and objective outcomes in the surgical arms. Observational studies indicate that the benefits peak at about 12 months and plateau or recede thereafter, but respiratory function remains

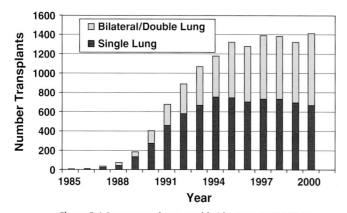

Figure 5.4 Lung transplants, worldwide, 1985–2000 [46]. Note that the reported transplantations done annually worldwide has numbered about 1400 since 1996. More than half of lung transplants are single lung type.

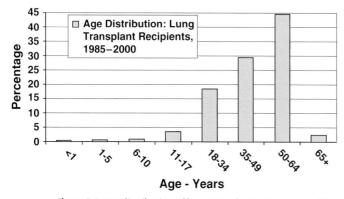

Figure 5.5 Age distribution of lung transplant recipients, worldwide, 1985–2000 [46]. Note that almost 45% of lung transplantations have been done on persons aged 50–64 years and that few transplantations have been done on persons older than 65 years.

above baseline for up to three to five years in some patients [31].

Comment

At this time it appears that in carefully selected patients, LVRS has a mortality of about 5–8% and about 70% of patients are helped substantially. It is not known with good confidence how long the improvement lasts (one would certainly not expect it to be indefinite). There is no information on the relative longevity of patients who have had LVRS versus medically treated patients. The question is whether information on longevity is necessary for patients and their doctors to make informed judgements on whether the *palliative* effects of LVRS are worthwhile. Palliative treatments of limited duration are regularly used in cancer treatment.

Lung transplantation

A brief history

The first lung transplantation in a human was performed in 1963 by James Hardy and colleagues [32]. Over the next 20 years approximately 20 lung transplantations were performed worldwide [33] with no survivals beyond a few months. Disruption of the bronchial anastomosis, which related largely to the use of high doses of corticosteroids given for immunosuppression, was a common problem. The modern era of lung transplantation began in the early 1980s with the addition of ciclosporin to the immunosuppressive regimen. Double lung transplantation by the sequential technique, usually done without cardiopulmonary bypass, was established by the late 1980s [31].

Analysis of the early experience [34,35] suggested that single lung transplantation (SLT) was not suitable for emphysema because hyperexpansion of the highly compliant native lung would occur. The mediastinum would shift towards the transplanted lung, with compression and resultant impairment of ventilation and gas exchange in the donor lung. This concept continued to be held into the 1980s. Consequently, SLT was first performed in the early 1980s for interstitial pulmonary fibrosis [36] and was not used for emphysema until after 1989 when Mal and coworkers in France [37] published a preliminary report of successful SLT for emphysema. The procedure was rapidly taken up by transplantation surgeons [38–43] and, although functional results are slightly better with double lung transplantation [44] and there is still some controversy on the use of SLT in younger patients [44,45], SLT has now become the most frequent method of transplantation for emphysema [46–48]. Scarce donor lungs are better utilized and cardiopulmonary bypass is not usually needed.

Hyperinflation of the native lung does indeed occur occasionally after SLT, with mediastinal shift toward the donor side and the development of severe ventilation–perfusion imbalance [49]. LVRS has been used to control encroachment of the hyperinflated native lung on the transplanted lung [49–51]. Preliminary reports of simultaneous SLT and lung volume reduction have also been published [43,52,53].

Between 1983 and 2000 11 283 lung transplants were performed worldwide; 4908 were bilateral/double lung transplants; 6375 were single lung transplants (Figure 5.4); 83.4% of all these lung transplantations were performed between 1995 and 2000. Figure 5.5 shows the age distribution of lung transplant recipients worldwide from 1985 to 2000. More than half of all lung transplantations were performed in persons aged less than 50 years; just under 45% of

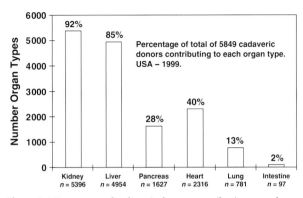

Figure 5.6 Percentage of cadaveric donors contributing to each organ type, USA, 1999 [54]. Note that lungs were contributed by only 13% of cadaveric donors, in sharp contrast to the contribution of kidneys by 92% and livers by 85% of cadaveric donors.

Table 5.1. Adult lung transplantation – indications, 1983–2000

	Single lung	Bilateral/double lung
Chronic obstructive pulmonary disease (COPD)	47	20.1
Interstitial pulmonary fibrosis	21	7.8
Cystic fibrosis	3	33.3
Alpha-1-antitrypsin deficiency COPD	11	9.8
Primary pulmonary hypertension	4	9.1
Miscellaneous	11	17.7
Retransplant	3	2.2
Total	100	100

Note: Values are percentage of total. Single lung ($n = 6375$); bilateral/ double lung ($n = 4908$); data from the Eighteenth Annual Heart/ Lung Transplant Registry Data Report, 2001 [46].

transplantations were in persons aged 50–64 years and few transplantations were done in persons older than 65 years [46].

In 1999, there was a total of 5849 cadaveric donors in the USA; only 13% of these donors contributed lungs for transplantation (Figure 5.6). Over the last 10 years, the total number of organs recovered has increased by 41%. In 1999, 1451 lungs were recovered for transplant. Only 8% of all lungs recovered in 1999 were either used for research or not used at all. Of the lungs recovered for transplant but not used, 50% were due either to organ damage or poor organ function. In 1999 there were 5074 patients on the waiting list for lung transplantation of whom 591 died while awaiting transplantation [54].

De Meester and colleagues [55] studied life expectancy and transplant effect, stratified by type of end-stage lung disease in the Eurotransplant experience. They observed the highest global mortality rates, defined as post-transplantation + waiting list deaths, for patients with pulmonary fibrosis and pulmonary hypertension (54% and 52%, respectively); emphysema patients had the lowest global mortality rate (38%). These authors recommended that allocation algorithms should be developed that would lessen the impact of waiting time and take into account the type of end-stage lung disease.

The special problems of lung transplantation

The lungs are fragile organs that are susceptible to infection, the hydrostatic effects of cardiac failure and increased capillary permeability following injury to the alveolar walls by a variety of different factors. As noted earlier, only 13% of cadaveric donors contribute lungs suitable for transplantation (Figure 5.6). There is a well-developed immune system in the lungs and they are more subject to rejection than any other solid organ [56]. Obliterative bronchiolitis, the major manifestation of chronic rejection, accounts for most of the late deaths from lung transplantation [57,58].

COPD: the commonest indication for lung transplantation

From the beginning, COPD has been the commonest indication for lung transplantation. Table 5.1 shows that, through 2000, usual COPD was the diagnosis in 47% of SLTs and COPD due to AAT deficiency accounted for an additional 11% of SLTs. Thus a total of 58% of all SLTs was done for COPD. On the other hand, cystic fibrosis accounted for one third of all bilateral/double lung transplantations and only 3% of SLTs.

Lung transplantation, survival and quality of life

Actuarial survival rates after lung transplantation are 77% at one year, 58% at three years and 44% at five years, not as good as after kidney, liver or heart transplantation (Table 5.2). Infection and acute rejection are the major causes of morbidity and mortality during the first year; infection and chronic rejection account for slower attrition thereafter. Chronic rejection, the development of the obliterative bronchiolitis syndrome, has occurred in 34–41% of recipients after the first year, is intractable to treatment and is the leading cause of death in long-term transplant

Table 5.2. Patient survival rates at one, three and five years

Organ/Donor Type	1 year survival, %(SE)	3 year survival, %(SE)	5 year survival, %(SE)
Kidney, cadaveric	94.8(0.2)	88.9(0.1)	81.8(0.2)
Kidney, living	97.6(0.2)	94.6(0.2)	91.0(0.2)
Liver	87.9(0.4)	79.2(0.3)	74.2(0.3)
Heart	85.5(0.6)	76.9(0.3)	69.8(0.4)
Lung	77.0(1.1)	58.1(0.7)	44.2(0.8)
Heart–Lung	60.0(5.3)	51.4(2.4)	41.7(2.5)

Note: SE, Standard error.
Source: UNOS Scientific Registry Data as of 5 September 2000 [52].

Table 5.3. Adult lung transplantation risk factors for one year mortality ($n = 9563$) and five year mortality ($n = 5050$)

Variable	1 year survival Odds Ratio	5 year survival Odds Ratio
PPH	1.5	
Female recipient	0.85	0.87
Emphysema/COPD	0.56	0.76
Alpha-1-antitrypsin deficiency	0.83	0.70
Recipient age – quadratic		
20 years	0.82	1.22
35 years	0.83	0.91
50 years	1.09	1.08
65 years	1.86	2.1
Recipient BMI – linear		
17	0.83	0.83
22	0.97	0.97
27	1.13	1.13
32	1.32	1.31

Note: PPH, primary pulmonary hypertension; COPD, chronic obstructive pulmonary disease; BMI, body mass index.
All values statistically significant, $p < 0.05$ [46].

survivors [59]. Female sex, COPD (both usual and AAT-COPD), increasing recipient age and body mass index are risk factors for successful lung transplantation, Table 5.3 [46]. Five year survival rates are similar for usual and AAT-COPD (Table 5.3).

Stavem and colleagues [60] did a cross-sectional postal survey of 31 lung transplant recipients and 15 candidates for transplantation. They used the St George's Respiratory Questionnaire, the Short Form 36 (SF-36) and the Hospital Anxiety and Depression Scale. They found improvement in transplantation survivors of most dimensions of health-related quality of life, using both lung-specific and general measures. Although quality of life and functional capacity are dramatically improved by lung transplantation, the need for closely supervised medical care and expensive drug regimens remains.

Complications of lung transplantation

In addition to infection and rejection, a long list of complications, mostly related to immunosuppression, adds substantially to the morbidity of patients who have received transplants. Complications include lymphoproliferative disorders and other cancers, osteoporosis, obesity, systemic hypertension, renal insufficiency and diabetes mellitus [59].

Indications for lung transplantation

Minimal indications for referral to a lung transplant programme are postbronchodilator FEV_1 < 25% predicted, chronic hypercapnia, pulmonary hypertension, rapidly declining lung function and recurrent acute exacerbations of COPD. Waiting times for transplantation are long (>1 year) and deaths during the waiting period are to be expected. The upper limit of age for SLT in COPD patients is 65 years.

Contraindications for lung transplantation

Relative contraindications include symptomatic osteoporosis, nutritional issues (ideal body weight <70 or >130%), substance abuse (alcohol, tobacco and narcotics) and psychosocial problems that have a high likelihood of impacting negatively on the patient's outcome. Absolute contraindications include major organ dysfunction, infection with human immunodeficiency virus (HIV), active malignancy, hepatitis B antigen positivity and hepatitis C with biopsy-proven liver disease [59,61].

Economics of lung transplantation

Only limited information is available on the economics of lung transplantation. In a pilot study of the first 25 lung transplantations at the University of Washington in Seattle [62]. Ramsey and colleagues reported that transplantation charges averaged $164 989. Average monthly charges post-transplant were $11 917 for year 1 and $4525 thereafter versus monthly charges of $3395 for waiting-list patients. Quality of life was significantly greater for patients receiving transplants than for waiting-list patients. Life expectancy was not different (5.89 versus 5.32 years respectively), although quality-adjusted life expectancy did improve significantly. After converting charges to costs, the incremental cost per quality-adjusted life-year gained (QUALY) was $176 817 for post-transplant patients as compared with waiting-list patients.

A Dutch medical technology assessment group has studied the cost-effectiveness of lung transplantation in the Netherlands [63,64]. They studied 425 patients referred for transplantation, of whom 57 underwent transplantation. The estimated cost per life-year gained was US$116 400 and cost per quality life-year gained was US$100 200. Costs per life-year gained for heart and liver transplantation in Netherlands programmes are considerably less, US$39 600 and US$32 400, respectively. The main reason for the differences is the higher number of life-years gained for heart and liver transplants, 10.5 and 7.6 years, respectively, as compared with 5.1 life-years for lung transplantation.

In brief, lung transplantation is a high cost procedure that is less cost-effective than heart or liver transplantation, although it greatly improves quality of life. Two thirds of care costs are incurred after transplantation, which replaces one expensive chronic disease with another. Marginal gains in life expectancy account for the limited cost-effectiveness of the procedure in comparison with other solid organ transplants.

Public policy implications of lung transplantation

At the beginning of the 21st century, all governments are grappling with rapidly escalating health care costs and the limited amount of the gross domestic product that can be spent on health care. These rising costs are due to many factors. Past successes of public health and health care initiatives have resulted in ever-increasing proportions of older people in the populations of developed countries and greater utilization of health care systems by these older persons. However, at least half of the increase in health care costs is due to the great increase over the last half-century of high technology, expensive, noncurative but life-lengthening and enhancing therapies. The development of high technology therapies, especially expensive drugs, is proceeding at an ever-increasing pace. A dilemma

arises because frequently the expensive high technology solution is often the only therapy for a particular group of people. While any one high cost therapy does not pose an impossible burden for a health care system, in aggregate, these costs put great pressure on the system.

The future of lung transplant for COPD

Consider lung transplantation for COPD. In 1994 there were about 3.7 million people between the ages of 45 and 64 years with COPD in the USA [2]. One per cent or 37 200 of these might potentially be candidates for lung transplantation. If the donor lungs were available, one quarter of them or 9300 might come to lung transplantation. Assuming an average five year survival for both transplanted and usual care patients, transplantation would result in additional charges to the health care system of $230 000 per patient in 1993 dollars, or an estimated total additional expenditure of 2.14 billion dollars. It is evident that the constraints on spending for health care, even in wealthy, developed countries, make lung transplantation an inappropriate solution for relieving the suffering of persons with end-stage COPD.

For the last few years only about 1400 donor lungs per year have been available worldwide (Figure 5.4). On 21 August 1998, the federal Department of Health and Human Services of the USA promulgated regulation 42 CFR, Part 482. This national organ and tissue donation initiative requires hospitals to report all deaths to their designated organ procurement organization; only trained specialists can offer organ donation to families; and finally hospitals must provide access to deceased patients' charts to ensure that all potential donors are identified. The intent of this initiative is to address the critical shortage of donor organs for the more than 5000 people in the USA waiting for lung transplant operations, of whom more than 10% will die before they received a transplant.

Because of the shortage of donor lungs, the high cost to the health care system of lung transplantation for emphysema has not become a major public policy issue. However, if donor lung availability were to increase by improved organ donation and preservation or by the advent of xenotransplantation [65] we could suddenly be faced with major new demands on the health care system. Some heart-wrenching choices would surely need to be made.

A number of drugs have been added to corticosteroids, azothioprine and ciclosporin, which were the basic immunosuppressive regimen. These include tacrolimus, mycophenolate mofetil, antithymocyte and antilymphocyte globulin and OKT3 (muromonab-CD3), monoclonal antibody to the CD3 component of T-cell receptors [48,59]. Additional agents are under development. Improvement in survival after transplantation by development of improved drugs for immunosuppression and for preventing obliterative bronchiolitis would also make lung transplantation a more attractive option for dealing with end-stage COPD. We may yet need to deal with how many transplants we can afford to do each year for patients with COPD.

Ethical issues

Close examination of the relative number of lung transplantations done for usual COPD versus AAT deficiency raises some interesting ethical issues. As noted in Table 5.1, 58% of lung transplantations worldwide were done for COPD; 81% were done for usual COPD, 19% for AAT-COPD. In developed countries, AAT deficiency accounts for < 1% of COPD cases. AAT-COPD becomes severe on average in the fifth decade of life rather than the seventh decade for usual COPD. Nevertheless as noted earlier, there were some 37 000 COPD patients < 65 years of age who were potential lung transplant patients in the USA. This suggests that pulmonologists may not be fulfilling their ethical obligation to inform patients of all possible therapeutic options. There may be an age bias in favour of younger patients on the part of physicians in referring patients for lung transplantation. For that matter, as an academic who lectures frequently on COPD, it is only recently that I have begun to include lung transplantation as a therapeutic option for end-stage COPD in my talks to physicians. In the USA and the UK, lung transplantation waiting times are long and the queue is kept to a first-come, first-served basis. Lung transplant surgeons may have a bias in favour of younger patients, which is subtly exercised after a donor lung becomes available and the choice must be made of who from the waiting list will receive the transplant.

Some have suggested that resources for managing end-stage COPD should be limited because tobacco smoking is the main risk factor for the disease and 'the disease is self-inflicted.' I consider this idea reprehensible – it is an ancient tenet of medicine that the sick must always be treated regardless of the cause of the illness. Consider first the process of starting to smoke. Most persons become addicted to smoking when they are young – in the second or third decade of life, when the consequences of smoking are so far in the future that they are given little credence by the young person. Peer pressures and the subtle influences of bill-board, print media and sponsored-event advertising, which are perfectly legal and are condoned by our society, far outweigh the knowledge that 'tobacco smoking may be bad for your health;' and besides, 'the bad effects on health will occur in someone else and not in me' [66].

Turning to a consideration of smoking cessation, some never-smokers believe that failure to stop smoking is just a matter of weakness on the part of the individual – a failure to have exercised sufficient will power. The facts belie this simplistic approach. Tobacco smoking is highly addictive by virtue of its content of nicotine [67]. In the Lung Health Study [68], 4000 smoking subjects with mild airflow obstruction received an intensive smoking-cessation regimen, including nicotine chewing gum, for five years. At the end of that time, 22% of the subjects were sustained quitters and 78% were still smoking. This small percentage of quitters at five years is the highest ever reported after any organized smoking-cessation effort, thus supporting the contention that tobacco smoking is highly addictive.

High technology medicine and health care costs

Lung transplantation epitomizes the dilemma of high technology medicine in the modern health care system. Despite its fearsome costs, lung transplantation frequently gives additional years of life to highly productive people whose contributions to society would otherwise be lost.

Continued support of research leading to enhanced understanding of disease mechanisms is strongly supported by medical schools, government and industry. Administrators, health care policy advisors and clinical managers must continue to grapple with the medical, ethical, political and legal issues that will permit the development of mechanisms for introducing new and expensive therapies only once they have been proven to be effective. We must also continue to grapple with the best ways of using those therapies once they have been introduced – using them only under circumstances in which they are proven effective and avoiding their use when they are marginally effective [28].

The developed world is engaged in the struggle of learning how to incorporate the phenomenal technological advances of the last century into our health care system in such a way that we can afford to pay for those advances. Despite the difficult problems, there is no going back. Who among us would be willing to give up the enormous advances brought by high technology medicine? There will be no easy solutions. Continuing involvement by insurers, health care providers, legislators, civil servants and by a public fully educated in the issues driving health care costs is most likely to develop a process that will lead to acceptable systems for delivering health care.

Acknowledgement

This work was supported by the US Department of Veterans' Affairs.

REFERENCES

1 American Thoracic Society. Standards for the diagnosis and care of patients with chronic obstructive pulmonary disease. American Thoracic Society. *Am J Respir Crit Care Med* 1995; **152**(5 Pt 2): S77–S121.

2 American Lung Association. Trends in chronic bronchitis and emphysma: morbidity and mortality. In *Epidemiology and statisitics unit report*; 2000. American Lung Association, New York.

3 World Health Organization. *World Health statistics annual, 1995*. WHO, Geneva, 1996.

4 Piquette CA, Rennard S, Snider GL. Chronic bronchitis and emphysema. In: Murray JF, Nadel JA, Mason RJ, Boushey HA Jr, eds. *Textbook of respiratory medicine*, 3rd edn. WB Saunders Co., Philadelphia, 2000: 1187–1246.

5 Tashkin DP, Altose MD, Bleeker ER, et al. The Lung Health Study: airway responsiveness to inhaled methacholine in smokers with mild to moderate airflow limitation. *Am Rev Respir Dis* 1992; **145**: 301–310.

6 Kanner RE, Connett JE, Altose MD, et al. Gender difference in airway hyperresponsiveness in smokers with COPD. *Am J Respir Crit Care Med* 1994; **150**: 956–961.

7 Hogg JC. Chronic obstructive pulmonary disease: an overview of pathology and pathogenesis. *Novartis Found Symp* 2001; **234**: 4–19.

8 Retamales I, Elliott WM, Meshi B, et al. Amplification of inflammation in emphysema and its association with latent adenoviral infection. *Am J Respir Crit Care Med* 2001; **164**: 469–473.

9 Stoller JK. Clinical features and natural history of severe alpha 1-antitrypsin deficiency. Roger S. Mitchell Lecture. *Chest* 1997; **111**(6 Suppl): 123S–128S.

10 World Health Organization. Alpha 1-antitrypsin deficiency: memorandum from a WHO meeting. *Bull World Health Organ* 1997; **75**: 397–415.

11 Silverman EK. Genetics of chronic obstructive pulmonary disease. *Novartis Found Symp* 2001; **234**: 45–58; discussion 58–64.

12 Perlmutter DH. Liver injury in alpha 1-antitrypsin deficiency. *Clin Liver Dis* 2000; **4**: 387–408, vi.

13 Eriksson S, Carlson J, Velez R. Risk of cirrhosis and primary liver cancer in alpha1-antitrypsin deficiency. *N Engl J Med* 1986; **314**: 736–739.

14 Alpha-1 Antitrypsin Deficiency Registry Study Group. Survival and FEV1 decline in individuals with severe deficiency of alpha1-antitrypsin. *Am J Respir Crit Care Med* 1998; **158**: 49–59.

15 Wencker M, Banik N, Buhl R, Seidel R, Konietzko N. Long-term treatment of alpha1-antitrypsin deficiency-related pulmonary emphysema with human alpha1-antitrypsin. Wissenschaftliche Arbeitsgemeinschaft zur Therapie von Lungenerkrankungen (WATL)-alpha1-Antitrypsin Study Group. *Eur Respir J* 1998; **11**: 428–433.

16 Seersholm N, Wencker M, Banik N, et al. Does alpha1-antitrypsin augmentation therapy slow the annual decline in FEV1 in patients with severe hereditary alpha1-antitrypsin deficiency? Wissenschaftliche Arbeitsgemeinschaft zur Therapie von Lungenerkrankungen (WATL) Alpha1-Antitrypsin Study Group. *Eur Respir J* 1997; **10**: 2260–2263.

17 Dirksen A, Dijkman JH, Madsen F, et al. A randomized clinical trial of alpha(1)-antitrypsin augmentation therapy. *Am J Respir Crit Care Med* 1999; **160**(5 Pt 1): 1468–1472.

18 Lieberman J. Augmentation therapy reduces frequency of lung infections in antitrypsin deficiency: a new hypothesis with supporting data. *Chest* 2000; **118**: 1480–1485.

19 Sandford AJ, Pare PD. Genetic risk factors for chronic obstructive pulmonary disease. *Clin Chest Med* 2000; **21**: 633–643.

20 Snider GL. Clinical relevance summary: collagen vs elastin in pathogenesis of emphysema; cellular origin of elastases; bronchiolitis vs emphysema as a cause of airflow obstruction. *Chest* 2000; **117**(5 Suppl 1): 244S–246S.

21 Saetta M, Turato G, Maestrelli P, Mapp CE, Fabbri LM. Cellular and structural bases of chronic obstructive pulmonary disease. *Am J Respir Crit Care Med* 2001; **163**: 1304–1309.

22 Ferguson GT. Chronic obstructive pulmonary disease: progress nevertheless [editorial]. *Hosp Pract (Off Ed)* 1995; 30(12): 11–13.

23 Steiner MC, Morgan MD. Enhancing physical performance in chronic obstructive pulmonary disease. *Thorax* 2001; **56**: 73–77.

24 Heffner JE. Role of pulmonary rehabilitation in palliative care. *Respir Care* 2000; **45**: 1365–1371; discussion 1371–1375.

25 Celli BR. Pulmonary rehabilitation for COPD. A practical approach for improving ventilatory conditioning. *Postgrad Med* 1998; **103**: 159–160, 167–168, 173–176.

26 Mahler DA. Pulmonary rehabilitation. *Chest* 1998; **113**(4 Suppl): 263S–268S.

27 Hill NS. Noninvasive ventilation in chronic obstructive pulmonary disease. *Clin Chest Med* 2000; 21: 783–797.

28 Snider GL. Reduction pneumoplasty for giant bullous emphysema. Implications for surgical treatment of nonbullous emphysema. *Chest* 1996; **109**: 540–548.

29 Brantigan OC, Kress MB, Mueller EA. The surgical approach to pulmonary emphysema. *Dis Chest* 1961; **39**: 485–501.

30 Cooper JD, Trulock EP, Triantafillou AN, et al. Bilateral pneumonectomy (volume reduction) for chronic obstructive pulmonary disease. *J Thorac Cardiovasc Surg* 1995; **109**: 106–119.

31 Berger RL, Celli BR, Meneghetti AL, et al. Limitations of randomized clinical trials for evaluating emerging operations: the case of lung volume reduction surgery. *Ann Thorac Surg* 2001; **72**: 649–657.

32 Hardy JD WW, Dalton ML, Walker GR. Lung homotransplantation in man: report of the initial case. *JAMA* 1963; **186**: 1065–1074.

33 Cooper JD. Current status of lung transplantation. *Transplant Proc* 1991; **23**: 2107–2114.

34 Stevens PM, Johnson PC, Bell RL, Beall AC, Jr, Jenkins DE. Regional ventilation and perfusion after lung transplantation in patients with emphysema. *N Engl J Med* 1970; **282**: 245–249.

35 Wildevuur CR, Benfield JR. A review of 23 human lung transplantations by 20 surgeons. *Ann Thorac Surg* 1970; **9**: 489–515.

36 Toronto Lung Transplant Group. Unilateral lung transplantation for pulmonary fibrosis. *N Engl J Med* 1986; **314**: 1140–1145.

37 Mal H, Andreassian B, Pamela F, et al. Unilateral lung transplantation in end-stage pulmonary emphysema. *Am Rev Respir Dis* 1989; **140**: 797–802.

38 Yacoub M, Khaghani A, Theodoropoulos S, Tadjkarimi S, Banner N. Single-lung transplantation for obstructive airway disease. *Transplant Proc* 1991; **23**: 1213–1214.

39 Kaiser LR, Cooper JD, Trulock EP, Pasque MK, Triantafillou A, Haydock D. The evolution of single lung transplantation for emphysema. The Washington University Lung Transplant Group. *J Thorac Cardiovasc Surg* 1991; **102**(3): 333–339; discussion 339–341.

40 Low DE, Trulock EP, Kaiser LR, et al. Morbidity, mortality, and early results of single versus bilateral lung transplantation for emphysema. *J Thorac Cardiovasc Surg* 1992; **103**: 1119–1126.

41 Briffa NP, Dennis C, Higenbottam T, et al. Single lung transplantation for end stage emphysema. *Thorax* 1995; **50**: 562–564.

42 Chacon RA, Corris PA, Dark JH, Gibson GJ. Comparison of the functional results of single lung transplantation for pulmonary fibrosis and chronic airway obstruction. *Thorax* 1998; **53**(1): 43–49.

43 Khaghani A, al-Kattan KM, Tadjkarimi S, Banner N, Yacoub M. Early experience with single lung transplantation for emphysema with simultaneous volume reduction of the contralateral lung. *Eur J Cardiothorac Surg* 1997; **11**: 604–608.

44 Sundaresan RS, Shiraishi Y, Trulock EP, et al. Single or bilateral lung transplantation for emphysema? *J Thorac Cardiovasc Surg* 1996; **112**(6): 1485–1494; discussion 1494–1495.

45 Bavaria JE, Kotloff R, Palevsky H, et al. Bilateral versus single lung transplantation for chronic obstructive pulmonary disease. *J Thorac Cardiovasc Surg* 1997; **113**: 520–527; discussion 528.

46 International Society for Heart and Lung Transplantation. The International Heart and Lung Transplant Registry, 2001 Report. Addison, TX. Website http://www.ishlt.org/

47 Bennett LE, Keck BM, Daily OP, Novick RJ, Hosenpud JD. Worldwide thoracic organ transplantation: a report from the UNOS/ISHLT International Registry for Thoracic Organ Transplantation. *Clin Transpl* 2000: 31–44.

48 Anyanwu AC, Rogers CA, Murday J. Where are we today with pulmonary transplantation? Current results from a national cohort. UK Cardiothoracic Transplant Audit Steering Group. *Transpl Int* 2000; **13**(Suppl 1): S245–S246.

49 Speziali G, McDougall JC, Midthun DE, et al. Native lung complications after single lung transplantation for emphysema. *Transpl Int* 1997; **10**: 113–115.

50 Venuta F, Boehler A, Rendina EA, et al. Complications in the native lung after single lung transplantation. *Eur J Cardiothorac Surg* 1999; **16**: 54–58.

51 Schulman LL, O'Hair DP, Cantu E, McGregor C, Ginsberg ME. Salvage by volume reduction of chronic allograft rejection in emphysema. *J Heart Lung Transplant* 1999; **18**: 107–112.

52 Todd TR, Perron J, Winton TL, Keshavjee SH. Simultaneous single-lung transplantation and lung volume reduction. *Ann Thorac Surg* 1997; **63**: 1468–1470.

53 Kroshus TJ, Bolman RM III, Kshettry VR. Unilateral volume reduction after single-lung transplantation for emphysema. *Ann Thorac Surg* 1996; **62**: 363–368.

54 UNOS 1990–2000. 1999 Annual report of the US Scientific Registry of Transplant Recipients and the Organ Procurement and Transplantation Network: transplant data 1989–1998. (2000, February 21). HHS/HRSA/OSP/DOT and UNOS, Rockville, MD, and Richmond, VA. (www.unos.org)

55 De Meester J, Smits JM, Persijn GG, Haverich A. Listing for lung transplantation: life expectancy and transplant effect, stratified by type of end-stage lung disease, the Eurotransplant experience. *J Heart Lung Transplant* 2001; **20**: 518–524.

56 Trulock EP III. Lung transplantation for COPD. *Chest* 1998; **113**(4 Suppl): 269S–276S.

57 Scott JP, Higenbottam TW, Sharples L, et al. Risk factors for obliterative bronchiolitis in heart–lung transplant recipients. *Transplantation* 1991; **51**: 813–817.

58 Schlesinger C, Veeraraghavan S, Koss MN. Constructive (obliterative) bronchiolitis. *Curr Opin Pulm Med* 1998; **4**: 288–293.

59 Trulock EP. Lung transplantation. *Am J Respir Crit Care Med* 1997; **155**: 789–818.

60 Stavem K, Bjortuft O, Lund MB, Kongshaug K, Geiran O, Boe J. Health-related quality of life in lung transplant candidates and recipients. *Respiration* 2000; **67**: 159–165.

61 Maurer JR, Frost AE, Estenne M, Higenbottam T, Glanville AR. International guidelines for the selection of lung transplant candidates. The International Society for Heart and Lung Transplantation, the American Thoracic Society, the American Society of Transplant Physicians, the European Respiratory Society. *Transplantation* 1998; **66**: 951–956.

62 Ramsey SD, Patrick DL, Lewis S, Albert RK, Raghu G. Improvement in quality of life after lung transplantation: a preliminary study. The University of Washington Medical Center Lung Transplant Study Group. *J Heart Lung Transplant* 1995; **14**: 870–877.

63 Al MJ, Koopmanschap MA, van Enckevort PJ, et al. Cost-effectiveness of lung transplantation in the Netherlands: a scenario analysis. *Chest* 1998; **113**: 124–130.

64 van Enckevort PJ, TenVergert EM, Bonsel GJ, et al. Technology assessment of the Dutch Lung Transplantation Program. *Int J Technol Assess Health Care* 1998; **14**: 344–356.

65 Cooper DK, Keogh AM, Brink J, et al. Report of the Xenotransplantation Advisory Committee of the International Society for

Heart and Lung Transplantation: the present status of xeno-transplantation and its potential role in the treatment of end-stage cardiac and pulmonary diseases. *J Heart Lung Transplant* 2000; **19**: 1125–1165.

66 Stewart M. The effect of advertising on tobacco consumption in OECD countries. *Int J Advertising* 1993; **12**: 155–180.

67 Schelling T. Addictive drugs: the cigarette experience. *Science* 1992; **255**: 430–433.

68 Anthonisen NR, Connett JE, Kiley JP, et al. Effects of smoking intervention and the use of an inhaled anticholinergic bronchodilator on the rate of decline of FEV1; The Lung Health Study [see comments]. *JAMA* 1994; **272**: 1497–1505.

6

Alpha-1-antitrypsin deficiency

Duncan C. S. Hutchison

King's College Hospital and Guy's, King's and St Thomas' School of Medicine, London, UK

Introduction

Alpha-1-antitrypsin (AAT) deficiency is a hereditary disorder associated with the onset of disabling emphysema at a relatively early age. The condition was first recognized by the Swedish workers Laurell and Eriksson [1], who observed a severe deficiency of the alpha-1-globulin fraction in a number of sera undergoing routine biochemical examination. The main protein in this fraction was already recognized to be a proteinase inhibitor, known as 'alpha-1-antitrypsin'. Laurell and Eriksson therefore coined the term 'alpha-1-antitrypsin deficiency' to describe the condition.

AAT has a much wider spectrum of antiproteolytic activity than its name implies and its most important action appears to be the inhibition of the powerful elastase found within the polymorphonuclear leukocytes. In the most severe form of the deficiency (subjects homozygous for protease inhibitor (PI) type Z), the serum AAT may be only 10–20% of normal and the pulmonary elastin may then be degraded by the unopposed action of the elastase. Alternative names for the inhibitor have therefore been introduced such as alpha-1-protease inhibitor, but the more familiar name AAT will be used here.

The Pi system

Advances in electrophoretic methods indicated that AAT forms a polymorphic system with a large number of possible biochemical variants; these are known collectively as the Pi system, the abbreviation standing for 'protease inhibitor'. Over 90 different AAT variants have been described using the method of isoelectric focusing in polyacrylamide gels. The nomenclature has thus become extremely complex; briefly, the variants are designated by a capital letter corresponding to their mobility by the isoelectric focusing method with the addition of a name or number if necessary. The methods and variants have been reviewed in detail elsewhere [2–4]. The common variant is known as type M which has four or more subtypes, in themselves probably of no clinical significance. For any given phenotype there is a wide range in the serum level so the phenotype should be established by isoelectric focusing in every case.

Geographical distribution

The abnormal PiZ gene is found predominantly in those of European stock and is very rare in Asian and African populations. The mutation is thought to have arisen in Scandinavia and in Europe the gene frequency is highest on the northwestern seaboard of the continent [5]. The prevalence of the type Z homozygote in the UK is about 1 in 3000 which is similar to that in Americans of European descent.

Clinical features of AAT deficiency

Of the commoner abnormal phenotypes, homozygotes of type Z have been most frequently associated with emphysema. Their clinical, physiological and radiological features were originally described by Eriksson [6] and these observations have been confirmed many times [7–9]. Progressively severe shortness of breath on exertion is the most important symptom; this may occur as early as 30 years of age or may only appear in patients of over 70. The physiological features are very similar to those of emphysematous patients of normal phenotype and include expiratory airflow limitation (attributable to loss of pulmonary elastic recoil), reduction in carbon monoxide transfer factor and increase in residual volume. The vital capacity and arterial blood gases usually deteriorate only in the later stages of the disease.

The average rate of decline in FEV$_1$ in type Z subjects is very much faster than the normal rate of 30 mL/year. In a British study [10], the rate of decline in patients followed for a number of years was 55 (standard deviation, SD 53) mL per year and similar results were obtained in the USA [11] and in Denmark [12].

In type Z homozygotes, cigarette smoking has a severe effect upon lung function and upon prognosis [6–8]. In Swedish subjects of this phenotype, the cumulative probability of survival was shown to be very considerably reduced in comparison with the normal population, smokers being at particular risk [13]. Considerable deterioration has usually occurred before symptoms oblige the patient to seek medical advice.

Radiographical features

The most striking feature is the predominant destruction of the lower zones of the lung, which is seen in over 90% of those with an abnormal radiograph, in contrast to the upper zone and to more uniformly distributed disease commonly found in emphysema of normal phenotype [6,9]. The lower zones may be more severely affected because of the greater blood flow per unit volume in that region, consistent with the prevailing view that the pulmonary damage is brought about by elastase released from circulating neutrophils. In pathological terms, AAT deficiency is associated with the panlobular form of emphysema [6,14].

Other phenotypes and lung disease

The great majority of patients with emphysema are current or ex-smokers of the normal MM phenotype. Heterozygotes of type SZ have a serum AAT concentration of about one third of the normal value and might thus appear to be at risk. In one study [15], however, all the SZ individuals with emphysema had a history of smoking and this phenotype in itself probably carries little or no extra risk of emphysema.

AAT deficiency and liver disease

An association between the homozygous type Z phenotype and hepatitis in newborn infants was first described by Sharp et al. [16]. Globular inclusion bodies consisting of the abnormal Z type of AAT are seen within the hepatocytes of subjects with the ZZ phenotype. A minority (probably fewer than 15%) of type ZZ newborn infants develop hepatitis and

some of these die in infancy or develop cirrhosis in childhood [17,18].

An autopsy study of Pi type Z adults in Sweden revealed that 50% had evidence of cirrhosis, a rate very much higher than that of controls [19]. Few patients presenting with emphysema have clinical evidence of cirrhosis [8], though this possibility should be considered carefully when one is assessing patients for transplant surgery. Many liver transplantations for this disorder have been carried out in both children and adults.

Nonsurgical treatment of emphysema in AAT deficiency

Treatment for the advanced case is limited. Abandonment of cigarette smoking will slow up the rate of decline in lung function in both AAT-deficient [10] and nondeficient patients [20].

AAT replacement therapy

AAT replacement therapy has been available for many years [21] and it has been claimed from two unrandomized trials that such therapy can reduce the rate of decline in lung function [22, 23]. Both of these trials had serious drawbacks [24] and the only double-blind randomized controlled trial to date [25] has shown that AAT replacement therapy had no significant influence on the rate of decline in any measure of lung function, though there was a marginal advantage ($p = 0.07$) in terms of lung density measured by computed tomography scanning.

This result is of interest, though it would be reasonable to expect AAT replacement therapy to produce a definite reduction in the rate of lung function decline similar to the effect of abandoning cigarette smoking [10]. One could argue for a larger study, but, even so, it seems likely that long-term intravenous AAT administration would only be worthwhile if started long before the advent of clinical symptoms.

This concept is illustrated in a model situation (Figure 6.1A,B) where death is assumed to occur when the forced expiratory volume in 1 s (FEV$_1$) falls to 0.3 L. Figure 6.1A then indicates that fully effective treatment starting at the age of 30 would lead to an extra 20 or more years of life, and starting at age 50 to an extra 10 years. Figure 6.1B, on the other hand, shows that less effective treatment starting at the age of 30, would reduce the additional life expectancy to 10 years and, starting at 50, to an extra three years only.

The detection of Pi Z individuals at such an early stage would require some form of population screening with

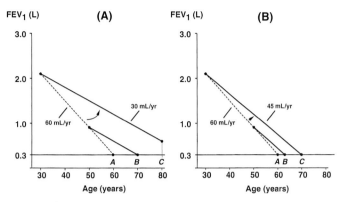

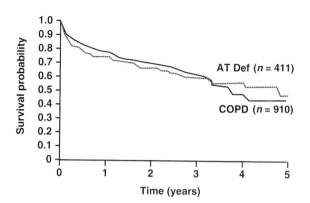

Figure 6.1 Theoretical model of AAT replacement therapy. Dashed line (A,B): untreated rate of decline in FEV_1 at 60 mL/yr over a 30 year period, starting at FEV_1 of 2.1 L or 70%P. Continuous lines: after treatment. (Panel A) Treatment reduces rate of decline to a normal rate of 30 mL/yr. (Panel B) Treatment results in a half-way correction of the FEV_1 slope to 45 mL/yr. Points *A*, *B* and *C* (Panels A and B): age of arrival at FEV_1 equal to 0.3 L in untreated case (point *A*) and after commencement of treatment at age 50 years (point *B*) and at age 30 (point *C*). (Reproduced from Hutchison DCS, Cooper D on behalf of the British Theracic Society. Alpha-1-antitrypsin deficiency: smoking, decline in lung function and implications for therapeutic trials. *Resp Med* 2002; **96**: 872–880. By courtesy of Elsevier Science Ltd.)

Figure 6.3 Actuarial survival after lung transplantation for AAT deficiency (AT Def) emphysema versus non-deficient COPD. (After Fig 4, Trulock EP, Cooper JD. Chap 25, Lung transplantation for alpha1AT-deficiency emphysema: In: *Alpha 1-antitrypsin deficiency*, ed Crystal RG. By courtesy of Marcel Dekker Inc.)

Lung transplantation

Records of the St Louis International Lung Transplant Registry [26] indicate that the total number of recorded lung transplants increased from less than 100 in 1988 to nearly 800 in 1993. By that time, a total of 361 lung transplantations had been performed for AAT deficiency, representing 13% of the total number of lung transplantations to that date. By 1997, the number had climbed to 673, compared with 1924 cases of non-AAT-deficient chronic obstructive pulmonary disease (COPD); 60% of the 673 cases received a single lung transplant (SLT), 34% a bilateral lung transplant (BLT) and only 6% a heart–lung transplant [27].

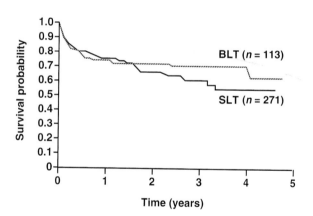

Figure 6.2 Actuarial survival for single (SLT) versus bilateral lung transplantation (BLT) in emphysema due to AAT deficiency. (After Fig 5, Trulock EP, Cooper JD. Chap 25, Lung transplantation for alpha1AT-deficiency emphysema: In: *Alpha 1-antitrypsin deficiency*, ed Crystal RG. By courtesy of Marcel Dekker Inc.)

Survival after lung transplantation

With respect to AAT deficiency, Trulock [26] reviewed the overall position, noting a 75% survival at one year for both procedures. At four years, survival was about 55% for SLT and slightly better for BLT at 60% (Figure 6.2). The five year post-transplantation survival for both AAT deficiency and nondeficient COPD was about 50%, without any important difference between the two groups (Figure 6.3). The deficiency state does not therefore appear in itself to have any obvious bearing on postoperative survival.

For COPD in general, the causes of postoperative death have been analysed by Trulock [27] and the figures are probably applicable to AAT deficiency itself. Early deaths were due to infection or graft failure and 38% of late deaths (more than one year after operation) were due to bronchiolitis obliterans, which remains the most important factor limiting long-term survival in all types of patient.

much labour and expense. Strategies for gene therapy have been suggested but any benefits lie some way in the future. The management of end-stage emphysema due to AAT deficiency will thus fall to transplant centres for some time to come.

Single or bilateral transplant?

A debate on the appropriate procedure for end-stage emphysema has been in progress for some time. Initially, it was felt that SLT in this condition would lead to overinflation of the remaining emphysematous lung, resulting in compression of the transplanted lung and of other organs. This does not necessarily happen and further experience shows that it occurs mainly in the presence of disease such as chronic rejection in the transplanted lung. SLT is a simpler and shorter procedure than BLT and one which makes donor lungs available to more recipients; it has a lower operative complication rate than BLT, an advantage to the older or higher risk patient [26].

BLT, on the other hand, has the advantage that lung function can be restored to near normal, whereas SLT can restore function to half the normal level at best. BLT can thus provide a better reserve against postoperative problems, which may have a favourable effect upon long-term survival.

In practice, Sundaresan et al. [28] preferred BLT to SLT, using the latter mainly for older patients and those of small stature. The majority of their AAT-deficient patients therefore had the bilateral procedure; five year survival was somewhat better in BLT but not significantly so. Another group [29,30], had a similar policy, of using BLT for all AAT-deficient patients and for all emphysematous patients under the age of 60, the five year survival for BLT being 61.9% and for SLT 57.4%, again a nonsignificant difference.

The evidence thus suggests that BLT has a modest advantage over SLT but it is difficult to compare the two procedures due to the different selection criteria and the important factor that the BLT group are on average some five years younger. Bronchiolitis obliterans, the main factor influencing survival, had a similar incidence of 22% in both BLT and SLT [30].

Comparison of survival in transplant and waiting-list patients

This has proved somewhat difficult to assess as a controlled trial has not been accepted as an ethical procedure. In comparisons of patients who have received transplants with those remaining on a waiting list, lung transplantation appears to confer little or no survival benefit in end-stage emphysema at two years of follow-up [31,32]. The authors noted that analysis is difficult owing to numerous underlying assumptions; in particular a number of units have a policy of early listing of emphysematous patients because of the long waiting time, a factor that could bias such studies in favour of waiting-list patients. This aspect has been reviewed in detail by Corris [33]. AAT deficiency has not

been assessed separately, but the same considerations are likely to apply.

Quality of life was nevertheless much improved [27] and most patients expressed satisfaction with their decision to have a transplant. At the two year follow-up point, 30% of the patients were working full-time. Likewise quality of life three or more years after transplantation was much improved [34], though in this respect BLT offered considerably better health status than SLT. It has been calculated, however, that owing to the limited supply of donor lungs only about one third of those needing a lung transplant are likely to receive it [35].

Choosing the optimum time for transplantation

One's natural desire would be to carry out transplantation at the moment when the expected survival time is substantially greater with the operation than without it. Predicting the optimal time for transplantation is unfortunately far from easy. Seersholm et al. [36] derived an exponential formula relating two year mortality to FEV_1 as percentage of the predicted value (%P). The two year mortality following lung transplantation [26] was found to be 0.35 (65% survival), which would correspond to an FEV_1 %P of about 20% using the above formula, but the 95% confidence limits for mortality rate are too wide (±0.15) for satisfactory prediction in the individual case.

In the British Thoracic Society survey of AAT deficiency [8] there were a large number of cases with very poor lung function and a poor prognosis. In all cases where FEV_1 %P was less than 40%, death was caused by, or was closely related to, emphysema. The nearest FEV_1 to the date of death was recorded in 108 cases who died without having had a lung transplant (British Thoracic Society, unpublished data). The peak value for FEV_1 was in the range 21–40%P (Figure 6.4). Thus over 60% of AAT-deficient patients would have died before reaching an FEV_1 of 20%P. To attempt prediction on the basis of FEV_1 alone is therefore unsatisfactory on the available evidence. Hypoxaemia and cor pulmonale are also likely to be important adverse factors.

Guidelines for referral for transplantation

The following guidelines for timing the referral have been suggested [27]: FEV_1 (after bronchodilator) <25% predicted; resting arterial oxygen pressure (PaO_2) <60 mmHg (8 kPa); hypercapnia; pulmonary hypertension; rapidly declining FEV_1; or life-threatening exacerbations. In 1994 the median waiting time for lung transplantation was 548 days (1.5 years) a period that must be taken into account when planning the referral. Many patients with AAT deficiency

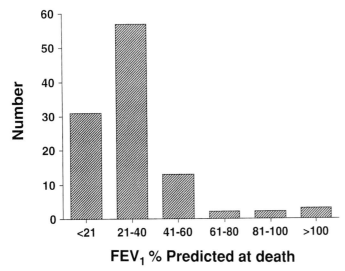

Figure 6.4 FEV_1 as percentage of predicted value (%P) in 108 AAT-deficient patients who died during the British Thoracic Society survey. In all cases where FEV_1 %P was less than 40%, emphysema was the main cause of death. Patients who died after lung transplantation are not included. (Unpublished data from British Thoracic Society survey, with permission.)

are relatively young compared to those with other forms of COPD and are thus somewhat better candidates for lung transplantation. Contraindications to transplantation [27] are similar to those in use for other disorders. They include other serious life-threatening conditions, significant coronary artery disease, drug or alcohol dependency and active smoking. Ventilator-dependent patients have a higher postoperative mortality.

Lung volume reduction surgery

While lung transplantation is now recognized to be the ultimate line of treatment for end-stage emphysema, there are other surgical possibilities. Lung volume reduction surgery (LVRS) has been proposed as an alternative to transplantation, or as a 'bridge' whereby the time for definitive transplant could be postponed, an important factor considering the shortage of donor lungs. This policy has been successful in the much commoner non-AAT-deficient type of emphysema, where the surgery focuses on the upper zones of the lungs, the site of the main lesions [37].

Cassina et al. [38] carried out LVRS in 12 AAT-deficient patients (operating on the lower zones) and compared the results with those of the usual upper zone surgery in non-AAT-deficient patients. The improvements in the nondeficient patients were significantly greater and were sustained for at least two years whereas the AAT-deficient patients

returned to their original preoperative lung function in only 12 months. Bavaria et al. [39] likewise reported an unsatisfactory outcome with LVRS in two out of three AAT-deficient patients. Gelb et al. [40], however, found that, in four AAT-deficient patients, LVRS relieved dyspnoea and provided modest physiological improvement for two to three years associated with increases in lung elastic recoil. This approach therefore has some limitations, but a place clearly still remains for the traditional bullectomy in patients with very large bullae compressing other parts of the lung or causing mediastinal shift [41,42].

Postoperative AAT replacement therapy

The postoperative administration of AAT replacement therapy has been debated, one side of the argument being that additional damage to the graft might occur simply as a result of the deficiency state. Against this concept is the fact that, for both SLT and BLT, there is no significant difference in survival time between AAT-deficient and non-AAT-deficient patients [26] and that emphysema usually takes 20–30 years to develop even in smokers, a time period far in excess of the conceivable lifetime of any transplanted lung. Nevertheless, repeated episodes of infection or rejection might accelerate this process.

To address this question, King et al. [43] studied the free elastase activity in bronchoalveolar lavage fluid obtained from AAT-deficient patients at intervals posttransplantation. No such activity was found, provided that the patients remained well without postoperative infection or rejection. In this study, seven patients had these complications at some stage, but only three actually showed free elastase activity. At present, therefore, there does not appear to be a strong case for administration of AAT replacement therapy, which would add very considerably to the costs of the procedure. Further study does, however, seem to be required.

Acknowledgements

The author is most grateful to the members of the British Thoracic Society who supplied data from AAT-deficient patients and to the Society for permission to use unpublished material.

REFERENCES

1 Laurell CB, Eriksson S. The electrophoretic alpha1-globulin pattern of serum in alpha1-antitrypsin deficiency. *Scand J Clin Lab Invest* 1963; **15**: 132–140.

2 Fagerhol MK, Cox DW. The Pi polymorphism: genetic, biochemical and clinical aspects of human alpha1-antitrypsin. *Adv Hum Genet* 1981; **11**: 1–62.

3 Brantly M, Nukiwa T, Crystal RG. Molecular basis of alpha-1-antitrypsin deficiency. *Am J Med* 1988; **84**(Suppl 6A): 13–31.

4 Norman MR, Mowat AP, Hutchison DCS. Molecular basis, clinical consequences and diagnosis of alpha-1 antitrypsin deficiency. *Ann Clin Biochem* 1997; **34**: 230–246.

5 Hutchison DCS. Alpha$_1$-antitrypsin deficiency in Europe: geographical distribution of Pi types S and Z. *Respir Med* 1998; **92**: 367–377.

6 Eriksson S. Studies in alpha1-antitrypsin deficiency. *Acta Med Scand* 1965; 177(Suppl 432): 1–85.

7 Kueppers F, Black LF. Alpha$_1$-antitrypsin and its deficiency. *Am Rev Respir Dis* 1974; **110**: 176–194.

8 Tobin MJ, Cook PJL, Hutchison DCS. Alpha$_1$-antitrypsin deficiency: the clinical and physiological features of pulmonary emphysema in subjects homozygous for Pi type Z: a survey by the British Thoracic Association. *Br J Dis Chest* 1983; **77**: 14–27.

9 Gishen P, Saunders AJS, Tobin MJ, Hutchison DCS. Alpha-1-antitrypsin deficiency: the radiological features of pulmonary emphysema in subjects of Pi type Z and Pi type SZ. *Clin Radiol* 1982; **33**: 371–377.

10 Hutchison DCS. The natural history of alpha1-protease inhibitor deficiency. *Am J Med* 1988; **84**(Suppl 6A): 3–12.

11 Brantly ML, Paul LD, Miller BH, et al. Clinical features and history of the destructive lung disease associated with alpha-1-antitrypsin deficiency of adults with pulmonary symptoms. *Am Rev Resp Dis* 1988; **138**: 327–336.

12 Evald T, Dirksen A, Keittelmann S, et al. Decline in pulmonary function in patients with alpha 1-antitrypsin deficiency. *Lung* 1990; **168**(Suppl): 579–585.

13 Larsson C. Natural history and life expectancy in severe alpha1-antitrypsin deficiency, Pi Z. *Acta Med Scand* 1978; **204**: 345–351.

14 Thurlbeck WM, Henderson JA, Fraser RG, Bates DV. Chronic obstructive lung disease: a comparison between clinical, roentgenologic, functional and morphologic criteria in chronic bronchitis, emphysema, asthma and bronchiectasis. *Medicine* (Baltimore) 1970; **49**: 81–145.

15 Hutchison DCS, Tobin MJ, Cook PJL. Alpha$_1$-antitrypsin deficiency: clinical and physiological features in heterozygotes of Pi type SZ. A survey by the British Thoracic Association. *Br J Dis Chest* 1983; **77**: 28–34.

16 Sharp HL, Bridges RA, Krivit W, Freier EF. Cirrhosis associated with alpha1-antitrypsin deficiency: a previously unrecognised inherited disorder. *J Lab Clin Med* 1969; **73**: 934–939.

17 Sveger T. The natural history of liver disease in alpha-1-antitrypsin deficient children. *Acta Paediat Scand* 1988; **77**: 847–851.

18 Hussain M, Mieli-Vergani G, Mowat AP. Alpha1-antitrypsin deficiency and liver disease: clinical presentation, diagnosis and treatment. *J Inherit Metabol Dis* 1991; **14**: 497–511.

19 Eriksson S, Carlson J, Velez R. Risk of cirrhosis and primary liver cancer in alpha-1-antitrypsin deficiency. *N Engl J Med* 1986; **314**: 736–739.

20 Hughes JA, Hutchison DCS, Bellamy D, et al. The influence of cigarette smoking and its withdrawal on the annual rate of change of lung function in pulmonary emphysema. *Quart J Med* 1982; **51**: 115–124.

21 Gadek JE, Klein HG, Holland PV, Crystal RG. Replacement therapy of alpha-1-antitrypsin deficiency. Reversal of protease–antiprotease imbalance within the alveolar structures of PiZ subjects. *J Clin Invest* 1981; **68**: 1158–1165.

22 McElvaney NG, Stoller JK, Buist AS, et al. Baseline characteristics of enrollees in the National Heart, Lung and Blood Institute Registry of alpha 1-antitrypsin deficiency. *Chest* 1997; **111**: 394–403.

23 Seersholm N, Wencker M, Banik N, et al. Does alpha-1-antitrypsin augmentation therapy slow the annual decline in FEV-1 in patients with severe hereditary alpha-1-antitrypsin deficiency? *Eur Respir J* 1997; **10**: 2260–2263.

24 Hutchison DCS, Hughes MD. Alpha-1-antitrypsin replacement therapy: will its efficacy ever be proved? *Eur Respir J* 1997; **10**: 2191–2193.

25 Dirksen A, Dijkman JH, Madsen F, et al. A randomised clinical trial of α_1-antitrypsin augmentation therapy. *Am J Respir Crit Care Med* 1999; **160**: 1468–1472.

26 Trulock EP. Lung transplantation for alpha-1-antitrypsin deficiency emphysema. *Chest* 1996; **110**(Suppl): 284S–294S.

27 Trulock EP. Lung transplantation for COPD. *Chest* 1998; **113** (Suppl): 269S–276S.

28 Sundaresan RS, Shiraishi Y, Trulock EP, et al. Single or bilateral transplantation for emphysema? *J Thorac Cardiovasc Surg* 1996; **112**: 1485–1495.

29 Bavaria JE, Kotloff R, Palevsky H, et al. Bilateral versus single lung transplantation for chronic obstructive pulmonary disease. *J Thorac Cardiovasc Surg* 1997; **113**: 520–528.

30 Pochettino A, Kotloff RM, Rosengard BR, et al. Bilateral versus single lung transplantation for chronic obstructive pulmonary disease: intermediate-term results. *Ann Thorac Surg* 2000; **70**:1813–1818.

31 Hosenpud JD, Bennett LE, Keck BM, et al. Effect of diagnosis on survival benefit of lung transplantation for end-stage lung disease. *Lancet* 1998; **351**: 24–27.

32 Geertsma A, Ten Vergert EM, Bonsel GJ, et al. Does lung transplantation prolong life? A comparison of survival with and without transplantation. *J Heart Lung Transplant* 1998; **17**: 511–516.

33 Corris PA. Lung transplantation for chronic obstructive pulmonary disease: an exercise in quality rather than quantity? *Thorax* 1999; **54**(Suppl 2): S24–S27.

34 Anyanwu AC, McGuire A, Rogers CA, Murday AJ. Assessment of quality of life in lung transplantation using a simple generic tool. *Thorax* 2001; **56**: 218–222.

35 Geertsma A, TenVergert EM, De Boer WJ, Van der Bij W. The need for lung transplantation in the Netherlands. *Transpl Int* 1997; **10**: 457–461.

36 Seersholm N, Dirksen A, Kok-Jensen A. Airways obstruction and two year survival in patients with severe alpha$_1$-antitrypsin deficiency. *Eur Respir J* 1994; **7**: 1985–1987.

37 Cooper JD, Patterson GA, Sundaresan RS, et al. Results of 150 consecutive bilateral lung volume reduction procedures

in patients with severe emphysema. *J Thorac Cardiovasc Surg* 1996; **112**: 1319–1330.

38 Cassina PC, Teschler H, Konietzko N, et al. Two-year results after lung volume reduction surgery in alpha$_1$-antitrypsin deficiency versus smoker's emphysema. *Eur Respir J* 1998; **12**: 1028–1032.

39 Bavaria JE, Pochettino A, Kotloff RM, et al. Effect of volume reduction on lung transplant timing and selection for chronic obstructive pulmonary disease. *J Thorac Cardiovasc Surg* 1998; **115**: 9–18.

40 Gelb AF, McKenna RJ, Brenner M, et al. Lung function after bilateral lower lobe lung volume reduction surgery for alpha1-antitrypsin emphysema. *Eur Respir J* 1999; **14**: 928–933 [Erratum in *Eur Respir J* 2000; **15**: 817].

41 Mineo TC, Pompeo E, Simonetti G, et al. Unilateral thorascopic reduction pneumoplasty for asymmetric emphysema. *Eur J Cardiothorac Surg* 1998; **14**: 33–39.

42 Kuno R, Kanter KR, Torres WE, Lawrence EC. Single lung transplantation followed by contralateral bullectomy for bullous emphysema. *J Heart Lung Transplant* 1996; **15**: 389–394.

43 King MB, Campbell EJ, Gray BH, Hertz MI. The proteinase–antiproteinase balance in alpha-1-proteinase inhibitor-deficient lung transplant recipients. *Am Rev Respir Crit Care Med* 1994; **149**: 966–971.

7

Bronchiectasis

Mary T. Keogan

Papworth Hospital, Cambridgeshire, UK

Introduction

Bronchiectasis is characterized by chronic dilatation and inflammation of bronchi, which may result from numerous defects in host defences, infectious or toxic insults to the lung or chronic pulmonary inflammation resulting from a variety of conditions. Diagnosis is based on high resolution computed tomography (CT) findings of bronchial dilatation and bronchial wall thickening. Until recently bronchial dilatation has been considered irreversible, but recent data suggest that at least some regression of 'chronic' changes is possible [1]. Cystic fibrosis (CF) is the most common underlying cause of bronchiectasis; however, as this is discussed in detail elsewhere, this chapter will focus on non-CF bronchiectasis. The true incidence of non-CF bronchiectasis is unknown, but this condition is almost certainly underdiagnosed due to a low index of suspicion.

Patients with bronchiectasis commonly present with chronic sputum production; however, episodic haemoptysis in the absence of infection or discrete episodes of respiratory infection with intervening symptom-free periods are seen in a minority of patients. The clinical course is highly variable, with some patients remaining stable for several years and others progressing to respiratory failure. At present little is known about the factors that determine the rate of disease progression in bronchiectasis. Despite extensive investigation, an underlying cause cannot be identified in over 50% of patients [2]. However, identification of a cause where possible may have a profound influence on management and aggressive treatment of the underlying cause may prevent or delay the need for transplantation in some patients. In those patients where transplantation is necessary, on-going treatment of the underlying cause of bronchiectasis is likely to delay or prevent recurrence in the allograft.

This chapter summarizes normal lung defences and the impact of transplantation on these defences, and will then focus on the known causes of bronchiectasis, which should be assessed during a transplant work-up to facilitate specific management, both pre- and post-transplantation.

Normal lung defences

It has been estimated that as many as 50 000 viable bacteria are inhaled daily; however, most people remain healthy most of the time. This is due to the highly effective local defences in the lung, and the rapid response of the normal immune system. The main stages of lung defence include the mucociliary elevator, immune exclusion and immune elimination.

Mucociliary elevator

Inhaled particles including viable organisms are trapped in a layer of mucus produced by specialized cells in the airway epithelium. The layer of mucus, which lines the airways, is normally transported towards the oropharynx by the rapid, coordinated beat of the cilia present on the ciliated respiratory epithelium. The effectiveness of this defence mechanism depends on the presence of mucus in the correct amount and of an appropriate composition, and normal cilia, which beat at an appropriate frequency in a coordinated fashion. The ability of the mucociliary elevator to remove particles is compromised by increased viscosity of mucus as seen in CF, or hypersecretion of mucus, as well as abnormalities of the cilia.

Following transplantation, reduced ciliary beat frequency in the allograft has been reported [3], although partial recovery appears to occur in the months following

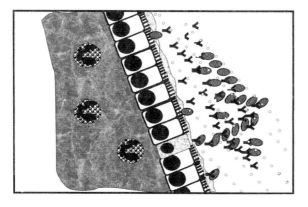

○ defensins

◄ immunoglobulins

● bacteria

Figure 7.1 Immune exclusion is a non-inflammatory process whereby components of the innate and adaptive immune response prevent organisms adhering to and infecting the airways. Defensins and secreted immunoglobulin molecules, usually of the IgA isotype prevent bacteria from adhering to the epithelium, which consists predominantly of ciliated epithelial cells. This is the main airway defence mechanism in health.

transplantation [4]. The data reported so far, however, are based on video photometry of mucosal biopsies and the clinical significance of the reduction in frequency observed post-transplantation (approximately 20–30%) remains to be evaluated. Little is known about the rheology of the mucus in transplanted lungs in humans; however, in a canine model of lung transplantation, mucous rigidity was increased following both autotransplantation and allotransplantation [4,5]. It is also of interest to note that in patients receiving transplants for lung diseases other than CF, expression of the cystic fibrosis transmembrane regulator (CFTR) is reduced in remodelled epithelium [6]. As CFTR plays a pivotal role in the regulation of mucus osmolarity, these findings raise the possibility that the quality of mucus secreted in the transplanted lung may be adversely affected.

Immune exclusion

Immune exclusion is the process whereby the immune system prevents the entry of organisms into the airways and lung tissues (Figure 7.1). This is a noninflammatory process and involves constituents of both the innate and adaptive immune systems.

Secreted components of the innate immune defence include lysozyme and defensins. Defensins are found in

neutrophil azurophilic granules, constituting 5–7% of the total protein content of neutrophils, in addition to which they are also produced by macrophages and epithelial cells [7,8]. Defensins are antimicrobial, cationic peptides that cause lysis of several pathogenic organisms within the airways. Normal function of the defensin system appears to require airway mucus of the appropriate salt concentration for optimal activity, and salt-dependent inactivation has been demonstrated in cystic fibrosis [9]. Little is known about secretion or function of defensins following transplantation.

Secretory immunoglobulin (Ig)A is the principal isotype of immunoglobulin secreted in the normal airway, and it is actively secreted across the respiratory epithelium in association with the secretory piece. IgM may be also be secreted by a similar mechanism and in the lower airways and alveolar lining fluid IgG is also found. Neutralizing antibodies, which bind to key adhesion molecules on the inhaled organisms, prevent binding and subsequent entry of organisms into or through the epithelium. Protection from both bacterial and viral infections may be provided by such neutralizing antibody. Organisms that are neutralized by antibody in the airway become trapped in the airway mucus and are subsequently removed by the mucociliary elevator. In healthy subjects, antibody produced locally in the lung is thought to be predominantly responsible for immune exclusion. The process of immune exclusion allows the neutralization and removal of potential pathogens in a noninflammatory way.

There are relatively few patient data about the ability of transplanted lungs to produce antibody. However, it is well documented that lungs transplanted from an asthmatic donor can result in asthma in the recipient, suggesting that local immune function in the lungs is sufficient to produce and maintain an asthmatic response independent of the systemic immune system, and that the transplanted lungs can continue to produce antibody indefinitely [10]. Following donor vaccination, continued production of antigen-specific antibody in transplanted lung tissue has been demonstrated in a canine model for almost one year post-transplantation [11]. However, marked depletion of submucosal IgA- and IgG-bearing plasma cells has been shown in allografts of subjects who experienced rejection, whereas subjects who had not had rejection episodes had only a mild reduction in these cells compared to normal controls [12]. Although more detailed studies are needed, the data obtained so far suggest that local immunoglobulin production is probably almost normal in allografts unless rejection has occurred.

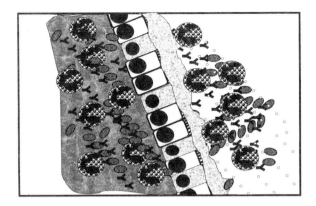

○ defensins
◄ immunoglobulins
🦠 bacteria

Figure 7.2 Immune elimination is an inflammatory process whereby the immune system eliminates organisms that have adhered to, and infected, the airway. Antibody molecules activate complement and neutrophils and other inflammatory cells migrate into the airway wall. The epithelium is damaged and the proportion of ciliated cells is reduced, with an increase in mucus production. Sputum becomes purulent due to the presence of neutrophil contents and debris. When this process occurs infrequently, it is consistent with recovery; however, when it is chronic or recurrent, airway damage will result. Local airway defences are impaired due to loss of ciliated epithelium and excessive mucus production, which predisposes to further episodes of infection.

Immune elimination

When potential pathogens succeed in entering the airway epithelium despite the above defence mechanisms, the normal immune system mounts a concerted attack to eliminate the organism (Figure 7.2). The immune mechanisms involved differ in response to infections with bacteria and viruses or other intracellular pathogens. This process results in airway inflammation, which may be regarded as the 'cost' of localizing and clearing the organism. However, when this process becomes chronic or is repeated frequently, airway damage and bronchiectasis may ensue.

Immune elimination of bacteria requires the integrity of the humoral immune response. Following activation of appropriate B lymphocytes, virtually always with help from T lymphocytes, B cells mature into antibody-producing plasma cells. Protective antibodies are frequently directed against surface epitopes of the invading organism, and activate complement via the classical pathway (IgG and

IgM), or the alternative pathway (IgA). Antibody and complement are capable of killing some bacteria, and complement deficiencies may be associated with recurrent infections. Complement also acts synergistically with antibodies in opsonizing bacteria – that is, flagging them for ingestion and killing by neutrophils. Complement activation products together with bacterial products and inflammatory cytokines attract neutrophils to the site of infection. Normal neutrophil function requires the ability to adhere to the endothelium, undergo chemotaxis in response to bacterial products, complement fragments and chemokines, phagocytosis and generate reactive oxygen intermediates to kill ingested organisms. Defects in all aspects of neutrophil function have been described and, although rare, are associated with recurrent infections and bronchiectasis.

Immune elimination of viruses and other intracellular pathogens requires the integrity of natural killer cells and cytotoxic T lymphocytes. Natural killer cells are part of the innate immune response and lyse virally infected cells, following downregulation of major histocompatibility complex (MHC) class I or other key ligands on the cell surface, during viral infection. Cytotoxic T cells recognize virally infected cells when viral peptides are presented on the cell surface in the context of MHC class I molecules. Virus-specific cytotoxic T cells then kill the infected cells either by activating programmed cell death (apoptosis) via the Fas pathway, or by discharge of granule contents, which include pore-forming proteins and granzymes (proteases that digest target cell proteins), causing necrosis. Defects in T-cell function are usually associated with viral, fungal, mycobacterial and other opportunistic infections and have only been associated with bronchiectasis in a small number of cases.

Immunosuppression following transplantation is heavily weighted towards the suppression of T-lymphocyte function, which greatly impairs the ability of the immune system to eliminate intracellular pathogens. A further factor that may impair immune elimination of intracellular pathogens is mismatch of MHC class I alleles. The recipients' T-cell repertoire is selected during T-cell education in recipient thymus, where the process of positive selection leads to survival of T lymphocytes capable of reacting with recipient MHC and apoptosis of other T lymphocytes. If the donor and recipient do not share at least some MHC class I alleles, then the recipient may not have T cells capable of reacting to, and lysing, virally infected donor cells. This would contribute to persistence of viral infection in the allograft, by a mechanism that is independent of the effects of immunosuppression.

Suppression of T-lymphocyte function leaves patients susceptible to viral, fungal and other opportunistic infections. However, additionally, suppression of T-lymphocyte function impairs T-cell help for B cells, and so possibly decreases antibody production in response to T-cell-dependent antigens. There is little information on antigen-specific antibody production post-transplantation. In patients with acquired immune deficiency syndrome (AIDS) T-cell help for B cells is severely diminished, but, despite this, adults with AIDS cope relatively well with bacterial pathogens, suggesting that B-cell memory is highly effective, even with severely diminished T-cell help. In children, loss of T-cell help for B cells appears to be clinically much more significant and recurrent bacterial infections are a frequent problem in paediatric human immunodeficiency virus (HIV) infection. Antibody production in response to a polysaccharide vaccine (Pneumovax II) in paediatric heart transplant recipients is reduced among younger recipients, with responses in older children being fairly well preserved, suggesting the impact of post-transplantation immunosuppression on the developing immune system is more significant [13].

The direct effect of azathioprine on B lymphocytes is relatively weak; however, mycophenolate mofetil is a more potent B-cell immunosuppressant, an effect which is being exploited in a number of antibody-mediated autoimmune disorders. Increased use of mycophenylate mofetil in renal transplantation has not been associated with a significant increase in bacterial infections; however, the effect of this agent on bacterial infections in lung transplantation requires careful evaluation.

Maintenance immunosuppression following lung transplantation is not known to significantly inhibit neutrophil function. However, in the early post-transplantation period when high doses of corticosteroids are used, neutrophil function will be somewhat impaired. Sulphonamides reduce the neutrophil respiratory burst; however, routine co-trimoxazole prophylaxis is unlikely to impair neutrophil function to a clinically relevant degree.

Pathogenesis of bronchiectasis

The pathogenesis of bronchiectasis is poorly understood. However, defects in host defence, or an infectious, toxic or inflammatory insult are all factors thought to be capable of initiating the process. At present we do not understand why apparently similar insults resolve in some individuals with no sequelae, but lead to chronic airway damage in others. During acute episodes of airway infection, the resultant inflammation impairs local lung defences in the area of injury. Impaired local defences predispose to further episodes of infection and more airway inflammation and damage. In some subjects this leads to progressive lung damage, eventually leading to respiratory failure. This cyclical process of self-perpetuating airway injury has been termed the vicious cycle of inflammation [14].

This hypothesis suggests that there are a number of possible aspects of the pathogenesis of bronchiectasis at which therapeutic intervention may be directed. In some patients, an underlying and ongoing cause of bronchiectasis may be identified and treated. However, if bronchiectasis is already established, additional treatment directed at control of infection and airway inflammation may be essential to halt or slow progression of the airway damage. Even when no precise cause can be identified with our current knowledge, or when the only identified cause cannot be reversed or treated, considerable symptomatic improvement, as well as an improvement in lung function can be achieved with physiotherapy, appropriate use of antibiotics and control of airway inflammation.

Underlying causes of bronchiectasis

The frequency with which an underlying cause for bronchiectasis is found varies greatly from series to series; however, in the Lung Defence Clinic at Papworth Hospital, Cambridgeshire, UK, a recent review of 150 patients with bronchiectasis demonstrated an underlying cause in almost half [2]. The most common causes are defects in lung defences; however, pulmonary inflammation from a variety of causes can also lead to bronchiectasis in susceptible individuals. A number of patients may have more than one underlying cause for developing bronchiectasis, and therefore investigation should be systematic, and not stop when a single possible cause is identified. In our series, the underlying cause(s) identified had significant, specific, implications for treatment in 15% of subjects [2]. There are no data on the effect of the underlying cause of bronchiectasis on outcome following transplantation. However, it would appear prudent to continue appropriate treatment for the underlying cause(s) of bronchiectasis following transplantation to prevent or delay recurrence in the allograft. The causes of bronchiectasis that we identified which were common in our patients, and those which have implications for management in post-transplantation patients, are discussed below.

Defects in lung defences

Hypogammaglobulinaemia
Hypogammaglobulinaemia is characterized by reduced levels of all classes of immunoglobulins, to a greater or

lesser degree. Hypogammaglobulinaemia may be primary, or secondary to lymphoid malignancies, drugs or protein loss. Primary hypogammaglobulinaemia includes both genetic and acquired disorders. Hypogammaglobulinaemia is readily diagnosed by measurement of immunoglobulins and examination of protein electrophoresis.

The commonest cause of primary hypogammaglobulinaemia is common variable immunodeficiency (CVI), a poorly understood and heterogeneous disorder that can present at any age from early childhood to old age [15]. In addition to recurrent infections, a subgroup of patients with CVI develop granulomatous inflammation in the lungs and other organs that may mimic sarcoidosis. Respiratory failure may be due to this inflammation and resultant fibrosis in addition to bronchiectasis. Recurrence of granulomatous pulmonary inflammation despite post-transplantation immunosuppression has been reported [16].

Genetic causes of hypogammaglobulinaemia include X-linked hypogammaglobulinaemia, in which a defective B-cell tyrosine kinase, Btk, prevents maturation of B cells, leading to profound deficiency of immunoglobulins. CD40 ligand deficiency, previously known as hyper-IgM syndrome is now recognized as a combined B- and T-cell immunodeficiency. CD40 ligand deficiency is also an X-linked disorder where a defect in CD40 ligand, which plays a pivotal role in the interaction between B cells and helper T cells, prevents effective class switching and maturation of the antibody response. Patients produce IgM, often in large amounts, but fail to produce IgA or IgG. In addition to hypogammaglobulinaemia and recurrent bacterial infections, patients are at risk of *Pneumocystis carinii* pneumonia and other opportunistic infections due to defective T-cell function [17]. Hypogammaglobulinaemia may also be the presenting feature of X-linked lymphoproliferative disease, where a defect in SLAM-associated protein (SAP) results in a combined immunodeficiency and a particular susceptibility to Epstein–Barr virus [18].

In patients with hypogammaglobulinaemia, diagnosis is frequently delayed and structural lung disease may already be present at the time of diagnosis. While aggressive immunoglobulin replacement and treatment of infections greatly slow the progression of disease in these patients, established bronchiectasis at diagnosis is a poor prognostic factor. Patients with X-linked lymphoproliferative disease have a particularly high risk of lymphoid malignancy; however, the risk of lymphoid malignancy is also increased in CVI disease and CD40 ligand deficiency. At present there are few data on how the risk of lymphoid malignancy is affected by post-transplantation immunosuppression, but the risks may be synergistic.

Hypogammaglobulinaemia can also be secondary to lymphoid malignancies, thymoma, drug therapy or protein loss. In patients with severe protein loss from either the gut or kidney, measured levels of immunoglobulins may be decreased. However, these patients often have relatively little problem with bacterial infection, as they are capable of producing antigen-specific antibody when challenged by infection. In contrast patients with B-cell malignancies may experience recurrent infections with only moderate decreases in immunoglobulin levels. Hypogammaglobulinaemia is commonly associated with chronic lymphocytic leukaemia and low grade B-cell lymphomas. These malignancies frequently run an indolent course; patients may experience considerable morbidity and even mortality due to the secondary immunodeficiency. Replacement therapy with intravenous immunoglobulin has been shown to decrease the frequency of severe infection in these patients [19]. Multiple myeloma is also associated with suppression of nonparaprotein immunoglobulin production with recurrent infection, and immunoglobulin replacement therapy may be of benefit in some patients. Thymomas are associated with immune dysregulation, which may be manifest as hypogammaglobulinaemia, autoimmunity or both. Thymomas are removed, as they may be malignant or cause local obstructive problems; however, this does not improve associated immunodeficiency and replacement therapy is required. Established bronchiectasis in patients with secondary hypogammaglobulinaemia associated with chronic lymphocytic leukaemia and thymoma is well recognized and adequate immunoglobulin replacement therapy may improve respiratory function as well as improving symptoms and quality of life.

Drug therapy, particularly with phenytoin and other anticonvulsants and penicillamine and other disease-modifying antirheumatic drugs may also cause a reversible hypogammaglobulinaemia. However, on occasions, diagnosis is delayed and bronchiectasis may be established.

In patients with hypogammaglobulinaemia who require lung transplantation, continued and intensive immunoglobulin replacement is required. Clinical experience in patients with established lung disease who have not received a transplant has shown that giving infusions more frequently and maintaining higher trough levels may be of benefit in reducing morbidity. Such strategies may also be effective post-transplantation if recurrent infections develop or following the development of obliterative bronchiolitis.

Selective IgA deficiency, IgM deficiency and IgG subclass deficiency

Selective IgA deficiency is common, affecting approximately 1 in 600 blood donors. It is generally thought that only a minority of patients with IgA deficiency experience recurrent infections, suggesting that many patients can compensate adequately for the loss of IgA [20]. However, many epidemiological studies of this condition have been cross-sectional with no follow-up, and the apparently benign nature of this condition has recently been questioned [21]. Infections appear to be more frequent in patients who have an associated IgG subclass deficiency, or in those who are unable to make an adequate antibody response following antigen challenge (see below). IgA deficiency is also associated with a significant increase in the prevalence of allergy and autoimmunity. Patients with IgA deficiency may become sensitized to IgA and thereafter are at risk of severe allergic reactions if transfused with blood products from non-IgA deficient donors.

Replacement of IgA is not possible, as IgA aggregates cause complement activation and severe anaphylactoid reactions. Immunoglobulin for replacement therapy consists of IgG with variable amounts of contaminating IgA. Patients with IgA deficiency are at risk of severe allergic reactions when treated with standard immunoglobulin preparations; however, low-IgA preparations can be successfully used for long-term intravenous immunoglobulin replacement [22]. Additionally, subcutaneous immunoglobulin infusions have been associated with a lower frequency of serious adverse events than intravenous immunoglobulin infusions and in a small number of patients have been reported to induce unresponsiveness to IgA [23].

Selective IgM deficiency is defined as a level of IgM less than 200 mg/L and normal levels of other immunoglobulins. This disorder is heterogeneous both clinically and at the laboratory level. It has been associated, in some subjects, with severe sinopulmonary infections and bronchiectasis. In some subjects there is a failure to respond to vaccinations, and in this group immunoglobulin replacement therapy may be of value.

Deficiencies of all of the immunoglobulin subclasses have been described in patients with recurrent sinopulmonary infection and bronchiectasis. Deficiency of IgG1, the predominant IgG subclass is almost always associated with low total IgG levels. Deficiency of IgG2 is usually but not always associated with IgA and IgG4 deficiency. These patients are frequently unable to mount an antibody response to test vaccination, particularly to polysaccharide antigens. IgG3 deficiency may also occur alone or in association with other subclass deficiency. The frequency with which IgG subclass deficiencies are found in patients with bronchiectasis varies considerably and methodological aspects of assays and the normal ranges used may explain some of the discrepancy [24,25]. In our group's experience, isolated deficiency of IgG subclasses was found infrequently in bronchiectasis patients [2].

The selective absence of the immunoglobulin heavy chain constant region genes for IgG1, IgG2 and IgA1 has been reported in healthy individuals. Combined deficiencies in the sets of genes for IgG1, IgA1, IgG2 and IgG4 have also been reported in healthy individuals and defects in genes encoding IgG1, IgG2 and IgA1 in others. These observations demonstrate the redundancy in the immune system, and argue against the idea that individual IgG subclasses have unique and essential functions. Rather, IgG subclass deficiencies may be markers of dysfunction of the immune system, which is more important than the absence of immunoglobulin molecules of a given subclass per se. Management of patients with IgG subclass deficiency relies initially on antibiotic therapy; however, intravenous immunoglobulin may be of value in severely symptomatic patients.

Specific antibody deficiency/defective antibody production

An inability to produce specific antibody despite normal or even elevated levels of immunoglobulins and normal IgG subclasses has been well documented. Many such individuals remain well, but increasing recognition of susceptibility to recurrent sinopulmonary infection, bronchiectasis and invasive infection with encapsulated bacteria has led to the recognition of specific antibody deficiency with normal immunoglobulin levels as an immunodeficiency [20]. There is considerable variation within this group of patients, with some subjects unable to respond to both protein and polysaccharide antigens, while others fail to respond to polysaccharides only. In some subjects only responses to specific polysaccharides may be affected. Patients frequently present with recurrent sinopulmonary infection; however, recurrent pneumococcal sepsis has also been reported. In our series of patients with bronchiectasis, isolated defective antibody production was found in 4% of subjects, while a further 4% of subjects with bronchiectasis had defective antibody production associated with some reduction in levels of IgA or IgG subclasses [2].

By definition, these patients have normal levels of immunoglobulins and therefore will not be diagnosed on routine immunoglobulin measurement. Test vaccination is required to evaluate qualitative function of the humoral immune system. Both protein and polysaccharide antigens may be used, although abnormalities in the response to polysaccharide antigens are most frequently found. Responses to Pneumovax II are measured most frequently, although Meningovac and typhoid polysaccharide vaccines are potential alternatives. Vaccination with *Haemophilus influenzac* type B (HiB) was frequently used; however, pure polysaccharide vaccines to HiB are no longer available in the UK. Protein vaccines in common use for test vaccination include tetanus and diphtheria. Serum is collected prior to, and two to four weeks post, vaccination and specific antibody levels measured by enzyme-linked immunosorbent assay (ELISA).

There are many anecdotal reports of beneficial responses to intravenous immunoglobulin in this condition. However, a trial comparing immunoglobulin therapy with optimal antibiotic and physiotherapy regimens is currently being conducted and should provide evidence on which to base therapeutic decisions. Many patients with bronchiectasis and defective antibody production respond well to physiotherapy and prophylactic antibiotics.

Following transplantation, these patients will continue to have an increased risk of infection. Additionally the risk of invasive sepsis needs to be considered, and this may be increased during the perioperative period, or during periods of augmented immunosuppression for episodes of rejection.

Other immunodeficiencies

The most common immunodeficiencies found in patients with bronchiectasis are the qualitative or quantitative defects in antibody function detailed above. Defects in neutrophil function, although rare, may result in bronchiectasis. Chronic granulomatous disease (CGD) is a genetically heterogeneous defect in the neutrophil NADPH-oxidase that generates the neutrophil respiratory burst. Affected patients are particularly susceptible to infections with catalase-positive organisms, including *Staphylococcus aureus*, *Pseudomonas aeruginosa*, *Burkholderia cepacia* as well as *Aspergillus* infections. Bronchiectasis may also result from neutrophil dysfunction in the hyper-IgE syndrome, where bacterial infection generates an ineffective IgE response rather than effective opsonizing antibodies.

T-cell immunodeficiency often causes a severe combined immunodeficiency, and many patients die from acute opportunistic infection, or undergo curative bone marrow transplantation, before chronic organ damage such as bronchiectasis results. However patients with chronic mucocutaneous candidiasis (CMC), a relatively less severe T-cell defect, demonstrate particular susceptibility to *Candida* infection, as well as recurrent bacterial infections in many cases. Bronchiectasis has been reported in the CMC subgroup with recurrent bacterial infections. Bronchiectasis has also been reported in the majority of patients with a specific T-cell immunodeficiency in which peptide presentation in MHC class I molecules is prevented due to a defective TAP (transported associated with antigen presentation) complex [26]. In this condition bronchiectasis may be associated with a necrotizing granulomatous vasculitis, which is highly destructive, resembles Wegener's granulomatosus but is anti-neutrophil cytoplasm antibody (ANCA) negative.

Bronchiectasis has been reported in a small percentage of HIV-positive subjects, usually following severe pulmonary infection such as mycobacterial infection, *Pneumocystis carinii* or recurrent pneumonia [27]. It is unclear whether the bronchiectasis is the direct result of the previous infection, or whether defective T-cell help for B cells impairs antibody quality to produce a qualitative humoral defect. Patients with HIV-associated bronchiectasis have been reported to have a particularly rapid deterioration in respiratory function [28].

Abnormalities of ciliary function

The prototypic ciliary dyskinesia, Kartagener's syndrome, is characterized by sinusitis, bronchiectasis, situs inversus and infertility in males. Ultrastructural studies of cilia in this syndrome show that absence of the dynein arms renders cilia immotile. A number of less well-characterized defects in ciliary function have been described, and are associated with recurrent sinopulmonary infection and bronchiectasis. These conditions have been grouped as the primary ciliary dyskinesias. This syndrome has even been reported with ultrastructurally and functionally normal cilia where abnormal orientation prevents the coordinated beat required to move mucus effectively [29].

Screening tests for ciliary abnormalities include the saccharin test, where a pellet of saccharin is placed on the inferior turbinate and the time taken for the subject to taste saccharin is recorded. This time is prolonged in the ciliary dyskinesias. An alternative approach is to take brushings from the inferior turbinate and examine the ciliary movement under phase contrast microscopy or using video photometry. Abnormalities in either test may be due to nasal inflammation, and so should be undertaken after resolution of any local infection and treatment of nasal allergies. Patients with abnormal screening tests require more detailed investigation including ultrastructural studies of cilia [30,31].

Patients with the ciliary dyskinesias require meticulous attention to bronchial drainage, as well as aggressive treatment of infections with antibiotics. Following transplantation, ciliary function will remain abnormal above the anastomosis and continued physiotherapy is likely to be essential to prevent recurrence in the transplanted lung. Persistent sinusitis may continue to be troublesome in the post-transplantation period, and may provide a reservoir of resistant organisms.

Atypical presentations of cystic fibrosis

This chapter has focused on non-CF bronchiectasis, as CF is discussed elsewhere in this book (see Hodson, Chapter 8).

However, in a series of 150 patients referred to an adult bronchiectasis clinic, two had definite CF with a further two patients having probable CF [2]. Relatively mild cases of CF have been increasingly reported, and it is now well documented that several CFTR mutations may be associated with normal sweat test results [32].

The incidence of CFTR gene mutations is significantly increased in bronchiectasis patients, compared with the normal population, raising the possibility that CFTR mutations may play a role in bronchiectasis possibly in concert with other factors [33].

Inflammatory disorders

Allergic bronchopulmonary aspergillosis

Aspergillus is a ubiquitous fungus, and can provoke powerful hypersensitivity reactions in predisposed individuals. Allergic bronchopulmonary aspergillosis (ABPA) is characterized by eosinophil-dominated inflammation in the bronchial wall and lung, which can be highly destructive and was originally described as causing bronchiectasis particularly involving the proximal airways. More recent CT studies have queried the value of the pattern of bronchiectasis in distinguishing between idiopathic and specific types [34]. ABPA is seen frequently in patients with asthma or CF but may also present in patients with no history of lung disease.

Differentiation between sensitization to *Aspergillus* and ABPA may be difficult in some patients; however, we have seen a number of patients with bronchiectasis who do not fulfil diagnostic criteria for ABPA but whose symptoms and pulmonary function respond dramatically to steroid therapy [M. Pasteur, D. Bilton & M. Keogan, unpublished observations]. No single test is diagnostic of this condition; however, combinations of positive skin prick tests to *Aspergillus*, elevated total IgE, elevated *Aspergillus*-specific IgG and IgE, eosinophilia and positive sputum cultures or sputum eosinophilia may indicate the presence of this condition.

Steroid therapy of ABPA results in improvements in lung function and symptoms, and may reduce lung destruction. Post-transplantation immunosuppression controls ABPA poorly, and recurrence may be seen within the first year post-transplantation. Additional steroids may be useful in reducing bronchial inflammation and preventing or delaying recurrence.

Connective tissue diseases and inflammatory bowel disease

A small percentage of patients who develop inflammatory bowel disease develop bronchiectasis, although the

mechanism underlying this clinically well established observation remains unclear. Post-transplantation immunosuppression generally controls inflammatory bowel disease well, and recurrence of bronchiectasis in this setting has not been reported post-transplantation.

Rheumatoid disease and the connective tissue diseases may all be associated with interstitial lung disease and bronchiectasis. Transplantation may become necessary due to pulmonary fibrosis or occasionally due to severe bronchiectasis. Additionally patients with the CREST syndrome (calcinosis, Raynaud's Phenomenon, oesophageal dysmotility, sclerodactyly and telangiectasia) and scleroderma are at risk of pulmonary hypertension. Rheumatoid disease and the lupus-like disorders are usually well controlled by post-transplantation immunosuppression. In contrast however, CREST and scleroderma are poorly controlled by standard immunosuppressive regimens, and high dose steroids may exacerbate some features of scleroderma, particularly renal disease.

Pulmonary injury

Gastro-oesophageal reflux

Gastro-oesophageal reflux (GOR) is common, but in a minority of subjects leads to structural lung disease. Identification of anaerobes or Gram-negative bacilli should increase suspicion of GOR. Clinical history is an insensitive indicator of the presence of reflux, and traditional barium imaging studies are also relatively insensitive. Oesophageal pH monitoring as well as isotope imaging may improve detection of this condition.

Treatment with proton pump inhibitors with or without a gastrointestinal prokinetic agent often produces dramatic symptomatic improvement, although the long-term effect of such treatment on progression of bronchiectasis in these subjects has not been recorded.

Post-transplantation, GOR will persist, and may be significantly worse in the early postoperative period. There are no trials of management of pre-existing gastro-oesophageal reflux post; transplantation however, intuitively, on-going treatment of GOR would appear advisable.

Postinfectious bronchiectasis

Previous severe pulmonary infection, often whooping cough or measles, is frequently proposed as the underlying cause of bronchiectasis. However, in over half of the patients in whom this explanation is offered, infections at anatomical sites outside the lungs are present, raising the possibility that the severe childhood infection was the initial manifestation of a defect in host defence. In some subjects, severe childhood infection may be the insult that initially damaged the lung, but it may be the first clinical indication of an underlying subtle defect in lung defence. In our series of bronchiectasis patients, 43% gave a history of severe pneumonia pre-dating their chronic respiratory symptoms; of these almost a third gave a history of chronic rhinosinusitis, suggesting a more generalized defect in host defence, while in a further third of patients another specific cause for bronchiectasis was found [2]. Thus, even when a history of antecedent pulmonary infection is present, full investigation for other underlying causes may still influence management. With the success of vaccination against common childhood infectious disease, the incidence of bronchiectasis secondary to childhood infection should decrease even further.

Following tuberculosis, severe bronchiectasis can occur in affected areas of the lung. Investigation of possible mycobacterial infection is clearly essential prior to transplantation. Appropriate chemoprophylaxis should be given if previous tuberculosis is proven or suspected.

Management of bronchiectasis

Management of bronchiectasis is aimed at controlling infection and reducing inflammation in the lung. Regular physiotherapy combining postural drainage and active cycle breathing techniques targeted at areas of disease involvement may help to reduce infection and control symptoms in many patients. Treatment of exacerbations requires antibiotics chosen with knowledge of the individuals' infecting organism(s), and at higher dose and for a longer duration than isolated chest infections in subjects with normal lungs. In subjects with frequent exacerbations, regular oral or nebulized antibiotics may greatly improve symptoms and quality of life; however, there are no randomized controlled trials evaluating the effect of such therapy on respiratory function or disease progression. In patients with defects in host defence such antibiotic therapy is frequently required.

Where bronchiectasis is localized, surgical resection of the involved segment or lobe may provide symptomatic relief. However, there are no long-term follow-up studies of patients following surgery, and therefore the relapse rate is unknown. Before surgery is contemplated, full investigation should be undertaken for known nonlocalized causes of bronchiectasis, which if present would be expected to cause a high rate of recurrence. As surgery will make future transplantation more difficult, this type of treatment should probably be reserved for patients with localized disease who have severe symptoms despite optimal medical therapy and still have an adequate respiratory

reserve. In patients with defects in lung defences, additional specific therapy may be of benefit in preventing development or slowing progression of bronchiectasis. There is a paucity of data on which to base such treatment in the post-transplantation period. However, as many of the defects in lung defences and other inflammatory insults will persist, after transplantation specific therapy is likely to be of value in the circumstances discussed above.

Transplantation for noncystic fibrosis bronchiectasis

Thirty-two patients received lung transplants for bronchiectasis at Papworth Hospital prior to June 1998. Twenty-four patients received a heart–lung transplant, six received double lung transplants and two single transplants (one because of an obliterated pneumonectomy space and one who had had previous surgery and would not accept blood products for religious reasons). There are several factors that would be expected to adversely affect outcomes in this group – older age at transplantation, underlying immune defects, previous surgery and chronic colonization with resistant organisms at the time of transplantation.

In the group receiving transplants for bronchiectasis as a whole, 70% were alive at one year, 47% at three years and 37% at five years. However, survival in the group who received heart–lung transplants for bronchiectasis did not differ from that in patients given transplants because of other indications.

Conclusions

Bronchiectasis is the final common pathway of many disease processes. Intensive investigation is worth while, yielding a diagnosis of the underlying cause in two thirds of patients. This information frequently affects management and may prevent or delay the need for transplantation. In patients who require transplantation, on-going treatment of the underlying cause may prevent or delay recurrence of bronchiectasis in the allograft. In patients with bronchiectasis who require transplantation bilateral lung replacement is usually required. Survival is comparable to that of other transplant recipients.

Acknowledgements

I would like to thank Dr Diana Bilton and Dr Keith McNeil for many stimulating discussions in this area over many years. I would also like to acknowledge the contribution of all the staff of the Lung Defence Clinic in Papworth Hospital.

REFERENCES

1 Bertolani MF, Marotti F, Bergamini BM, et al. Extraction of a rubber bullet from a bronchus after 1 year: complete resolution of chronic pulmonary damage. *Chest* 1999; **115**: 1210–1213.

2 Pasteur M, Helliwell SM, Houghton SJ, et al. An investigation into causative factors in patients with bronchiectasis. *Am J Respir Crit Care Med* 2000; **162**: 1277–1284.

3 Veale D, Glasper PN, Gascoigne A, Dark JH, Gibson GJ, Corris PA. Ciliary beat frequency in transplanted lungs. *Thorax* 1993; **48**: 629–631.

4 Marelli D, Paul A, Nguyen DM, et al. The reversibility of impaired mucociliary function after lung transplantation. *J Thorac Cardiovasc Surg* 1991; **102**: 908–912.

5 Paul A, Marelli D, Shennib H, et al. Mucociliary function in autotransplanted, allotransplanted and sleeve resected lungs. *J Thorac Cardiovasc Surg* 1989; **98**: 523–528.

6 Brezillon S, Hamm H, Heilmann M, et al. Decreased expression of the cystic fibrosis transmembrane conductance regulator protein in remodelled airway epithelium from lung transplanted patients. *Hum Pathol* 1997; **28**: 944–952.

7 Lehrer RI, Ganz T. Defensins: endogenous antibiotic peptides from human leukocytes. *Ciba Foundation Symp* 1992; **171**: 276–290.

8 Hiratsuka T, Nakazato M, Date Y, et al. Identification of human beta-defensin-2 in respiratory tract and plasma and its increase in bacterial pneumonia. *Biochem Biophys Res Commun* 1998; **249**: 943–947.

9 Goldman MJ, Anderson GM, Stolzenberg ED, Kari UP, Zasloff M, Wilson JM. Human beta-defensin-1 is a salt sensitive antibiotic in lung that is inactivated in cystic fibrosis. *Cell* 1997; **88**: 553–560.

10 Corris PA, Dark JH. Aetiology of asthma: lessons from lung transplantation. *Lancet* 1993; **341**: 1369–1371.

11 Bice DE, Williams AJ, Muggenburg BA. Long-term antibody production in canine lung allografts: implications in pulmonary immunity and asthma. *Am J Cell Mol Biol* 1996; **14**: 341–347.

12 Hruban RH, Beschorner WE, Baumgartner WA, et al. Depletion of bronchus-associated lymphoid tissue associated with lung allograft rejection. *Am J Pathol* 1988; **132**: 6–11.

13 Gennery AR, Cant AJ, Spickett GP, et al. Effect of immunosuppression after cardiac transplantation in early childhood on antibody response to polysaccharide antigen. *Lancet* 1998; **351**: 1778–1781.

14 Cole PJ. Inflammation: a two-edged sword – the model of bronchiectasis. *Eur J Respir Dis* 1986; **147**: 6–15.

15 Hammarstrom L, Vorechovsky I, Webster D. Immunodeficiency review: selective IgA deficiency and common variable immunodeficiency. *Clini Exp Immunodef* 2000; **120**: 225–231.

16 Hill AT, Thompson RA, Wallwork J, Stableforth DE. Heart–lung transplantation in a patient with end stage lung disease due to common variable immunodeficiency. *Thorax* 1998; **53**: 622–623.

17 Levy J, Español-Boren T, Thomas C, et al. Clinical spectrum of X-linked hyper-IgM syndrome. *J Pediatr* 1997; **131**: 47–54.

18 Nelson DL, Terhorst C. Immunodeficiency review. X-linked lymphoproliferative disease. *Clin Exp Immunol* 2001; **122**: 291–295.

19 Griffiths H, Brennan V, Lea J, Bunch C, Lee M, Chapel H. Crossover study of immunoglobulin replacement therapy in patients with low-grade B-cell tumors. *Blood* 1989; **73**: 366–368.

20 IUIS. Primary immunodeficiency diseases. Report of an IUIS Scientific Committee 1. *Clin Exp Immunol* 1999; **118**(Suppl. 1): 1–28.

21 Lilac D, & Sewell WAC. IgA deficiency: what we should – or should not – be doing. *J Clin Pathol* 2001; **54**: 337–338.

22 Cunningham-Rundles C, Zhou Z, Mankatious S, Courter S. Long-term use of IgA-depleted intravenous immunoglobulin in immunodeficienct subjects with anti-IgA antibodies. *J Clin Immunol* 1993; **13**: 272–278.

23 Sundin U, Nava S, Hammarstrom L. Induction of unresponsiveness against IgA in IgA-deficient patients on subcutaneous immunoglobulin infusion therapy. *Clin Exp Immunol* 1998; **112**: 341–346.

24 De Garcia J, Rodrigo MJ, Morell F, et al. IgG subclass deficiencies associated with bronchiectasis. *Am J Respir Crit Care Med* 1996; **153**: 620–625.

25 Hill SJ, Mitchell JL, Burnett D, Stockley RA. IgG subclasses in the serum and sputum from patients with bronchiectasis. *Thorax* 1998; **53**: 463–468.

26 Gadola SD, Moins-Teisserenc HT, Trowsdale J, Gross WL, Cerundolo V. Immunodeficiency review: TAP deficiency syndrome. *Clin Exp Immunol* 2000; **121**: 173–178.

27 Monteverde A, González A, Fernandez A, Del Valle E, Micele C, Laplunme H. Bronchiectasia in HIV-positive patients. *Medicina (B Aires)* 1999; **59**: 67–70.

28 Bard M, Coudere LJ, Saimot AG, et al. Accelerated obstructive pulmonary disease in HIV infected patients with bronchiectasis. *Eur Respir J* 1998; 1998; **11**: 771–775.

29 Rayner CF, Rutman A, Dewar A, Greenstone MA, Cole PJ, Wilson R. Ciliary disorientation alone as a cause of primary ciliary dyskinesia syndrome. *Am J Respir Crit Care Med* 1996; **153**: 1123–1129.

30 Bush A, Cole P, Hariri M, et al. Primary ciliary dyskinesia: diagnosis and standards of care. *Eur Respir J* 1998; **12**: 982–988.

31 Tsang KWT, Zheng L, Tipoe G. Ciliary assessment in bronchiectasis. *Respirology* 2000; **5**: 91–98.

32 Rosenstein BJ, Cutting GR. The diagnosis of cystic fibrosis: a consensus statement. Cystic Fibrosis Foundation Consensus Panel. *J Pediatr* 1998; **132**: 589–595.

33 Girodon E, Cazeneuve C, Lebargy F, et al. CFTR gene mutations in adults with disseminated bronchiectasis. *Eur J Human Genet* 1997; **5**: 149–155.

34 Reiff DB, Wells AU, Carr DH, Cole PJ, Hansell DM. CT findings in bronchiectasis: limited value in distinguishing between idiopathic and specific types. *Am J Roentgenol* 1995; **165**: 261–267.

8

Cystic fibrosis

Margaret E. Hodson

Royal Brompton Hospital, London, UK

Introduction

The disease

Cystic fibrosis (CF) is an inherited disease characterized by malabsorption, bronchopulmonary sepsis and a high sweat sodium concentration. The inheritance is by a Mendelian recessive gene. The abnormal CF gene primarily controls abnormalities of sodium and chloride transport. A functionally defective chloride channel in the apical membrane of the epithelial cell leads to loss in luminal salt and water in the airways. This predisposes to lung infection and bronchiectasis. Secondary bacterial infection can stimulate the host immunological response and there is an excess production of mediators from neutrophils, macrophages and lymphocytes. This all stimulates mucus production and further damages the airway [1]. Respiratory disease is the major cause of morbidity and mortality in CF [2]. When the disease was first described in l938, 80% of babies died within the first year of life [3] but now 50% of patients in the UK survive to 31.5 years [4]. Survival in North America is similar [5]. One of the best predictors of death in CF patients is a forced expiratory volume in 1 s (FEV$_1$) [6]. Although the survival for patients with CF has improved significantly in recent decades, many young people are still dying of end-stage respiratory failure and it is for them that the advent of lung transplantation has been a very significant advance.

Special challenges of CF for the transplant team

Patients with CF are often malnourished due to malabsorption. They often have coexisting liver disease, may be diabetic and may have infection present in the upper respiratory tract. Patients are usually colonized by *Pseudomonas aeruginosa* and/or *Staphylococcus aureus* but may be colonized by other more challenging organisms such as *Aspergillus fumigatus*, *Burkholderia cepacia*, *Stenotrophomonas maltophilia* or methicillin-resistant *Staphylococcus aureus* (MRSA)) and some of these organisms may be relatively drug resistant. In the postoperative period there may be problems with salt loss and small bowel obstruction. Malabsorption means that patients may need much higher doses of immunosuppressives, such as ciclosporin A, and the levels are more difficult to control, needing more careful monitoring. The higher doses of immunosuppressive drugs required also increase the cost of transplantation. Many patients have coexisting pleural disease that makes the transplantation procedure more difficult and may lead to heavy blood loss. Patients may have coagulation problems associated with vitamin K malabsorption.

The CF patient is, however, young and extremely well motivated. The families and friends are used to providing support and the patient is very familiar with hospitals and hospital procedures. The patients are used to following complicated medical regimens.

Transplantation for CF

More than 1000 CF patients with end-stage lung disease have now undergone transplantation [7]. The surgical options include (1) heart–lung transplantation (HLT), (2) double lung transplantation (DLT), (3) bilateral single lung transplantation (BSLT), (4) single lung transplantation (SLT), and (5) lobar transplantation from living donors. There are many more patients with CF who need lung transplantation than there are organs available and, in many centres, as many as 40–50% die while on the waiting list because of a lack of donor organs.

Table 8.1. Selection criteria

Indications
Deteriorating chronic respiratory failure despite good medical
    treatment
Severely impaired quality of life
Patient must want a transplant

Strong contraindications
Psychosocial instability
Active mycobacterial or *Aspergillus* infection
Infection outside the respiratory tract
Pulmonary bacterial pathogens resistant to all available
    antibiotics
Methicillin-resistant *Staphylococcus aureus* not confined to the
    respiratory tract
Other end organ failure or malignant disease
Gross malnourishment
Less than 10 years of age or older than 50 years
High dose corticosteroids
Smoking or addiction to drugs or alcohol
Previous pleurectomy or talc pleurodesis
Severe liver dysfunction
Preoperative ventilation involving intubation

Selection criteria

Indications (Table 8.1)

When a patient is first referred for transplantation it is important that the clinician makes absolutely certain that he or she has had the best available medical treatment. Some patients may not have been doing appropriate chest physiotherapy or may not have had the advantage of treatment with dornase alfa or inhaled antibiotics. In this situation, medical treatment should be maximized before the patient is considered for transplantation. Patients should be accepted for transplantation only when they have a severely impaired quality of life, as there is a significant morbidity and mortality associated with this procedure and there is also a shortage of donor organs. Not all patients want a transplant. Patients should be gently informed of the advantages and disadvantages of transplantation and then the small numbers who do not want to proceed any further should have their wishes respected. Most patients are not accepted onto the transplant list until they have a life expectancy of less than 18 months with conventional treatment, although this is difficult to judge. The most commonly used criteria are a forced expiratory volume in 1 s (FEV_1) of <30% predicted, an arterial oxygen saturation (SaO_2) when the patient is stable of 90% or less, or

increasing frequency of exacerbations of infection. Most of these patients will be oxygen dependent at the time they are accepted for transplantation.

Strong contraindications

Patients who are psychosocially unstable would not be able to comply properly with postoperative medication and follow-up and therefore would not do well. If patients are psychosocially unstable then attempts should be made to improve the situation before there is further consideration for transplantation. Patients with active mycobacteria or infection with *A. fumigatus* should be treated before consideration of transplantation. Infection outside the respiratory tract should be aggressively treated. Most patients have one or more organisms in their sputum and many transplant centres would accept patients only if the organism is sensitive to an antibiotic that could be used at the time of transplantation. Centres differ in their response to *B. cepacia* and MRSA. We would accept patients with *B. cepacia* as long as the organism was sensitive to one of the available antibiotic groups (see also Chapters 12 and 20). Patients with MRSA confined to the respiratory tract are accepted, but those who have the organism on their skin or epithelial surfaces are not accepted until it is cleared. Patients with other end organ failure or malignant disease are not accepted. Patients with gross malnourishment should have this corrected before being accepted onto the waiting list. Patients of less than 10 years of age seem to have more trouble with chronic rejection, and certainly there seem to be more psychological problems for them and their families than are seen in older patients. Due to the shortage of donor organs, patients over the age of 50 years are only rarely accepted.

Corticosteroids should be 10 mg/day or less as higher doses affect airway healing. Patients addicted to drugs, alcohol or smoking are not accepted and patients with previous pleurectomy or talc pleurodesis are at very high risk due to their tendency to bleed heavily at the time of surgery. Patients with limited abrasion pleurodesis and other chemical pleurodesis have not, in the author's experience, proved major problems. Patients with severe liver dysfunction may not be suitable for lung transplantation unless a liver is available at the same time and this undoubtedly increases the risks. Patients intubated and ventilated do poorly after transplantation and probably should not be accepted. However, patients preoperatively ventilated with nasal intermittent positive pressure ventilation (NIPPV) may do very well, and this form of ventilation is not a contraindication to transplantation [8].

Table 8.2. Investigations

Test	Remarks
Height	
Weight	
Chest measurements	
Lung function	Review previous results
Blood gases	
Exercise test	6 minute walk
Radiology	Chest radiography, CT scan, X-ray sinuses and teeth
Haematology	HB, ESR, WBC, platelets
	Blood group
	Coagulation tests
Biochemistry	Urea and electrolytes
	Sugar
	Immunoglobulins
	Creatinine clearance
	Liver function tests
Serology	CMV, EBV, hepatitis A, B and C, toxoplasma, herpes simplex and zoster
	HIV
Microbiology	Urine – MSU, 24 hour protein
	Skin – swab for MRSA
Cardiac	ECG, echocardiogram, 24 hour tape, cardiac catheter in some patients
Reports	Psychological, social, ENT, dental

Note: CT, computed tomography; HB, haemoglobin; ESR, erythrocyte sedimentation rute; WBC, white blood cell count; CMV, cytomegalovirus; EBV, Epstein–Barr virus; HIV, human immunodeficiency virus; MSU, midstream urine; MRSA, methycillin-resistant *Staphylococcus aureus*; ECG, electrocardiogram; ENT, ear, nose and throat.

Preoperative assessment

Medical

The investigations are summarized in Table 8.2. A detailed history must be taken, both from the patient and the family. The patient's height and weight are recorded and full pulmonary function tests are performed. These are reviewed together with lung function tests over the previous years. It is also important to check that the patient has been taking the best possible medical treatment. In a series of 79 patients transplanted for CF at the time of being accepted for surgery the mean FEV_1 was 22% predicted, and the mean forced vital capacity (FVC) 35% predicted. When patients were breathing air, PaO_2 (arterial oxygen pressure) was 6.8 kPa and $PaCO_2$ (arterial CO_2 pressure)

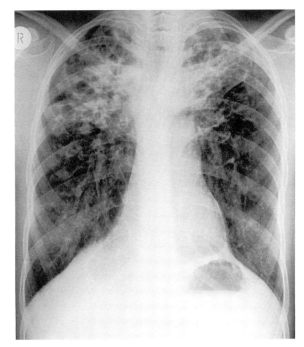

Figure 8.1 Chest X-ray film of an adult with cystic fibrosis showing extensive bilateral shadowing and fibrosis, particularly in the upper zones.

6.8 kPa (51 mmHg). Most patients were unable to work or attend school or college and most required continuous or intermittent oxygen [9]. Kerem et al. showed that in 673 CF patients with an FEV_1 of <30% predicted and a PaO_2 below 55 mmHg (7.3 kPa) or a $PaCO_2$ above 50 mmHg (6.7 kPa) there was a mortality rate of over 50% in a two year period [6]. They concluded that measurement of FEV_1 was the most sensitive predictor of mortality. They considered patients with an FEV_1 of below 30% predicted should be considered as candidates for lung transplantation.

Chest radiograph and CT scan should be performed (Figures 8.1 and 8.2). This enables the clinician to assess the severity of the pulmonary disease and the presence of any complications. Many patients have extensive pleural disease, which means that the operative procedure will be more difficult and more blood products are necessary. The presence of a mycetoma would also be a source of anxiety as the presence of *Aspergillus* in the pleural cavity of an immunosuppressed patient is a worrying situation. Patients have a sinus X-ray and full ear, nose and throat (ENT) and dental assessment. It is important that any sources of sepsis are dealt with as effectively as possible before transplantation. In some patients limited ENT work can be done in the preoperative period and major procedures have to be

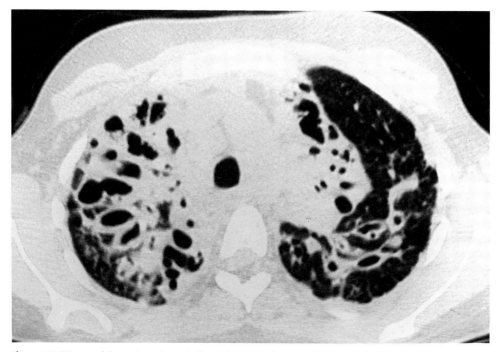

Figure 8.2 CT scan of the patient shown in Figure 8.1. Extensive bronchiectasis and pleural disease are present.

delayed until the patient has been successfully transplanted. Coagulation studies should be performed and any abnormality corrected before surgery. Patients with CF often have a prolonged prothrombin time which can be corrected by administering vitamin K. Full blood count should be performed and the blood group established. A full biochemistry screen including urea, electrolytes, blood sugars, immunoglobulin, creatinine clearance, and liver function tests should be performed and if any of these are abnormal further investigations are required. Routine serology includes testing for cytomegalovirus (CMV), Epstein–Barr virus (EBV), hepatitis, toxoplasma, herpes simplex and zoster, and human immunodeficiency virus (HIV). Microbiological studies include detailed sputum examination for bacterial pathogens, mycobacteria and fungi. Sensitivity of organisms should be determined both at time of assessment and at regular intervals when the patient is on the waiting list. Urine should be cultured and a 24 hour protein titre measured. Skin and epithelial surfaces should be swabbed for MRSA. Electrocardiogram, echocardiogram and 24 hour tape are performed. If a patient is receiving a BSLT or DLT it is important to make certain their own hearts are healthy. Detailed cardiac assessment is also essential for patients undergoing heart–lung transplantation who may donate their heart to another patient via the domino procedure [10]. As most of these patients are young and malabsorb fats the incidence of coronary artery

disease is so low that we do not routinely request coronary angiograms.

Psychosocial

It is vital that both the patient and the family are seen by a psychiatrist or psychologist experienced in the field of CF. Often a clinician or senior nurse who has known the patient or family for years can provide useful information. It is essential to make certain that their understanding of the issues and expectations are realistic. Written information should be given to the patient and family about the procedure and the survival results. The patient should have a stable personality and be of sufficient intelligence to understand what transplantation involves. Any psychiatric illness should be fully treated before the patient is accepted for transplantation. The patient should understand that there is a shortage of donor organs and the fact that not everyone on the waiting list gets a transplant. She/he should also understand that transplantation is not a 'cure' for CF. The patient will still have a CF body but will exchange CF lungs for transplanted lungs. If all goes well the quality of life will improve significantly as will the time taken for treatment, but the patient will be required to take immunosuppressive agents for the rest of his or her life and will require regular medical supervision. Patients should be allowed to discuss fully their feelings about receiving organs from another human being during this period. An experienced social worker should interview the patient and significant other. There are often important financial problems involved for a patient who is being assessed for transplantation. They may not have worked for a number of years and their parents may have had to take time off work to care for them. Patients may have to travel a considerable distance from their home to a CF transplant centre and this also causes added expense. The family members may wish to stay in the hospital adjacent to the patient during the time of assessment and should certainly be present at the time of surgery and early postoperative period. All this has financial implications. The social worker may be able to provide help from government resources or may need to refer the family to an appropriate charity fund. In some countries where private insurance is the major source of funding for health care, transplant surgery may not be fully covered. These patients and their families have a tremendous problem and would need help in raising the appropriate funding.

Spiritual issues

A patient being considered for transplantation realizes that they are seriously ill and that their life expectation without transplantation is severely limited. Even in the Western materialistic society when faced with the possibility of death many patients benefit from discussions with an appropriate spiritual counsellor. This person may be the hospital chaplain, the local rabbi or mullah. Indeed, a well-informed hospital chaplain can be a very useful member of the transplant team, not only supporting the patients while they wait for transplantation, but also caring for the relatives over the operative period. He is sometimes also required to support relatives who have lost their loved ones either while on the waiting list or following surgery.

Matching criteria

The major matching criteria are blood group, CMV status and the patient's size. In the UK, in the event of two patients matching identically then usually the sickest patient goes first. If the patients are equally sick then the patient who has been longest on the waiting list goes first. In some countries, however, more priority is given to the length of time the patient has been on the waiting list rather than the disease severity. In the author's opinion this is not ideal as it encourages patients to go on the waiting list long before it is necessary and probably some patients receive a transplant before they medically need it. This is inappropriate, as it is not a procedure without risk.

Outcome of assessment

The assessment period includes providing the patient and family with information about the advantages, disadvantages and risks of transplantation and completing the detailed assessments outlined above. If at the end of the assessment there is no contraindication for transplantation and the patient positively wishes to have a transplant she/he can then be placed on the waiting list. It is interesting that very few CF patients decline an offer for transplantation even when they are told very clearly the mortality and morbidity statistics. These young people realize that it is a real chance for them to survive, although they know it may be only for a limited period.

Time on the waiting list

Infection

Patients should be kept under close observation while waiting for transplantation. They should be seen at least once a month and more often if necessary. Regular sputum microbiology should be performed so the clinicians are aware of the organisms present and their sensitivities when an organ becomes available. Careful monitoring of FEV_1, FVC and arterial oxygen saturations are essential so that everything possible can be done to keep the patient as fit as possible. The patient and family should be encouraged to contact the physician at any time if there is a change in their condition. If there is any increase in the patient's sputum volume, or she/he develops a temperature the physician should be contacted at once and appropriate antibiotic therapy should be given. During this time nearly all patients are using inhaled antibiotics to try to reduce the bacterial load in the sputum.

Respiratory failure

If the patient is hypoxic, oxygen therapy should be given but care should be taken to check the carbon dioxide level as many of these patients get a degree of carbon dioxide retention. Patients who develop carbon dioxide retention should have any exacerbation of infection treated extremely promptly and may also be helped by aminophylline, which is a respiratory stimulant, and protriptylline in a dose of 5 mg twice daily can also be helpful. Some patients will benefit from a small dose of oral steroids, which act to reduce the bronchoconstriction and mucosal oedema. During an acute exacerbation, infusions of aminophylline or terbutaline may help to maintain acceptable blood gases. If patients deteriorate in spite of these measures, the results from intubation are not good and this treatment should probably be avoided as there are not enough donor organs for all patients on the tranpslant waiting list. However, if a patient's condition deteriorates then nasal intermittent positive pressure ventilation should be used [8] as many patients have successfully received transplants following this treatment. It is very cost effective, allows the patient to continue to communicate with relatives and does not require an intensive care unit bed. It is easier to maintain nutrition and muscle strength of patients nasally ventilated than when a patient is intubated.

Nutrition

Many patients accepted for transplantation are underweight. This may be largely due to malabsorption or inappropriate enzyme replacement therapy. However, as the patient's respiratory function deteriorates they use more calories because the respiration rate is higher and there are increasing episodes of sepsis. A breathless patient is also less able to eat, reducing the calorie intake. Initially good dietetic counselling should be given. The patient should be encouraged to eat regularly with snacks between main meals. If, however, the patient is extremely breathless and very malnourished, a gastrostomy tube should be inserted and it is possible, by this route, for the patient to eat what they wish during the day and to receive an extra 2000 calories at night [11].

Mobility

It is important that, during the waiting period, patients have as good a quality of life as possible. They should be encouraged to leave the house, if necessary using a wheelchair with oxygen attached or in a car driven by a family member or friends, and again oxygen can be taken with them. Muscle strength should be maintained as far as possible and some patients benefit from an exercise bike at home. However, many of these patients are severely hypoxic and it might be appropriate that the exercise is only done with oxygen. Initially, it should be monitored by a physiotherapist with an oxygen saturation meter to make sure any exercise prescribed does not cause dangerous hypoxia.

Psychosocial support

When patients are first accepted on to the waiting list there is usually a period of euphoria. As the weeks and months go by they begin to think 'Will an organ become available for me in time?'. Sometimes depression sets in which needs appropriate counselling and treatment. Both the patients and relatives should have access to hospital staff by telephone at any time to discuss problems and any questions they may have. Patients get to know other patients on the waiting list and transplant support groups can be helpful.

Communication

Patients in our centre are issued with a long-range pager. This enables them to live as normal a life as possible and not sit at home waiting for the telephone to ring. The patients must make certain they can be contacted at any time should an organ become available. During the period of assessment they will have been advised to keep a bag packed and to be ready to leave for the transplant centre within 20 minutes of receiving a call. The patient and their family should know the mode of transport to be used and exactly what they have to do when an organ becomes available. It is our policy to encourage the patients to wait in their own home, but in larger countries it may be essential that patients relocate adjacent to the transplant centre. This can cause other psychosocial challenges.

Surgery

Donor selection

The usual criteria for donor selection are shown in Table 8.3. The commonest cause of brain death in donors is trauma and brain injury. The gas exchange should be normal, i.e. a PaO_2 of >15 kPa (112 mmHg) with a fraction of O_2 in inspired gas (F_1O_2) of 35%. Ideally there should be no pulmonary infection. However, normal pulmonary infection can be treated in the recipient and lungs should not be rejected out of hand due to localized infection. Prolonged mechanical ventilation is undesirable. The donor's condition must be stablized while the organ procurement teams are in transit. Pulmonary preservation can be achieved by

Table 8.3. Usual criteria for donor selection

---

1. No significant cardiac or pulmonary injury
2. <55 years of age
3. Nonsmoker
4. Clear chest radiograph
5. Normal gas exchange
6. No significant infection
7. Normal electrocardiogram for HLT

Note: HLT, heart–lung transplant.

several techniques (see Chapters 13 and 14). For heart–lung transplantation, the heart is preserved with cold blood potassium cardioplegia solution and the organs are transported in cold donor blood and packed in ice. Ideally the ischaemic time should be less than five hours. This time is measured from the end of ventilatory support for the donor until reperfusion of the transplanted organs is achieved.

Matching of recipient and donor

This is based on ABO blood group compatibility, size and CMV antibody status. In some centres, the potential recipients are also screened for preformed antibodies against a panel of human leukocyte antigens (HLAs) (see Chapter 17). Ideally, the donor lungs should be slightly smaller than the recipient's chest. CMV can be a major problem following transplantation [12]. CMV infection can be transmitted via the organ or the blood products. CMV-negative patients should have CMV-negative blood and organs if possible. All patients should be carefully screened for CMV antigenaemia following transplant surgery.

Surgical procedure

Heart–lung transplantation (HLT)

Heart–lung transplantation was the first operation used for CF patients. There is a tracheal, aortic and right atrial anastomosis. There is a low incidence of airway problems following this operation and many patients donate their heart to another patient via the domino procedure. In a series of 103 domino procedures performed at our centre, 58 of the hearts were from CF patients (see Chapter 14).

Double lung transplantation (DLT)

This involves tracheal, pulmonary arterial and pulmonary venous (left atrial) anastomosis. Initially, the results of this enbloc procedure gave poor results and there were particular problems with airways [13]. It is no longer used.

Bilateral single lung transplantation (BSLT)

In addition to pulmonary arterial and venous anastomosis, bibronchial anastomoses are performed. This procedure offers the advantage that airway healing is less impaired as the bronchus obtains some of its blood supply from the neighbouring hilum. Results of BSLT are encouraging and many CF patients now receive this procedure, particularly in North America. In the UK, approximately 50% of patients receive heart–lung and 50% bilateral lung transplants.

Single lung transplantation (SLT)

This is not a suitable procedure for CF patients who have sepsis in both lungs. Its only application is in the occasional patient, post-transplantation, who develops severe obliterative bronchiolitis that does not respond to increased immunosuppression and who has no infection. Some of these patients have been treated successfully with SLT.

Lobar transplantation from living donors

Following bilateral pneumonectomy the recipient receives bilateral sequential transplant of a lower lobe from each of two living donors [14]. Early results indicate satisfactory short-term results. However, there are very important clinical, psychosocial and legal issues involved with the donors and very careful evaluations must take place. No pressure must be put on parents or healthy siblings to become donors. If a parent has more than one CF child, they may donate only once and they must not be put in the position of having to choose between their children.

Immunosuppression

The most commonly used immunosuppressive agents in CF patients are ciclosporin, azathioprine and prednisolone (see Chapter 18). Ciclosporin A acts by inhibiting the synthesis of interleukin 2, preventing clonal expansion of T-helper cells. It is given with the premedication in a dose of 6–10 mg/kg and thereafter the dosage to maintain levels of 300 ng/mL (whole blood monoclonal antibody assay) for the first three months; 250 ng/mL for three months to one year, and thereafter 200 ng/mL. If the patient's renal function deteriorates and the serum creatinine rises to an excess of 200 μmol/L, ciclosporin is reduced or stopped and immunosuppression is achieved with steroids or other immunosuppressive agents. Major side effects of ciclosporin are nephrotoxicity, hepatotoxicity, hypertension, hypercalaemia, convulsions, gum hypertrophy and hirsutism. Azathioprine is an antimetabolite which effects cellular proliferation of both B and T cells. It is administered orally 4 mg/kg preoperatively and 2 mg/kg per day postoperatively. It is discontinued if there is leukopenia with a blood white count of $<4 \times 10^9$/L, or thrombocytopenia. It can occasionally cause liver dysfunction and pancreatitis. Methylprednisolone is given intravenously in a dose of 1 g preoperatively and 125 mg daily for the first three postoperative days. Some clinicians prescribe prednisolone for the first three postoperative months, gradually reducing the dose to 0.2 mg/kg per day after two weeks. Some transplant centres maintain patients on long-term low dose prednisolone. Methylprednisolone is also used as the treatment of choice for episodes of acute rejection. Other immunosuppresive agents that are being used in some patients include tacrolimus and mycophenolate mofetil.

Intensive care management

Some patients who do well may be fit for discharge from the intensive care unit to a high dependency unit within 48 hours of transplantation. The average patient, however, will stay four to five days and the occasional patient who develops complications may be in intensive care for a number of weeks (see Chapter 15).

Immunosuppression

This should be maintained as outlined above. Particular care should be taken with the renal function and the dose of ciclosporin adjusted as appropriate. The dose of azathioprine is determined by monitoring the white count. If the patient develops fever, deteriorating pulmonary function as indicated by blood gases or abnormal shadowing on the chest X-ray, this should be carefully assessed. Likely causes are postoperative pulmonary oedema, infection, rejection or reperfusion injury. If the diagnosis is in doubt, fibreoptic bronchoscopy and transbronchial biopsy should be performed.

Mechanical ventilation

This should aim to maintain the blood SaO_2 at greater than 90%. The patient should be weaned from ventilation as soon as possible and early extubation is the goal.

Fluid balance and inotrophic support

The newly transplanted lungs are very sensitive to over hydration and fluid balance must be carefully monitored. Inotropic support and diuretic therapy is adjusted to maintain the mean pulmonary capillary wedge pressure at the lowest possible level to maintain satisfactory tissue perfusion and renal function.

Infection

Reverse barrier nursing is not routinely used but all staff should be careful with handwashing. Single rooms are desirable. Patients are prescribed antibiotics as indicated by their preoperative sputum culture together with flucloxacillin while drains and central lines are in situ.

Aminoglycosides are avoided whenever possible to reduce the possibility of synergy with ciclosporin promoting nephrotoxicity. Patients are prescribed nebulized colomycin administered by face mask in a dose of one megaunit twice daily for the first three postoperative months and thereafter one megaunit daily. This is because the patient retains CF mucosa in the upper respiratory tract, which has an affinity for *Pseudomonas*. Patients are given life-long prophylaxis against *P. carinii* and take either oral co-trimoxazole daily or nebulized pentamidine once a month. Patients also receive oral nystatin for the first three postoperative months to reduce the incidence of *Candida* infection and aciclovir to reduce the chances of viral infections.

Nutrition

As soon as the bowel sounds return the patient should be given an oral feed via a nasogastric tube or gastrostomy if one is in situ. An elemental diet is advisable at this stage so that pancreatic enzymes do not need to be administered. If the patient is very ill, then intravenous nutrition may become necessary.

Gastrointestinal

Any CF patient may develop meconium ileus equivalent or small bowel obstruction. This is particularly troublesome after transplantation as there is the additional problem of relative gut immobility following vagal nerve mobilization and relative dehydration. Patients should be given suppositories early and if the bowels do not function regular acetylcysteine and lactulose should be prescribed. If this is not effective gastrograffin should be given.

Physiotherapy

In the postoperative period, airways clearance may be hampered due to intubation, pain and discomfort, decreased mobility and denervated lungs. Prior to extubation regular suction of the lungs should be performed, and after extubation deep breathing and coughing with the help of a chest physiotherapist is very important to clear secretions. Mobility of the limbs should be maintained and the patient mobilized as quickly as possible.

Postoperative problems

There are problems common to all lung transplant recipients and those specific for CF patients.

Infection

This can be due to infection with bacteria, viruses, fungi or parasites (see Chapter 20). In a recent review of 141 CF patients receiving transplants, bacterial infection accounted for 81% of all infective episodes, *Pseudomonas* being the most common. Viral infection accounted for 9%, CMV being the commonest organism, and fungal and protozoal infection accounted for 10%. Of infective episodes, 89% were confined to the respiratory tract. Infection is a very significant cause of mortality after lung transplantation (K. Gyi, M.E. Hodson, M. Yacoub et al., unpublished observations). Bacterial infection is commonest in the first six months after transplantation and then decreases significantly. *Pseudomonas aeruginosa* is the commonest bacterium isolated but there is a significant incidence of infection with *S. aureus* and *Haemophilus influenzae* [15]. Bacterial infection should be treated with the appropriate antibacterial agent avoiding, whenever possible, drugs that are known to be nephrotoxic. Great care should be taken with aminoglycosides. The commonest viral pathogen is CMV, which should be treated with ganciclovir and CMV-specific gammaglobulin if the response to ganciclovir alone is inadequate or there is severe infection. Some centres give all patients prophylaxis with ganciclovir after transplantation, whereas others monitor for evidence of CMV and treat pre-emptively when there is evidence of infection even without clinical symptoms (see Chapter 21). *Aspergillus fumigatus* is the most common fungal infection in this group of patients. Many patients have *Aspergillus* in their sputum preoperatively and all efforts should be made to clear this before surgery. If a patient is known to have an *Aspergillus* problem, he/she should be treated with inhaled amphotericin and oral itraconazole after surgery for at least one month. Other patients should be carefully monitored for evidence of *Aspergillus* infection and sputum samples or bronchoalveolar lavage samples should be cultured for this organism. If it is isolated, itraconazole and inhaled amphotericin should be given immediately and, if there is any evidence of invasion either on computed tomography (CT) scan, or bronchoscopy and biopsy, then immediate liposomal amphotericin should be given.

The incidence of *P. carinii* pneumonia has dropped markedly since the introduction of regular prophylaxis with co-trimoxazole. If it occurs, high dose co-trimoxazole for three weeks is indicated.

The presenting symptoms in patients developing infection may be cough, with or without purulent sputum, dyspnoea, pyrexia or a gradual reduction in exercise tolerance, lung function and oxygen saturation. The chest X-ray may be normal but often at this stage shows interstitial shadowing. It is vitally important to identify the organism responsible and in most cases bronchoscopy with bronchoalveolar lavage and transbronchial biopsy is indicated. In addition to culture for common bacteria, viruses and fungi as outlined above, the specimen should be studied for *Mycobacterium tuberculosis*, *Legionella pneumophilia*, *Candida albicans*, *Mycoplasma pneumonia* and *Nocardia*, all of which infect lung transplant patients from time to time.

Rejection

Acute rejection typically occurs 10–14 days postoperatively and is fairly common for the first three months. The patient may present with increased breathlessness, pyrexia, cough and reduced lung function. The chest radiograph may show interstitial shadowing or pleural effusion. Diagnosis should be by transbronchial biopsy and may demonstrate perivascular cuffing with mononuclear cells. Treatment is by intravenous methylprednisolone, usually commencing with 1 g daily for three days. This is supplemented by oral prednisolone in gradually reducing dosage. A few patients with particularly aggressive rejection may require additional treatment, for example antithymocyte globulin or OKT3 (see Chapters 16 and 20).

Lymphoproliferative disorders

These can be disorders of the T- or B-cell type. The patient may be asymptomatic and abnormalities are noted on routine chest X-ray, or there may be a rash, lymphadenopathy or a palpable mass. It is essential that these masses are biopsied. B-cell disorders are usually associated with EBV. Antibodies to this virus may be demonstrated in the patient's serum. Treatment consists of reducing immunosuppression and treatment with high dose aciclovir for B-cell disorders. B-cell disorders may respond to reducing immunosuppression alone. In some patients the lymphoma may become aggressive and require conventional chemotherapy. The prognosis in these cases is poor, although the prognosis of patients who respond to reducing immunosuppression is usually good (see Chapters 23 and 24).

Grand mal seizures

These may occur in up to 10% of patients and are usually due to metabolic causes such as high ciclosporin levels, hyponatraemia, hypoklycaemia, hypermagnesaemia or hypokalaemia. If a metabolic cause is not immediately identified a CT scan is indicated to exclude cerebal haemorrhage, infarction or infection. If it is safe to do so a lumbar puncture may be necessary to exclude infection.

Obliterative bronchiolitis

This is the major late complication of lung transplant recipients. The patient develops progressive airflow obstruction and may present with cough or deterioration in lung function. The cumulative probability (70% confidence interval) of having this complication at one, two and three years postsurgery are 17% (12–23), 23% (16–29) and 48% (38–59) [15] (see Chapters 19 and 23).

The term obliterative bronchiolitis (OB) is now used for patients who have histological confirmation of airway obliteration, which the majority do not have as the disease is patchy. Bronchiolitis obliterans syndrome (BOS) is diagnosed by progressive airways obstruction after excluding infection or large airway complications as a cause of pulmonary dysfunction [16]. Onset may be as early as six months old. Median age of onset in CF patients attending our centre is 18 months. Treatment consists of augmenting immunosuppression with intravenous followed by oral steroids. If the condition is not arrested, tacrolimus can be substituted for ciclosporin and mycophenolate for azathioprine. In some cases, total lymphoid irradiation is given. Other new drugs such as sirolimus are being investigated for the treatment of this condition. A proportion of patients will stabilize but many will have a relentless decline in lung function and unless they can receive another transplant, the condition will be fatal. The aetiology of this condition is uncertain. It has been suggested that it follows repeated episodes of acute rejection or viral infection, which may facilitate MHC class II expression on the epithelium and endothelium in the graft.

Further research is urgently needed to determine the aetiology of this condition, methods of prevention and effective treatment.

Miscellaneous problems

Airways complications

Eleven per cent of our CF patients have required treatment for airway complications. The incidence is higher in patients undergoing double lung transplantation than those receiving heart–lung transplants. Airway obstruction may result in granulation tissue and stenosis and may be present in the trachea or bronchus. Treatment consists of cryotherapy, dilatation procedures, stent incision or occasionally retransplantation.

Complications of immunosuppression

Ciclosporin may be associated with renal impairment, hirsutism, gum hypertrophy, hypertension, lymphoproliferative disorders and grand mal fits. Azathioprine may cause bone marrow suppression, jaundice and pancreatitis and the dose may have to be reduced if there is a significant drop in white blood cell count. Particular care is necessary if the patient is also prescribed allopurinol. Steroid side effects include obesity, hypertension, osteoporosis, diabetes mellitus and increased susceptibility to infection.

Other medications may affect immunosuppressive therapy. Itraconazole, ketaconazole, fluconazole and erythromycin increase plasma ciclosporin levels whereas anticonvulsants and antituberculosis drugs may reduce the plasma levels. It is important whenever these drugs are used that the blood levels of the immunosuppressive agents are carefully monitored. Ciclosporin and tacrolimus given long term in the majority of patients cause progressive renal impairment and some patients may require dialysis. Amphotericin, aminoglycosides, lincosamides and nonsteroidal anti-inflammatory agents can potentiate renal impairment and great care must be given when these are prescribed together with immunosuppressive agents.

Coronary artery disease

In a review of 140 CF patients who underwent transplantation monitored over a 12 year period, only two patients developed coronary artery disease [15]. This is probably because of the low lipid levels in these patients due to malabsorption.

Long-term nephrotoxicity and hypertension

There is a gradual rise in creatinine levels over time following transplantation. A small proportion of patients will need dialysis, although many can be managed for considerable periods of time by gentle reduction in immunosuppression. A proportion of patients will develop hypertension (blood pressure persistently higher than 140/90). Hypertension usually responds to a calcium antagonist or an alpha-blocker drug.

Specific CF-related problems

Upper respiratory tract infection

The CF patient who has had a successful lung transplantation still has CF affecting mucosa in the upper airways and sinuses and typically these are colonized by *Pseudomonas aeruginosa*. Colistin sulphate should be given by inhalation life long to protect the transplanted lungs. Infection in the sinuses should be treated aggressively including surgical treatment if necessary. Polyps may respond to local steroid therapy but if not they should be surgically removed.

Malnutrition

After the early postoperative period, patients commence oral feeding with appropriate pancreatic enzymes and most of them put on weight. A few patients will require the continuation of feeding by a nasogastric tube for some time.

Malabsorption of ciclosporin

Ciclosporin is lipophilic and is poorly absorbed in patients with CF. It is routinely given twice daily but in some patients it may need to be given three times daily with a calcium antagonist to elevate blood levels. Patients with CF need very careful monitoring of ciclosporin A levels and will require much higher doses than other lung transplant patients.

Diabetes mellitus

A considerable proportion of adults with CF have diabetes mellitus. Following the stress of transplantation and the use of steroids, a number of additional patients develop diabetes, which is usually easily controlled with oral agents or insulin.

Salt loss

Patients with CF lose excess salt in their sweat; as intensive care units and hospital wards are often very hot it is important to make sure the patients do not become salt depleted; careful monitoring of electrolytes is essential.

Liver disease

Many adult patients with CF have liver disease and those with very severe disease will require heart–lung and liver transplantation. However, the majority of these patients tolerate lung transplantation without exacerbation of liver problems. However, liver function should be carefully monitored and it should be remembered that azathioprine and ciclosporin are potentially hepatotoxic.

Intestinal obstruction

Patients with CF are liable to develop small bowel obstruction (meconium ileus equivalent). However, in the author's experience it appears to be most common immediately after transplantation. This may be due to manipulation of the vagus nerve, dehydration, the use of analgesics and changes in diet. However, it is a disaster if a postoperative patient needs a laparotomy. Patients should therefore be very carefully monitored as soon as they return from the operating theatre and if their bowels do not work regularly appropriate action with lactulose, acetylcysteine, gastrograffin and enemas should be instituted.

Long-term care

Patients with CF who have received lung transplantation will require follow-up both for their multisystem CF and their lung transplant. Ideally this should be done in one clinic with personnel who are expert in both transplantation and cystic fibrosis. If not, patients should attend two centres who communicate efficiently with one another. Patients are reviewed at clinic frequently after discharge and then monthly for about one year. After that attendance can usually be reduced to every three to six months. It is, however, vital that they attend a local hospital for routine haematological and biochemical monitoring and measurement of levels of immunosuppressive agents. Due to malabsorption in CF, monitoring of levels should be done at least monthly. All results are faxed to the transplant centre and any changes in treatment are made as appropriate. Patients should be familiar with the use of home spirometry and keep a diary. They should record daily their temperature, FEV_1, FVC and medication taken. If there is a 15% reduction in lung function over two days, or development of cough, pyrexia or breathlessness, they should contact the transplant centre immediately for medial evaluation. Patients are encouraged to return to work and lead as active a life as possible. Many of them participate in sports.

Quality of life

Clinicians caring for patients with CF who undergo successful lung transplantation are in no doubt that many of the patients have a greatly improved quality of life (Figure 8.3). Many patients return to full time higher education or employment, go on overseas holidays, marry and a few have children. There are also a number of scientific studies showing that the quality of life is improved after transplantation [17,18].

Results

In spite of multisystem disease, patients with CF have survival rates comparable to other diagnostic groups after transplantation [19]. The largest series of heart–lung transplantation for CF has been carried out in the UK [9]. Actuarial survival was 69% to one year, 52% to two years, and 49% to three years. A 12 year follow-up of the same centre of 113 heart–lung transplant patients showed one year survival 72%, two year 54%, five years 51% and 10 years 37%. Comparable data have been reported from Stanford University, California [20]. Bilateral lung transplantation is the most

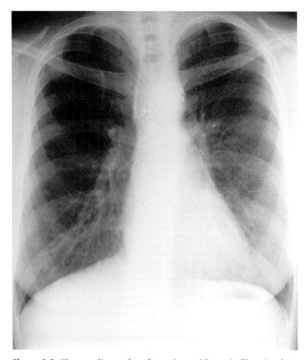

Figure 8.3 Chest radiography of a patient with cystic fibrosis who received a transplant 11 years ago. Patient has near normal lung function and is living a normal life.

commonly employed transplant procedure for CF patients worldwide. Egan reported 75% one year and 57% two year survival after bilateral lung transplantation [21]. The ISHLT International Registry for one, two and three year survival shows 70%, 62% and 53%, respectively, for bilateral lung transplantation [22]. Patients with major intrapleural intervention, for example pleurectomy and talc pleurodesis, may have a less favourable outcome. There have been a number of reports of patients transplanted after conventional ventilation [23] but the outcome is often unsatisfactory. Using noninvasive positive pressure ventilation as a bridge to transplantation in CF patients with ventilatory failure, the outcome is at least as good as in nonventilated patients [8] and in the more recent analysis of our patients there is a trend towards better survival.

Combined lung and liver transplantation for patients with CF is also feasible [24], but it is difficult to find the number of organs required by these patients and in the author's unit the mortality is certainly higher than in lung transplantation alone. Transplantation for patients with MRSA confined to their sputum and without skin or mucosal involvement, and patients with *B. cepacia* in their sputum, is feasible [9]. However, it may be associated with a higher mortality [25,26]. Pretransplant body mass index does not influence post-transplantation survival [27] and no

evidence was found that clinical status prior to transplant has any effect on post-transplantation survival of children with CF [28]. Central nervous system complications have been reported more frequently in CF patients than in other lung transplant recipients [29].

Retransplantation is possible. The problem is shortage of donor organs and a higher mortality than the first transplantation procedure. Patients may receive second transplants for obliterative bronchiolitis, airway complications, bronchiectasis or primary graft failure. Some centres offer heart–lung or bilateral single lung, but increasingly for patients with obliterative bronchiolitis single lung transplantation is the only option. Actuarial survival for retransplantation at one year was 45% in the Harefield/Brompton series of 20 CF patients undergoing redo procedures.

One year actuarial survival following living lobe transplantation for CF is 70% [14]. FEV_1 and FVC of approximately 70% predicted at the end of one year has been reported. The long-term outcome of this procedure remains to be determined.

Challenges

The major problems facing lung transplantation for CF patients is the shortage of donor organs and obliterative bronchiolitis. The shortage of donor organs can be addressed in each country by making certain that relatives are requested to make organs available whenever a suitable patient is diagnosed as brain dead. However, even if this is done the numbers of organs available would not be sufficient to meet the need. At least 50% of CF patients who want transplantation are dying while on waiting lists. The more widespread use of living lobe transplantation may be one way forward and results from European centres are awaited. It has been suggested that the number of transplants may also be increased by using bilateral lobal transplantation with bi-partitioning of the left donor lung and bilateral transplantation of the two lobes for children and small adults [30]. An attempt to overcome the shortage of organs by using animal organs for human transplantation (xenografting) is being made but it will be a number of years before this is a practical alternative. Hyperacute rejection may be a major problem in transplantation across species. There is also concern about the possible transmission of infection from animals to humans.

Obliterative bronchiolitis needs intensive research to find ways of preventing its occurrence and to improve methods of treatment for patients who develop this complication. A number of immunosuppressive treatments are being intensively studied in the hope of preventing this very serious complication, for example tacrolimus, mycophenolate mofetil, sirolimus and total lymphoid irradiation.

It is also essential when transplanting a CF patient to get the timing of surgery right. There is a significant mortality and one does not wish to operate too early, but on the other hand if one leaves it too long one may find oneself with a patient who is too ill for transplantation or one who dies while on the waiting list. Some evidence exists that overemphasis on the FEV$_1$ on timing of referral may adversely effect survival. Other facts, such as oxygen requirements, rate of deterioration of lung function, microbiology, quality of life and frequency of antibiotics should be considered [31].

Conclusions

Lung transplantation for CF has come of age. Long-term survival (over 15 years) is achievable with good lung function and quality of life. It has been shown that there is a higher survival benefit in patients with CF who are transplanted than in other patients with end-stage disease, such as emphysema and interstitial lung disease [32]. It is essential therefore that CF patients receive their appropriate share of the cadaveric organ pool and that live lobar transplantation becomes more widely available for this group of patients. Data from Papworth Hospital [33], Great Ormond Street Hospital (presented BTS 1998) and our own unit shows that there is a definite survival advantage of up to 70% for patients on the transplant waiting list who receive a transplant as compared with those who do not receive a donor organ.

REFERENCES

1 Alton EWFW. *Cystic fibrosis.* In Hodson ME, Geddes DM, eds. *Cystic fibrosis.* Chapman & Hall, London, 1995: Chap. 3.

2 Penketh AR, Wise A, Mearns MB, Hodson ME, Batten JC. Cystic fibrosis in adolescents and adults. *Thorax* 1987; **42**: 526–532.

3 Andersen DH. Cystic fibrosis of the pancreas and its relation to celiac disease. A clinical and pathological study. *Am J Dis Children* 1938; **56**: 344–399.

4 Dodge JA, Morison S, Lewis PA, et al. Incidence, population and survival of cystic fibrosis in the UK 1968–95. *Arch Dis Child* 1997; **77**: 493–496.

5 Cystic Fibrosis Foundation Patient Registry 1995. *Annual Data Report*, Bethesda, MD, USA. August 1996. FitzSimmons SC.

6 Kerem E, Reisman J, Corey M, Canny GJ, Levison H. Prediction of mortality in patients with cystic fibrosis. *N Engl J Med* 1992; **326**: 1187–1191.

7 Vankaskas JR, Mallory GB. Lung transplantation in cystic fibrosis; concensus conference statement. *Chest* 1998; **113**: 217–226.

8 Hodson ME, Madden BP, Steven MH, Tsang VT, Yacoub MH. Non-invasive mechanical ventilation for cystic fibrosis patients: a bridge to transplantation. *Eur Respir J* 1991; **4**: 524–527.

9 Madden BP, Hodson ME, Tsang V, Radley-Smith R, Khaghani A, Yacoub MY. Intermediate-term results of heart–lung transplantation for cystic fibrosis. *Lancet* 1992; **339**: 1583–1587.

10 Yacoub MH, Banner NR, Khaghani A, et al. Heart–lung transplantation for cystic fibrosis and subsequent domino heart transplantation. *J Heart Transplant* 1990; **9**; 459–467.

11 Poole S, McAlweenie A, Ashworth F. Cystic fibrosis. In: Hodson ME, Geddes DM, eds. *Cystic Fibrosis*, Arnold, London, 2000: Chap. 19b.

12 Hutter JA, Wreghitt T, Scott JP, et al. The importance of cytomegalovirus in heart–lung transplant recipients. *Chest* 1989; **95**; 627–631.

13 Patterson GA, Todd TR, Cooper JD, et al. Airway complications after double lung transplantation. *J Thorac Cardiovasc Surg* 1990; **99**; 14–21.

14 Starnes VA, Barr M, Cohen R, et al. Living lobar lung transplantation experience: intermediate results. *J Thorac Cardiovasc Surg* 1996; **112**; 1284–1291.

15 Madden BP, Kamalvand K, Chan CM, Khaghani A, Hodson ME, Yacoub M. The medical management of patients with cystic fibrosis following heart–lung transplantation. *Eur Respir J* 1993; **6**; 965–970.

16 Cooper JD, Billingham M, Egan T, et al. A working formulation for the standardisation of nomenclature and for clinical staging of chronic dysfunction in lung allografts. *J Heart Lung Transplant* 1993; **12**: 713–716.

17 Caine N, Sharp ES, Smith R, et al. Survival and quality of life of cystic fibrosis patients before and after heart–lung transplantation. *Transplant Proc* 1991; **23**: 1203–1204.

18 Squier HC, Ries AL, Kaplan RM, et al. Quality of well-being predicts survival in transplantation candidates. *Am J Respir Crit Care Med* 1995; **152**: 2032–2036.

19 Yankaskas JR, Mallory GB, the Consensus Committee. Lung transplantation in cystic fibrosis: consensus conference statement. *Chest* 1998; **113**: 217–226.

20 Sarris GE, Smith JA, Shunway NE, et al. Long-term results of combined heart–lung transplantation for cystic fibrosis. *J Heart Lung Transplant* 1997; **16**; Abstract 230.

21 Egan TM, De Herbeck FC, Mill MR, et al. Lung transplantation for cystic fibrosis; effective and durable therapy in a high risk group. *Ann Thoracic Surg* 1998; **66**: 337–346.

22 Hosenpud JD, Bennett LE, Keck BM, Fiol B, Novick RJ. The Registry of the International Society of Heart and Lung Transplantation: 14th Official Report – 1997. *J Heart Lung Transplant* 1997; **16**; 691–712.

23 Flume PA, Egan TM, Westerman JH, et al. Lung transplantation for mechanically ventilated patients. *J Heart Lung Transplant* 1994; **13**: 15–21.

24 Coeutil JP, Houssin DP, Soubrane O, et al. Combined lung and liver transplantation in patients with cystic fibrosis. *J Thorac Cardiovasc Surg* 1995; **110**: 1415–1423.

25 Aris RM, Gilligan PH, Newinger IP, et al. The effects of pan-resistant bacteria in cystic fibrosis patients on lung transplant outcomes. *Am J Respir Crit Care Med* 1997; **155**: 1699–1704.

26 Chaparro C, Maurer J, Gutierrez C, et al. Infection with *Burkholderia cepacia* in cystic fibrosis – outcome following lung transplantation. *Am J Respir Crit Care Med* 2001; **163**: 43–48.

27 Snell GI, Banetts K, Bartolo J, et al. Body mass index as a predictor of survival in adults with cystic fibrosis referred for lung transplantation. *J Heart Lung Transplant* 1998; **17**: 1097–1103.

28 Aurora P, Gassas A, Ehtishar S, et al. No evidence that clinical status prior to transplant has any effect on the post-transplant survival of children with cystic fibrosis. *Eur Respir J* 2000; **16**; 1061–1064.

29 Goldstein AB, Goldstein LS, Perl MK, et al. Cystic fibrosis patients with and without central nervous system complications following lung transplantation. *Pediatr Pulmonol* 2000; **30**: 203–206.

30 Couetil JP, Tolan MJ, Loulnet DF, et al. Pulmonary bipartitioning and lobar transplantation: a new approach to donor organ shortage. *J Thorac Cardiovasc Surg* 1997; **113**: 529–537.

31 Doershuk CF, Stern RC. Timing of referral for lung transplantation for cystic fibrosis – over emphasis on FEV_1 may adversely affect overall survival. *Chest* 1999; **115**: 782–787.

32 Hosenpud JD, Bennett LE, Keck BM, et al. Effect of diagnosis on survival benefit of lung transplantation for end-stage lung disease. *Lancet* 1998; **351**; 24–27.

33 Sharples L, Hathaway T, Dennis C, et al. Prognosis of patients with cystic fibrosis awaiting heart and lung transplantation. *J Heart Lung Transplant* 1993; **12**: 669–673.

9

Diffuse lung disease

R. M. du Bois

Royal Brompton Hospital and Imperial College of Science, Technology and Medicine, London, UK

Introduction

Diffuse lung disease (DLD) is a term that embraces a wide variety of disorders characterized by inflammation, damage and fibrosis in the acinar regions of the lungs. Formerly known as interstitial lung disease, the new term more properly embraces the concept that the pathological process can involve the air space as well as the interstitium. Strategies to improve understanding and treatment of these diseases have become clearer over recent years because of a better understanding of their molecular basis and clinicopathophysiological definition. Two areas in which significant advances have been made are molecular genetics (that will inform molecular epidemiological approaches – genotype) and the effects of new imaging and other technologies in diagnostic protocols (that have improved disease pattern recognition – phenotype).

Genotype

There are over 200 specific diffuse lung diseases including those characterized by granulomatous and fibrosing histopathology. The aetiology of some of these diseases is known, whereas for others it is not. For example, occupational exposure to beryllium can cause a chronic granulomatous disease that is clinically and histologically indistinguishable from sarcoidosis. A disease resembling cryptogenic fibrosing alveolitis (CFA) can be caused by exposure to asbestos, and exposure to cobalt may cause interstitial pneumonia and fibrosis. Other agents that are known to produce diffuse lung disease include some therapeutic drugs and radiation. General environmental risk factors for diseases of unknown aetiology have been identified, including exposure to dusts, cigarette smoking, sex, age and race [1,2]. For example, systemic sclerosis occurs predominantly in females (9:1; female:male) whereas sarcoidosis occurs predominantly in the 30–40 year age range and is more aggressive in patients of Afro-Caribbean descent than in Caucasians. Exposure to wood or metal dusts and cigarette smoking increase the relative risk of developing CFA.

Remarkably, exposure to similar amounts of environmental agents does not induce diffuse lung disease in all individuals and apparently trivial exposure to these agents can result in disease. This suggests that genetic predisposition may be important in disease development.

We have identified specific candidate genes, on the basis of a knowledge of the mechanisms that produce lung injury and fibrosis, that may be of particular importance in diffuse lung disease (Table 9.1) [3]. To investigate the complex genetics of these polymorphisms, we have devised a series of polymerase chain reaction (PCR) plates that allow us to group candidate genes of interest, with polymorphic loci such that multiple genetic polymorphisms can be identified simultaneously. The plates consist of groups of genes whose polymorphisms are of relevance to fibrosing lung diseases.

All of the selected candidate genes either have well-recognized and reported polymorphisms or have polymorphisms that have been identified by our group. This has allowed us to get a more rapid insight into polymorphic loci in diffuse (fibrosing) lung diseases in candidate genes of relevance to the fundamental pathophysiology of the disease. Of the candidate genes that might be studied, those of particular interest include the major histocompatibility complex (MHC), early cytokine genes and genes that modulate injury and repair.

Table 9.1. Candidate genes with known polymorphisms in diffuse lung disease

Cytokines
IL-1α, IL-1β, IL-4, IL-6, IL-10, TNF-α, LT-α, IFN-α/β receptor, TNF receptor, IL-1 receptor antagonist

Antigen presenting genes
HSP, TAP1, TAP2, LMP2, LMP7, HLA-DMA, HLA-DMB

Chemokine receptors
Duffy, CCR2, CC-CKR-5

MHC classes I and II

Adhesion molecules/Co-stimulating molecules
CD2, Pecam-1, L-selectin, E-selectin, ICAM-1, CTLA-4, E-cadherin, platelet glycoprotein 1b-α (CD42b)

Growth factors
Fibronectin, TGF-β

Proteases
Matrix metalloproteases

Note: IL, interleukin; TNF, tumour necrosis factor; LT, leukotriene; IFN, interferon; ICAM, intercellular adhesion molecule; CTLA, cytotoxic lymphocyte-associated protein; TGF, transforming growth factor.

Fibrosing lung disease

Cryptogenic fibrosing alveolitis
Of the diffuse lung diseases that result in lung fibrosis, CFA is the most life threatening and one of the most frequent; it is of unknown cause and has a relatively late age of onset. The pathogenesis of CFA involves chronic accumulation of inflammatory and effector cells, predominantly macrophages and neutrophils, in the lower respiratory tract resulting in respiratory failure and death in over half of its victims in less than three years. There are identifiable risk factors for development of the disease that include environmental exposure to dusts, chemicals and cigarette smoking. It is clear that not all individuals sharing a common environment develop the disease and, therefore, genetic predisposition may be important, although the precise mode of inheritance has not been defined.

It has long been recognized that there is a familial form of idiopathic pulmonary fibrosis. Some studies have confirmed that individuals in different generations have the usual interstitial pneumonia of histopathology that, by the newly defined criteria, is truly idiopathic pulmonary fibrosis. However, such phenotypic definition is not true for all pedigrees. A US initiative has begun to enrol a number of families with lung fibrosis and it is hoped that, by combining linkage analysis with subsequent fine mapping, key genetic factors will be elucidated.

In a recent report, a mutation in the gene for surfactant protein C was reported in a mother and her infant offspring, both of whom had diffuse lung disease (mother had desquamative interstitial pneumonia, daughter nonspecific interstitial pneumonia) [4]. This mutation produced a substitution at base 1728 at the junction of exon 4 and intron 4, and resulted in a decreased or absent protein in both individuals' lungs. Subsequent studies have identified several mutations in this gene in sporadic interstitial lung disease in children. In adults there have been no genetic studies in families.

One area of the genome that is central to the immune response is the short arm of chromosome 6 wherein reside a number of immune response genes most notably the MHC human leukocyte antigen (HLA) loci (Figure 9.1). Studies of the association between genes of the MHC complex and CFA have produced inconsistent results. Association between CFA and genes of the MHC complex therefore remains controversial. However, CFA is characterized by

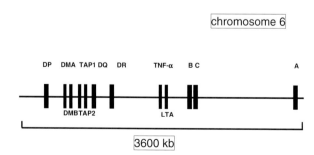

Figure 9.1 MHC class II region on the short arm of chromosome 6. Within this region are important class II loci as well as the antigen processing genes *DMA*, *DMB*, *TAP1* and *TAP2*.

inflammation, damage and progressive fibrosis in the acinar regions of the lungs. Therefore genes that influence the processes of inflammation, wound healing and repair may play a role in the development and progression of this disease.

There have been few studies that have identified susceptibility factors for the development of sporadic idiopathic pulmonary fibrosis. In one report of case association studies from two cohorts of patients in the UK and Italy differences in the interleukin 1 (IL-1) receptor antagonist (at +2018) and tumour necrosis factor alpha (TNF-α) (at −308) genes were reported but not confirmed by the same authors in a third patient cohort from New Mexico.

Our group has been unable to confirm this observation but has, however, been able to identify associations between severity of disease and candidate cytokines. Our approach has been to study the genes involved in the 'early' cytokine pathway. These genes include the IL-1 and TNF clusters [5]. We have described associations between polymorphisms at different loci and severity of lung function, allowing for disease duration. The severity of gas transfer impairment appears to be associated with a combination of an IL-6 intron 4 region polymorphism, particularly when combined with the C allele at position 1690 of the TNF-RII gene. In the case of IL-1, a number of genes and their receptors together with the natural antagonist are located on chromosome 2 at 2q12–14.2. Severity of gas transfer deficit appears to be particularly linked to the T polymorphism at −889 of the IL-1α gene: there were lesser degrees of involvement in polymorphisms in genes both telomeric and centromeric to IL-1α.

To date there have been no descriptions of associations between growth factor genes and either disease susceptibility or progression. Further appropriate targets would be genes that affect the balance of control within the lung including oxidant/antioxidant, proteases/antiproteases, Th1/Th2, angiogenic/angiostatic pathways and pro- and anticoagulation pathways.

Scleroderma

Scleroderma is a spectrum of relatively uncommon diseases ranging from localized skin disease to systemic sclerosis (SSc). Fibrosing alveolitis is one of the most common features of SSc and some degree of pulmonary fibrosis is found in the majority of patients at postmortem. SSc is considered to be an autoimmune disease and therefore the candidate genes of first choice have been those encoded by the MHC. Initial studies of the MHC loci in systemic sclerosis indicated increased frequency of specific MHC class I and class II alleles [6]. Subsequent studies showed a stronger association with HLA-DQ7 and DQ5

than with HLA-DR alleles and suggested that DR associations were due to linkage disequilibrium. This lack of concordance between studies may be attributed to geographical and environmental variability, ethnic variability or clinical heterogeneity. A variety of environmental agents are known to induce SSc-like pulmonary disease including D-penicillamine, tryptophan, bleomycin and pentazocine and the industrial agents vinyl chloride, benzene, toluene and trichloroethylene. Silica exposure increases the odds ratio of SSc, and silicosis increases the rate even further. Toxic oil syndrome occurred in Madrid in 1981 following the ingestion of an adulterated cooking oil that contained rapeseed oil denatured with aniline. This provoked a scleroderma-like syndrome with pulmonary involvement. The association with silicone breast implants is unproven.

Geographical variability also may result in the presence of different environmental triggers but also in differences in the gene pool of a given population. A further complicating factor may be heterogeneity of disease diagnosis that could result in a lack of consistency with respect to disease subsetting. For example, in a subset of patients with systemic sclerosis in association with pulmonary fibrosis (FASSc), it has been shown that the presence of the HLA-DR3/DR52a alleles and the anti-DNA topo-isomerase antibody (anti-Scl-70) confers a 16.7-fold excess risk for the development of pulmonary fibrosis compared with SSc patients without these risk factors [7]. The HLA-DPB1 1301 allele at another class II locus, HLA-DP, has been shown to be associated with *Scl-70* expression and we have developed a rapid PCR technique to type DP [8,9] (Figure 9.2). Such genetic diversity might at least partially explain the different susceptibility of individuals to the profibrotic effect of environmental agents and/or local immune reactions in the lung interstitium.

Pulmonary hypertension

Pulmonary hypertension may be seen in rheumatological diseases, normally as a consequence of diffuse lung disease. In addition, in scleroderma pulmonary hypertension can occur without diffuse lung disease, which is similar to primary pulmonary hypertension.

Primary pulmonary hypertension may also be seen alone (without rheumatological disease) and does not appear to segregate with any ethnic group but there is an increase in the female to male ratio 1.7:1. There is evidence of common ancestry in sporadic primary pulmonary hypertension, which suggests a genetic basis for the disease and also that familial primary pulmonary hypertension may be more common than previously recognized (see Chapter 2). It has also been reported that in families with pulmonary hypertension, successive generations are more likely to

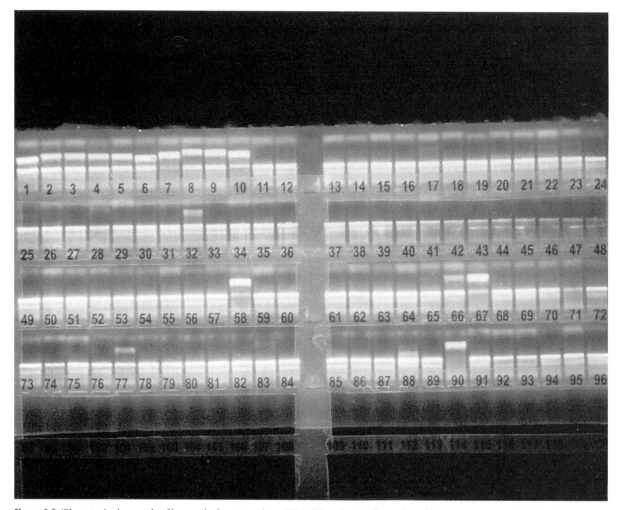

Figure 9.2 'Phototyping' example of human leukocyte antigen (HLA) DP typing. Each numbered lane represents an individual primer pair. The pattern of positive response determines the HLA DPB and HLA DPA alleles. In this 96 well reaction, a degree of redundancy is built into the system to provide highly accurate individual DP typing in a single PCR plate (courtesy Dr F. Gilchrist).

develop the disease at an earlier age (genetic anticipation). Pulmonary hypertension in scleroderma as a consequence of lone vascular disease is normally found in patients with limited, rather than diffuse, SSc. Anticentromere antibodies have been detected in 43% of patients with limited SSc, and this suggests a possible immunogenetic association, although they are not absolutely predictive of pulmonary hypertension. This is supported by the observation that pulmonary hypertension in scleroderma in adults is associated with an increased frequency of HLA-DR52. Since this pulmonary hypertension may be regarded as an autoimmune disease, the candidate genes of interest have also been those of the MHC. Differences in the frequency of HLA alleles has been found in children (HLA-DR3, DR52, DQ2) with primary pulmonary hypertension and adults with familial primary pulmonary hypertension. These data

would be consistent with the concept that there is a complex genetic basis to pulmonary hypertension, but it is clear that further studies, particularly of polymorphisms of genes whose products impact on the vasculature, are still required to determine the exact nature of that predisposition. It has been suggested that transforming growth factor beta (TGF-β) may play a role in pulmonary vascular hypertension via its action on fibroblasts and matrix deposition. In this regard a recent study has shown that genetic polymorphisms within the promoter region of TGF-β_1 may be associated with myocardial infarction and hypertension.

Granulomatous lung diseases

There is strong evidence for a genetic component to the development of sarcoidosis that comes from familial clustering of the disease; families with two or more members affected are more common than would be expected from the incidence of sarcoidosis in the general population. For example, in a study of familial sarcoidosis in Ireland, 10% of individuals with sarcoidosis had siblings with the disease [10]. In observations of sarcoidosis in twins, monozygotic twins are more concordant for the disease than dizygotic twins, suggesting a significant genetic component to the disease in addition to environmental influences.

Also, there are a number of studies that have shown that relatives of individuals with sarcoidosis are more likely to develop the disease [11]. This risk can be quantified as a ratio of disease prevalence in siblings or family members of individuals with sarcoidosis to the prevalence of the disease in the general population. This relative risk varies from 8 to 73 across various populations [11–13]. In further support of a genetic predisposition to disease is the finding of high levels of genetic heterogeneity that implies varying contributions of genetic and environmental factors to the initiation and/or progression of disease. The MHC region is the most logical region for study in a disease that is antigen driven and recent studies in familial and nonfamilial disease have shown this to be the case. In particular, HLA-DR12, 14, 15 and 17 have been associated with disease susceptibility but HLA-DR1 and 4 with 'protection' [14]. There remain important differences across ethnic boundaries, stressing the importance of studying matched cohorts and controls. Candidate genes other than those in the MHC complex that may be important in the development and progression of the disease include genes for antigen processing proteins (*TAP*) [15], cytokines and their receptors, comprising early proinflammatory cytokines and their receptors (TNF and TNF receptor (TNFR), IL-1 and IL-1R, IL-1RA), those associated with Th1 and Th2 profiles such as IL-2 and IL-2R, interferon gamma (IFN-γ) and IFN-γR, IL-4 and IL-4R, IL-10 and IL-10R, IL-12 and IL-12R and genes for profibrotic factors such as IL-6, TGF-β and IL-13. These genes all have known or suspected polymorphic loci and are relevant to the process of granuloma formation and fibrosis.

Molecular genetics and disease prognosis

Although a single or primary aberrant gene has not been identified in any diffuse lung disease, finding genetic associations such as those described above will allow the identification of patients who are more likely to develop diffuse lung disease and, importantly, more severe lung disease that will therefore provide a marker or markers of a poor prognosis and the probable need for transplantation in the future. Early clinical intervention in such cases would also be of considerable benefit for the patient by targeting novel therapies at an early stage.

Phenotype

Diffuse lung diseases are responsible for roughly 4000 deaths each year in England and Wales. CFA has increased over the last decade worldwide and death rates match the increase in disease prevalence [16]: in the UK about 2000 individuals and in the USA about 2500–10 000 people die each year of CFA [16–18]. The imprecision of the numbers reflects differences in coding practices in the USA, together with inaccuracies in notification. These death rates exceed those from asthma and cystic fibrosis but CFA is underdiagnosed in life and misclassified at death. It seems likely that this is because there exist no agreed strategies for the diagnosis and treatment of diffuse lung diseases. In addition, there have been few prospective studies of the effects of treatment on outcome and those that have been completed comprise small numbers of patients. There are a number of reasons why the management of diffuse lung disease is so inconsistent.

A misconception exists that all diffuse lung diseases can be considered as a single entity. Using terms such as 'interstitial lung disease' or 'pulmonary fibrosis' as diagnoses exacerbates this: the individual diseases included within the term(s) have specific pathogeneses, natural history and likely responsiveness to treatment. Because of this misconception, many physicians equate all diffuse lung disease as having the same outcome as CFA, in which high death rates occur. Lastly, few patients with any of the less common diffuse lung diseases are seen in any but the most specialized unit.

More precise disease classification will aid studies of causation, predisposition and trials of treatment. Recent statements and guidelines have clarified phenotype more specifically. This can best be appreciated by referring to Figure 9.3, in which the four main groupings of the diffuse lung diseases are defined. From these, the idiopathic interstitial pneumonias are the most important, including CFA (idiopathic pulmonary fibrosis), the most lethal member of this group. From Figure 9.4 it can be seen that there are six entities that fall within the general classification of idiopathic interstitial pneumonias and all

Diffuse Parenchymal Lung Disease

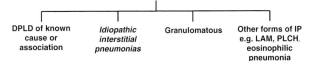

| DPLD of known cause or association | *Idiopathic interstitial pneumonias* | Granulomatous | Other forms of IP e.g. LAM, PLCH, eosinophilic pneumonia |

Figure 9.3 Diffuse parenchymal lung disease (DPLD): broad groupings. LAM, lymphangioleiomyomatosis; PLCH, pulmonary Langerhans cell histiocytosis; IP, interstitial pneumonia.

Diffuse Parenchymal Lung Disease

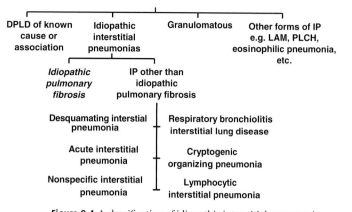

Figure 9.4 A classification of idiopathic interstitial pneumonias. LAM, lymphangioleiomyomatosis; PLCH, pulmonary Langerhans cell histiocytosis; IP, interstitial pneumonia.

Diagnostic Process in DPLD

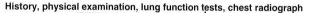

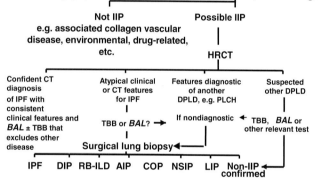

Figure 9.5 Diagnostic algorithm for idiopathic interstitial pneumonias. IIP, idiopathic interstitial pneumonia; HRCT, high resolution computed tomography; BAL, bronchoalveolar lavage; TBB, transbronchial biopsy; DPLD, diffuse parenchymal lung disease; PLCH, pulmonary Langerhans cell histiocytosis; IPF, idiopathic pulmonary fibrosis (synonymous with cryptogenic fibrosing alveolitis); DIP, desquamative interstitial pneumonia; RB-ILD, respiratory bronchiolitis-associated interstitial lung disease; AIP, acute interstitial pneumonia; COP, cryptogenic organizing pneumonia; NSIP, nonspecific interstitial pneumonia; LIP, lymphocytic interstitial pneumonia.

of these have at one time or another been mistaken for CFA.

Controversy exists about the use and role of a number of investigations in the staging of diffuse lung disease. We adopt the algorithm shown in Figure 9.5. This includes a number of key or controversial components, particularly the role of bronchoalveolar lavage, high resolution computed tomography, radionuclide imaging and surgical lung biopsy.

Bronchoalveolar lavage

This technique is used by only approximately 10% of UK physicians in the diagnostic evaluation of patients with suspected diffuse lung disease whereas the investigation is much more prevalent in the rest of the world, especially Europe [19]. The main reasons are lack of local expertise and the failure of those who do believe in the technique to demonstrate unequivocally that it provides added value to the patient.

In occupationally induced diseases, opportunistic infection that can mimic diffuse lung disease, and drug-induced disease, lavage can be diagnostic. The same is true of rarer diseases such as alveolar proteinosis (electron microscopical (EM) appearance) and Langerhans cell histiocytosis (CD1a+ cells) [20]. In other forms of diffuse lung disease, the predominance of lymphocytes or granulocytes on differential cell counting helps to provide a signpost to the type of disease process present. In granulomatous disease, lymphocytes predominate: in CFA, granulocytes (neutrophils and/or eosinophils) are the most numerous cells present [21]. BAL is particularly useful if the cell differential is discordant with other clinical or investigative features. In suspected CFA, large numbers of lymphocytes (>20%) should alert the clinician to another diagnosis, for example rheumatological lung complications or granulomatous disease. In selected situations, bronchoalveolor lavage (BAL) taken together with other indices may make diagnosis sufficiently secure to preclude the need for biopsy. This is very helpful if comorbid conditions, disease severity or frailty increase the risk of biopsy to unacceptable levels, especially in suspected CFA.

The important role of BAL and its untapped potential is illustrated by a recent publication by Drent et al. in which BAL data from a large cohort of 277 patients with cryptogenic fibrosing alveolitis, sarcoidosis and extrinsic allergic alveolitis was studied. A logistics regression equation was constructed, using a number of lavage indices as variables to provide the most likely diagnosis [22]. This equation was then used to test diagnostic prediction in a second population of 128 patients from a different hospital and was found to be accurate in 94.5% of patients. This sort of approach could be applied to derive likelihood ratios for the diagnosis of specific diseases for different lavage profiles and be further used to quantify the added advantage of performing a particular diagnostic test – evidence-based medicine. It must, however, always be used in the context of all other clinical and investigational data.

High resolution computed tomography

High resolution computed tomography (HRCT) has transformed the evaluation of diffuse lung disease [23–27]. The whole of both lungs can be 'sampled'. HRCT is more sensitive and specific than chest radiography in the diagnosis of early diffuse lung disease, especially with a high level of confidence. Information on prognosis can also be obtained. A predominantly groundglass pattern of infiltration is generally associated with a more cellular inflammatory process, confirmed subsequently by histopathological analysis of lung, and is usually predictive of probable responsiveness to treatment in all diffuse diseases, but there are some pitfalls [28]. Fine fibrosis can share this pattern and be mistaken for cellular disease. There are, however, clues in the image that will allow the more experienced observer to avoid this mistake. In fine fibrosis, the small airways are pulled open if the groundglass pattern is due to fibrosis but this is not seen when it is due to inflammation. CT can be of value even when the lung appears to be 'end stage' in diseases such as sarcoidosis, asbestosis, CFA and extrinsic allergic alveolitis because the pattern, even at late stages, is often indicative of a particular disease process [29]. This can be enormously helpful if it suggests that there is an external trigger causing ongoing inflammation and injury as the removal of this environmental factor may prevent progressive, terminal decline in pulmonary function.

^{99m}TcDTPA clearance

The clearance of ^{99}technetium-labelled diethylene diamine penta-acetic acid (DTPA) has been introduced into the list of diagnostic tools in recent years. It has proved to be of value in the detection of subtle diffuse lung disease and in the prediction of likely disease progression in CFA occurring alone but especially in systemic sclerosis, extrinsic allergic alveolitis and sarcoidosis. Nebulization of the isotope and carrier molecule to particles of 2–3 μm in size allows alveolar targeting. The isotope is cleared from the lungs rapidly where there is inflammation in the lower respiratory tract and airways by comparison with normal individuals where the isotope is retained in the lung for longer periods. In SSc, persistently normal clearance times will predict disease stability over a period up to five years following the second of two measurements performed a year apart [30]. Patients who have persistently normal clearance rarely lose more than 10% lung vital capacity over a subsequent three to five year period whereas individuals whose clearance, having started abnormal, becomes nor-

mal are more likely to show a significant improvement in pulmonary function subsequently. It is in the persistently rapid group that those whose lung function declines are found. This test is therefore a prediction of future events rather than a correlation with lung function improvement or deterioration. Cigarette smoking enhances clearance through inflamed airways and measurements are not a reflection of parenchymal disease in this situation and should not be performed in current smokers. Cessation of smoking for one month or longer restores the interpretability of the test.

Lung biopsy

Lung biopsy is required if a precise diagnosis cannot be made after all other investigations have been performed unless the patient's general condition precludes the procedure, for example severe respiratory failure or uncontrolled heart failure [19]. The biopsy route is determined by the pattern of abnormality: some diseases are centred around the airways and have such characteristic histopathology in small samples that transbronchial biopsy is the correct approach; more peripheral disease requires a surgical biopsy so that sufficient material can be obtained to determine the spatial arrangement of the pathological changes that are essential for precise diagnosis. Video-assisted thoracoscopic biopsy, which has a number of advantages – time of postoperative intubation, in-patient stay, immediate postoperative complications and expense – is now the operation of choice unless more detailed lung examination is required in which case limited thoracotomy is performed.

The need for guidelines

Too often diffuse lung diseases are diagnosed on the basis of 'clinical' features but HRCT has demonstrated how inaccurate this approach is. Now that newer clinicopathological entities have been identified with better outcomes, it is clear that a precise diagnosis is crucial for proper patient management.

A second problem is errors in diagnostic grouping. A good example of this is the diffuse lung diseases seen in systemic disorders such as the rheumatological diseases, which are often grouped with lone CFA in scientific and clinical studies. There have been several recent studies that have shown that the pathophysiology and outcome of CFA occurring in the context of rheumatological disease is quite different from lone CFA and there is therefore no justification in failing to identify these diseases individually.

To address the question of minimum data sets for the diagnosis and management of diffuse lung diseases, a number of working parties have been set up. The European Respiratory Society (ERS) together with the American Thoracic Society (ATS) has defined CFA [18] and will shortly issue a statement on the idiopathic interstitial pneumonias. In the UK the British Thoracic Society (BTS) has published guidelines for management of diffuse lung diseases [19].

It is hoped that these statements will encourage respiratory physicians to use agreed criteria for the diagnosis of diffuse lung disease. This may necessitate some investigations being performed in specialist centres but this is inevitable and arguably desirable when some techniques are available only in centres where the experience in treating these disease(s) is located. This model of cooperative management has already been applied to cancer in the UK, where all hospitals that wish to manage patients with cancer are required to fulfil certain minimum criteria and also to have an association with a specialist cancer centre. This model should also be adopted for diffuse lung disease.

Treatment

There have been few good controlled studies of treatment of diffuse lung diseases. Reasons for this include: difficulty in recruiting appropriate numbers of patients to give the study sufficient power; variable criteria of disease definition; selection of clear outcome measures; and entry of patients at a time when they have an opportunity to benefit, i.e. giving treatment before the disease has reached end stage. Despite this, there are some data to support the use of certain types of treatment for some of these disorders. Commonly used first-line treatments for a variety of diffuse lung diseases are shown in Table 9.2. The situation is most difficult in the fibrosing lung conditions. Here, it is commonly believed by many physicians that treatment cannot help patients with fibrosing lung diseases and that it may do more harm than good. The result is that treatment is withheld in the early stages when there is most opportunity to benefit. This view is now being challenged since HRCT and biopsy reviews have demonstrated clearly defined subsets of disease that have hitherto been considered as 'fibrosing alveolitis'. This has implications for treatment response and survival. In those patients with predominant fibrosis, up to 10% of patients will show a physiological improvement but in many of the remainder pretreatment deterioration is arrested. This arrest of decline must be considered to be a positive response to treatment. The belief that there is no treatment for 'fibrosing alveolitis' and other less common forms of diffuse lung disease is too nihilistic. The result is that no attempt is made to treat the problem until the patient is severely limited by symptomatology, at which point a small dosage of therapy is given with the aim to 'minimize' the likelihood of side effects. The result of this is of course that the patient does not improve and the self-fulfilling prophecy has been realized. It is now increasingly well recognized that the only hope of achieving a successful outcome in diseases such as CFA is to start therapy early at a time when there is significant respiratory reserve retained and before any further increment in the burden of disease produces a disproportionate increase in symptoms.

Good quality evidence of treatment efficacy is also needed. This will result from properly controlled prospective clinical trials that will require sufficient numbers of patients to be recruited into multi-national coordinated studies. A number of international studies testing novel therapies are underway and include IFN-γ, pirfenidone, and N-acetylcysteine. It will then be possible finally to answer the questions about response to therapy using in the first instance the drugs that are currently available. The template for these studies would then be available, based on a platform of sound logic and outcome analysis, to test the newer more specific therapies that are undoubtedly going to emerge in the near future from clinical scientific molecular biological studies.

This approach necessitates well-defined disease phenotypes, identified by the guidelines set out by the ATS, ERS, and BTS working parties. The ATS/ERS joint statement on cryptogenic fibrosing alveolitis makes specific recommendations with regard to treatment strategies and monitoring. This regimen is a modification of the ATS/ERS guidelines on treatment [18], in which a combination approach was also recommended:

- Corticosteroid therapy (prednisone or equivalent) at a dose of 0.5 mg/kg (lean body weight, LBW) per day orally for 4 weeks, 0.25 mg/kg (LBW) per day for 8 weeks, and then tapered to 0.125 mg/kg daily or 0.25 mg/kg (LBW) every other day as initial therapy for idiopathic pulmonary fibrosis. (LBW is the ideal weight expected for a patient of this age, sex, and height), together with either:
- Azathioprine at 2–3 mg/kg (LBW) per day to a maximum dose of 150 mg/day orally. Dosing should begin at 25–50 mg/day and increase gradually, by 25 mg increments, every 7–14 days until the maximum dose is reached. Or
- Cyclophosphamide at 2 mg/kg LBW per day to a maximum dose of 150 mg/day orally. Dosing should begin at 25–50 mg/day and increase gradually, by 25 mg increments every 7–14 days until the maximum dose is reached.

For many patients with IPF and other DLDs there is a relentless decline in respiratory function despite optimum

Table 9.2. First-line treatments in diffuse interstitial lung disease

Disease	Treatment
Cryptogenic fibrosing alveolitis	Corticosteroids (low dose) *And* Azathioprine or cyclophosphamide (possibly using pulse intravenous treatment in acute exacerbations)
Desquamative interstitial pneumonia	Corticosteroids (high dose): stop smoking
Cryptogenic organizing pneumonitis (BOOP)	Corticosteroids (high dose)
Rheumatological diffuse lung disease	Corticosteroids (low dose) *And* Azathioprine or cyclophosphamide
Sarcoidosis	Corticosteroids
Extrinsic allergic alveolitis	Allergen avoidance ± corticosteroids
Langerhans cell histiocytosis	Stop smoking ?Prednisolone, ? penicillamine
Vasculitis	Corticosteroids (high dose) *And* Cyclophosphamide
Lymphangioleiomyomatosis	Progestogens

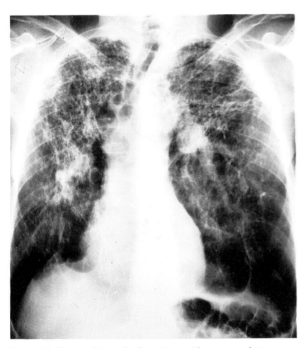

Figure 9.6 Chest radiograph of a patient with severe end-stage fibrotic sarcoidosis. This patient is now a transplantation candidate because of extensive irreversible lung fibrosis.

medical management (Figure 9.6). In this situation lung transplantation should be considered with single lung transplantation as the preferred operation. Because of the limited availability of donor organs, many patients die whilst awaiting a transplant, and, as most patients present over the age of 50 years, many will not be accepted onto a transplantation programme. It remains extremely difficult to state at what point transplantation should be recommended but should include a consideration of the patient's pattern of illness and the median survival for the disease. The likelihood of a patient being alive without transplantation should be set against that likelihood with transplantation. In practice, once gas transfer has reduced below 30% we refer patients with DLD for transplantation work-up. Patients with idiopathic interstitial pneumonia/cryptogenic fibrosing alveolitis should be referred earlier because of their poor prognosis (see Chapter 12).

Monitoring treatment response

In the ATS/ERS published guidelines, the following were recommended as monitoring guidelines:

A discernible objective response to therapy may not be evident until the patient has received >3 months of therapy. Consequently, in the absence of complications or adverse effects of the medications, combined therapy should be continued for at least 6 months. At that time, repeat studies should be performed to determine the response to therapy. The committee recommends that a combination of factors be used to assess the response to treatment and clinical course of IPF:

A **favourable (or improved)** response to therapy is defined by two or more of the following, documented on two consecutive visits over a 3- to 6-month period:

- A decrease in symptoms, specifically an increase in the level of exertion required before the patient must stop because of breathlessness or a decline in the frequency or severity of cough

- Reduction of parenchymal abnormalities on chest radiograph or HRCT scan
- Physiologic improvement defined by two or more of the following:
  - at least 10% increase in TLC [total lung capacity] or VC [vital capacity] (or at least 200-mL change)
  - at least 15% increase in single-breath DL_{CO} [diffusing capacity for carbon monoxide] (or at least 3 mL/min per mmHg)
  - an improvement or normalization of O_2 saturation (at least 4 percentage point increase in the measured saturation) or PaO_2 (at least 4-mmHg increase from the previous measurement) achieved during a formal cardiopulmonary exercise test.

A **stable (and presumed favourable)** response to therapy is defined by two or more of the following, documented on two consecutive visits over a 3- to 6-month period:
- 10% change in TLC or VC, or <200-mL change
- <15% change in DL_{CO}, or <3 mL min per mmHg
- no change in O_2 saturation (<4% increase) or PaO_2 (<4-mmHg increase) achieved during a formal cardiopulmonary exercise test.

A **failure** to respond to therapy (e.g., after 6 months of treatment) is defined as:
- an increase in symptoms, especially dyspnea or cough
- an increase in opacities on chest radiograph or HRCT scan, especially the development of honeycombing or signs of pulmonary hypertension
- evidence of deterioration in lung function in two or more of the following:
  - at least 10% decrease in TLC or VC (or at least 200-mL change)
  - at least 15% decrease in single-breath DL_{CO} (or at least 3-mL/min per mmHg change)
  - worsening (greater fall) of O_2 saturation (at least 4 percentage point decrease in the measured saturation) or rise in the $AaPO_2$ [alveolar–arterial oxygen gradient] at rest or during a formal cardiopulmonary exercise test (at least 4-mmHg increase from the previous measurement).

Summary

It is hoped that, with better understanding of genetic predisposition and disease triggers coupled with earlier recognition of disease and the development of more rational approaches to clinical phenotype, staging and management will improve outcome in these diseases. It would also be extremely useful to set up registries of diffuse lung disease internationally, with central coordination that would then facilitate truly international studies.

Sadly, however, there will undoubtedly be a number of patients for whom this strategy will be unsuccessful and we will continue to depend on transplantation to provide these individuals with the opportunity of life. The timing of referral is crucial so that sufficient time is allocated for the assessment process and the wait for a suitable donor.

REFERENCES

1 Hubbard R, Lewis S, Richards K, Johnston I, Britton J. Occupational exposure to metal or wood dust and aetiology of cryptogenic fibrosing alveolitis. *Lancet* 1996; **347**: 284–289.

2 Baumgartner KB, Samet JM, Coultas DB, et al. Occupational and environmental risk factors for idiopathic pulmonary fibrosis: a multicentre case-control study. Collaborating Centres. *Am J Epidemiol* 2000; **152**: 307–315.

3 Lympany PA, du Bois RM. Interstitial lung disease: basic mechanisms and genetic predisposition. *Monaldi Arch Chest Dis* 1997; **52**: 33–36.

4 Nogee LM, Dunbar AE III, Wert SE, Askin F, Hamvas A, Whitsett JA. A mutation in the surfactant protein C gene associated with familial interstitial lung disease. *N Engl J Med* 2001; **344**: 573–579.

5 Pantelidis P, Fanning GC, Wells AU, Welsh KI, du Bois RM. Analysis of tumor necrosis factor-alpha, lymphotoxin-alpha, tumor necrosis factor receptor II, and interleukin-6 polymorphisms in patients with idiopathic pulmonary fibrosis. *Am J Respir Crit Care Med* 2001; **163**: 1432–1436.

6 Welsh KI, Black CM. Environmental and genetic factors in scleroderma. In: Jayson MIV, Black CM, eds. *Systemic sclerosis: scleroderma*, John Wiley and Sons Ltd., Chichester, 1988: 33–47.

7 Briggs DC, Vaughan RW, Welsh KI, Myers A, du Bois RM, Black CM. Immunogenetic prediction of pulmonary fibrosis in systemic sclerosis. *Lancet* 1991; **338**: 661–662.

8 Gilchrist FC, Bunn C, Foley PJ, et al. Class II HLA associations with autoantibodies in scleroderma: a highly significant role for HLA-DP. *Genes Immun* 2001; **2**: 76–81.

9 Gilchrist FC, Bunce M, Lympany PA, Welsh KI, du Bois RM. Comprehensive HLA-DP typing using polymerase chain reaction with sequence-specific primers and 95 sequence-specific primer mixes. *Tissue Antigens* 1998; **51**: 51–61.

10 Brennan NJ, Crean P, Long JP, FitzGerald MX. High prevalence of familial sarcoidosis in an Irish population. *Thorax* 1984; **39**: 14–18.

11 McGrath DS, Daniil Z, Foley P, et al. Epidemiology of familial sarcoidosis in the UK. *Thorax* 2000; **55**: 751–754.

12 Rybicki BA, Harrington D, Major M, et al. Heterogeneity of familial risk in sarcoidosis. *Genet Epidemiol* 1996; **13**: 23–33.

13 Rybicki BA, Maliarik MJ, Major M, Popovich J Jr, Iannuzzi MC. Epidemiology, demographics, and genetics of sarcoidosis. *Semin Respir Infect* 1998; **13**: 166–173.

14 Foley PJ, McGrath DS, Puscinska E, et al. HLA-DRB1 position 11 residues are a common protective marker for sarcoidosis. *Am J Respir Cell Mol Biol* 2001; in press.

15 Foley PJ, Lympany PA, Puscinska E, Zielinski J, Welsh KI, du Bois RM. Analysis of MHC encoded antigen-processing genes TAP1 and TAP2 polymorphisms in sarcoidosis. *Am J Respir Crit Care Med* 1999; **160**: 1009–1014.

16 Hubbard R, Johnston I, Coultas DB, Britton J. Mortality rates from cryptogenic fibrosing alveolitis in seven countries. *Thorax* 1996; **51**: 711–716.

17 Selman M, King TE, Pardo A. Idiopathic pulmonary fibrosis: prevailing and evolving hypotheses about its pathogenesis and implications for therapy. *Ann Intern Med* 2001; **134**: 136–151.

18 Idiopathic pulmonary fibrosis: diagnosis and treatment. International consensus statement. *Am J Respir Crit Care Med* 2000; **161**: 646–664.

19 The diagnosis, assessment and treatment of diffuse parenchymal lung disease in adults. *Thorax* 1999; **54**,(Suppl 1).

20 Drent M, Jacobs JA, Wagenaar SS. Bronchoalveolar lavage. In Olivieri D, du Bois RM, eds. *Interstitial Lung Diseases*, European Respiratory Monographs, 2000: 63–78.

21 Costabel U. *Atlas of bronchoalveolar lavage*. Chapman & Hall, London, 1998.

22 Drent M, van Nierop MA, Gerritsen FA, Wouters EF, Mulder PG. A computer program using BALF-analysis results as a diagnostic tool in interstitial lung diseases. *Am J Respir Crit Care Med* 1996; **153**: 736–741.

23 Hartman TE, Swensen SJ, Hansell DM, et al. Non-specific interstitial pneumonia: variable appearance at high-resolution chest CT. *Radiology* 2000; **217**: 701–705.

24 Müller NL, Miller RR. Computed tomography of chronic diffuse infiltrative lung disease: part 2. *Am Rev Respir Dis* 1990; **142**: 1440–1448.

25 Müller NL, Miller RR. Computed tomography of chronic diffuse infiltrative lung disease. Part 1. *Am Rev Respir Dis* 1990; **142**: 1206–1215.

26 Hansell DM. Imaging the lungs with computed tomography. *IEEE Eng Med Biol Mag* 2000; **19**: 71–79.

27 Hansell DM. High-resolution computed tomography and diffuse lung disease. *J R Coll Physicians Lond* 1999; **33**: 525–531.

28 Wells AU, du Bois RM. Prediction of disease progression in idiopathic pulmonary fibrosis. *Eur Respir J* 1994; **7**: 637–639.

29 Primack SL, Hartman TE, Hansell DM, Müller NL. End-stage lung disease: CT findings in 61 patients. *Radiology* 1993; **189**: 681–686.

30 Wells AU, Hansell DM, Harrison NK, Lawrence R, Black CM, du Bois RM. Clearance of inhaled ^{99m}Tc-DTPA predicts the clinical course of fibrosing alveolitis. *Eur Respir J* 1993; **6**: 797–802.

10

Explant pathology

Susan Stewart

Papworth Hospital, Cambridgeshire, UK

Introduction

Lung transplantation is now a well-established successful surgical treatment for a range of pulmonary diseases for which no alternative therapies exist in the advanced stages [1]. Lung transplantation can take the form of combined heart–lung, bilateral or single lung grafts and is performed for four main categories of lung disease. These are obstructive, restrictive, suppurative and vascular diseases, the latter including both primary and secondary causes [1]. Lung transplantation has enabled the surgical pulmonary pathologist to study whole lungs without the superimposed agonal complications seen in autopsy specimens. The availability of these fresh lungs has proved a valuable resource for research into a range of pulmonary diseases as well as allowing detailed histopathological study. Lung transplantation has also promoted interest in so called 'end-stage' lung diseases, with a greater drive for accurate diagnosis before referral for assessment of potential candidates [2–5]. This chapter examines aspects of the impact of lung transplantation on the diagnosis of pulmonary conditions and research into their aetiology encouraged by this material.

Accuracy of referral diagnosis

Diagnosis of parenchymal lung disease prior to referral for transplantation will have been made on clinical, radiological and/or histopathological criteria. Some patients may have had biopsy material in the form of transbronchial or open lung samples but this may have been obtained relatively late in the course of the disease when specific features are no longer present. Examination of the explanted lungs has enabled more accurate diagnoses to be made in many cases and effectively constitutes an audit of the thoracic

medical practice of both the referring and specialist transplant centres. In addition, in this highly selected group of patients, examination of the explanted lungs may reveal co-existent supplementary diagnoses that may not have been considered prior to transplantation.

An extensive review of explanted lungs over a 10 year period at Papworth Hospital, Cambridgeshire, UK, examined 109 heart–lung, 65 single lung and 9 double lung explants [6] (Tables 10.1 and 10.2). This study excluded patients with the referral diagnosis of primary or secondary pulmonary hypertension or other forms of pulmonary vascular disease. However, patients with cystic fibrosis and other forms of bronchiectasis were included. Wherever possible the lungs had been inflated with perbronchial formalin, improving fixation and assessment of gross morphology. Some lungs, however, were received in a collapsed state, had been dissected around the hilum or showed occlusion of major airways by purulent secretions precluding inflation fixation. The study of explanted lungs requires adequate sampling, which include an average of 10 standard blocks per lung with major airways, apical, peripheral and central portions of upper and lower lobes, middle lobe or lingula, and hilar nodes and vessels. Further blocks are always taken of focal abnormalities including nodules, cysts or areas of necrosis. As well as haemotoxylin and eosin routine staining combined Perls elastic van Gieson stains are liberally used, with special stains for organisms performed as indicated. Immunohistochemical methods are reserved for selected cases which include Langerhans cell histiocytosis and lymphangioleiomyomatosis.

The referral diagnosis used in this audit was available from a clinical summary produced at the time of assessment for transplantation. In the early phases of the transplant programme, the clinical, functional and radiological work-up for each patient was far from uniform. In particular

Table 10.1. Summary of referral diagnosis; 183 explanted lungs

Referral diagnosis	Heart–lung ($n = 109$)	Single lung ($n = 65$)	Double lung ($n = 9$)
Cystic fibrosis	65 (5)		1
Pulmonary fibrosis	8 (4)	16 (3)	
Emphysema	16 (2)	39 (6)	4
Bronchiectasis	14 (5)	1 (1)	4
Sarcoidosis	4 (1)	3 (2)	
LCH	2	1	
Re Tx OB		2	
Others		3	
Totals	109 (17)	65 (12)	9

Note: LCH, Langerhans cell histiocytosis; Re Tx OB, retransplantation because of obliterative branchiolitis.

Table 10.2. Accuracy of referral and explant diagnoses in lung transplantation

Diagnosis	Single lung		Double lung		Heart–lung	
	Total	Discrepancy	Total	Discrepancy	Total	Discrepancy
COPD	23	3	17	4	7	2
AAT deficiency	10	1	13	4	5	1
Pulmonary fibrosis	29	8	8	0	1	0
Bronchiectasis	0	0	7	1	9	3
CF	0	0	10	1	37	1
Sarcoidosis	0	0	0	0	3	2
Other	5	1	1	0	0	0
Total	67	13 (19%)	56	10 (18%)	62	9 (14%)

Note: COPD, chronic obstructive pulmonary disease; AAT, alpha-1-antitrypsin; CF, cystic fibrosis.

high resolution computed tomography (HRCT) was performed only on some of the more recent patients in this 10 year cohort. Significant discrepancies between the final pathological diagnosis on the explanted lungs and the referral diagnosis were assessed, excluding features of histopathological interest only, such as tumourlets. This large study demonstrated a significant discrepancy rate of 19% for single lung explants and 16% for heart–lung explants between the referral and explant diagnosis. Tuberculosis (TB) and sarcoidosis were the commonest novel diagnoses. The discrepancy rate was similar in the various lung transplant groups but the significance in single lung patients with a remaining native lung was likely to be greater. Patients identified as being at risk of pulmonary mycobacterial or fungal infection in view of unsuspected explant pathology may require appropriate treatment or prophylaxis in the postoperative period. Therefore discrepancies can influence patient management [6].

The significance of the discrepancy rate is difficult to assess in the absence of similar studies from other transplant centres and, although it seems relatively high in a group of highly monitored patients, it is comparable to discrepancies revealed by autopsy studies comparing clinical and final pathological diagnoses [7]. The demonstration of a significant discrepancy rate has improved practice in both the referring hospitals and the transplant centre itself. In the case of the pulmonary interstitial diseases any biopsy material available is now reviewed at the transplant centre at the time of assessment so that the previous tissue diagnosis can be confirmed, modified or refuted. It may be necessary to obtain further biopsy material or initiate a first biopsy. This allows for a more informed decision on suitability for transplantation, taking account of prognosis and the most appropriate form of lung transplant for a particular candidate. It also ensures that conditions with a possibility of recurrence in the graft can be discussed fully, the commonest being sarcoidosis [8–10], which as yet is not of clinical significance. Recurrence of uncommon conditions such as lymphangioleiomyomatosis [11–13] or Langerhans cell histiocytosis can jeopardize the graft [14,15]. Patients whose diagnosis is still uncertain or who may have an occupational element raising medicolegal issues and patients posing a risk of infection can be clearly identified at the assessment process. The explanted lungs can then be dealt with appropriately at the time of transplantation so that maximum diagnostic information can be obtained, including from submission of fresh tissue for culture or specialized molecular methods. This is not without difficulty, however, as many explants become available outside working hours.

A re-audit of the accuracy of referral and histopathological explant diagnosis was performed recently on a cohort of patients receiving transplants over a six year period. The number of explanted lungs was 185, which was comparable to the first audit. The explant diagnosis was again compared with clinical information on the referral and assessment letters, which contained more detailed information as a result of the first audit and its recommendations. Thirty-two significant discrepancies were identified, including revision of the primary diagnosis and significant novel and unsuspected diagnosis. All the major referral categories of end-stage lung disease included discrepancies, the highest rate being in chronic obstructive airways disease, alpha-1-antitrypsin (AAT) deficiency, pulmonary fibrosis and sarcoidosis. The overall discrepancy rate was 17% and, as previously, was higher in the single lungs than in the combined heart–lung grafts. The commonest unsuspected finding was the supplementary diagnosis of sarcoidosis, previously unsuspected TB and *Aspergillus* disease. The primary referral diagnosis was not confirmed in 10 cases, mainly in the pulmonary fibrosis patients, where there is still difficulty in diagnosis and classification despite improvements in diagnostic imaging and the more liberal use of lung biopsy. The utility of lung biopsy for diagnosis of idiopathic pulmonary fibrosis is still a matter for debate. In this re-audit, biopsy had contributed to more accurate diagnosis of usual interstitial pneumonia and identified some further asbestos-related cases. This re-audit emphasized the continuing importance of sarcoidosis, TB and *Aspergillus* as unsuspected, novel and supplementary diagnosis in lung transplant patients. The implications for postoperative management are greatest in single lung recipients with a native lung in situ. Awareness of sarcoidosis in the explant is important for the interpretation of granulomas in the new graft, where this condition may recur, although meticulous exclusion of opportunistic infection is needed before a diagnosis of recurrent disease is possible [8,16,17].

The accuracy of referral diagnosis is important in relation to the suitability and type of transplant, anticipation of postoperative complications, identifying pulmonary conditions as part of a systemic disease [18–20] and being alert to the possibility of recurrence in the graft. Rarely, examination of the explanted lung may highlight a diagnostic pitfall,

as was the case in a female recipient in whom metastatic endometrial stromal sarcoma masqueraded as pulmonary lymphangioleiomyomatosis [21]. Unsuspected infections may require additional treatment. Above all, the assessment of outcomes for the wide range of conditions now successfully treated with lung transplantation can only be done accurately with validation of the primary diagnosis and any supplementary diagnosis [1].

Pulmonary interstitial disease

Pulmonary fibrosis

Patients with advanced pulmonary fibrosis constitute a significant proportion of referrals and eventual transplants [1]. In the past these have been treated with combined heart–lung grafts but are now more commonly treated with a single graft, leaving a fibrotic native lung in situ. Cryptogenic fibrosing alveolitis (CFA) is becoming commoner in the UK, although it is still an uncommon condition and has a poor prognosis, which has not been improved significantly by medical therapy [22]. In the USA, idiopathic pulmonary fibrosis (IPF) is an increasingly common cause of life-threatening respiratory failure affecting approximately 30 per 100000. Patients with IPF are usually elderly, but only those under 65 years of age are referred for consideration of lung transplantation. The clinical syndrome of IPF represents a histopathological spectrum of lung inflammation and fibrosis and it is important to assess lung tissue for an accurate diagnosis. The histological classification of IPF has recently been modified by Katzenstein and Myers [23] to include usual interstitial pneumonia (comparable to CFA in the UK), desquamative interstitial pneumonia, acute interstitial pneumonia and nonspecific interstitial pneumonia (UIP, DIP, AIP and NSIP, respectively). UIP is characterized by temporal heterogeneity, interstitial fibrosis with honeycombing and fibroblastic foci whereas DIP is characterized by temporally uniform inflammation without honeycombing or fibroblastic foci but with striking intra-alveolar macrophage accumulation. NSIP is also temporally uniform, with marked inflammation and infrequent fibroblastic foci, and is characterized by a much better prognosis than UIP [23–25]. Such a classification clearly requires an open biopsy, transbronchial lung biopsy having no role except in excluding possible mimics such as sarcoidosis or lymphangitis carcinomatosa. It may be advisable to obtain more than one open lung biopsy in order that established and less involved areas of lungs can be sampled and compared. High resolution computed tomography (HRCT) offers a noninvasive technique for examining the entire lung fields and has been suggested by radiologists to have a high specificity. This view is not always shared by pulmonary pathologists, who are aware of discrepant cases, and it is important that at least some centres, probably those also functioning as transplant centres, should continue to biopsy and correlate with HRCT and assess any response to therapy [22,26]. Of course, if lung biopsy is the 'gold standard' for diagnosis it is imperative that histopathologists use standard criteria and demonstrate intra- and interobserver agreement. Accurate diagnosis of pulmonary fibrosis is important, not just for transplantation (in a minority of cases) but also in relation to prognosis for the patient and suitability for new trials [27].

In our internal audit, transplant patients with a diagnosis of idiopathic pulmonary fibrosis requiring single lung transplantation had usual interstitial pneumonitis confirmed in eight cases, with appropriate clinical, radiological and biopsy appearances [6]. However, three cases thought to be usual interstitial pneumonitis showed sarcoidosis in the explanted lungs, one patient having plexiform pulmonary hypertension in addition. These patients had not undergone previous open or transbronchial biopsies, although one had noncaseating granulomas in a previous mediastinal lymph node biopsy that appeared to have been overlooked in the final referral process. The referrals for heart–lung transplantation for end-stage pulmonary fibrosis showed similar discrepancies. Out of eight patients, three had usual interstitial pneumonitis confirmed, three had extensive sarcoidosis in heart, lungs and lymph nodes and one of these patients had had a previous open lung biopsy specimen that was nonspecific. The eighth patient had ischaemic heart disease and pneumoconiosis, both of which were confirmed, but an unsuspected adenocarcinoma of the lung was also present. This could have been more significant in a single lung recipient's native lung rather than a combined heart–lung graft. The re-audit of explant diagnoses included 38 patients, of whom 29 underwent single lung transplantation. All the eight discrepancies were in single lung grafts and included three patients thought to have extrinsic allergic alveolitis but demonstrated at explant to have usual interstitial pneumonia. A further case thought to be extrinsic allergic alveolitis in a patient with coeliac disease was confirmed to be pulmonary fibrosis associated with the underlying condition rather than being due to hypersensitivity [28]. Of the concordant diagnoses, seven cases of UIP were diagnosed on clinical and radiological grounds without biopsies and a further nine had UIP confidently diagnosed on open or thoracoscopic biopsies prior to referral. One criterion used in the assessment of accuracy of pulmonary fibrosis in the second audit was the distinction between usual inter-

stitial pneumonia and non-UIP, as described in a recent study by Hunninghake et al., [29] where the term IPF is restricted to UIP, which is the most common idiopathic interstitial pneumonia and has the worst prognosis. A further conundrum in the explant diagnosis of usual interstitial pneumonitis is the significance of previous asbestos exposure and this is another reason for extensive sampling. To date we have not seen asbestos bodies in patients transplanted for 'idiopathic' pulmonary fibrosis thought to be within the 'background' range. However, in one patient with a combined UIP/DIP reaction with asbestos bodies, recurrence of DIP in the transplanted single lung was refractory to treatment and may have been related to asbestos remaining in the affected native lung.

Sarcoidosis

Lung transplantation for respiratory failure caused by sarcoidosis is an uncommon outcome of this condition, occurring in fewer than 10% of affected patients [30]. Study of the explant organs of this subgroup is important to document the pathological process albeit end-stage (Figures 10.1 and 10.2). As already alluded to in this chapter, the diagnosis of sarcoidosis pretransplantation is not straightforward. Improvement may be possible on appropriate therapy for sarcoidosis obviating or delaying the need for transplantation, so accurate diagnosis is essential to distinguish sarcoidosis from forms of pulmonary fibrosis with worse prognosis. Patients with pulmonary fibrosis, especially those with concomitant heart failure, may not be correctly identified as having sarcoidosis. Also sarcoidosis may be seen as a supplementary diagnosis, for example in patients with emphysema. In our internal audit study seven patients referred for lung transplantation (four heart–lung and three single lungs) had the diagnosis confirmed on four occasions. Misdiagnoses included UIP, pulmonary fibrosis with TB and pulmonary veno-occlusive disease (Figure 10.3) and these were associated with lack of preoperative tissue diagnosis [6]. Patients with end-stage severe sarcoidosis requiring lung transplantation with or without the heart universally show fibrosis and this is most often nodular, involving both upper and lower zones, and also associated with bullous change (Figure 10.4). The pathogenesis of the fibrosis may be related to transforming growth factor beta$_1$ (TGF-β_1) genotype in sarcoidosis [31]. Bronchiectasis was also a feature in some cases and indeed some patients referred for transplantation with severe bronchiectasis showed histological features of sarcoidosis as either a primary or a supplementary diagnosis. In addition to extensive fibrosis the sarcoid lung explants show differing numbers of bronchovascular and subpleural active granulomas and inactive

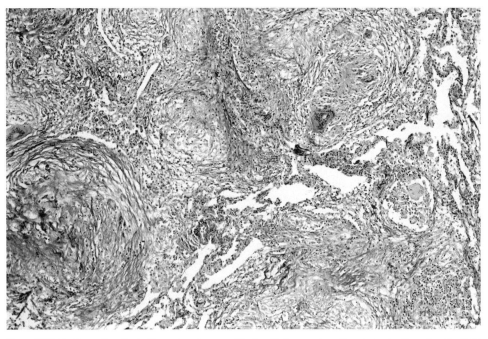

Figure 10.1 Sections of explanted lung showing sarcoidosis with frequent confluent giant cells and epithelioid granulomata with fibrosis at the periphery of these granulomata. Elastic van Gieson (EVG). Medium power.

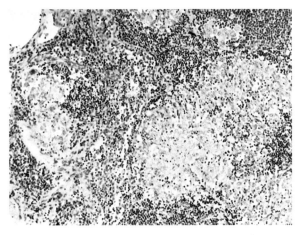

Figure 10.2 Lymph node showing noncaseating giant cell and epithelioid granulomas in the case of heart–lung transplantation for end-stage sarcoidosis. Haemotoxylin and eosin (H & E). High power.

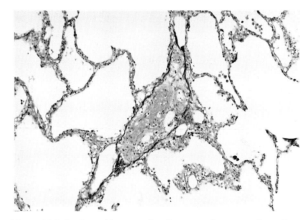

Figure 10.3 Explanted lung section from a patient transplanted for pulmonary hypertension and interstitial radiological changes. Many medium-sized veins show occlusion as seen in this vein by loose fibrous tissue with features suggestive of recanalization. Elsewhere the lung showed abundant haemosiderin pigment and fibrosis. EVG. Medium power.

Schaumann bodies which are embedded in dense fibrous tissue and are no longer identifiable as granulomatous. A particular feature is the presence of granulomatous vasculitis, where the sarcoidal granulomas involve periadventitial or mural tissue with destruction of normal vascular wall architecture and intimal occlusion [32]. The incidence of granulomatous vasculitis is known to be greater in open biopsy material than transbronchial biopsies due both to

sampling and the size of vessel examined and it is therefore not surprising that it should be easily found in whole explanted lungs (Figure 10.5). The liberal use of elastic stains highlights the extent of vascular involvement in this subgroup of severely affected patients and may explain the propensity to nodular scarring. Vascular occlusion, fibrosis and the effects of hypoxia may all contribute

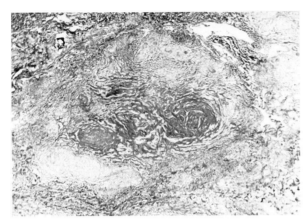

Figure 10.4 Part of a macroscopic nodule of fibrotic sarcoidosis from same case as in Figure 10.1, showing dense collagenous fibrosis in the centre of confluent granulomas. EVG. Medium power.

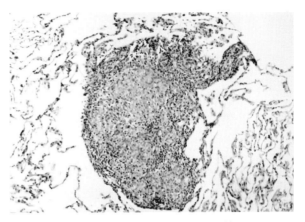

Figure 10.6 Transbronchial biopsy of transplanted lung in a patient with end-stage sarcoidosis showing recurrent disease. Meticulous exclusion of other, mainly infectious, causes of granulomatous pneumonitis is required before ascribing the new granulomata to recurrence. H & E. Medium power.

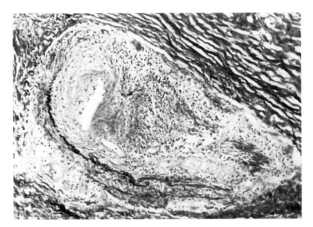

Figure 10.5 A case of nodular fibrotic sarcoidosis showing vascular involvement. The artery shown has dense adventitial fibrosis and medial destruction by granulomatous inflammation that has occluded the lumen. EVG. Medium power.

to pulmonary hypertension, which has often been noted preoperatively. Interestingly we have seen cases of pulmonary hypertension secondary to congenital heart disease in which numerous granulomas in a distribution typical of sarcoidosis have been present in lungs, heart and lymph nodes, implying that sarcoidosis is a supplementary condition in these patients. This observation is particularly interesting in relation to angiotensin converting enzyme (ACE) genotypes [33] and the increased ACE immunoreactivity demonstrated in the endothelium and neointima of patients with so-called primary pulmonary hypertension.

The re-audit of a subsequent cohort of patients revealed two incorrect diagnoses in the three cases referred as sarcoidosis for heart–lung transplantation in which the

diagnosis was not confirmed. Sarcoidosis was seen as an unsuspected supplementary diagnosis in 11 lung transplants most commonly in chronic obstructive airways disease and AAT deficiency patients.

Patients with documented sarcoidosis in explanted lungs have been shown in several studies to develop recurrent sarcoid granulomas in their grafts [2,8,34]. A diagnosis of recurrent disease can obviously be accepted only after meticulous exclusion of other causes, particularly infection by opportunistic pathogens (Figure 10.6). The recurrence in the graft as yet has not been related to graft loss or decreased function except in one case reported by Walker et al., [35] where the development of granulomas in the graft was associated with clinical deterioration necessitating retransplantation. The experience of lung transplantation for sarcoidosis is still small and longer follow-up, both clinical and histological, may further clarify the incidence and outcome of recurrent disease. The UK Heart–Lung Transplant Pathology Group is involved in multicentre data collection for sarcoidosis and transplantation and may be able to resolve these issues.

The relationship between *Mycobacterium tuberculosis* and sarcoidosis remains a conundrum and much work has been done with molecular techniques to elucidate this. Extensively monitored patients coming to transplantation for sarcoidosis with rigorous examination of the explanted lungs followed by long-term immunosuppression have not shown evidence of subsequent TB except in a rare case [6,36]. Mycobacterium *tuberculosis* was grown from one patient from transbronchial biopsies and lavage three years post-transplantation when obliterative bronchiolitis had developed.

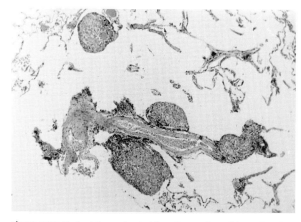

Figure 10.7 Patient transplanted for advanced smoking-related emphysema showing unsuspected concomitant sarcoidosis in his explanted lung. Enlarged air spaces are clearly seen, together with bronchovascularly distributed noncaseating granulomata. H & E. Low power.

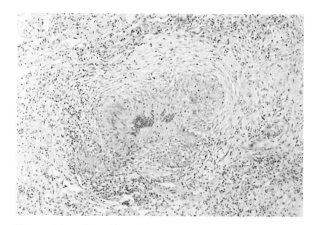

Figure 10.8 Explanted lung from patient with cystic fibrosis showing granulomatous inflammation with prominent giant cells replacing bronchiolar wall and occluding its lumen. Adjacent parenchyma showed many infiltrating eosinophils. Patient was also atopic and had no evidence of mycobacterial disease. No fungal hyphae are identified in this lesion but the most likely cause in this clinical setting is bronchocentric granulomatous mycosis. H & E. Medium power.

In patients with sarcoidosis as a supplementary diagnosis the question is raised but not yet answered as to whether sarcoidosis has exacerbated the primary condition to the point of developing end-stage lung disease and requiring transplantation, for example, combined sarcoidosis and emphysema (Figure 10.7). There may be additional airway pathology in cases of bronchiectasis or asthma with sarcoidosis. The supplementary diagnosis of sarcoidosis may also be associated with pulmonary vascular disease causing pulmonary hypertension of greater severity than that usually associated with a given primary condition, for example chronic obstructive airways disease or AAT deficiency-related emphysema. Pathological study of these explanted organs suggests that the vascular changes are out of proportion to the extent and duration of hypoxia in some patients, raising the possibility of other predisposing influences such as ACE genotype [33] or even the pulmonary hypertensive gene described elsewhere in this book (Trembath and Harrison, Chapter 2).

Cystic fibrosis

The majority of transplants performed for end-stage cystic fibrosis at our institution have been combined heart–lung grafts with a few double lung transplants. The explanted lungs allow a rare opportunity to examine severe cystic fibrosis uncomplicated by terminal pneumonia. They have revealed a range of additional pathological findings that are related partly to the condition of the surgically explanted lung and partly to the longer survival achieved by aggressive childhood therapy deferring the age of transplantation into adulthood. A very striking feature has been the wide

disparity in macroscopic and microscopic severity of disease in this group of patients with clinically defined end-stage disease. Variation is particularly noticed in relation to the size, frequency and distribution of cysts, the amount of relatively uninvolved aerated parenchyma, the extent of fibrosis and indeed the extent of suppurative occlusion of major airways at the time of operation. In some patients the obstruction of the airways is so complete as to beg the question of how the patient was surviving at all (and it should be remembered that transplantation is not performed at the time of pneumonic or infectious exacerbations). Other histological features of granulomatous inflammation, giant cells, asthmatic changes of basement membrane thickening, eosinophils and smooth muscle hyperplasia and the presence of *Aspergillus* are also highly variable correlates in some patients with known eosinophilia, allergic bronchopulmonary aspergillosis or previous pneumothoraces. In an initial study of 66 explanted lungs for cystic fibrosis, *Aspergillus* was identified in two patients in whom the largest cavities were 4 and 9 cm, respectively [6]. Also bronchocentric granulomatous mycosis most likely related to *Aspergillus* was identified in a further three patients (Figure 10.8). One or more of giant cells, granulomas, eosinophils, cysts, and cavities were present in 46 of the 66 patients. A subsequent study showed one unsuspected *Aspergillus* infection and one bronchocentric granulomatous mycosis in 47 patients, and 20 cases with giant cells, granulomas suggestive of *Aspergillus* colonization but without histological demonstration of fungus. The

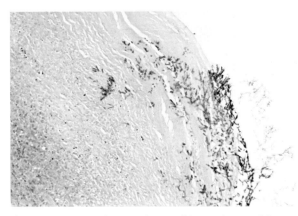

Figure 10.9 Section of an apical cyst wall in a patient receiving a transplant for cystic fibrosis. The wall is clearly invaded by fungal organisms. Grocott methanamine silver. Medium power.

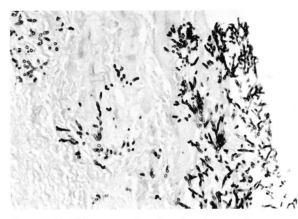

Figure 10.10 Higher power view of previous figure to show branching dichotomous hyphae with septa having the appearance of *Aspergillus*. Grocott stain.

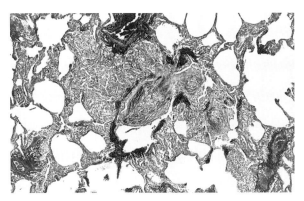

Figure 10.11 Explanted lung from patient with cystic fibrosis showing a subtotal occlusion of a bronchiole by dense collagenous fibrous tissue. Obliterative bronchiolitis can occur in cystic fibrosis as a strictly bronchiolar lesion or in the form of bronchiolitis obliterans organizing pneumonia. It is easily overlooked without liberal use of connective tissue stains and extensive sampling. EVG. Low power.

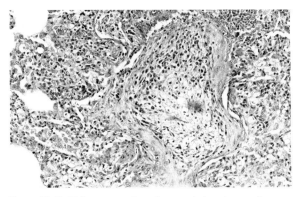

Figure 10.12 Higher power view of a granulation tissue polyp plugging a bronchiole in cystic fibrosis. This lesion is less fibrotic than that shown in Figure 10.11 and potentially reversible. The accompanying alveolar inflammation indicates that this is part of an organizing pneumonia. The adjacent alveoli show frequent foamy macrophages consistent with proximal small airway obstruction. H & E. High power.

identification of *Aspergillus* (Figures 10.9 and 10.10) or histological features strongly suggestive of *Aspergillus* infection or colonization are important in view of the high risk of invasive *Aspergillus* disease in the postoperative period. There is a particular risk to the airway anastomosis if it is not adequately vascularized and residual *Aspergillus* infection in the pleural space in patients with numerous adhesions can pose a threat. One patient with cavities, giant cells, eosinophils and apical adhesions all suggestive of *Aspergillus* in the explant, developed invasive *Aspergillus* into the subclavian artery with fatal dissemination and intrathoracic haemorrhage. Reporting of the explant histopathology in cystic fibrosis patients should therefore be performed expediently so that patients at risk of postoperative *Aspergillus* infection can be identified.

A further rather unexpected feature in cystic fibrosis explants is the extent of involvement of small airways with a fibro-obliterative process (Figures 10.11 and 10.12), either isolated to the airways, i.e. obliterative bronchiolitis, or as part of organizing pneumonia of a BOOP (bronchiolitis obliterans organizing pneumonia) pattern. This has rekindled interest in the small airways in the pathogenesis of cystic fibrosis, where the clinical features tend to be dominated by the large airway inflammation and ectasia. Small airways disease related to bronchiectasis is recognized in other pathological settings, most notably in the transplantation setting of obliterative bronchiolitis (OB) of chronic rejection. Here patients with OB show evidence of bronchiectasis by computed tomography relatively early in their course and can be clinically dominated by large airway sepsis in the late stages of chronic lung rejection.

The availability of stored explanted cystic fibrosis lungs has supported research into pathogenesis as well as providing detailed histopathological descriptions. One of the suggested mechanisms for the inflammation in cystic fibrosis is an imbalance between neutrophil elastase and proteinase inhibitors, the most important of which is AAT. Deficiency of AAT is associated with early onset panlobular emphysema in smokers, bronchiectasis [37] and asthma [38], and has been linked to cryptogenic fibrosing alveolitis [39,40].

Approximately 12% of the UK population have the common S and Z deficiency alleles, with plasma AAT concentrations in a homozygote of 60% and 10%, respectively, when compared to the normal M homozygote. A recent study showed that cystic fibrosis patients with mild to moderate AAT deficiency unexpectedly had significantly better lung function than nondeficient patients [41]. Another study, by Döring et al. [42], also shows that AAT deficiency was not associated with more severe lung disease in paediatric patients despite significantly earlier colonization with *Pseudomonas aeruginosa*. These studies on living patients may have been biased by not including the most severely affected patients, who had either died or had received a transplant. Using formalin-fixed lung tissue from 72 patients with cystic fibrosis who had undergone heart–lung or double lung transplantation at Papworth Hospital and blood spots for seven cystic fibrosis patients who had died in childhood from their lung disease, we were able to perform polymerase chain reaction (PCR) amplification of both Z and S AAT phenotypes. Two patients were found to be heterozygous with a Z allele and four for the S allele, which is not significantly different from the incidence in the normal population of 4% and 8%, respectively. These data support the previous findings that deficiency of AAT is not associated with more severe pulmonary disease and cystic fibrosis and indeed may be associated with milder lung disease. The archiving of explanted material in this highly monitored group of patients will be invaluable in exploring the possible mechanisms by which mild to moderate deficiency phenotypes of AAT could protect against cystic fibrosis lung disease, for example by linkage with other protective mutations.

Pulmonary emphysema

Emphysema often in association with chronic bronchitis is a common indication for lung transplantation [1]. In many centres combined heart–lung grafts were used until single and double lung transplantation became established several years later. Emphysema was considered an

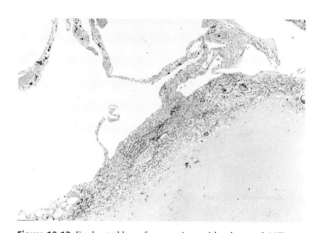

Figure 10.13 Explanted lung from patient with advanced AAT deficiency-related emphysema and a necrotic granulomatous focus with giant cells and epithelioid cells. Acid-fast bacilli were present (not shown) confirming this to be unsuspected tuberculosis. H & E. Medium power.

appropriate condition for single lung replacement, with the beneficial effect on donor organ utilization. However, as emphysema is a bilateral disease the remaining native lung can cause significant problems with infection, and with pneumothoraces or with hyperinflation with compression of the transplanted lung. The latter phenomenon particularly occurs when the graft itself is compromised by the development of OB. In some cases lung reduction surgery is required to deal with the native lung. The complications related to the native lung have led to consideration of bilateral lung transplantation for emphysema and this is particularly indicated in AAT deficiency-related emphysema, in which single lung transplant recipients have a significantly worse survival.

In our institution we have noted several unexpected findings in explanted lungs. Previously unsuspected TB has been seen (Figure 10.13), with greater implication for single than bilateral or heart–lung recipients, as a possibility of TB in the remaining native lung has to be considered. Other cases have shown bronchovascularly distributed noncaseating granulomas with the features of sarcoidosis and associated with sarcoid granulomas in hilar lymph nodes. We have also seen a case with additional unsuspected allergic bronchopulmonary *Aspergillus* infection.

Explanted lungs with emphysema, in common with other conditions are made available for examination when the disease is in an advanced but not agonal stage. By definition the patients are not suffering from an acute complication such as pneumonia or thromboembolism at the time of transplantation surgery and examination of these lungs provides insights not available in autopsy material.

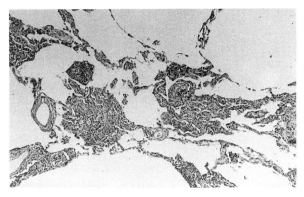

Figure 10.14 Explanted lung from patient with AAT deficiency-related emphysema showing enlargement of air spaces and interstitial inflammation with some intra-alveolar macrophage accumulation. This inflammatory process was present in all lung lobes, often being quite diffuse. H & E. Low power.

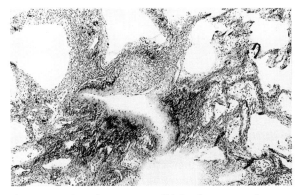

Figure 10.16 Granulomatous vasculitis in a lung removed at heart–lung transplantation for presumed pulmonary fibrosis with pulmonary hypertension. Sarcoidosis of heart, lungs and nodes was diagnosed and granulomatous vasculitis is one contributory cause to the pulmonary hypertension by vascular occlusion. EVG. Low power.

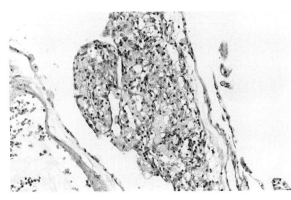

Figure 10.15 Higher power view of interstitial infiltrate shown in Figure 10.14 demonstrating macrophages, some foamy and others pigmented. H & E.

Particularly in the AAT deficiency-related emphysematous lungs, the degree of inflammatory change is usually very striking (Figures 10.14 and 10.15). The disease appears far from 'burnt out' and the interstitium, both in irreversibly damaged and less affected areas, can show large numbers of macrophages. These predominate over neutrophils except in small foci where acute inflammation is present, most likely due to subclinical infection. The persistence of such intense inflammation at an advanced stage of the disease raises the possibility of effective treatment strategies for patients at presentation. One such strategy is the replacement of AAT [43]. Emphysema in patients without AAT deficiency is usually less overtly inflammatory in the explanted organs, but this can be very variable.

A further variable feature is the degree of pulmonary vascular abnormality in patients with advanced emphysema. Many have striking intimal longitudinal smooth muscle

and medial hypertrophy but in others the pulmonary vessels can appear within normal limits for the patient's age. The severity of the patient's condition may be related to the degree of pulmonary vascular disease as well as the percentage destruction of alveolar tissue. It is possible to speculate that the risk of developing pulmonary arterial abnormalities apparently out of proportion to the parenchymal disease may be genetic in nature. The availability of well-documented explanted emphysematous lungs may be a useful tool in elucidating this further.

Pulmonary hypertension

Lung transplantation, both with and without the heart, has been offered for pulmonary hypertension of both primary and secondary origin. Patients with pulmonary hypertension secondary to congenital heart disease (with and without previous surgical correction) and patients with end-stage thromboembolic pulmonary hypertension generally have their diagnosis confirmed on an examination of the organs removed at transplantation. Chronic thromboembolic pulmonary hypertension is now treated surgically by pulmonary thromboendarterectomy and we no longer see explanted lungs for this condition. As mentioned earlier in this chapter, occasionally concomitant sarcoid granulomas in heart, lungs and lymph nodes are found and may be either coincidental or pathogenetically significant (Figure 10.16). A significant number of patients transplanted for pulmonary hypertension have idiopathic so-called primary plexogenic pulmonary hypertension and the major cardiothoracic transplant centres have collected

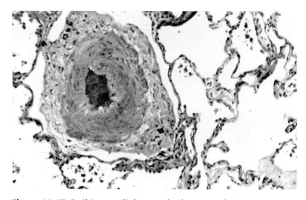

Figure 10.17 Striking medial muscular hypertrophy in an explanted primary pulmonary hypertension lung. The increased muscular thickness is circular in orientation. H & E. Medium power.

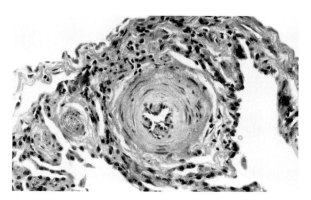

Figure 10.18 Concentric laminar intimal fibrosis with luminal narrowing in an arteriole from a patient with primary pulmonary hypertension. H & E. High power.

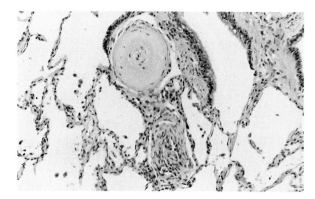

Figure 10.19 Totally occluded arteriole with concentric laminar fibrosis from same patient as used for Figure 10.18. The lesion is less cellular and is associated with a plexiform lesion adjacent, which is very cellular. H & E. Medium power.

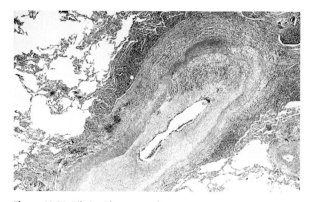

Figure 10.20 Fibrinoid segmental necrotizing arteritis in a patient with severe primary pulmonary hypertension leading to transplantation. Frequent plexiform lesions were present in both lungs. This form of arteritis is only seen in advanced severe disease. EVG. Low power.

significant numbers of these unusual and fascinating lungs. Liberal sampling of these lungs is essential to appreciate the range of vascular lesions. Adult patients generally have easily found plexiform lesions with concentric laminar fibrosis, intimal fibrosis and medial hypertrophy in many vessels (Figures 10.17, 10.18 and 10.19). Patients coming to transplantation have often been maintained on chronic epoprostenol (prostacyclin) infusions, extending their survival to the point of transplantation. This may explain the severity of the lesions seen and the identification of grade 6 lesions of true fibrinoid arteritis, which are rarely seen in other material (Figure 10.20) [44]. There is increasing focus on the cellular and molecular pathogenesis of idiopathic primary pulmonary hypertension and the use and abuse of appetite suppressants may further increase the incidence of this potentially fatal form of pulmonary hypertension [45,46]. Animal models do not reproduce the morphological features of human pulmonary hypertension, making it imperative that the human tissue available through transplantation is adequately studied. The development of the hallmark intimal, medial and plexiform lesions depends on vascular remodelling [47], and many studies have concentrated on the role of the pulmonary endothelial cells in the pathogenesis of severe pulmonary hypertension [48]. Endothelial cell proliferation is the hallmark lesion of several forms of severe pulmonary hypertension, including primary (idiopathic), familial, liver cirrhosis, human immunodeficiency virus (HIV) and congenital heart malformations. The plexiform lesions seen readily in these conditions consist of intravascular cellular clusters with capillary type lumina and are often present at branching points of small pulmonary arteries and arterioles. They have been proposed to represent an abnormal form of intravascular angiogenesis [49–51]. It has been suggested that plexiform lesions form at the site of focal fibrinoid necrosis of the vessel wall (to be distinguished from the true fibrinoid necrotizing arteritis or grade 6 lesion) and multiple levels through blocks of explanted pulmonary hypertensive lung tissue may be required to demonstrate healed acellular hyaline segments representing such damage. Cell-specific markers have also demonstrated the endothelial nature of the onion-skin type concentric laminar obliteration of pulmonary artery branches. The relationship between concentric laminar fibrosis and plexiform lesions may not be one of progression as implied by the Heath–Edwards grading system [44]. It is quite striking that they are present in differing proportions in primary pulmonary hypertension explants and concentric laminar fibrotic lesions are usually outnumbered by plexiform lesions. This observation is interesting in relation to work done by Cool et al. [52–53], who showed an intimate juxtaposition between plexiform and concentric obliterative lesions in primary pulmonary hypertension by computer-aided three-dimensional reconstruction. Both lesions occurred a few micrometres distal to branch points of the parent pulmonary arteries. Plexiform lesions occurred as sole lesions but concentric obliterative lesions appeared only proximal to, and associated with, plexiform lesions. Thus, unlike Heath and Edwards [44] and Wagenvoort and Mooi [54], who proposed that plexiform lesions occurred at a later stage than concentric laminar fibrotic or obliterative lesions, Cool et al. propose that it is just as likely that concentric lesions represent the later stage [53]. This is a further example where the study of explanted human tissue can advance our understanding of pathogenesis and evolution of the plexiform lesions hopefully leading to better clinical staging and more effective treatment strategies.

The identification of a familial gene for primary pulmonary hypertension on chromosome 2, together with the burgeoning evidence of phenotypic alterations of the endothelial cell in severe pulmonary hypertension, may translate into successful therapeutic intervention for both primary and secondary forms of the disease [55–57] (see Chapters 1–4). The value of explanted tissue and the further stimulus to the study of pulmonary hypertension provided by the therapeutic advances of epoprostenol and lung transplantation cannot be overemphasized in both familial and sporadic cases [58]. Using explanted primary hypertensive lungs including familial cases, with unused donor lungs as controls, it has been possible to study the expression of the gene for bone morphogenetic protein receptor type II (BMPR2) and TGF-β type I and II receptors in this condition. Heterozygous germline mutations

involving the gene encoding BMPR-II, which is a member of the TGF-β superfamily of receptors, have been found to underlie many cases of both familial and sporadic plexogenic pulmonary hypertension. Normal lungs show BMPR-II predominantly in vascular endothelial cells at all levels of the pulmonary vasculature and this can be demonstrated by both in situ hybridization and immunohistochemistry. BMPR2 is also seen on some vascular and bronchial smooth muscle and on the brush border of airway epithelium. In explanted lungs of primary pulmonary hypertension, in addition to endothelial staining, BMPR2 mRNA and protein expression was also observed in the myofibroblasts comprising intimal lesions and on endothelial cells lining the vascular channels of plexiform lesions. TGF-β receptors type I and II co-localized predominantly to vascular endothelium, with only weak staining of underlying smooth muscle but airway epithelial staining was also prominent. In primary pulmonary hypertension TGF-βRI immunostaining is prominent on endothelial cells and myofibroblasts but TGF-βRI was almost absent in intimal lesions including endothelial cells and absent from plexiform lesions. Thus using explanted primary pulmonary hypertensive lungs it has been possible to demonstrate TGF-βRI and RII co-localizing to vascular endothelium in the normal pulmonary circulation, with reduced expression of TGF-βRII subtype in plexiform and intimal lesions of primary pulmonary hypertension and to show BMPR2 expression in endothelial cells of the normal pulmonary circulation and in the intimal and plexiform lesions of primary pulmonary hypertension. Evidence is emerging that germline and/or somatic mutations in key cell growth regulatory genes play a role in the development of idiopathic sporadic and familial pulmonary hypertension. It has been shown in other studies that monoclonal endothelial cell proliferation is present in primary but not secondary pulmonary hypertension [59,60].

In the absence of appropriate animal models, pulmonary arteries in patients with end-stage pulmonary hypertension are an ideal model with which to evaluate changes in angiotensin converting enzyme (ACE) expression in human vascular tissue as these vessels are characterized by active remodelling. The lung endothelial tissue is a rich source of ACE and this can be studied both in normal lung tissue obtained at the time of lung transplantation from donors and also in lungs resected from patients with end-stage primary pulmonary hypertension. Schuster et al. [61] compared the immunoreactivity for ACE in pulmonary artery and lung parenchymal tissue from eight patients with end-stage primary pulmonary hypertension with the reactivity seen in normal donor lungs. The

ACE immunoreactivity was markedly and consistently increased in the endothelium and subendothelial neointimal regions of the elastic pulmonary arteries from the patients with primary pulmonary hypertension when compared with normal pulmonary arteries. In addition, immunoreactivity in normal muscular pulmonary arteries was usually less than that of surrounding capillary endothelial cells in contrast to patients with primary pulmonary hypertension, where the muscular pulmonary artery intensity was comparable to that of surrounding alveolar capillaries. This study using explanted material provided evidence for the first time that ACE expression can be altered in human vascular tissue associated with vascular remodelling. It is hypothesized in this study that increased angiotensin 2, which is generated locally by ACE, can stimulate vascular smooth muscle proliferation in the intimal tissue together with fibroblast growth factor, which in itself can induce increased ACE expression in response to injury.

Madden et al. [62], studied 20 patients undergoing heart–lung transplantation for end-stage primary pulmonary hypertension to examine any correlation between the histopathology, ultrastructure, pulmonary endocrinology and clinical manifestations of the disease. They found that length of clinical history and clinical evidence of severe disease are not necessarily associated with advanced histopathology. Plexiform lesions were seen in 15 of the 20 patients that were cellular in nine and mature in six. The remaining five patients showed intimal proliferation and/or muscularization of pulmonary arterioles with preplexiform changes including prominent myofibroblasts in the intima of small pulmonary arteries and arterioles. In the absence of particular clinical features predicting histological appearance, the duration of disease did correlate with occlusion of pulmonary veins thought to represent adaptation to sustained elevation of pulmonary arterial pressure and was more marked in female than in male patients. The presence of small contracted muscular pulmonary arteries did not imply responsiveness to vasodilators, the mean pulmonary artery pressure tended to be lower in patients with increased numbers of pulmonary endocrine cells and higher in those with reduced numbers.

Conclusion

Lung transplantation in its various combinations has been a successful development in the treatment of end-stage parenchymal and pulmonary vascular disorders. This therapeutic modality has given hope to patients with end-stage pulmonary disease and has an enormous impact on the interest in lung disease both in the primary condition leading to transplantation and in the subsequent behaviour of the transplanted lung. Study of the explanted lungs as well as being a useful audit tool for the quality of thoracic medicine has also contributed to advances in our understanding of the pathogenesis of lung diseases by providing the essential morphological substrate for many molecular and genetic studies. This histological underpinning of research will continue to be important in future studies and the localization of cell-specific markers and genotypic and phenotypic alterations is very likely to have an impact on therapy for both pre- and post-transplant conditions [63–67].

REFERENCES

1 Hosenpud JD, Bennett LE, Keck BM, Boucek MM, Novick RJ. The Registry of the International Society for Heart and Lung Transplantation: 17th Official Report – 2000. *J Heart Lung Transplant* 2000; **19**: 909–931.

2 Nunley DR, Hattler B, Keenan RJ, et al. Lung transplantation for end-stage pulmonary sarcoidosis. *Sarcoidosis Vasc Diffuse Lung Dis* 1999; **16**: 93–100.

3 Semenzato G, Agostini C. Lung transplantation in sarcoidosis: lesions learned from immunology. *Sarcoidosis Vasc Diffuse Lung Dis* 1999; **16**: 21–23.

4 Nonn RA, Garrity ER Jr. Lung transplantation for fibrotic lung diseases. *Am J Med Sci* 1998; **315**: 146–154.

5 Barbers RG. Lung transplantation in interstitial lung disease. *Curr Opin Pulm Med* 1995; **1**: 410–415.

6 Stewart S, McNeil K, Nashef SAM, Wells FC, Higenbottam TW, Wallwork J. Audit of referral and explant diagnoses in lung transplantation: a pathologic study of lungs removed for parenchymal disease. *J Heart Lung Transplant* 1995; **14**: 1173–1186.

7 Sonderegger-Iseli K, Burger S, Muntwyler J, Salomon F. Diagnostic errors in three medical eras: a necropsy study. *Lancet* 2000; **355**: 2027–2031.

8 Stewart S. The pathology of lung transplantation. *Sem Diag Pathol* 1992; **9**: 210–219.

9 Bjortuft O, Foerster A, Boe J, Geiran O. Single lung transplantation as treatment for end-stage pulmonary sarcoidosis: recurrence of sarcoidosis in two different lung allografts in one patient. *J Heart Lung Transplant* 1994; **13**: 24–29.

10 Johnson BA, Duncan SR, Ohori NP, et al. Recurrence of sarcoidosis in pulmonary allograft recipients. *Am Rev Respir Dis* 1993; **148**: 1373–1377.

11 O'Brien JD, Lium JH, Parosa JG, Deyoung BR, Wick MR, Trulock EP. Lymphangiomatosis recurrence in the allograft after single-lung transplantation. *Am J Respir Crit Care Med* 1995; **151**: 2033–2036.

12 Bittman I, Dose TB, Müller C, Dienemann H, Vogelmeier C, Löhrs U. Lymphangiomatosis: recurrence after single lung transplantation. *Hum Pathol* 1997; **26**: 1420–1423.

13 Nine JS, Yousem SA, Paradis IL, Keenan R, Griffith BP. Lymphangioleiomyomatosis: recurrence after lung transplantation. *J Heart Lung Transplant* 1994; **13**: 714–719.

14 Gabbay E, Dark JH, Ashcroft T, et al. Recurrence of Langerhans' cell granulomatosis following lung transplantation. *Thorax* 1998; **53**: 326–327.

15 Habib SB, Congleton J, Carr D, et al. Recurrence of recipient Langerhans' cell histiocytosis following bilateral lung transplantation. *Thorax* 1998; **53**: 323–325.

16 Müller C, Briegel J, Haller M, et al. Sarcoidosis recurrence following lung transplantation. *Transplantation* 1996; **61**: 1117–1119.

17 Carre P, Rouquette I, Durand D, et al. Recurrence of sarcoidosis in a human lung allograft. *Transplant Proc* 1995; **27**: 1686.

18 Yeatman M, McNeil K, Smith JA, et al. Lung transplantation in patients with systemic diseases: an eleven-year experience at Papworth Hospital. *J Heart Lung Transplant* 1996; **15**: 144–149.

19 Levine SM, Anzueto A, Peters JI, Calhoon JH, Jenkinson SG, Bryan CL. Single lung transplantation in patients with systemic disease. Chest 1994; **105**: 837–841.

20 Pigula FA, Griffith BP, Zenati MA, Dauber JH, Yousem SA, Keenan RJ. Lung transplantation for respiratory failure resulting from systemic disease. *Ann Thoracic Surg* 1997; **64**: 1630–1634.

21 Mahadeva R, Stewart S, Wallwork J. Metastatic endometrial stromal sarcoma masquerading as pulmonary lymphangioleiomyomatosis. *J Clin Path* 1999; **52**: 147–148.

22 Egan J. Pharmacologic therapy of idiopathic pulmonary fibrosis. *J Heart Lung Transplant* 1998; **17**: 1039–1044.

23 Katzenstein AL, Myers JL. Idiopathic pulmonary fibrosis. To biopsy or not to biopsy. *Am J Respir Crit Care Med* 2001; **164**: 185–186.

24 Katzenstein AL, Fiorelli RF. Nonspecific interstitial pneumonia/fibrosis. Histological features and clinical significance. *Am J Surg Pathol* 1994; **18**: 136–147.

25 Bjoraker JA, Ryu JH, Edwin MK, et al. Prognostic significance of histopathologic subsets in idopathic pulmonary fibrosis. *Am Respir Crit Care Med* 1998; **157**: 199–203.

26 Gay SE, Kazerooni EA, Toews GB, et al. Idiopathic pulmonary fibrosis. Predicting response to therapy and survival. *Am J Respir Crit Care Med* 1998; **157**: 1063–1072.

27 Ziesche R, Hofbauer E, Wittmann K, et al. A preliminary study of long-term treatment with interferon γ-1b and low-dose prednisolone in patients with idiopathic pulmonary fibrosis. *N Engl J Med* 1999; **341**: 1264–1269.

28 Edwards C, Williams A, Asquith P. Bronchopulmonary disease in coeliac patients. *J Clin Pathol* 1985; **38**: 361–367.

29 Hunninghake GW, Zimmerman MB, Schwartz DA, et al. Utility of a lung biopsy for the diagnosis of idiopathic pulmonary fibrosis. *Am J Respir Crit Care Med* 2001; **164**: 193–196.

30 Hillerdal G, Nou E, Osterman K, et al. Sarcoidosis: epidemiology and prognosis. *Am Rev Respir Dis* 1984; **130**: 29–30.

31 Rosen Y, Moon S, Huang C-T, Lyons HA. Granulomatous pulmonary angiitis in sarcoidosis. *Arch Pathol Lab Med* 1977; **101**: 170–174.

32 Takemura T, Matsui Y, Saika S, Mikami R. Pulmonary vascular involvement in sarcoidosis. A report of 40 autopsy cases. *Hum Pathol* 1992; **23**: 1216–1223.

33 McGrath DS, Foley PJ, Petrek M, et al. ACE gene I/D polymorphism and sarcoidosis pulmonary disease severity. *Am J Respir Crit Care Med* 2001; **164**: 197–201.

34 Judson MA. Lung transplantation for pulmonary sarcoidosis. *Eur Respir J* 1998; **11**: 738–744.

35 Walker S, Mikhail G, Banner N, et al. Medium term results of lung transplantation for end stage pulmonary sarcoidosis. *Thorax* 1998; **53**: 281–284.

36 Klemen H, Husain AN, Cagle PT, Farrity ER, Popper HH. Mycobacterial DNA in recurrent sarcoidosis in the transplanted lung – a PCR-based study on four cases. *Virchows Arch* 2000; **436**: 365–369.

37 King MA, Stone JA, Diaz PT, et al. α_1-Antitrypsin deficiency: evaluation of bronchiectasis with CT. *Radiology* 1996; **199**: 137–141.

38 Colp C, Pappas J, Moran D, et al. Variants of α_1-antitrypsin in Puerto Rican children with asthma. *Chest* 1993; **103**: 812–815.

39 Geddes DM, Webley M, Brewerton DA, et al. Alpha-1 antitrypsin phenotypes in fibrosing alveolitis and rheumatoid arthritis. *Lancet* 1997; **ii**: 1049–1051.

40 Hubbard R, Baoku Y, Kelsheker N, et al. Alpha-1 antitrypsin phenotypes in patients with cryptogenic fibrosing alveolitis: a case-control study. *Eur Respir J* 1997; **10**: 2881–2883.

41 Mahadeva R, Westerbeek RC, Perry DJ, et al. Alpha1-antitrypsin deficiency alleles and the Taq-I G→A allele in cystic fibrosis lung disease. *Eur Respir J* 1998; **11**: 873–879.

42 Döring G, Krogh-Johannsen H, Weidinger S, et al. Allotypes of α_1-antitrypsin in patients with cystic fibrosis, homozygous and heterozygous for deltaF608. *Pediatr Pulmon* 1994; **18**: 3–7.

43 Stoller JK. Augmentation therapy for severe α_1-antitrypsin deficiency: is the jury still out on a trial? *Thorax* 1998; **53**: 1007–1009.

44 Heath D, Edwards JE. The hypertension of pulmonary vascular disease. A description of six grades of structural changes in the pulmonary arteries with special reference to congenital cardiac septal defects. *Circulation* 1958; **18**: 533–547.

45 Voelkel NF. Appetite suppressants and pulmonary hypertension. *N Engl J Med* 1997; **335**: 609–616.

46 Voelkel NF, Clarke WR, Higenbottam T. Obesity, dexfenfluramine, and pulmonary hypertension. *Am J Respir Crit Care Med* 1997; **155**: 786–788.

47 Botney MD, Bahadori L, Gold LI. Vascular remodeling in primary pulmonary hypertension. *Am J Pathol* 1994; **114**: 285–295.

48 Fishman AP. Etiology and pathogenesis of primary pulmonary hypertension. A perspective. *Chest* 1998; **114**: 242S–247S.

49 Tuder RM, Lee S-D, Cool CC. Histopathology of pulmonary hypertension. *Chest* 1998; **114**: 1S–6S.

50 Tuder RM, Wang J, Lee SD, et al. Vascular endothelial growth factor (VEGF) expression in normal and remodeled pulmonary arteries in severe pulmonary hypertension. *Am J Respir Crit Care Med* 1997; **155**: A627.

51 Tuder RM, Groves B, Badesch DB, et al. Exuberant endothelial cell growth and elements of inflammation are present

in plexiform lesions of pulmonary hypertension. *Am J Pathol* 1994; **144**: 275–285.

52 Cool C, Voelkel FN, Tuder RM. Three-dimensional reconstruction of the plexiform lesions in pulmonary hypertension. *Am J Repir Crit Care Med* 1996; **153**: A85.

53 Cool CD, Kennedy D, Voelkel NF, et al. Pathogenesis and evolution of plexiform lesions in pulmonary hypertension associated with scleroderma and human immunodeficiency virus infection. *Hum Pathol* 1997; **28**: 434–442.

54 Wagenvoort CA, Mooi MJ. Controversies and potential errors in the histological evaluation of pulmonary vascular disease. In: Wagenvoort CA, Denolin H, eds. *Pulmonary circulation, advances and controversies.* Elsevier Science Publishing, New York, 1989: 7–26.

55 The International PPH Consortium, Lane KB, Machado RD, Pauciulo MW, et al. Heterozygous germ-line mutations in *BMPR2*, encoding a TGF-β receptor, cause familial primary pulmonary hypertension. *Nature Genet* 2000; **26**: 81–84.

56 Thomson JR, Machado RD, Pauciulo MW, et al. Sporadic primary pulmonary hypertension is associated with germline mutations of the gene encoding BMPR-II, a receptor member of the TGF-β family. *J Med Genet* 2000; **37:** 741–745.

57 Machado RD, Pauciulo MW, Thomson JR, et al. BMPR2 haploinsufficiency as the inherited molecular mechanisms for primary pulmonary hypertension. *Am J Hum Genet* 2001; **68**: 92–102.

58 Pietra GG, Edwards WD, Kay JM, et al. Histopathology of primary pulmonary hypertension. A qualitative and quantitative study of pulmonary blood vessels from 58 patients in the National Heart, Lung and Blood Institute, Primary Pulmonary Hypertension Registry. *Circulation* 1989; **80**: 1198–1206.

59 Lee SD, Shroyer KR, Markham NE, Cool CD, Voelkel NF, Tuder RM. Monoclonal endothelial cell proliferation is present in primary but not secondary pulmonary hypertension. *J Clin Invest* 1998; **101**: 927–934.

60 Tuder RM, Radisavljevic Z, Shroyer KR, Polak JM, Voelkel NF. Monoclonal endothelial cells in appetite suppressant-associated pulmonary hypertension. *Am J Respir Crit Care Med* 1998; **158**: 1999–2001.

61 Schuster DP, Crouch EC, Parks WC, Johnson T, Botney MD. Angiotensin converting enzyme expression in primary pulmonary hypertension. *Am J Respir Care Med* 1996; **154**: 1087–1091.

62 Madden BP, Gosney J, Coghlan JG, et al. Pretransplant clinico-pathological correlation in end-stage primary pulmonary hypertension. *Eur Respir J* 1994; **7**: 672–678.

63 Kalassian KG, Doyle R, Kao P, Ruoss S, Raffin TA. Pulmonary perspective. Lymphangioleiomyomatosis: new insights. *Am J Respir Crit Care Med* 1997; **155**: 1183–1186.

64 Selman M, King TE Jr, Pardo A. Idiopathic pulmonary fibrosis: prevailing and evolving hypothesis about its pathogenesis and implications for therapy. *Ann Intern Med* 2001; **134**: 136–151.

65 Mahadeva R, Stewart S, Bilton D, Lomas DA. Alpha-1-antitrypsin deficiency alleles and severe cystic fibrosis lung disease. *Thorax* 1998; **53**: 1022–1024.

66 Myers JL. NSIP, UIP and the ABCs of idiopathic interstitial pneumonias. *Eur Respir J* 1998; **12**: 1003–1004.

67 Brézillon S, Hamm H, Heilmann M, et al. Decreased expression of the cystic fibrosis transmembrane conductance regulator protein in remodeled airway epithelium from lung transplanted patients. *Hum Pathol* 1997; **28**: 944–952.

Part 2

Lung transplantation

11

Overview

Magdi H. Yacoub and Emma J. Birks

Harefield Hospital, Harefield, Middlesex, UK

Introduction

Lung transplantation has been shown to be an effective means of treating a variety of conditions including pulmonary vascular and parenchymal lung disease. Despite many advances in lung transplantation over the preceding decades there are still many challenges that need to be addressed if lung transplantation is to achieve its full potential.

The scarcity of organs suitable for transplantation

The shortage of donor organs remains an on-going difficulty, with the number of transplants performed continuing to fall in the UK [1] and elsewhere. It is therefore increasingly important to improve public awareness of the need for organ donation and develop strategies to optimize the number of cadaveric donors and explore alternative strategies.

Abu Dhabi declaration

At the recent organ transplantation congress in Abu Dhabi, delegates came to the conclusion that there are a considerable number of patients who would benefit from organ transplantation in every country. The Congress felt there is currently no adequate alternative therapy for most of these patients except transplantation. Sending patients from one country to another for transplantation is impractical because each country has a donor problem of its own. Therefore it is important for each country to start its own organ transplant programme. For this purpose cooperative effort is required, which includes the public, government, media, heath care professionals and religious leaders. There is a need to establish a voluntary foundation to support research in, and practice of, transplantation. The input and guidance of religious leaders and ethics committees are an essential part of this venture. The meeting recognized the vital role of government in providing a regulatory framework and financial support for transplantation, contributing to the establishment of local and regional coordination teams, and supporting organ donation as well as research into transplantation.

Donor management

Management of the potential organ donor after brain death needs to be improved in order to prevent the development of infection and organ dysfunction, which may prevent subsequent transplantation; continued research into the mechanisms of organ dysfunction and their potential reversibility is of increasing importance [2,3,4] (see Chapter 15). The potential to use lungs from nonheart-beating cadavers for transplantation is being explored [5–8].

Living lobar lung transplantation

Living related or unrelated lobar transplantation is now being used at a small number of centres [9,10] including our own. The procedure consists of removal of the recipient lungs and implantation of right and left pulmonary lobes each obtained from a separate volunteer organ donor. Potentially this method will be associated with shorter ischaemic times, better matched organs and will increase the supply of donor lungs. Importantly these organs will not have been subjected to injury known to occur during and after brain death and therefore may be less likely to develop dysfunction and/or rejection [11].

Xenotransplantation

In theory, xenotransplantation can supply a potentially unlimited source of donor organs. However, there are many problems that need to be addressed before clinical application to the lung can be considered. These include the following:

1 There is a lack of knowledge of organ-specific xenogeneic lung tissue behaviour.
2 Although the creation of transgenic pig organs expressing human decay-accelerating factor (DAF) or membrane cofactor protein (MCP) has partially solved hyperacute rejection, the problems of vascular rejection, cell-mediated rejection and chronic rejection remain largely undefined.
3 The fact that intensive pharmacological immunosuppression may be needed, with its attendant risks, means strategies for inducing specific immune tolerance may be required as a safer alternative [12]. Despite intensive research this approach has not yet developed to the point where it is ready for clinical application.
4 There is a risk of cross-species infection particularly after a report that pig enterovirus can infect human cells [13], in contradiction to previous findings [14].

Although none of these problems are totally insurmountable they will require concerted research effort, with adequate funding and time to solve them in a way that is acceptable to all parties concerned as well as to public opinion [15].

Lung transplant surgery

Preoperative management

Careful preoperative assessment and optimal management of the recipient prior to transplantation are important factors which will contribute to a successful outcome (see Chapter 12). Intravenous or inhaled epoprostenol (prostacyclin) has been used with increasing success to reduce the pulmonary artery pressure and maintain patients with primary or secondary pulmonary hypertension whilst waiting for lung transplantation [16] (see Chapter 1).

The use of mechanical ventilatory support prior to transplantation (such as nasal positive pressure ventilation and its variants [17]) serves to improve quality of life and can maintain some patients waiting for transplantation [18]. Some patients may require full ventilation (see Chapter 15); in the future development of an 'artificial lung' may provide a method to bridge patients to transplantation or even become an alternative to lung transplantation (see Chapter 29).

Donor selection

The criteria for donor selection vary between transplant centres. At Harefield Hospital, the criteria currently include an age of less than 60 years, no history of significant cardiopulmonary disease, and preferably no history of smoking. Lung function, as assessed by arterial blood gases and ventilation requirements, is of paramount importance. An arterial oxygen pressure (PaO$_2$) of more than 12 kPa (90 mmHg), with a fraction of oxygen in inspired gas (F$_I$O$_2$) of less than 35% or a PaO$_2$ of more than 35 kPa (260 mmHg) on l00% oxygen is considered satisfactory. Minute ventilation and airway pressure to maintain a normal arterial CO$_2$ pressure (PaCO$_2$) level should be within the normal range.

There should be no significant consolidation or contusion within the lung parenchyma. Potential donors with extensive shadowing on the chest radiograph are considered unsuitable. The length of mechanical ventilation is an important factor in influencing the incidence of pulmonary infection, but we do not set a specific time limit and each potential donor is considered on an individual basis. Prior to organ harvesting, the donor is given a cocktail of intravenous antibiotics. Tracheal cultures are taken and, where necessary, the recipient is started on appropriate antibiotic therapy after transplantation. Neurogenic pulmonary oedema may be seen in brain-dead potential organ donors. A history of neurogenic oedema has not been regarded as a contraindication to organ harvesting provided the radiological changes have resolved and pulmonary gas exchange is adequate.

For combined heart and lung transplantation, cardiac function must also be satisfactory, with either no, or minimal, inotropic support being provided. When donors are receiving large doses of inotropic support, the cause is often intravascular volume depletion and the situation should be re-evaluated following volume expansion with colloid solutions.

The donor must be screened for potential transmissible disease, particularly hepatitis B and C and antibodies to the human immunodeficiency virus (HIV). We do not accept donors from high risk groups for HIV infection because of the danger of missing an early infection in the window period before an antibody response develops. The recipient's cytomegalovirus (CMV) status is determined serologically, and we attempt to use CMV-negative donors for

CMV-negative recipients to reduce the risks of postoperative CMV infection (see Chapter 21).

Donor recipient matching

Approximate matching of donor and recipient chest size is required to prevent problems of cardiac compression, pulmonary collapse, or persistent pleural effusions postoperatively. A number of size-matching techniques are used by different centres, including measurement of thoracic dimensions on the chest radiograph and the matching of donor lung volume (predicted on the basis of height and weight) to recipient lung volume. The technique used at our centre has been based on a series of external chest cage measurements on both donor and recipient.

ABO blood group compatibility is considered essential. We do not match for Rh blood group (see Chapter 24). At present we try to prospectively match for human leukocyte antigens (HLAs). Retrospective analysis of our data suggests that HLA class I matching does not influence survival following heart–lung transplantation, but there was a trend for class II (DR) matching to influence survival [19]. The presence of lymphocytotoxic antibodies in potential transplant recipients appeared to be associated with a lower survival after transplantation, but a positive lymphocytotoxic cross-match between the donor and recipient did not appear to affect the survival [19]. However, we now consider a prospective cross-match a contraindication. Strategies for dealing with this problem need to be developed.

Organ retrieval and preservation

The first clinical distant organ procurement was performed in our centre in June 1985. The technique consists of cooling the donor organs using a portable cardiopulmonary bypass machine, which can be transported to the donor's hospital. Bypass is established by cannulating the ascending aorta and right atrium. Systemic cooling is commenced and, when the donor heart fibrillates spontaneously, the left ventricle is vented at the apex to prevent distension. Cooling is then continued on bypass until a core temperature lower than 10 °C is achieved. During this time lung cooling continues owing to flow to the bronchial circulation and, to some extent, to the pulmonary arterial system. Surface cooling of the lungs can also be achieved with cold donor blood. The circulation is then arrested. This technique has allowed us to successfully preserve the donor organs for well over five hours and has allowed organ procurement

from as far afield as Spain, Greece, and Austria for transplantation in the UK (see Chapter 14).

Other centres have used alternative methods of organ preservation. The pulmonary flush technique is currently the preservation method in widest clinical use. The method involves infusing a cold hypertonic crystalloid solution directly into the pulmonary artery (see Chapter 13).

Choice of operation

Several types of lung transplantation are performed. The choice of operation depends on the nature of the patient's pulmonary condition, the likely availability of donor organs and, to some extent, the preference of the individual transplant team (see Chapters 13 and 14). In our centre we have generally performed heart–lung transplantation for patients with cystic fibrosis or primary pulmonary hypertension in order to avoid problems of postoperative pulmonary oedema. In addition this approach can generate a 'domino' heart with a primed right ventricle for transplantation into a patient with high pulmonary pressures requiring heart transplantation (see Chapter 14). Some other centres perform bilateral or single lung transplantation respectively for these patients [20] (see Chapter 13). We also perform heart–lung transplantation for Eisenmenger's atrial or ventricular septal defects and complex congenital disorders. For emphysema, bronchiectasis and fibrosing alveolitis single or bilateral lung transplantation is currently performed. Whereas other centres prefer single lung transplantation for obstructive lung disease [21] and bronchiectasis, if possible we prefer to do bilateral lung transplantation, although this option is limited by the decreasing number of donor organs. Bilateral lung transplantation has the advantage of avoiding compression of the transplanted lung by the native lung postoperatively (which can also be dealt with by single lung transplantation in combination with volume reduction of the native lung), pulmonary oedema in the transplanted lung, and infection of the transplanted lung by the native lung. Combining this procedure with revascularization with the internal mammary artery [22] may improve tissue healing by improving the blood supply to the new lung.

Domino heart transplantation

Heart–lung transplantation offers a unique source of hearts from live donors [23,24] and has many advantages as well as some potential problems. Apart from expanding the supply of donor organs, domino hearts offer several benefits: the heart has not been subjected to the process of brain death, which is known to have a potentially damaging effect; the transplant team have had the opportunity to perform detailed preoperative examination and potential for prospective HLA matching between donor and recipient. In addition, the presence of varying degrees of right ventricular hypertrophy in some of these hearts can be extremely useful for patients with potentially reversible elevation of pulmonary vascular resistance, which can be a major risk factor in orthotopic cardiac transplantation from a cadavaric donor [25]. Although ventricular hypertrophy is a normal adaptive response to haemodynamic load that tends to normalize wall stress, with the passage of time it almost always results in pathological changes in the heart, which includes structural molecular and functional changes in myocardial cells, blood vessels, and fibrous framework [26–28]. The resulting systolic and diastolic dysfunction is partially or completely reversible following correction of the haemodynamic load, as in the case of domino operations. This is due to the close interaction between ventricular function and afterload and the fact that the pulmonary vascular resistance of the recipient is chosen to be slightly lower than that in the donor. Furthermore, following transplantation the drop in left atrial pressure results in slow (over a period of months) but almost complete resolution of pulmonary vascular disease, which is reversible if the primary cause was pulmonary venous hypertension [29].

In the domino heart, reports have tended to concentrate on concerns about right ventricular function in the short and long term. We have observed that left ventricular performance, particularly during the early or postoperative period, may be critically compromised. This could be due to a variety of reasons, which include ventriculo-ventricular interaction [30] and afterload mismatch. The hypertrophied abnormal right ventricle ceases to contribute positively to left ventricular function. Instead it compresses the left ventricle and affects its function through the abnormal interventricular septum and other mechanisms [30]. Apart from the intrinsic impairment in left ventricular function, gross mismatch between right and left ventricular output can result if a heart from a severely pulmonary hypertensive donor is transplanted into a recipient with minor or no elevation of pulmonary vascular resistance; this could produce a precipitous rise in left atrial pressure and possibly pulmonary oedema. We therefore believe that it is essential to choose the pulmonary vascular resistance of the recipient to be only slightly lower than that of the donor and to monitor left atrial pressure directly during the periopera-

tive period, with the realization that right atrial pressure may have to be allowed to drop to very low levels to prevent pulmonary oedema. In addition, early discontinuation of intermittent positive pressure ventilation should be allowed only if left atrial pressure is consistently low. The majority of domino hearts are from patients with cystic fibrosis and other parenchymal lung conditions who tend to have only mild to moderate pulmonary hypertension and resulting right ventricular hypertrophy, and can therefore be used for patients with mildly elevated pulmonary vascular resistance while reserving hearts from patients with pulmonary arterial hypertension for recipients with moderate to severe increase in pulmonary resistance (in excess of 8 units) due to left heart failure.

Although the medium- and long-term survival of recipients of domino hearts are at least as good as those receiving cadavaric hearts, the haemodynamic performance of the domino hearts, particularly in the long term, needs to be studied further. The same haemodynamic principles apply to patients with pulmonary hypertension who undergo bilateral lung transplantation. In this case the imbalance function between the hypertrophied right and left ventricles can predispose to pulmonary oedema in the transplanted lungs.

Infection

Infection remains a major cause of early as well as late death. Causes include bacteria, viruses, fungi and protozoa with bacterial pneumonia, CMV pneumonitis and invasive aspergillosis being the most problematic [31]. Early detection and improvements in therapy are important [32] (see Chapters 20 and 21). Under normal conditions the bronchial epithelium contributes to host defence through mucosal secretions and mucociliary action. We have previously shown that following lung transplantation without bronchial revascularization these functions are impaired [33]. Direct bronchial revascularization could maintain these functions. This is supported by our findings of infrequent bouts of infection following single lung transplantation with bronchial revascularization [22].

Bronchial healing

Ischaemia of the bronchial wall, particularly at the site of anastomosis can cause necrosis of the bronchial wall, with resulting dehiscence, or excessive granulation that can progress to fibrous stricture. Although several surgical and pharmacological interventions have resulted in reduction in the incidence and severity of these complications, it continues to be a cause of morbidity following single lung or bilateral lung transplantation [34]. Some of the surgical procedures designed to increase the blood supply to the lung by indirect means have been shown to be ineffective. Colquhoun et al. [35] in 1994 reported an incidence of 10.6% bronchial anastomotic complications. This occurred despite the fact that they have used a bronchial wrap in 68.1% of the cases. We have found in a prospective clinical trial that wrapping the anastomoses with omentum or an internal mammary artery pedicle does not improve bronchial healing after single lung transplantation [36]. We have also found that direct arterial bronchial circulation using the internal mammary artery virtually abolishes anastomotic problems [22].

Bronchiolitis obliterans

The most important factor limiting long-term survival and quality of life after lung transplantation is bronchiolitis obliterans syndrome (BOS). Bronchiolitis obliterans is a diffuse, concentric, luminal narrowing of the terminal bronchioli thought to be due to chronic allograft rejection. It occurs in a patchy but extensive distribution and results in a progressive loss of vital capacity and forced expiratory volume in 1 s (FEV_1) with an obstructive airflow pattern. It affects up to 55% of patients at five years after transplantation [37] and the pathogenesis remains poorly understood (see Chapter 19).

Bronchiolitis obliterans is a multifactorial disease. The three main factors thought to contribute to its occurrence are immunological damage, recurrent infection (viral or otherwise) and ischaemia of the bronchioli. Risk factors for the development of BOS include acute rejection, HLA mismatch [38], anti-HLA antibodies [39], CMV pneumonitis, donor/recipient CMV mismatch [40] and postoperative airways ischaemia [40].

Some of the factors contributing to BOS could be influenced by direct revascularization of the bronchial artery. Immunological damage could be modulated as the bronchial arteries supply the donor hilar and intrapulmonary lymph nodes and so enhance their viability, which in turn could increase the likelihood of the development of graft-versus-host disease and a mixed allogeneic chimerism. We have also found a low incidence of BOS in our series of patients who have undergone bronchial revascularization [22], but a larger number of patients need to be followed for a longer amount of time to confirm this observation.

Post-transplant function

Our studies have shown a pattern of respiration and a response to exercise which, although not normal, appears to be adequate for a good quality of life [41–44]. Further studies to define the role of reinnervation in changing the physiology of the transplanted organ are needed [45,46].

Conclusions

Lung transplantation can provide patients with advanced pulmonary disease with a good level of rehabilitation and excellent quality of life. Overall one, three and five year survival rates in the International Society for Heart and Lung Transplantation Registry are: 74%, 60% and 50% for bilateral sequential and double lungs; 74%, 57% and 46% for single lungs; and 63%, 50% and 42% for heart–lungs, respectively [21]. However, the benefits that can be obtained by lung transplantation are currently limited by the scarcity of organs suitable for transplantation and the long-term problem of bronchiolitis obliterans.

REFERENCES

1 United Kingdom Transplant Support Service Authority. *Thoracic Organ Transplant Audit.* UKTSSA, Bristol 2001.

2 Birks EJ, Owen V, Burton P, et al. Tumour necrosis factor-α is expressed in donor heart and predicts right ventricular failure after human heart transplantation. *Circulation* 2000; **102**: 326–331.

3 Birks EJ, Burton PB, Owen V, et al. Elevated tumor necrosis factor-alpha and interleukin-6 in myocardium and serum of malfunctioning donor hearts. *Circulation* 2000; **102**: III352–III358.

4 Birks EJ, Yacoub MH, Burton PBJ, et al. Activation of apoptotic and inflammatory pathways in dysfunctional donor hearts. *Transplantation* 2000; **70**: 1498–1506.

5 Loehe F, Mueller C, Annecke T, et al. Pulmonary graft function after long-term preservation of non-heart-beating donor lungs. *Ann Thorac Surg* 2000; **69**: 1556–1562.

6 Egan TM. Non-heart-beating lung donors: yes or no? *Ann Thorac Surg* 2000; **70**: 1451–1452.

7 Shimada K, Kondo T, Okada Y, et al. Lung transplantation from non-heart-beating donors. *Transplant Proc* 2000; **32**: 279–280.

8 Fukushima N, Shirakura R, Chang J, et al. Successful multiorgan transplants from non-heart-beating donors using percutaneous cardiopulmonary support. *Transplant Proc* 1998; **30**: 3783–3784.

9 Barr ML, Schenkel FA, Cohen RG, et al. Recipient and donor outcomes in living related and unrelated lobar transplantation. *Transplant Proc* 1998; **30**: 2261–2263.

10 Starnes VA, Barr ML, Cohen RG, et al. Living-donor lobar lung transplantation experience: intermediate results. *J Thorac Cardiovasc Surg*. 1996; **112**: 1284–1290.

11 Wilhelm MJ, Pratschke J, Beato F, et al. Activation of the heart by donor brain death accelerates acute rejection after transplantation. *Circulation* 2000; **102**: 2426–2433.

12 Birmingham K. Merger signals shift in xenotransplantation research. *Nature Med* 2000; **6**: 1195.

13 Van der Laan LJW, Lockey C, Griffeth BC, et al. Infection by porcine endogenous retrovirus after islet xenotransplantation in SCID mice. *Nature* 2000; **407**: 90–94.

14 Paradis K, Langford G, Long Z, et al. Search for cross-species transmission of porcine endogenous retrovirus in patients treated with living pig tissue. *Science* 1999; **285**: 1236–1241.

15 Griffiths PD. Xenotransplantation: one trotter forward, one claw back. *Lancet* 2000; **356**: 1049–1050.

16 Mikhail G, Gibbs J, Richardson M, et al. An evaluation of nebulized prostacyclin in patients with primary and secondary pulmonary hypertension. *Eur Heart J* 1997; **18**: 1499–1504.

17 Elliott MW, Simonds AK, Carroll MP, Wedzicha JA, Branthwaite MA. Domiciliary nocturnal nasal intermittent positive pressure ventilation in hypercapnic respiratory failure due to chronic obstructive lung disease: effects on sleep and quality of life. *Thorax* 1992; **47**: 342–348.

18 Bott J, Carroll MP, Conway JH, et al. Randomised controlled trial of nasal ventilation in acute ventilatory failure due to chronic obstructive airways disease. *Lancet* 1993; **341**: 1555–1557.

19 Festenstein H, Banner N, Smith J, et al. The influence of HLA matching and lymphocytotoxic antibody status on survival in heart–lung allograft recipients receiving cyclosporin and azathioprine. *Transplant Proc* 1989; **21**: 797–798.

20 Bando K, Armitage JM, Paradis IL, et al. Indications for and results of single, bilateral and heart–lung transplantation for pulmonary hypertension. *J Thorac Cardiovasc Surg* 1994; **108**: 1056–1065.

21 Hertz MI, Taylor DO, Trulock EP, et al. The Registry of the International Society for Heart and Lung Transplantation: 19th official report – 2002. *J Heart Lung Transplant* 2002; **21**: 950–970.

22 Yacoub M, Al-Kattan KM, Tadjkarimi S, Eren T, Khaghani A. Medium term results of direct bronchial arterial revascularisation using IMA for single lung transplantation (SLT with direct revascularisation). *Eur J Cardiothorac Surg* 1997; **11**: 1030–1036.

23 Yacoub MH, Khaghani A, Aravot D, et al. Cardiac transplantation from live donors. *J Am Coll Cardiol* 1988; **11**: 102A.

24 Cavarocchi NC, Badellino M. Heart–lung transplantation. The domino procedure. *Ann Thorac Surg* 1989; **38**: 130–133.

25 Kirklin JK, Naftel DC, Kirklin JW, et al. Pulmonary, vascular resistance and the risk of heart transplantation. *J Heart Transplant* 1988; **7**: 331–336.

26 Doering CW, Jalil JE, Janicki JS, et al. Collagen network remodelling and diastolic stiffness of the left ventricle with pressure overload hypertrophy. *Cardiovasc Res* 1988; **22**: 686–695.

27 Scheuer J, Buttrick P. The cardiac hypertrophic response to pathological and physiological overload. *Circulation* 1986; **75**: 163–168.

28 Wong K, Boheler KR, Petrou M, Yacoub MH. Pharmacological modulation of pressure overload hypertrophy changes in ventricular function, extracellular matrix and gene expressions. *Circulation* 1997; 96: 2239–2246.

29 Khaghani A, Santini F, Dyke CM, Onuzu O, Radley-Smith R, Yacoub MH. Heterotopic cardiac transplantation in infants and children. *J Thorac Cardiovasc Surg* 1997; **113**: 1042–1049.

30 Yacoub MH. Two hearts that beat as one. *Circulation* 1995; **92**: 16–161.

31 Trulock EP. Lung transplantation. *Am J Resp Crit Care Med* 1997; **155**: 789–818.

32 Oldenburg N, Lam KM, Khan MA, et al. Evaluation of human cytomegalovirus gene expression in thoracic organ transplant recipients using nucleic acid sequence-based amplification. *Transplantation* 2000; **70**: 1209–1215.

33 Read RC, Shanker S, Rutman A, et al. Ciliary beat frequency and structure of recipient and donor epithelia following lung transplantation. *Eur Resp J* 1991; **4**: 796–801.

34 Patterson GA, Todd TR, Cooper JD, Pearson FG, Winton TL, Maurer J. Airway complications after double lung transplantation. *J Thorac Cardiovasc Surg* 1990; **99**: 14–21.

35 Colquhoun IW, Gascoigne AD, Au J, Corris PA, Hilton CJ, Dark JH. Airway complications after pulmonary transplantation. *Ann Thorac Surg* 1994; **57**: 141–145.

36 Khaghani A, Tadjkarimi S, Al-Kattan K, et al. Wrapping the anastomosis with omentum or an internal mammary artery pedicle does not improve bronchial healing after single lung transplantation: results of a randomised clinical trial. *J Heart Transplant* 1994; **13**: 767–773.

37 Boehler A, Estenne M. Obliterative bronchiolitis after lung transplantation. *Curr Opin Pulm Med* 2000; **6**: 133–139.

38 Sundaresan S, Mohanakumar T, Smith MA, et al. HLA-A locus mismatches and development of antibodies to HLA after lung transplantation correlate with the development of bronchiolitis obliterans syndrome. *Transplantation* 1998; **65**: 648–653.

39 Smith MA, Sundaresan S, Mohanakumar T, et al. Effect of development of antibodies to HLA and cytomegalovirus mismatch on lung transplantation survival and development of bronchiolitis obliterans syndrome. *J Thorac Cardiovasc Surg* 1998; **116**: 812–820.

40 Bando K, Paradis IL, Similo S, et al. Obliterative bronchiolitis after lung and heart–lung transplantation. An analysis of risk factors and management. *J Thorac Cardiovasc Surg* 1995; **110**: 4–13; discussion 13–14.

41 Banner NR, Lloyd MH, Hamilton RD, Innes JA, Guz A, Yacoub MH. Cardiopulmonary response to dynamic exercise after heart and combined heart–lung transplantation. *Br Heart J* 1989; **61**: 215–223.

42 Banner NR, Williams TDM, Patel N, Chalmers J, Lightman SL, Yacoub MH. Altered cardiovascular and neurohormonal responses to head-up tilt after heart–lung transplantation. *Circulation* 1990; **82**: 863–871.

43 Shea SA, Horner RL, Banner NR, et al. The effect of human heart–lung transplantation upon breathing at rest and during sleep. *Respir Physiol* 1988; **72**: 131–150.

44 O'Brien BJ, Banner NR, Gibson S, Yacoub MH. The Nottingham Health Profile as a measure of quality of life following combined heart and lung transplantation. *J Epidemiol Commun Health* 1988; **42**: 232–234.

45 Springall DR, Polak JM, Howard L, et al. Persistence of intrinsic neurones and possible phenotypic changes after extrinsic denervation of human respiratory tract by heart–lung transplantation. *Am Rev Respir Dis* 1990; **141**: 1538–1546.

46 Wharton J, Polak JM, Gordon L, et al. Immunohistochemical demonstration of human cardiac innervation before and after transplantation. *Circ Res* 1990; **66**: 900–912.

12

Patient selection and indications for lung transplantation

Janet R. Maurer

CIGNA HealthCare, Bloomfield, Connecticut, USA

Introduction

Selection of appropriate candidates for lung transplantation, as it is for all solid organ transplantation, remains one of the most important elements of a successful outcome. Since the number of patients awaiting organs continues to significantly exceed the number of donor organs, it is important to ensure that patients who have far advanced pulmonary disease, but are otherwise medically appropriate, are selected. Optimal outcomes also require careful preoperative medical management. This chapter will address general health and disease-related selection criteria, elements of the selection process, medical management prior to transplantation and the selection of type of transplant.

General medical health

Transplant surgery itself is a major stressor for any patient with pulmonary failure; it is much more so when immunosuppressive medications have been started. In this milieu, comorbidities, even those which otherwise may seem trivial, can have an important negative impact on outcome.

In general, potential transplant candidates should be in excellent health except for their advanced lung disease. Since most of the patients who present for lung transplantation, however, are between 40 and 65 years old [1], it is not surprising that many have at least one comorbidity. In addition, the nature of many of the diseases/causes from which patients develop end-stage pulmonary disease, i.e. systemic illness such as cystic fibrosis or scleroderma, smoking-related chronic obstructive pulmonary disease (COPD), are such that comorbidities are expected as part of the entire picture.

Comorbidities that are optimally treated and, as a result, are well controlled such that they are unlikely to impact on the grafted lung or other vital organs are generally acceptable in the lung transplant candidate. These might include, for example, diabetes mellitus, which can be present in 25% or more of adult cystic fibrosis patients [2]. Diabetes is also often present in patients with other diseases who are using steroids. In the absence of demonstrable nephropathy, ischaemic cardiomyopathy, gastroparesis or other end-organ damage, well-controlled diabetes has not been identified as a poor outcome prognosticator. Other common illnesses, such as hypertension, peptic ulcer disease, and diverticulosis would be handled in a similar fashion. If, on the other hand, a potential candidate has diabetes that is volatile, with frequent large fluctuations in glucose values despite aggressive management, or a patient has hypertension that requires three or more drugs for control, postoperative management would probably be extremely difficult. It is important to ensure that optimal medical management has been attempted in these situations. Apparent poor control of hypertension, for example, may actually be a result of suboptimal dosing of medications, poor patient education or even use of suboptimal medications. Some diseases that have periods of exacerbation and remission need to be assessed on a case-by-case basis. Inflammatory bowel disease is an example of a disease which, depending on its course in a specific patient may be of little consequence to the patient's ultimate transplantation outcome or, alternatively, may be a major negative risk factor.

Those comorbidities that are more often themselves associated with poor quality of life and a less successful post-transplant outcome include symptomatic metabolic bone disease, nonambulatory status, obesity or significant weight loss, on-going psychosocial problems, on-going substance abuse, thoracic cage deformity with fixation, colonization with resistant organisms, and ongoing high dose or long-term steroid use. Each of the listed comorbidities can potentially be addressed and, if successfully treated, may render the patient a transplantation candidate. Conditions that are amenable to treatment should always be addressed before a life-saving transplant is denied to the patient.

Metabolic bone disease

Although not clearly identified as a major factor in lung transplantation outcomes until the mid-1990s, metabolic bone disease now has been widely recognized for its morbidity in this population and is the subject of several studies. It has been shown that more than half of patients with diagnoses of cystic fibrosis and COPD have significant osteopenia or osteoporosis when evaluated for transplantation. In a recent prospective study of pre- and post-lung transplantation patients, a fall in bone mineral density of about 5% was shown in both femoral neck and lumbar spine within 6–12 months of transplantation. This change was associated with fractures in 18% of the patients [3]. Two other studies have demonstrated the benefit of bisphosphonate pamidronate – which was delivered intravenously every three months for one to two years – or hormone replacement therapy in reducing the rate of bone loss or actually improving bone density in the early post-transplantation period. Only one of the studies, however, showed a difference in the rate of post-transplantation fractures [4,5]. These data along with other earlier studies support the detection and treatment of metabolic bone disease as early as possible in the lung transplant candidate. A new recombinant form of parathyroid hormone, PTH (1–34), has been shown in multiple studies to be a strong stimulus to bone formation and probably will soon be available. It may have a role in 'recovering' patients who are noncandidates because of severe metabolic bone disease.

Nonambulatory status

Nonambulatory status in itself is associated with increased bone mineral loss and on-going deconditioning. However, it also identifies patients who lack motivation, are significantly depressed, do not understand the benefits of on-going exercise or who are very end stage. These are all markers of poor outcome. Patients who are depressed, unmotivated or lack understanding of their disease can often become reasonable transplant candidates when these issues are identified and managed appropriately. Patients who are essentially terminal or who are ventilator dependent, on the other hand, are less likely to be salvageable. Ventilator dependency represents the highest risk for early death post-transplantation according to the United Network for Organ Sharing (UNOS)/International Society

for Heart and Lung Transplantation Registry data [1]. In addition to the poorer outcomes reported for this group of patients, published data show prolonged periods of ventilation postoperatively and significantly longer hospital stays [6].

Poor nutritional status

Poor nutritional status, usually defined as ideal body weight less than 70% predicted or more than 130% predicted, are usually considered to be risk factors for poor outcome. Recent literature in lung transplants supports this concern [7]. The same study and two others have identified low body weight as a potential post-transplant survival risk factor [7–9]. Others, however, have not found this to be the case. At any rate, nutrition is one area where a significant impact – either by regular food supplementation or by strict dieting and exercise as the case may require – can often be made. Thus, optimal, or at least improved, nutrition ought to be a goal for preoperative patients. Uncorrected morbid obesity, because of its operative and other associated comorbidities, remains a relative contraindication.

Unresolved or untreated psychosocial issues and substance abuse

The disruption of normal life style and family interrelationships that accompany chronic illness make psychosocial issues virtually universal. Some patients will have, in addition to the situational changes associated with their disease, pre-existing mental or interpersonal problems that can become exacerbated by the transplantation process and make postoperative compliance and health maintenance a challenge. At the least, a psychosocial evaluation should be completed on all potential candidates and should include a psychiatric examination covering current and past mental health, compliance with past and current treatment regimens, history of substance use and abuse, assessment of current cognitive status, an assessment of the patient's interpersonal and intrapersonal resources and liabilities and an interview of the patient's support system [10]. As with the medical assessment of the potential candidate, areas of need that can be successfully addressed are often identified. These often include untreated anxiety or depression, which are easily addressed with therapy or medication. Substance abuse issues with narcotics, alcohol or tobacco must also be addressed, as patients should be free from such drugs for at least six months prior to consideration for transplantation. Poorly responsive psychiatric issues or refusal by the patient to comply with treatment regimens bode poorly for postoperative compliance with the required complex medical programmes and should be considered contraindications to transplant candidacy.

Thoracic cage deformity with fixation

Patients with progressive musculoskeletal diseases often are not transplant candidates because of the likelihood that the disease will progress after transplantation and impair ability to cough, breathe deeply, and adequately clear secretions. However, patients with primarily bony deformations may present a different problem. Kyphoscoliosis can present as respiratory failure with little intrinsic lung disease simply because of the chest deformity and fixation of the bones causing profound hypoventilation. The assessment of a patient becomes much more difficult when there is underlying lung disease accompanying significant kyphoscoliosis because the relative contribution of each process to the respiratory failure may be difficult to assess. This situation may require special studies to assess mobility of the chest cage, maximum voluntary ventilation and other manoeuvres before a decision regarding the potential benefit of transplant can be made.

Colonization with resistant organisms

The issue of resistant organisms is an ever-changing scenario in the selection of transplant recipients. Some types of candidates for lung transplantation, those with bronchiectasis and cystic fibrosis, are *always* colonized with pathogenic organisms and other types of candidate, such as those with obstructive lung disease and pulmonary fibrosis, *may be* colonized with pathogenic organisms. Depending upon how many courses of antibiotics these patients have received, the colonizing organisms may be highly resistant to antibiotic treatment. Initial concerns about the risk of disseminated infection in the face of postoperative immunosuppression in these patients has been significantly modified as transplant centres have gained more experience. Practically speaking, nearly all patients with bronchiectasis (including cystic fibrosis patients) harbor resistant bacterial organisms. A growing body of data suggests that when the bulk of the resistant organism load is removed, as is the case in bilateral lung transplantation, in most cases patient survival is not compromised. Specific data have been published relative to resistant species of *pseudomonal* organism [11]. The one type of resistant organism that has clearly been reported to have a negative impact upon outcome is *Burkholderia cepacia*, where in several series colonized patients appear to have a 40–60% death rate, mostly in the early postoperative period [12]. All *Burkholderia* strains may not have the same level of

virulence, however, with those at particular risk probably harbouring genomovar-3 [13]. Future selection of candidates may include specific genetic typing of their strains of *B. cepacia* to assess risk. Colonization with other types of hard-to-treat organisms, particularly fungi and atypical mycobacteria, has not been reported to result in disseminated infection in the postoperative period – with two exceptions. Early reports of *Candida* colonization in donors identified as a specific survival risk for recipients, but there have been no subsequent studies reproducing this experience [14]. *Aspergillus* species colonization may be much more significant. Many centres have documented the morbidity and mortality associated with *Aspergillus* infection [15–17]. Nevertheless it is not clear whether preoperative colonization, particularly if the recipient receives a bilateral transplant and appropriate postoperative prophylaxis, confers a particular survival risk. Thus, the impact of *Aspergillus* colonization on a specific patient's candidacy for transplantation should be considered in the context of the patient's overall situation.

High dose or long-term steroid use

In the early years of lung transplantation, the use of steroids was considered a contraindication. This is no longer the case [18–19], but the long-term use of steroids remains a problem primarily because of the morbidity resulting from this type of treatment. Steroid morbidity includes osteoporosis, hypertension, hyperglycaemia, myopathy, obesity and skin fragility. Referring physicians are encouraged to taper steroids as much and as quickly as possible, preferably to dosages less than or equivalent to 15–20 mg prednisone.

Medical contraindications to lung transplantation

Nonpulmonary organ failure

Generally the presence of significant nonpulmonary vital organ dysfunction is a contraindication to lung transplantation. The problem becomes determining 'significant organ dysfunction'. Of particular concern is renal disease because one of the primary toxicities of the required calcineurin immunosuppressant (either tacrolimus or ciclosporin) in lung transplantation is nephrotoxicity [20]. Since the majority of lung recipients have as much as a 40% fall in creatinine clearance within a few months of transplantation, creatinine clearances of at least 50% predicted are usually required for lung transplant candidates.

The importance of coronary disease has changed considerably since the early era of lung transplantation. From being considered an absolute contraindication, the thinking about coronary artery disease has evolved so that transplant candidates may have limited treated or treatable coronary disease or one which can be addressed pretransplantation or at the time of transplantation. It is imperative that left ventricular function be normal or near normal. In some limited circumstances, patients with combined lung disease and ventricular dysfunction may be candidates for heart–lung transplantation.

Hepatic function is also important in lung transplantation outcomes. Occult cirrhosis can become manifest with the stress of surgery and the overall impact of the transplantation process. Thus it is important to take a careful history to elicit prior alcohol abuse and to test for evidence of hepatitis B and C. Evidence of persistent hepatitis B antigenaemia is usually a contraindication to transplantation. A history of previous significant alcohol use or evidence of hepatitis C infection should trigger a liver biopsy to assess the extent of liver damage present. Significant fibrosis/cirrhosis generally contraindicates lung transplantation. Two specific diagnoses, cystic fibrosis and alpha-1-antitrypsin deficiency, often have associated liver disease as part of the underlying illness. In these patients if the history suggests any liver disease a liver biopsy may be indicated to assess the extent of damage. Portal hypertension in any case would be a contraindication to lung transplantation.

HIV infection

In the International Criteria for the Selection of Lung Transplant Candidates, the presence of human immunodeficiency virus (HIV) infection was deemed an absolute contraindication to lung transplantation. In the current era of multidrug treatment of HIV with both antiretroviral agents and protease inhibitors, this thinking has changed somewhat. Several liver and heart transplantations have been performed on experimental protocols with satisfactory early and intermediate term results [21]. This has led to a rethinking of the approach to patients with HIV. At present, probably the best approach is to assess each case on an individual basis, taking into account the extent of HIV-related health issues and the progression of the underlying process. At the very least, the virus should have been undetectable in the patient's blood for a sustained period of time.

Malignancy

A history of malignancy is not uncommon, but problematic in dealing with transplant candidates for any solid organ. Immunosuppression removes one of the primary defences of the cancer victim against the disease. The primary question is how remote is remote enough? Generally, at least two years should have elapsed since there was any evidence of malignancy according to data reported by Penn [22], who for many years kept the only registry of post-transplant malignancy. His data, which were probably somewhat incomplete as they depended on voluntary reporting, also suggest a high recurrence rate for certain types of tumour, including lymphomas, most carcinomas of the breast, prostate or colon or large (>5 cm) symptomatic renal carcinomas [23]. The exceptions to a required disease-free waiting period are basal and squamous cell carcinoma of the skin, which, if they recur, are easily visible and can be quickly removed.

Disease-specific issues and selection criteria

Unlike with most other solid organ transplants, the underlying diagnosis is important in determining when a patient should be selected as a lung transplant candidate. Emphysema patients, for example, generally have slowly progressive disease and often live extended periods of time with very poor functional capacity before they die; thus they can be selected when very ill and still survive to transplantation. Pulmonary fibrosis patients, in contrast, often have a relentlessly progressive course with death in three to five years, no matter what therapeutic intervention is tried and must be selected relatively early in the disease or miss the window for transplantation. Other diseases such as cystic fibrosis and pulmonary hypertension may create more difficulty in prognosis if state of the art care, which can alter progressive functional loss, is given. Primary pulmonary hypertension or secondary pulmonary hypertension are fundamentally different from the other types of diagnosis coming to lung transplantation because they involve primarily the pulmonary vasculature and not the parenchyma. The use of novel vasodilator therapy in the past decade in these patients has changed their prognosis by at least temporarily allaying symptoms and prolonging life. This therapy has reset the threshold haemodynamics for determining when to list patients, but it has been difficult to determine appropriate new parameters. As a result, a number of patients have died on intravenous vasodilator treatment because of being listed too late. It should be kept in mind that patients are generally chosen for lung transplantation when they are considered to be within two years of dying from their illness. This reflects the facts that patients are often very disabled, with poor quality of life by this point in their diseases, and the wait for a donor organ at many transplant centres is up to two years. In this section I will review the current published criteria and emerging

Table 12.1. Disease-specific criteria for transplant candidate selection

Cystic fibrosis/bronchiectasis
FEV_1 < 30% predicted *or*
FEV_1 > 30% predicted *and* any of the following:
- Rapid FEV_1 deterioration
- Rapid weight loss
- Increased numbers of hospitalizations
- Massive haemoptysis
- PCO_2 > 55 mmHg or PO_2 < 55 mmHg (7.3 kPa)

High risk: female; paediatric or adolescent

Obstructive lung disease
FEV_1 < 25% predicted *and/or*
PCO_2 > 55 mmHg (7.3 kPa) with pulmonary hypertension/cor pulmonale

Cryptogenic pulmonary fibrosis
Symptomatic disease: includes *any* symptom including rest or exercise desaturation *or*
    exercise dyspnoea
Desaturation should be reassessed every three months.
Transplant-eligible candidates often have:
    VC < 60–70% predicted
    DLCO < 50–60% predicted

Pulmonary hypertension
NYHA class III or IV while on adequate epoprostenol (or equivalent) vasodilator
Worsening functional capacity/cor pulmonale despite increased doses of vasodilator

Eisenmenger's syndrome
Progressive symptoms: NYHA class III or IV

Paediatric cardiopulmonary disease
Optimum management with continued NYHA class III or IV *and/or* cor pulmonale, cyanosis,
    falling cardiac output

Note: FEV_1, forced expiratory volume in 1 s; VC, vital capacity; DLCO diffusing capacity for
carbon monoxide; NYHA, New York Heart Association.
Source: Adapted from ref. 25.

data when available for selection of patients with the four general types of pulmonary disease.

Cystic fibrosis and bronchiectasis

The overwhelming bulk of patients referred with the pathology of bronchiectasis are suffering from cystic fibrosis. Occasionally patients with other causes of bronchiectasis such as ciliary dyskinesia syndromes or postinfectious disease are referred, but the numbers are so small that no good data exist to predict survivals. Thus, data derived from cystic fibrosis populations are generally applied to any bronchiectatic patient.

Cystic fibrosis patients have been the largest single group to receive living donor grafts. In that operation two donors are used and each donates a lower lobe. Initial patients receiving these grafts were chosen very late in their disease in what many consider beyond the transplantation window.

However, now most of these candidates are chosen according to the same criteria as those candidates destined for cadaver grafts.

The current criteria were derived from a landmark paper on the epidemiology of cystic fibrosis published by Kerem et al. in 1992 [24]. This study reported the longitudinal follow-up of a large, relatively constant group of cystic fibrosis patients and was able to correlate pulmonary function parameters with risk of death within certain time periods. The pulmonary function and arterial blood gas parameters were strongly predictive of an approximate risk of death within two years once they reached certain levels (Table 12.1). Other points that were made in this study were that low body weight (<70% weight-for-height ratio), female sex and poor pulmonary function occurring at a younger age were predictive of poor survival.

The Kerem et al. [24] criteria have come under some criticism from other cystic fibrosis centres. The fact that the population reported upon was a fairly homogeneous population has been cited as a potential weakness for that population may not fairly represent the broader cystic fibrosis population in North America, Europe or other continents. In point, it has been noted that the Toronto population has a relatively high rate of colonization with *B. cepacia*, which as noted previously has been associated with rapid deterioration and higher mortality in some groups of cystic fibrosis patients. While this same organism is a known colonizer in some UK cystic fibrosis populations, it is much less common in US cystic fibrosis populations. The importance of this difference is unclear, however, since the overall life expectancy of the Toronto population was longer than that of the average US cystic fibrosis population.

Following the publication of the selection criteria in 1998 [25], two single centre studies challenged the use of pulmonary function data as a primary criterion for selection. In these populations, patients with forced expiratory volume in 1 s (FEV$_1$) values of < 30% but without *B. cepacia* colonization, the median survival ranged from 3.9 to 4.6 years [26,27]. In paediatric patients, another study argued, the 30% cutoff might be too low and a 50% FEV$_1$ might be a better predictor of two year survival [28].

In the wake of this controversy, authors have tried to use other criteria such as exercise data, haemodynamic data and the presence of comorbidities such as diabetes to better define a poor prognostic group. None of these approaches has as yet defined a better system than that of the criteria defined by Kellem et al. [24] for selecting cystic fibrosis patients with poor prognoses. Perhaps the best chance of refining the current criteria is through the use of models in which a number of variables from each individual patient is used to predict survival. One of these models has worked with the US Cystic Fibrosis Foundation Patient Registry to identify nine separate parameters that appear to affect five year mortality [29]. These include FEV$_1$ percentage predicted, age, gender, weight-for-age, pancreatic sufficiency, diabetes mellitus, *Staphylococcus aureus* infection, *B. cepacia* infection and annual number of acute exacerbations. Most of these parameters are acknowledged in the Kerem et al. study, but their relative contributions to survivorship are not precisely documented. While this model is detailed and it remains to be proven in clinical practice, it does underscore the complexity of the disease. Hopefully this, or other models like it, will help in more precise identification of the most appropriate transplant candidates.

A final factor not accounted for in any model is the changing management of the disease. While the great strides in improved life expectancy that occurred since the 1960s have certainly slowed in the last 10 years, many new approaches to cystic fibrosis treatment have followed the discovery of the cystic fibrosis transmembrane regulator genetic defect. Genetic manipulation/therapy is almost certain to become clinically feasible in the near future, along with improvements in anti-inflammatory and antibiotic treatment. Advances in any or all of these may significantly impact on prognosis and delay or decrease the need for transplantation for these patients.

Nonbronchiectatic chronic obstructive disease

Obstructive lung disease constitutes approximately half of all lung transplant recipients because this type of pulmonary disease has a much higher prevalence in the general population than any of the other pulmonary diseases that cause death. In the US population alone each year more than 110 000 deaths are due to obstructive lung disease; approximately 350 die from cystic fibrosis [29,30]. Since such a small percentage of those who have advanced disease will ever receive a lung transplant and since there are a number of things that can be done to improve quality of life for these patients, it is imperative that medical management be optimized. This means that appropriate bronchodilator and anti-inflammatory airway therapy be utilized and the patient be thoroughly educated in proper usage. In addition most patients will benefit from a well-designed pulmonary rehabilitation programme with educational and nutritional aspects as well as the exercise portion [31]. The need for supplemental oxygen therapy should also be addressed and appropriate prescriptions for rest, exercise and sleep needs written. Sometimes the patient's quality of life is so improved by these measures that transplantation is deferred.

Volume reduction surgery in which the apical (most diseased) portions of both lungs are removed to improve the mechanical aspects of the respiratory system in patients with severe emphysema has been recently popularized as an alternative to lung transplantation for some patients [32–34]. Recent interim reports from a large prospective randomized trial in the USA, the National Emphysema Treatment Trial, however, has clearly shown a significant early mortality in the more severely ill patients [35]. Even with the uncertainty of what constitutes a good volume reduction candidate and the long-term outcomes of the procedure in general, volume reduction may be an attractive option to some patients. The reality is that lung transplant will not be an option for the vast majority of patients dying from emphysema; those who are transplanted have only a 50% chance of being alive in five years, the financial burdens of transplantation and the likelihood of immunosuppressive complications.

It is also important for COPD patients requesting a transplant to understand that data from the UNOS/International Heart and Lung Transplantation Society

Registry shows that transplantation does not confer a survival advantage to patients with their diagnosis [36]. The transplant team should communicate this to the patient. Transplantation does probably confer a significant functional improvement and therefore quality of life advantage to survivors.

The pulmonary function parameters for consideration of COPD patients for transplant are listed in Table 12.1. While the FEV_1 upper limit is 25% predicted, for practical purposes most patients receiving transplants have FEV_1 values under 20%. The exceptions are those patients who have significant hypoxaemia and hypercapnia with episodes of cor pulmonale. This constellation has been associated with a poorer prognosis and may occur with somewhat higher FEV_1 values.

Pulmonary fibrosis

Pulmonary fibrosis is fortunately much less common than obstructive lung disease, but it tends to be a relentlessly progressive disease, especially in the idiopathic or cryptogenic form, and has a much shorter course than most obstructive diseases. Pulmonary fibrosis is a heterogeneous group of processes. Those which most often come to transplantation are idiopathic or cryptogenic disease, familial disease, fibrotic hypersensitivity lung disease, asbestosis and fibrosis as part of a systemic disease. The most common systemic diseases are sarcoidosis, scleroderma, lymphangioleiomyomatosis (LAM) and histiocytosis X. The presence of a systemic disease poses added problems and issues for transplantation that will be discussed below.

Cryptogenic disease occurs generally in older patients with the mean age at diagnosis of late 50s to early 60s. Most studies of these patients document a mean survival of from 3.5 to 5 years from diagnosis. Numerous studies have sought to define the best prognostic criteria, but none has been very successful [37–39]. Compounding the difficulty in defining useful prognostic features is the difficulty in finding successful medical treatment. None of the currently available medical treatments – including corticosteroids, various other cytotoxic drugs or anti-inflammatories – appear to have better than a 20% chance of resulting in improvement or stabilization. Current studies assessing the potential for antifibrotic agents and interferons are ongoing.

Unfortunately time is often lost while futile treatments are being pursued in this cohort of patients. The criteria listed in Table 12.1 are meant to encourage early referral of patients, as the majority of these patients die before appropriate donors can be found. In general, pulmonary fibrosis patients who are not improving within a few months

of the start of medical therapy, or certainly those who are worsening, should be quickly referred to a transplant centre for evaluation. This referral process should not be delayed while different drug regimens are tried. Time is of the essence with these patients and most will die waiting for a graft even if referral has been early.

Since cryptogenic pulmonary fibrosis patients are often near the upper limits of age for lung transplantation and since they have often been subjected to prolonged immunosuppressive therapy, they are prone to other comorbidities related both to age and their former therapy. Toxicities of the immunosuppressive therapy include hypertension, osteoporosis, diabetes mellitus, haemorrhagic cystitis, and cataracts among others. Reduction of drug dosages to the minimal levels at which they are effective helps the patient to remain a suitable transplant candidate.

Other concerns include occult infection in areas of traction bronchiectasis or large cystic areas, indolent reactivation tuberculosis or fungal infection and coexistent lung carcinomas. These issues are best assessed by the use of computed tomography (CT) scans with high resolution cuts. Scans should be done at least yearly while the patient remains a transplant candidate.

Possibly the best management for the cryptogenic pulmonary fibrosis patient is pulmonary rehabilitation accompanied by adequate oxygen supplementation. This group of patients almost invariably has very high supplemental oxygen needs. The requirements at rest are often at least doubled with minimal exercise and it is critical to assess requirements with exercise to avoid critical and prolonged episodes of desaturation. The oxygen requirements also change rapidly and should be reassessed at rest and exercise at no longer than three month intervals.

In general the same criteria used for selection of patients with cryptogenic pulmonary fibrosis are used for patients with other diagnoses such as fibrotic hypersensitivity lung disease, drug-induced fibrotic disease, etc. (see Table 12.1). The same criteria are also used for patients with systemic diseases, but who are dying of pulmonary fibrosis. However, these patients pose some other issues as discussed below.

Systemic disease with pulmonary fibrosis

A number of systemic diseases involve the lung as a primary part of the disease. Most often the pulmonary manifestation that results in pulmonary failure is an interstitial inflammation that progresses to pulmonary fibrosis. The other common pulmonary process seen in systemic disease is pulmonary vascular involvement resulting in pulmonary hypertension; it will be discussed in the section on pulmonary hypertension, below.

Sarcoidosis is the most frequent underlying diagnosis of systemic-related pulmonary fibrosis. This, as well as most of the other systemic-related pulmonary fibrosis patterns, is different in both distribution and underlying histopathology from that of cryptogenic pulmonary fibrosis. In general, the systemic disease-related pulmonary fibrosis does not progress at the same relentless rate as that of cryptogenic disease. In fact, in diseases such as LAM, histiocytosis X or sarcoidosis, 15 or more years may elapse from the diagnosis until the patient reaches the end-stage of the disease. Pulmonary functions may be difficult to interpret in these diseases as they may be restrictive and obstructive or may be primarily obstructive! A common feature is often a marked reduction in diffusing capacity; yet reliable prognostic criteria for any of these diagnoses have not been developed. It is probably best to refer patients early who appear to have progressive disease despite appropriate medical therapy. 'Progression' might include increasing symptoms, the requirement for supplemental oxygen therapy or deteriorating pulmonary function including diffusing capacity.

Because these are all systemic diseases, it is important to assure that other end organs are not significantly impaired before proceeding to transplantation. In sarcoid patients, for example, both kidney and liver function should be carefully evaluated. In LAM patients, abdominal CT should be done to assess for the presence of any angiomyolipomas and their size.

The group of diseases referenced above have all been noted to recur in transplanted grafts. Sarcoidosis has been reported to recur most often [40], but both LAM and histiocytosis X as well as other, rarer diseases have also been reported. In most instances the diseases have been subclinical or have not resulted in recurrent pulmonary failure. Long-term follow-up of recurrent cases has not yet been documented.

The other major group of systemic diseases with pulmonary fibrosis as a feature are the autoimmune diseases. Scleroderma most often presents with pulmonary fibrosis, though mixed connective tissue disease and systemic lupus erythematosus may also have it as a feature. In these diseases, the pulmonary disease does not seem to progress as fast as in cryptogenic pulmonary fibrosis, but it is often the cause of death. In general, the same referral criteria as are used in the cryptogenic disease are useful.

Aside from the usual concerns regarding adequate renal and hepatic function in the setting of systemic disease, scleroderma presents other challenges. Many scleroderma patients have oesophageal and other gut motility dysfunction that can be of concern. Oesophageal reflux with aspiration is a potential threat to the transplant so a careful evaluation of oesophageal function and successful medical treatment of reflux is essential in scleroderma patients coming to transplantation. Since gastroparesis has been documented as a frequent postoperative complication in lung transplantation [41], oesophageal problems can be magnified, especially in the early post-transplant period. This risk requires both careful medical management and specialized nursing care.

Pulmonary hypertension

Pulmonary hypertension occurs as a 'primary' process without a clear cause, secondary to a variety of insults to the pulmonary vascular bed, and as a manifestation of systemic illness. Regardless of its aetiology, this disease is a major cause of morbidity and mortality in its victims. Until recent years, patients generally underwent a progressive downhill course; however, new vasodilators are achieving some inroads into treatment of this heterogeneous group of diseases and even better options are on the horizon.

Primary disease does not have a known cause, though recent genetic research, aided by specimens from the families with familial disease, may greatly improve our understanding of the pathogenesis [42]. In 1991, D'Alonzo and colleagues published data from the National Institutes of Health (NIH) Pulmonary Hypertension Registry that showed mean survival of all patients entering the registry was 2.8 years [43]. Since all of these patients had invasive haemodynamic studies, the authors were able to sort out 'good' and 'poor' haemodynamic prognostic data. These were used for several years as criteria for referral of patients for transplantation, and they were included in the 1998 'International Guidelines' [25]. In the past five years, however, the outlook for these patients has changed significantly with the widespread use of epoprostenol and the published haemodynamic data are no longer as useful. Epoprostenol has largely replaced calcium channel blockers and other oral vasodilators – though initial trials with these drugs may still be tried – and is considered the 'gold standard' of care because in most patients it both increases the functional capacity and may benefit survival [44]. Despite its apparent success, however, epoprostenol is far from being the perfect drug. Not only is it prohibitively expensive, it requires a complex continuous intravenous infusion system that is prone to complications, and dosages require regular escalation to maintain the desired effects. Nevertheless, patients often feel so much better on the drug that they request removal from the transplant waiting list.

One of the effects of eposprostenol's success as a treatment for pulmonary hypertension has been to make it more difficult to determine when patients are no longer responding to the drug and should be 'reactivated' on the transplant waiting list. Often precious time is wasted with attempts at dose escalation that are unsuccessful and the patient deteriorates and dies. Failure of a patient to respond in the usual fashion to an increase in dose of drug should be a warning sign to the treating physician. Other issues that might mandate earlier consideration for transplantation include multiple intravenous line infections or other complications of epoprostenol infusion.

In addition to epoprostenol, a synthetic, stable form of the drug called Remodulin, which is delivered as a continuous subcutaneous infusion, as well as several oral endothelin receptor antagonists, such as bosentan, and other oral drugs are under investigation and show promise in this disease. Nitric oxide also is a potent vasodilator and is in ongoing trials. Both Remodulin and Tracleer (bosentan) have gained regulatory approval in the USA. Occasionally, rapidly deteriorating patients have been offered a surgical procedure, atrial septostomy, with temporary relief of symptoms. One would hope that, in the next decade, a feasible long-term treatment for pulmonary hypertension will emerge and permanently remove this disease from those on the transplant waiting list.

Pulmonary hypertension in systemic disease

Pulmonary hypertension, like pulmonary fibrosis, is a common manifestation of systemic diseases such as scleroderma, CREST (calcinosis, Raynaud's phenomenon, oesophageal dysmotility, sclerodactyly and telangiectasis) syndrome, systemic lupus erythematosus, sarcoidosis, thromboembolic disease, veno-occlusive disease, capillary haemangiomatosis and some diet medication. In general, this disease is treated in the same manner as primary disease and has the same prognosis. It is imperative that, when available, any potential alternative treatments such as thromboendarterectomy in thromboembolic disease be explored.

Eisenmenger's syndrome

Pulmonary hypertension resulting from markedly increased blood flow through the lung, as occurs in many types of congenital heart disease, is known as Eisenmenger's syndrome. Interestingly the course of this disease is usually much longer than that of primary disease despite similar or even higher pulmonary pressure levels [45]. Prognostic indices for this group of patients are not well delineated and the role of vasodilator therapy is under investigation. Because of the lack of other good survival predictors, a functional classification of New York Heart Association (NYHA) class III or IV is usually used for listing;

however, because of the relatively prolonged survival of patients with severe disease, patients should be informed that a transplant might not confer a survival advantage.

Paediatric transplantation

End-stage pulmonary disease in the paediatric age group is generally either secondary to cystic fibrosis or cardiopulmonary vascular disease. Referral criteria are much harder to find for these patients, especially the very young children, because pulmonary function data may not be available and functional capacity is difficult to assess. Clinical course, blood gas data, rate of deterioration, and NYHA class III or IV status are useful parameters to use in making candidate decisions.

Investigations

Once identified as a potential candidate, the patient will need a series of investigations that measure vital organ function, previous exposure to infections that may be of importance postoperatively, and functional studies.

Blood work will include haematology and metabolic panels and arterial blood gases. In addition a series of serologies to determine exposure to Epstein–Barr virus, cytomegalovirus, hepatitis B, hepatitis C and HIV are necessary. Individual centres may require other serologies as well. Tissue typing will be done later, once the patient is determined to be a suitable candidate.

A 24 hour creatinine clearance will be done in patients with systemic diseases and may be done in other patients as well.

Imaging studies will include a DEXA (dual-energy X-ray absorptometry) scan to assess bone mineral density and an echocardiogram to assess cardiac function. Many centres require stress echocardiograms or cardiac catheterization in patients over 40 with risk factors for coronary artery disease. Recent recommendations from the American College of Cardiology are that coronary arteriography be limited to the latter high risk group [46].

Studies of pulmonary status include pulmonary functions, ventilation–perfusion scans, and CT scan of the chest, usually with high resolution images. CT studies are invaluable in better characterizing the lung disease and distribution, pleural and mediastinal abnormalities and unsuspected parenchymal nodules, bronchiectasis or cystic areas.

Other essential evaluations include the psychosocial, financial and nutritional. In each of these areas, potential sources of stress/abnormality that might result in an unsuccessful outcome should be identified and addressed.

Pretransplantation management

Once all information has been gathered regarding a potential candidate, the transplant team will meet and decide on the person's candidacy. Once a patient is selected for transplantation, the process is just beginning. Someone on the team, often a transplant coordinator, needs to educate the candidate about the details of the transplant process from start to finish. This educational process will need to be repeated at least every three months. Each member of the team should participate in this process in his or her interactions with the patient. It is often the case that certain needs are identified in candidates that require input during the waiting period. These might include, for example, osteopenia requiring medication or depression or anxiety requiring psychotherapy or medication, or a high body mass index requiring weight loss. Interventions to address all outstanding issues must be put in place and followed-up in the pretransplant period. Most patients should be placed in a regular exercise or rehabilitation programme to maintain as high a functional level as possible. To ensure that a candidate follows the suggested interventions and remains functional, regular preoperative visits to the transplant centre should be arranged. While different centres handle these visits in different ways, periodic reassessment of exercise capability, oxygen requirements and overall psychosocial and nutritional status are valuable. Patients waiting more than a year may require other repeat tests such as the CT scan and cardiac stress exam.

Which transplant for whom

There are three different types of lung grafts – unilateral, bilateral and heart–lung – however, the small number of heart–lung blocks that are available in North America essentially restricts the use of heart–lung transplantation to patients with irreparable heart disease. However, in Europe, heart–lung transplantation is used for a wider range of indications.

Bilateral transplant

All patients with bilateral lung infection require bilateral transplants. Pulmonary hypertension patients often also receive bilateral transplants in part because they often have a somewhat rocky early postoperative course. In theory most other patients would be adequately served by uni-

lateral grafts including pulmonary fibrosis patients, obstructive lung disease patients and most patients who have pulmonary failure in the setting of systemic disease. However, a number of bilateral grafts are done for these diseases and, in fact, the second highest number of patients receiving bilateral grafts are obstructive lung disease patients [1]. Some of these are performed because of colonization of the patient with potentially pathogenic organisms, for example *Aspergillus* species, or because of the age of the patient. However, many are performed because the surgeon feels the patient will do better with two lungs.

Unilateral grafts

Unilateral grafts represent slightly more than half of the transplantations performed each year [1]. Most unilateral grafts go to COPD patients and pulmonary fibrosis patients. The advantages of a unilateral transplant are that it is easier and quicker to perform, usually does not require placing the patient on bypass and potentially results in twice as many patients receiving lung grafts. There are significant disadvantages, however, to unilateral transplantation. The first of these is the native lung. Native lungs with abnormal architecture have been implicated in many complications that can result in the death of the patient. These range from overinflation, to pneumothorax, to life-threatening infection, to bronchogenic carcinoma [47,48]. In addition, recent data from the International Registry document a better survival for patients with bilateral grafts beginning at about three years post-transplantation [49].

Summary

Lung transplants have the poorest outcomes of all solid organ transplantations. Patient selection is the single most important factor in the eventual success of the transplant. To be a successful lung transplant recipient, the patient with advanced lung disease must be in general good health, be motivated to undertake the gruelling transplant process and psychologically capable of coping with the prolonged stress of the evaluation, surgery and postoperative period. This requires careful, extensive mental, nutritional, financial and medical evaluation and the support of the entire transplant team.

REFERENCES

1 Hosenpud JD, Bennett LE, Keck BM, et al. The Registry of the International Society for Heart and Lung Transplantation: 18th official report – 2001. *J Heart Lung Transplant* 2001; **20**: 805–815.

2 Yankaskas JR, Aris R. Outpatient care of the cystic fibrosis patient after lung transplantation. *Curr Opin Pulm Med* 2000; **6**: 551–557.

3 Spira A, Gutiérrez C, Chaparro C, et al. Osteoporosis and lung transplantation: a prospective study. Chest 2000; **117**: 476–481.

4 Trombetti A, Gerbase MW, Spiliopoulos A, et al. Bone mineral density in lung-transplant recipients before and after graft: prevention of lumbar spine post-transplantation-accelerated bone loss by pamidronate. *J Heart Lung Transplant* 2000; **19**: 736–743.

5 Aris RM, Lester GE, Renner JB, et al. Efficacy of pamidronate for osteoporosis in patients with cystic fibrosis following lung transplantation. *Am J Respir Crit Care Med* 2000; **162**: 941–946.

6 Meyers BF, Lynch JP, Battafarano RJ, et al. Lung transplantation is warranted for stable, ventilator-dependent recipients. *Ann Thorac Surg* 2000; **70**: 1675–1678.

7 Madill J, Gutiérrez C, Grossman J, et al. Nutritional assessment of the lung transplant patient: body mass index as a predictor of 90-day mortality following transplantation. *J Heart Lung Transplant* 2001; **20**: 288–296.

8 Sharples L, Hathaway T, Dennis C, et al. Prognosis of patients with cystic fibrosis awaiting heart and lung transplantation. *J Heart Lung Transplant* 1993; **12**: 669–674.

9 Plochl W, Pezawas L, Artemiou O, et al. Nutritional status, ICU duration and ICU mortality in lung transplant recipients. *Intensive Care Med* 1996; **22**: 1179–1185.

10 Dew MA, Switzer GE, DiMartini AF, et al. Psychosocial assessments and outcomes in organ transplantation. *Prog Transplant* 2000; **10**: 239–261.

11 Aris RM, Gilligan PH, Neuringer IP, et al. The effects of pan-resistant bacteria in cystic fibrosis patients on lung transplant outcome. *Am J Resp Crit Care Med* 1997; **155**: 1699–1674.

12 Chaparro C, Maurer J, Gutiérrez C, et al. Infection with *Burkholderia cepacia* in cystic fibrosis: outcome following lung transplantation. *Am J Respir Crit Care Med* 2001; **163**: 43–48.

13 Clode FE, Kaufmann ME, Malnick H, Pitt TL. Distribution of genes for putative transmissibility factors among epidemic and nonepidemic strains of *Burkholderia cepacia* from cystic fibrosis patients in the United Kingdom. *J Clin Microbiol* 2000; **38**: 1763–1766.

14 Zenati M, Dowling RD, Dummer JS, et al. Influence of the donor lung on development of early infections in lung transplant recipients. *J Heart Lung Transplant* 1990; **9**: 502–508.

15 Grossi P, Farina C, Fiocchi R, Dalla Gasperina D. Prevalence and outcome of invasive fungal infections in 1,963 thoracic organ transplant recipients: a multicenter retrospective study. Italian Study Group of Fungal infections in Thoracic Organ Transplant Recipients. *Transplantation* 2000; **70**: 112–116.

16 Nunley DR, Ohori P, Grgurich WF, et al. Pulmonary aspergillosis in cystic fibrosis lung transplant recipients. *Chest* 1998; **114**: 1321–1329.

17 Husni RN, Gordon SM, Longworth DL, et al. Cytomegalovirus infection is a risk factor for invasive aspergillosis in lung transplant recipients. *Clin Infect Dis* 1998; **26**: 753–755.

18 Shafers H-J, Wagner TOF, Demertzis S, et al. Preoperative corticosteroids: a contraindication to lung transplantation? *Chest* 1992; **102**: 1522–1525.

19 Colquhoun IW, Gascoigne AD, Au J, et al. Airway complications after pulmonary transplantation. *Ann Thorac Surg* 1994; **57**: 141–145.

20 Zaltzman JS, Pei Y, Maurer J, et al. Cyclosporine nephrotoxicity in lung transplant recipients. *Transplantation* 1992; **54**: 875–878.

21 Gow PJ, Pillay D, Mutimer D. Solid organ transplantation in patients with HIV infection. *Transplantation* 2001; **72**: 177–181.

22 Penn I. Overview of the problem of cancer in organ transplant recipients. *Ann Transplant* 1997; **2**: 5–6.

23 Penn I. Evaluation of transplant candidates with pre-existing malignancies. *Ann Transplant* 1997; **2**: 14–17.

24 Kerem E, Reisman J, Corey M, et al. Prediction of mortality in patients with cystic fibrosis. *N Engl J Med* 1992; **326**: 1187–1191.

25 Maurer J, Frost A, Estenne M, et al. International guidelines for the selection of lung transplant candidates. *J Heart Lung Transplant* 1998; **17**: 703–709.

26 Doershuk C, Stern R. Timing of referral for lung transplantation for cystic fibrosis. *Chest* 1999; **115**: 782–787.

27 Milla C, Warwick W. Risk of death in cystic fibrosis patients with severely compromised lung function. *Chest* 1998; **113**: 1230–1234.

28 Robinson W, Waltz DA. FEV_1 as a guide to lung transplant referral in young patients with cystic fibrosis. *Pediatr Pulmonol* 2000; **30**: 198–202.

29 National Center for Health Statistics: Leading causes of death. National Vital Statistics Reports **48** (11). Website: www.cdc.gov/nchs/fastats/lcod.htm

30 Fiel S, FitzSimmons S, Suhidlow D. Evolving demographics of cystic fibrosis. *Semin Respir Crit Care Med* 1994; **15**: 349–355.

31 Ries AL, Kaplan RM, Limberg TM, et al. Effects of pulmonary rehabilitation on physiologic and psychosocial outcomes in patients with chronic obstructive pulmonary disease. *Ann Intern Med* 1995; **122**: 823–832.

32 Cooper JD, Paterson GA, Sundaresan RS, et al. Results of 150 consecutive bilateral lung volume reduction procedures in patients with severe emphysema. *J Thorac Cardiovasc Surg* 1996; **112**: 1319–1330.

33 McKenna RJ Jr, Brenner M, Gelb AF, et al. A randomized prospective trial of stapled lung reduction versus laser bullectomy for diffuse emphysema. *J Thorac Cardiovasc Surg* 1996; **111**: 317–322.

34 Gelb AF, McKenna RJ Jr, Brenner M, et al. Lung function 5 yr after lung volume reduction surgery for emphysema. *Am J Respir Crit Care Med* 2001; **163**: 1562–1566.

35 National Emphysema Treatment Trial Research Group. Patients at high risk of death after lung-volume-reduction surgery. *N Engl J Med* 2001; **345**: 1075–1083.

36 Hosenpud JD, Bennett LE, Keck BM, et al. Effect of diagnosis on survival benefit of lung transplantation for end-stage lung disease. *Lancet* 1998; **351**: 24–27.

37 Hanson D, Winterbauer RH, Kirtland SH, et al. Changes in pulmonary function test results after one year of therapy as predictors of survival in patients with idiopathic pulmonary fibrosis. *Chest* 1995; **108**: 305–310.

38 Schwartz DA, Helmers RA, Galvin JR, et al. Determinants of progression in idiopathic pulmonary fibrosis. *Am J Respir Crit Care Med* 1994; **149**: 450–454.

39 Douglas WW, Ryu JH, Swensen SJ, et al. Colchicine versus prednisone in the treatment of idiopathic pulmonary fibrosis. A randomized prospective study. Members of the Lung Study Group. *Am J Respir Crit Care Med* 1998; **158**: 220–225.

40 Padilla ML, Schilero GJ, Teirstein AS. Sarcoidosis and transplantation. *Sarcoidosis Vasc Diffuse Lung Dis* 1997; **14**: 16–22.

41 Berkowitz N, Schulman LL, McGregor C, Markowitz D. Gastroparesis after lung transplantation. Potential role in postoperative complications. *Chest* 1995; **108**: 1602–1607.

42 Thomas AQ, Gaddipati R, Newman JH, Loyd JE. Genetics of primary pulmonary hypertension. *Clin Chest Med* 2001; **22**: 477–491.

43 D'Alonzo GE, Barst RJ, Ayers SM, et al. Survival in patients with primary pulmonary hypertension. *Ann Intern Med* 1991; **115**: 343–349.

44 Higenbottam T, Butt AY, McMahon A, et al. Long-term intravenous prostaglandin (epoprostenol or iloprost) for treatment of severe pulmonary hypertension. *Heart* 1998; **80**: 151–155.

45 Hopkins WE, Ochoa LL, Richardson GW, et al. Comparison of the hemodynamics and survival of adults with severe primary pulmonary hypertension or Eisenmenger syndrome. *J Heart Lung Transplant* 1996; **15**: 100–105.

46 Scanlon PJ, Faxon DP, Audet AM, et al. ACC/AHA guidelines for coronary angiography. A report of the American College of Cardiology/American Heart Association Task Force on practice guidelines (Committee on Coronary Angiographies). Developed in collaboration with the Society for Cardiac Angiographies and Interventions. *J Am Coll Cardiol* 1999; **33**: 1756–1824.

47 Arcsoy SM, Harsh C, Christie JD, et al. Bronchogenic carcinoma complicating lung transplantation. *J Heart Lung Transplant* 2001; **20**: 1044–1053.

48 McAdams HP, Erasmus JJ, Palmer SM. Complications (excluding hyperinflation) involving the native lung after single-lung transplantation: incidence, radiologic features, and clinical importance. *Radiology* 2001; **218**: 233–241.

49 Meyer DM, Bennett LE, Novick RJ, Hosenpud JD. Single vs bilateral, sequential lung transplantation for end-stage emphysema: influence of recipient age on survival and secondary endpoints. *J Heart Lung Transplant* 2001; **20**: 935–941.

13

Single and bilateral lung transplantation

John Dark

The Freeman Hospital, Newcastle upon Tyne, UK

Historical background

Success with clinical single lung transplantation was first described by the Toronto group in 1986 [1]. They built on a huge programme of experimental work going back almost 40 years. The basic surgical steps of lung transplantation had been set out by Metras in 1949 [2], much of the physiology being described in a series of experiments coming from the laboratory of Frank Veith in New York. The first human lung transplantation was performed as early as 1963 by Hardy [3]. This case was indeed notable because it demonstrated early function of a lung from a nonheart-beating donor. Other landmarks during the 1970s included an appreciation of the difficulties of ventilation–perfusion (VQ) mismatch in the setting of emphysema [4], and a patient in Belgium who lived for over six months, the latter demonstrating the physiological advantage of giving patients with restrictive disease a transplant [5]. The other theme running through these initial attempts was the problem of bronchial healing [5].

The Toronto group ascribed their success to solution of the bronchus problem (by wrapping with an omental pedicle), and an emphasis on case selection. They realized the advantages of giving a transplant to patients with fibrotic disease and the importance of adequate preoperative rehabilitation.

Evolution of isolated lung transplantation

Fibrotic disease is the ideal indication for a single lung transplant because both ventilation and perfusion are directed towards the graft. The very earliest attempts to perform single lung transplant for emphysema had been unsuccessful because of the preferential ventilation of the much more compliant native lung. However, by 1988, Mal

and colleagues in Paris demonstrated successful outcome and had shown that the VQ mismatch was only a problem if there was dysfunction of the transplanted lung [6]. Emphysema, either smoking induced or related to alpha-1-antitrypsin deficiency, is now the commonest indication for single lung transplantation.

In North America, where organ allocation practices have severely hampered the availability of heart–lung blocs, isolated lung transplantation has been used extensively for patients with pulmonary vascular disease. The first report was from the Toronto group, who performed a single lung transplantation simultaneously with closure of a patent ductus arteriosus in 1988 [7]. The technique was subsequently extended to patients with primary pulmonary hypertension, with excellent results in some hands [8]. The debate about the most appropriate procedure for these patients continues [9,10].

During the mid-1980s, heart–lung transplantation was applied to patients with a variety of different parenchymal lung diseases [11]. For those with sepsis, and to a lesser extent emphysema, removal of both lungs was felt to be mandatory. It was rapidly realized that inclusion of the heart provided an excellent blood supply, through coronary to bronchial collaterals, to the distal trachea, but was otherwise unnecessary. Tracheal healing in these heart–lung transplant patients was usually reliable. The first alternative technique to be described was en bloc double lung transplantation, initially in the laboratory [12] and then in a clinical series [13]. However, further experience revealed a number of drawbacks. There was an incidence of serious tracheal complications (often dehiscence) in at least 20% of patients, even with the use of omentopexy [14]. The extensive mediastinal dissection resulted in functional cardiac dennervation, even when the native heart was retained [15]. Finally there was a definite cardiac morbidity, arising out of the need for aortic cross-clamping and cardioplegic arrest for construction of the atrial anastomosis. By the early 1990s, the en bloc double lung transplant procedure had been virtually abandoned, except by teams such as those in London or Copenhagen in Europe and the Mayo Clinic in the USA. These surgeons preserved the major bronchial arteries at the time of organ retrieval and performed subsequent bronchial revascularization using either the internal mammary artery or a segment of saphenous vein [16]. The technique never became popular: it was technically demanding, time consuming and could be accompanied by excessive blood loss. Although tracheal healing was excellent when the revascularization was successful, a failed bronchial artery anastomosis could well result in airway dehiscence. While there was some evidence that ciliary function was improved in the immediate postoperative period, there is no suggestion that the risk of obliterative bronchiolitis is altered by reducing bronchial ischaemia. Indeed, there is no evidence that significant bronchial ischaemia, other than occasionally in the bronchus intermedius on the right-hand side, occurs except outwith the lung parenchyma.

The next step in the evolution of the paired lung transplant was to perform the bronchial anastomoses closer to the lung parenchyma, but still through the posterior mediastinum. This, the so called bi-bronchial technique, was championed by French surgeons and appeared to give good results [17].

The definitive procedure, entitled sequential single or bilateral lung transplantation, was finally evolved by Pasque and colleagues from St Louis, USA [18]. As the name implies, the operation is effectively two single lung transplants, performed with the anastomosis at hilar level. This approach was coupled with the adoption of a 'clam-shell' rather than a sternotomy incision. The bilateral anterior thoracotomies joined in the middle across the sternum give an excellent view to the whole pleural space and make division of the often dense, vascular, pleural adhesions in patients with inflammatory lung disease relatively straightforward. By means of this very extended incision, the operation could be performed without cardiopulmonary bypass, although the advantages of this strategy are now less obvious.

Bilateral lung transplantation has continued to evolve with descriptions of its performance through a median sternotomy [19], and most recently via two limited anterior thoracotomies [20]. This latter is particularly appropriate for the patients with obstructive lung disease who rarely have significant pleural adhesions.

A further adaptation of the bilateral lung technique was with the use of living donors. The first description of a lobar, as opposed to whole lung, transplant, came in 1991 and included reference to a live donor [21]. The technique

has been developed by Starnes and his colleagues in Los Angeles [22]. Most recipients are children or small adults with cystic fibrosis. Complementary (left and right) lower lobes are removed from *two* donors. Results have been a little disappointing, perhaps because many of the procedures were performed urgently on ventilator-dependent or moribund patients. A one year survival of only 72% is recorded [22]. There is, however, some evidence that the cause of late death is rarely obliterative bronchiolitis, but usually sepsis [23]. It has been implied that rejection is less of a problem, and that these patients are over-immunosuppressed.

Case selection, choice of bilateral or single lung transplant

Isolated lung transplantation can be applied to any pulmonary condition with acceptable cardiac function. There are four diagnostic categories to be considered: fibrotic disease, emphysema, septic lung disease or bronchiectasis, and pulmonary hypertension from a variety of subtypes. Indications for lung transplant in these areas have already been discussed (Maurer, Chapter 12).

Fibrotic lung disease

The logical advantages of a single lung transplant in this setting were established early and this remains the procedure of choice. A degree of pulmonary hypertension almost invariably accompanies end-stage fibrosing alveolitis; the use of marginal donor lung in this setting is fraught with risk. Anxieties about a marginal lung might be the only reason for considering a bilateral lung transplant in the fibrotic patient. In practice this is rarely done.

There are a number of series with long-term follow-up, and late function is at least as good as for any of the other conditions of transplantation [24]. The VQ mismatch sometimes seen late after single lung transplantation for pulmonary hypertension is virtually never a problem. Ventilation remains directed to the transplanted lung even after the development of obliterative bronchiolitis.

Obstructive lung disease

Patients with emphysema of various kinds predominate as the commonest indication in single lung transplantation and, increasingly, in bilateral lung transplantation [25]. A contralateral lung may be a source of sepsis, either from existing bronchiectasis or the colonization of bullae with pathogens such as *Aspergillus* [26]. A bilateral lung transplant is clearly required in these cases. In most recipients, however, the opposite lung is 'harmless' other than its predilection for air trapping overexpansion if the patient requires mechanical ventilation.

Comparisons between single lung transplantation and bilateral lung transplantation are difficult to make. The latter operation has in general been applied to younger and fitter recipients with emphysema and there are no randomized controlled trials. There are, however, a number of reports from single institutions and some interesting Registry data [25]. Spirometry is much better after paired lung transplantation, approaching normal, although functional measures such as the six minute walk test show little difference. At least in the early stages after transplantation, the patient's perception of functional wellbeing is excellent with single lung transplant. At a later stage, there is clear evidence of superior quality of life to match the better functional measures in the bilateral lung transplant patients [27]. This is evident up to at least 36 months posttransplantation. There are a number of papers suggesting an improved early survival for bilateral lung transplants. These groups describe particularly low mortality in bilateral lung transplant patients [28]. In Registry reports the advantages of having two lungs (rather than one) is apparent from about three years post-transplantation [25]. Presumably if bronchiolitis obliterans occurs and there is a fall in expiratory flow, this is better tolerated when the starting point is higher. Thus, from the point of view of the individual patient, bilateral lung transplantation is the best choice. There is better early function, longer survival and probably better quality of life for a longer period.

As these results have become apparent, there have also been the observations that, for chronic obstructive pulmonary disease patients in particular, transplantation did not prolong life. The Dutch lung transplant group could demonstrate no difference in survival amongst the patients receiving a transplant as compared with those remaining on the waiting list [29]. The great bulk of the patients in this experience suffered from emphysema. Hosenpud et al. analysed data from the United Network for Organ Sharing (UNOS) Registry [30]. He showed that patients with emphysema have a significantly lower attrition rate whilst on the waiting list for transplantation and that their posttransplant mortality rate was the same as pretransplantation. This contrasts with those patients with cystic fibrosis or fibrotic lung disease who clearly had a survival advantage from transplantation (Figure 13.1). The difference is accentuated in the USA, where waiting time is an important determinant of organ allocation. This favours the subgroup of patients for whom in some respects transplantation is less important. The principal gain from transplantation for patients with emphysema is *quality* of life; it is difficult to reconcile this with the demonstration that the best outcome

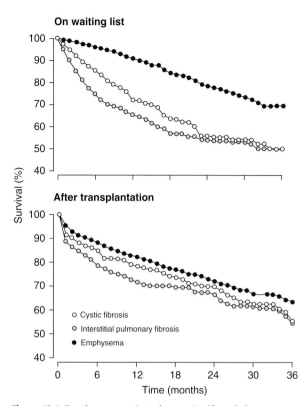

Figure 13.1 Emphysema patients have a significantly better survival on the waiting list than those with fibrotic disease of cystic fibrosis. The survival of the three groups after transplant is largely similar and in the case of emphysema is little different from the natural history of these patients. (Reproduced with permission from the *Lancet* 1998; **351**: 24–27. Hosenpud JD, Bednett LE, Keck BM, Edwards EB, Novick RJ. Effect of diagnosis on survival benefit of lung transplantation for end-stage lung disease.)

for this group of patients is achieved with the worst economy of donor organs.

Septic lung disease

Most of the patients in this category suffer from cystic fibrosis or other forms of bronchiectasis. Almost all will require removal of all the native lung tissue and the standard procedure is bilateral lung transplantation. Single lung transplantation and contralateral pneumonectomy has been described for cystic fibrosis but is only applicable in very rare circumstances [31].

Two centres in the UK have continued to utilize heart–lung transplantation with a subsequently 'domino' transplant of the recipient's heart. The results are excellent: the Harefield group reported 50% five year survival and 47% seven year survival in a group of 105 heart–lung transplant recipients. The early mortality rate fell towards 5%

in the late 1990s; these results are comparable with those achieved with bilateral lung transplant [32].

The outcome of the use of the recipient's heart in the domino procedure is excellent and probably better than that achieved with cadaver donor hearts [33]. These hearts have never been exposed to the effects of brain stem death and may have better early and late function. On the other hand, the heart–lung transplant recipient is disadvantaged. Denervation results in a measurable physiological impairment [34], (although of little clinical significance) and some of these patients will die as a result of accelerated graft coronary disease [35]. The heart–lung recipient is perhaps most disadvantaged when retransplantation is considered. The presence of graft coronary disease, often developing in parallel to obliterative bronchiolitis, will preclude relatively straightforward single or bilateral lung retransplantation. Heart and lung retransplantation, the indicated procedure, carries an exceedingly high mortality even in the most experienced hands [36] and is rarely performed.

Pulmonary vascular disease

Early descriptions of successful single lung transplant for pulmonary hypertension suggested a complete return to a normal haemodynamic state even with the vascular bed of a single lung [8,37]. Later reviews of large numbers of patients described higher mortality and poorer functional performance in single lung transplant recipients as compared with either bilateral lung transplant or heart and lung transplant recipients [10]. If obliterative bronchiolitis develops, there is likely to be gross VQ mismatch and severe symptoms from the resultant large physiological dead space: the native lung is ventilated but not significantly perfused [38].

The early postoperative management of the bilateral lung transplant recipient is more straightforward, probably because of the larger vascular bed. The consequences of implanting a substandard lung are clearly demonstrated in Figure 13.2. Mortality, both early and late, remains higher for this pulmonary vascular disease group, regardless of procedure [39].

Donor selection

There have been many recent developments in the understanding of the pathophysiology of brain stem death and how it affects the lung. There are two, possibly interlinked, mechanisms of lung damage. The abrupt rise in blood pressure following intense release of noradrenaline at the time of rising intracranial pressure may result in a stress injury to the pulmonary endothelium. In its most florid form, this presents as 'neurogenic pulmonary oedema'. In parallel

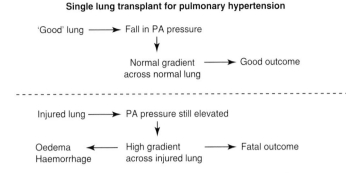

Single lung transplant for pulmonary hypertension

Figure 13.2 In the upper part, the large vascular bed of a "good" lung presents a low vascular resistance and results in a fall in pulmonary artery pressure. In the lower half, the injured lung represents a still elevated pulmonary vascular resistance so pulmonary pressure stays high. This is turn results in continuing damage to the lung and there is a vicious circle leading to a fatal outcome.

Table 13.1. Lung transplant donor selection criteria

Age < 65 years
ABO blood type compatibility
Clear chest radiograph
$PaO_2 > 40$ kPa (300 mmHg) on $F_1O_2 = 1.0$, PEEP 5 cmH$_2$O
Tobacco history – ignore
Absence of severe chest trauma
Absence of extensive lung contusion
No evidence of aspiration/sepsis
No previous cardiopulmonary surgery
If no airway mucosal inflammation at bronchoscopy, ignore positive sputum Gram stain and purulent secretions at bronchoscopy

there is a generalized cytokine release with involvement of a number of pathways and an inflammatory state that causes damage to a range of organs [40]. A degree of lung injury is probably always present in brain stem dead donors [41].

This inflammatory state compounds the other causes of lung injury, which include trauma, aspiration (with inadequate bronchial toilet) and infection, such that lungs can be removed from only about 20% of cadaver donors. PaO_2 (arterial oxygen pressure), measured during ventilation with an F_1O_2 (fraction of oxygen in inspired gas) of 1.0 with 5 cm PEEP (positive end-expiratory pressure), is currently our best determinant of lung viability [42]. Donor criteria are shown in Table 13.1. It should be noted that if there are unilateral radiographical changes, then patients who are more hypoxic may have a usable single lung on the other side. Selective measurement of pulmonary vein gases at the time of organ retrieval may identify these lungs [43].

Best management of the lung donor has to take into account the various physiological changes that follow brain stem death. Bronchial toilet and physiotherapy are clearly obvious, as is maintenance of body temperature. Excessive crystalline infusion (often recommended by renal transplant surgeons) should be avoided. Relatively modest changes in central venous pressure may result in a rapid deterioration of gas exchange, probably because of established endothelial damage [44]. Pressures from the left and right ventricles may be very different and monitoring with a pulmonary artery catheter is essential in all but the most stable patients [45]. There may be a conflict between maintenance of optimal perfusion of abdominal organs, avoidance of unnecessary catecholamines (from the point of view of the heart) and best management of the lungs by keeping the left atrial pressure low. There is also evidence that high dose steroids given early may reduce deterioration in the donor [46].

Organ retrieval and preservation

The final assessment of the lungs is made by the surgical team after opening the chest. Lung preservation is relatively straightforward, although there is an appreciation that pre-donation damage and events during reperfusion are crucial in determining the overall function of the donor lung. Preservation is achieved by flushing a cold solution through the pulmonary artery, preceded by epoprostenol (prostacyclin) to obtain maximum vasodilatation [47]. Topical cooling is also used, although the inflated lung is such a good insulator that most of the effect is obtained by the flushing solution. The most popular preservation solution has been the 'intracellular' (i.e. high potassium, low sodium) Euro-Collins solution borrowed from renal transplantation. Recent laboratory research and some initial clinical experience has suggested that a low potassium/dextran solution (Perfadex) is superior [48,49]. This solution is increasingly used in mainland Europe and North America.

Lungs are stored inflated and ischaemic times of up to eight hours are generally tolerated. There is, however, a correlation between early dysfunction and late dysfunction with obliterative bronchiolitis and ischaemic time. This is particularly the case for organs from older donors [25].

Surgical technique

Single lung transplant

In general, the side with worst function, as judged from an isotope perfusion scan, is chosen for the transplant. Exceptions would be the presence of extensive previous surgery, for instance pleurectomy or lobectomy on the site with the worst function. In these circumstances, the disadvantages of removing the best lung, perhaps with the need for cardiopulmonary bypass during the implantation, have to be balanced against the likely surgical difficulties on the other side.

The chest is opened through a standard thoracotomy, pleural adhesions divided and the hilar structures mobilized. One lung ventilation of the contralateral side should be instituted and trial clamping of the pulmonary artery performed. Almost all patients with emphysema and the majority of those with fibrotic disease can be maintained on one lung anaesthesia. Haemodynamic instability, particularly with evidence of right ventricular dysfunction, or a rising $PaCO_2$ (arterial carbon dioxide pressure) are the usual indications for the use of cardiopulmonary bypass [50].

If the patient is stable after 10 minutes of trial clamping, a standard extrapericardial pneumonectomy is performed, ligating or stapling the vascular structures and dividing the bronchus where it emerges from the mediastinum. A suitable length of pulmonary artery is mobilized to allow subsequent clamping division and anastomosis. Ligating the vascular structures at this stage avoids having to place clamps in a crowded operative field. The pericardium is opened around the pulmonary veins, which are mobilized to produce, after applying a side biting clamp, a suitable cuff of left atrium.

When the donor lung is brought into the field, the bronchus is trimmed as close as possible to the lung parenchyma, where it is vascularized by pulmonary to bronchial collaterals. Pulmonary artery and the left atrial cuff on the donor are trimmed appropriately then the lung is placed in the anterior part of the chest. Anastomosis begins with the bronchus and our own routine is a continuous polypropylene suture along a membranous portion and a series of figure of eight sutures anteriorly (Figure 13.3). Telescoping of the donor bronchus is avoided and indeed the aim is to ensure accurate apposition of the mucosal surfaces. Although telescoping has been popularized by some groups, and may reduce the risk of dehiscence, there is inevitably at least one ring of ischaemic cartilage incorporated within the airway that can subsequently lead to stenosis. The 'short donor bronchus' technique, with careful apposition of the two cut ends, results in a bronchial complication rate of less than 3% [51]. Dehiscence is now exceedingly rare, and the occasional fibrous stricture can be easily managed with dilatation or endobronchial stenting [52]. Wrapping the anastomosis with omentum, pericardium or intercostal muscle is unnecessary but we would

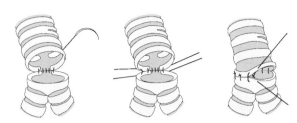

Figure 13.3 The donor bronchus is cut as short as possible. The anastomosis is performed with continuous polypropylene suture along the membranous portion and interrupted figure-of eight sutures anteriorly, aiming for precise apposition, not telescoping, of the two ends1

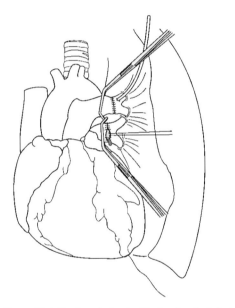

Figure 13.4 The lung is de-aired by leaving the left atrial suture line untied whilst a little blood is allowed to go through the lung. The left atrial clamp is then removed and the lung reperfused under controlled circumstances. A pulmonary artery monitoring line is placed and pulmonary artery clamp only partially released, to ensure pulmonary arterial pressure does not exceed 20 mmHg for the first 10 min of reperfusion.

routinely approximate peribronchial tissues over the suture line.

The corresponding atrial donor cuff on the donor lung is simply sutured to that on the recipient and the implantation completed with end-to-end anastomosis with the pulmonary artery. De-airing is performed by partially releasing the clamp on the pulmonary artery and allowing egress of air and blood from the left atrial anastomosis before tying the final suture. A pressure monitoring line is introduced into the pulmonary artery and

care taken to maintain a mean pulmonary artery pressure no greater than 20 mmHg (2.7 kpa) for the first 10 or 15 minutes of reperfusion (Figure 13.4). The lung is gently ventilated at this stage to encourage perfusion of as great a part of the pulmonary bed as possible. After pressure-controlled reperfusion, the cross-clamp is removed completely and the lung fully ventilated with 5 cm of PEEP. There may be some bleeding from the cut edges around the donor site (i.e. remnants of donor pericardium) but this is rarely of any consequence and indeed demonstrates the presence of pulmonary artery to bronchial collaterals. The chest is then simply closed over apical and basal drains.

Combined lung transplantation and lung volume reduction (LVRS)

If there are 'target areas' of poorly perfused lung on the side opposite to the transplant, there may be additional gain by performing simultaneous LVRS. Not only may it improve early function, but also reduce air trapping and overdistention of the native lung if prolonged ventilation is needed. Descriptions remain anecdotal [53]; any advantage seems offset by the morbidity in terms of extended surgery and air leak from the additional surgery.

Bilateral lung transplant

This procedure duplicates most of the above for both lungs. A standard clam-shell incision, through the fourth or fifth interspace (Figure 13.5), and dividing the sternum horizontally, gives superb access to all parts of the pleural cavity. It allows for ease of control of vascular adhesions that may accompany longstanding cystic fibrosis in particular. Sequential removal and implantation of the lung can be performed but requires very skilful anaesthetic management, with alternating one lung ventilation and often haemodynamic instability. The first lung is exposed to all the pulmonary blood flow while the second lung is implanted. If the heart has to be retracted during this latter process, the lung is squeezed between a vigorous right ventricle and intermittent elevations of left atrial pressure. A unilateral appearance of reperfusion injury on this first side, is often seen, despite the shorter ischaemic time. An alternative is to use cardiopulmonary bypass for both removal and implantation of the lungs and this is now the policy in our unit. Airway management is very straightforward and reperfusion can take place in a controlled fashion to the

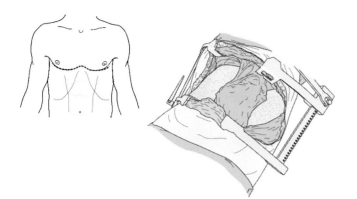

Figure 13.5 Bilateral anterior thoracotomy with division of sternum (the clam-shell incision) gives magnificent access to all parts of the chest.

whole pulmonary vascular bed. This strategy is of course essential when a double lumen tube cannot be placed (usually in a small recipient) and for lobar transplants.

If there are no pleural adhesions, as might be the case in patients with emphysema, then a separate anterior thoracotomy [20] or a sternotomy [19] have both been described for bilateral lung transplantation. These approaches have the advantages of less pain and less sternal instability, which can sometimes accompany the clam-shell incision.

Technical aspects of living donor lung transplantation

Almost all these procedures consist of a pair of lower lobes from separate donors implanted as a bilateral lung transplant. The key components of the donor operations have been well described [54]. The donated lobe must have enough of the key structures–bronchus, artery and vein – to allow implantation, but without jeopardizing the remaining structures. Patching of the residual pulmonary artery may be required, together with an imaginative approach to preserving the middle lobe bronchus on the right. Morbidity amongst donors has been modest [55], although there is a permanent reduction of lung function by about 20%.

Implantation of the lobes is always performed on cardiopulmonary bypass, and is relatively straightforward. The single vein on the lobe is anastomosed directly to the superior pulmonary vein stump in the recipient. Minimal tailoring of the bronchus and pulmonary artery may be required but anastomotic problems have been very rare.

Persistent fluid and air collections are a particular postoperative problem, because the lungs rarely fill the whole pleural space. Prolonged intercostal draining, often for weeks, is preferable to repeated reinsertion of drains.

Postoperative management – reperfusion injury

Features of oedema on chest X-ray, with hypoxia and poor compliance, are seen in between 10% and 25% of patients with lung transplants in the postoperative period. In its most florid form, there is a proteinaceous pulmonary oedema and also leakage of similar fluid into the pleural space. The pathogenesis is probably an endothelial damage which is initiated in the donor and exacerbated by interaction with neutrophils from the recipient and subsequent free-radical-mediated injury [42]. Progression to a full-blown adult respiratory distress syndrome is possible but can frequently be prevented. Attention to pressure-controlled reperfusion [56] and the use of inhaled nitric oxide (NO) together with modulators of neutrophil activation such as pentoxifillin may all ameliorate injury. NO has a beneficial effect when the injury occurs but has no proven advantage in terms of preventing injury. There is at least one report suggesting that the combination of NO and pentoxifillin dramatically decreases the incidence of reperfusion injury [57].

Inhaled NO in a dose of 20 ppm with positive end-expiratory pressure and avoidance of transfusion, are the mainstays of management. The majority of patients can be successfully brought through the acute phase using these techniques and early mortality after lung transplantation has fallen progressively over recent years [43].

Where reperfusion injury occurs in the emphysematous patient, the situation may be more complex. Air trapping in the contralateral lung prevents application of positive and expiratory pressure to the transplant, with the result that there is further alveolar collapse and further deterioration in compliance. This manifests itself as overinflation of the native lung and shrinkage or apparent 'compression' of the donor lung. The process is very much led by donor organ dysfunction and probably does not occur if the transplanted lung is in good condition. Because of trapping of ventilation by the underperfused native lung, there is a large physiological dead space, and satisfactory ventilation may be achieved only by the use of a double lumen tube and separate lung ventilation. The standard technique would be to apply PEEP and keep a modest tidal volume to the transplanted lung and simply insufflate oxygen into the other side. This normally results in re-expansion of the transplanted lung, shrinkage of the overinflated native lung and a return to satisfactory gas exchange. The double lumen tube can be exchanged for a single lumen tube and the patient weaned from the ventilator after 48–72 hours [58].

Conclusion

The isolated lung transplant can be applied to almost any end-stage respiratory condition. Difficult techniques have become standardized and early results in the hands of experienced groups can be excellent.

For some conditions, particularly fibrotic disease, the single lung remains the operation of choice. There is a trend towards increased usage of the bilateral lung transplant even in nonseptic conditions. This trend is supported by evidence of better results with marginal donors in the early period and later with lower mortality from obliterative bronchiolitis. Conciliation of these better results with less favourable organ utilization remains a major difficulty.

REFERENCES

1 Toronto Lung Transplant Group. Unilateral transplant for pulmonary fibrosis. *New Eng J Med* 1986; **314**: 1140–1145.

2 Metras H. Note preliminaire sur la graffe totale du poumon chez le chien. *Fr Acad Sci* 1950: 1176.

3 Hardy JD, Watts RW, Dalton ML, et al. Lung homotransplantation in man. *J Am Med Assoc* 1963; **186**: 1065–1074.

4 Stevens PM, Johnson PC, Bell RL, Beall AC, Jenkins DE. Regional ventilation and perfusion after lung transplantation in patients with emphysema. *New Engl J Med* 1970; **282**: 245–249.

5 Wildevuuer CRH, Benfield JR. A review of 23 lung transplantations by 20 surgeons. *Ann Thorac Surg* 1979; **9**: 489–515.

6 Mal H, Andreassian B, Pamela F, et al. Unilateral lung transplantation in end-stage pulmonary emphysema. *Am Rev Respir Dis* 1989; **140**: 797–802.

7 Fremes SE, Patterson GA, Williams WG, et al. Single lung transplantation and closure of patent ductus arteriousus for Eisenmenger's syndrome. Toronto Lung Transplant Group. *J Thorac Cardiovasc Surg* 1990; **100**: 1–5.

8 Pasque MK, Trulock EP, Kaiser LR, Cooper JD. Single lung transplantation for pulmonary hypertension: three month haemodynamic follow-up. *Circulation* 1991; **84**: 2275–2279.

9 Bando K, Armitage JA, Paradis IL, et al. Indications for and results of single, bilateral and heart lung transplantation for pulmonary hypertension. *J Thorac Cardiovasc Surg* 1994; **108**: 1056–1065.

10 Conte JV, Borja MJ, Patel CB, Yang SC, Jhaveri RM, Orens JB. Lung transplantation for primary and secondary pulmonary hypertension. *Ann Thorac Surg* 2001; **72**: 1673–1680.

11 Penketh A, Higgenbotham TW, Hakim M, Wallwork J. Heart and lung transplantation in patients with end-stage lung disease *Br Med J* 1987; **295**; 311–316.

12 Dark JH, Patterson GA, Al-Jihaihawi AN, Hsu H, Egan T, Cooper JD. Experimental en-bloc double lung transplant in dogs. *Ann Thorac Surg* 1986; **42**: 395–398.

13 Patterson GA, Cooper JD, Dark JH, et al. Experimental and clinical double-lung transplantation. *J Thorac Cardiovasc Surg* 1988; **95**: 70–75.

14 Patterson GA, Todd TR, Cooper JD, et al. Airway complications following double lung transplantation. *J Thorac Cardiovasc Surg* 1990; **99**: 14–20.

15 Schaefers HJ, Waxman MB, Patterson GA, et al. Cardiac innervation after double lung transplantation. Toronto Lung Transplant Group. *J Thorac Cardiovasc Surg* 1990; **99**: 22–29.

16 Petterson G, Norgaard MA, Arendrup H, et al. Direct bronchial revascularisation and en-bloc double lung transplanation – surgical techniques and early outcome. *J Heart Lung Transplant* 1997; **16**: 320–333.

17 Noirclerc MJ, Metras D, Vaillant A, et al. Bilateral bronchial anastomosis in double lung and heart lung transplantations. *Eur J Cardiothorac Surg* 1990; **4**: 314–317.

18 Pasque MK, Cooper JD, Kaiser LR, et al. Improved technique for bilateral lung transplantations: rationale and initial clinical experience. *Ann Thorac Surg* 1990; **49**: 785.

19 Macchiarini P, Ladurie FL, Cerrina J, Fadel E, Chapelier A and Dartevelle P. Clamshell or sternotomy for double lung or heart-lung transplantation? *Eur J Cardiothorac Surg* 1999; **15**: 333–339.

20 Meyers BF, Sundaresan RS, Guthrie T, Cooper JD, Patterson GA. Bilateral sequential lung transplantation without sternal division eliminates post-transplantation sternal complications. *J Thorac Cardiovasc Surg* 1999; **117**: 358–364.

21 Starnes VA, Barr ML, Cohen RG. Lobar transplantation: indications, technique and outcome. *J Thorac Cardiovasc Surg* 1994; **108**: 403–411.

22 Starnes VA, Barr ML, Rohen RG, et al. Living donor lobar lung transplantation experience: intermediate results. *J Thorac Cardiovasc Surg* 1996; **112**: 1284–1291.

23 Woo MS, MacLaughlin EF, Horn MV, et al. Bronchiolitis obliterans is not the primary cause of death in pediatric living donor lobar lung transplant recipients. *J Heart Lung Transplant* 2001; **20**: 491–496.

24 Chaparro C, Scavuzzo M, Winton T, Keshavjee S, Keston S. Status of lung transplant recipients surviving beyond five years. *J Heart Lung Transplant* 1997; **16**: 511–516.

25 Hosenpud JD, Bennett LE, Keck BM, et al: The Registry of the International Society for Heart and Lung Transplantation: Sixteenth official report. *J Heart Lung Transplant* 1999; **18**: 611–626.

26 Colquhoun IW, Gascoigne AD, Gould FK, Corris PA, Dark JH. Native pulmonary sepsis following single lung transplantation. *Transplantation* 1991; **52**: 931–933.

27 Sundaresan RS, Shiraishi Y, Trulock EP, et al. Single or bilateral lung transplantation for emphysema? *J Thorac Surg* 1996; **112**: 1485–1495.

28 Bavaria JE, Kotloff R, Palevsky H, et al. Bilateral versus single lung transplant for chronic obstructive pulmonary disease. *J Thorac Cardiovasc Surg* 1997; **113**: 520–528.

29 Geertsma A, van der Bij W, de Boer WJ, TenVergert EM. Survival with and without lung transplantation. *Transplant Proc* 1997; **29**: 630–631.

30 Hosenpud JD, Bednnett LE, Keck BM, Edwards EB, Novick RJ. Effect of diagnosis on survival benefit of lung transplantation for end-stage lung disease. *Lancet* 1998; **351**: 24–27.

31 Forty J, Hasan A, Gould FK, Corris PA, Dark JH. Single lung transplantation with simultaneous contralateral pneumonectomy for cystic fibrosis. *J Heart Lung Transplant* 1994; **13**: 727–730.

32 Yacoub MH, Gyi K, Khagani A, et al. Analysis of 10-year experience with heart-lung transplantation for cystic fibrosis. *Transplant Proc* 1997; **29**: 632.

33 Smith JA, Roberts M, McNeil K, et al. Excellent outcome of cardiac transplantation using domino donor hearts. *Eur J Cardiothorac Surg* 1996; 10628–10633.

34 Au J, Scott CD, Hasan A, et al. Bilateral sequential lung transplantation for septic lung disease: surgical and physiologic advantages over heart–lung transplantation. *Transplant Proc* 1992; **24**: 2652–2655.

35 Smith JA, Stewart S, Roberts M, et al. Significance of graft coronary disease in heart–lung transplant recipients. *Transplant Proc* 1995; **27**: 2019–2020.

36 Adams DH, Cochrane AD, Khaghani A, Smith JD, Yacoub M. Retransplantation in heart lung recipients with obliterative bronchiolitis. *J Thorac Cardiovasc Surg* 1994; **107**: 450–459.

37 Doig JC, Richens D, Corris PA, et al. Resolution of pulmonary hypertension after single lung transplantation. *Br Heart J* 1990; **64**: 72.

38 Levine SM, Jenkinson SG, Bryan CL, et al. Ventilation–perfusion irregularities during graft rejection in patients undergoing single lung transplantation for primary pulmonary hypertension. *Chest* 1992; **101**: 401–405.

39 Waddell T, Bennett L, Kennedy R, et al. Heart–lung or lung transplantation for Eisenmenger's syndrome. *J Heart Lung Transplant* 2002; **21**: 731–737.

40 Pratschke, J Wilhelm MJ, Kusaka M, et al. Brain death and its influence on donor organ quality and outcome after transplantation. *Transplantation* 1999; **67**: 343–348.

41 Fisher AJ, Dark JH, Corris PA. Improving donor lung evaluation–new approach to increase organ supply for lung transplantation. *Thorax* 1998; **53**: 818–820.

42 Fisher AJ, Donnelly SC, Hirani N, et al. Elevated levels of interleukin-8 in donor lungs is associated with early graft failure after lung transplantation. *Am J Respir Crit Care Med* 2001; **163**: 259–265.

43 Aziz T, El-Gamel A, Yonan N. Pulmonary vein gas analysis for assessment of donor lung function. *J Heart Lung Transplant* 2001; **20**: 225–255.

44 Pennefather SH, Bullock RE, Dark JH. The effect of fluid therapy on alveolar arterial oxygen gradient in brain-dead organ donors. *Transplantation* 1993; **56**: 1418–1422.

45 Pennefather SH, Bullock RE, Mantle D, Dark JH. Use of low dose arginine vasopressin to support brain-dead organ donors. *Transplantation* 1995; **59**: 58–62.

46 Follette DM, Rudich SM, Babcock WD. Improved oxygenation and increased lung recovery with high-dose steroid administration after brain death. *J Heart Lung Transplant* 1998; **17**: 423–429.

47 Kirk AJB, Colquhoun IW, Dark JH. Lung preservation: a review of current practice and future directions. *Ann Thorac Surg* 1993; **56**: 990–1000.

48 Keshavjee SH, Yamazaki F, Yokomise H, et al. The role of dextran 40 and potassium in extended hypothermic lung preservation for transplantation. *J Thorac Cardiovasc Surg* 1992; **103**: 314–325.

49 Fischer S, Matte-Martyn A, de Perrot M, et al. Low potassium dextran preservation solution improves lung function after human lung transplantation. *J Thorac Cardiovasc Surg* 2001; **121**: 594–596.

50 Triantafillou AN, Pasque MK, Huddleston CB, et al. Predictors, frequency, and indications for cardiopulmonary bypass during lung transplantation in adults. *Ann Thorac Surg* 1994; **57**: 1248–1251.

51 Wilson IC, Hasan A, Healy M, et al. Healing of the bronchus in pulmonary transplantation. *Eur J Cardiothorac Surg* 1996; **1**: 521–527.

52 Sudarshan CD, Dark JH. A technique for insertion of self-expanding tracheal and bronchial stents. *Ann Thorac Surg* 1999; **67**: 271–272.

53 Khaghani A, al Kattan KM, Tadjkarimi S, Banner N, Yacoub M. Early experience with single lung transplantation for emphysema with simultaneous volume reduction of the contralateral lung. *Eur J Cardiothorac Surg* 1997; **11**: 604–608.

54 Cohen RG, Barr ML, Schenkel FA, DeMeester TR, Wells WJ, Starnes VA. Living-related donor lobectomy for bilateral lobar transplantation in patients with cystic fibrosis. *Ann Thorac Surg* 1994; **57**: 1423–1428.

55 Battafarano RJ, Anderson RC, Meyers BF, et al. Preoperative complications after living donor lobectomy. *J Thorac Cardiovasc Surg* 2000; **120**: 909–915.

56 Clark SC, Sudarshan C, Khanna R, Roughan J, Flecknell PA, Dark JH. Controlled reperfusion and pentoxifylline modulate reperfusion injury after single lung transplantation. *J Thorac Cardiovasc Surg* 1998; **115**: 1335–1341.

57 Thabut G, Brugière O, Leseche G, et al. Preventive effect of inhaled nitric oxide and pentoxifylline on ischaemia/reperfusion injury after lung transplantation. *Transplantation* 2001; **71**: 1295–300.

58 Smiley RM, Navedo AT, Kirby T, et al. Postoperative independent lung ventilation in a single-lung transplant recipient. *Anaesthesiology* 1991; **74**: 1144–1148.

14

Combined heart and lung transplantation

Rosemary Radley-Smith, Asghar Khaghani and Nicholas R. Banner

Harefield Hospital, Harefield, Middlesex, UK

Introduction

Experimentation into the feasibility of heart–lung transplantation began about 60 years ago. Demikhov performed the operation in dogs but had no long-term survivors because of the development of abnormal respiratory patterns in the recipients [1]. Subsequently Castaneda performed the operation in primates and achieved long-term survivors [2]. Cooley carried out the first clinical heart–lung transplantation in 1968 in a 23 month old girl with a complete atrioventricular septal defect but she survived for only 14 hours [3]. In 1969 Lillehei performed transplantation on a 43 year old man with emphysema who survived 8 days [4]. In 1971 Barnard operated on another patient with chronic lung disease who survived 23 days [5].

The first human heart–lung transplantation that resulted in long-term survival was carried out in Stanford, USA, in 1981; the patient was a 45 year old woman with primary pulmonary hypertension [6]. The first heart–lung transplantation at Harefield Hospital, UK, was performed in 1983; our longest survivor is a woman diagnosed with primary pulmonary hypertension and operated on in 1984 at 14 years of age [7]; she is still alive with her original graft. By 1985, 14 centres worldwide were carrying out heart–lung transplantation, predominantly for pulmonary vascular disease [8].

The rationale for combined transplantation of the heart and the lungs was that patients with pulmonary hypertension usually have concomitant cardiac abnormalities either as the cause of the pulmonary hypertension (Eisenmenger's syndrome) or right ventricular hypertrophy and failure secondary to the pulmonary hypertension (as in primary pulmonary hypertension). The success of the combined procedure was partly due to improved tracheobronchial healing when the lungs were transplanted en bloc with the heart but was also due to the availability of ciclosporin, which had recently been introduced into clinical transplantation and which was a more potent and specific immunosuppressive agent [6].

During the same period attempts at isolated lung transplantation were also made. Hardy transplanted a single lung into a patient with carcinoma of the lung [9]. This patient survived for 18 days, dying of renal failure. The first single lung transplant with long-term survival was performed on a patient with pulmonary fibrosis in 1983 by Cooper in Toronto [10]. In 1988 the same group undertook the first successful single lung transplant in a patient with Eisenmenger's syndrome, with simultaneous closure of a patent ductus arteriosus [11]. This was followed shortly thereafter by small series of patients from Stanford [12] and Pittsburgh [13] in which repair of cardiac defects were performed simultaneously with single lung transplantation for pulmonary vascular disease. Since that time increasing numbers of patients, including children, with congenital heart disease and pulmonary vascular disease (Eisenmenger's syndrome) [14] have undergone similar operations [15–17].

Double lung transplantation was developed during the 1980s, initially for patients with parenchymal lung disease [18]. The initial technique used was that of transplantation of the two lungs en bloc. Three such operations were carried out at our centre in 1986 [19]. The early operations were associated with a high morbidity, predominantly from problems with the healing of the tracheal anastomosis and ischaemia in the airway of the donor lungs [20]. One approach to this problem was to revascularize the bronchial circulation of the donor lungs using an internal mammary graft [19]. Although this technique produced satisfactory healing, it made the operative procedure more complex and technical failure occasionally led to severe anastomotic complications; following the introduction of bilateral

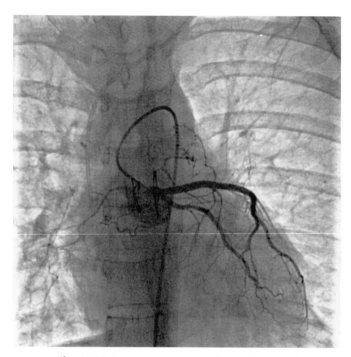

Figure 14.1 Coronary angiogram performed in a heart–lung transplant recipient, demonstrating filling of the bronchial circulation of the transplanted lungs from the coronary circulation of the transplanted heart.

sequential lung transplantation, the en bloc double lung transplant has been abandoned.

Although problems with bronchial anastomotic healing sometimes occurred in single lung transplants, modifications of the surgical technique have gradually reduced their frequency. This led to the introduction of bilateral sequential lung transplantation using bronchial anastomoses (essentially two single lung transplants performed as one operation in the same patient) [19,21–23].

The shortage of suitable donor organs and the consequent long waiting times for transplantation (especially in paediatric patients and small adults) led Starnes to introduce the technique of bilateral lobar transplantation [24]. This method was then developed to allow the use of lobes from two living donors [25]. This technique was initially applied to patients with parenchymal lung disease such as cystic fibrosis but subsequently it has also been used in infants with pulmonary hypertension [24]. This method potentially increases the number of lung transplantations that can be performed and it avoids the adverse effects of brain death and donor ventilation on the transplanted lung as well as reducing organ ischaemia time and providing the possibility of better human leukocyte antigen (HLA)

matching between the donors and the recipient. However, there continue to be some ethical concerns about the use of living donors for such lung transplants and this technique has not been widely applied [26].

Characteristics of the various lung transplant procedures

Heart–lung transplantation

This has the advantage of conceptual simplicity in removing all the diseased tissue which is replaced by the donor organs which are implanted en bloc. As the connection between the heart and lungs is maintained, the coronary-bronchial collaterals, which are an important source of blood supply to the donor airways, are preserved [27] (Figure 14.1). This reduces the risk of poor anastomotic healing due to airway ischaemia [28]. By using this operation for patients with Eisenmenger's syndrome, the need for an additional cardiac repair procedure is removed. Postoperatively both ventilation and perfusion are equally distributed to both lungs and cardiac function is relatively normal.

A disadvantage of heart–lung transplantation is that it puts a heavy demand on the supply of donor organs. This problem can be offset by the use of hearts from selected patients undergoing heart–lung transplantation for subsequent 'domino' heart transplantation [29]. Another potential problem is the risk of excessive bleeding related to the extensive nature of the surgery and the necessity for cardiopulmonary bypass and consequently for systemic heparinization. This can be a particular issue in patients with congenital heart disease because of adhesions from previous operations or the presence of collateral vessels. A previous thoracotomy has been shown to significantly increase the perioperative mortality [28,30,31]. Consequently, measures to promote haemostasis, such as the use of aprotinin during surgery and fibrin sealants, are often necessary [32]. Other limitations of the combined heart–lung transplant are concerns about cardiac denervation, particularly if a 'normal' heart has been removed as part of the procedure [33]; and the possibility of acute or chronic rejection of the heart as well as the lungs [34–37].

Transplantation of the lungs alone

The major advantage of isolated lung transplantation is that it uses fewer organs, thus shortening waiting times for individual patients. It also obviates the need for routine cardiac surveillance after transplantation. On the other hand, the range of conditions that can be addressed is reduced. If the heart is to be retained, its function should be as near normal as possible after transplantation. Therefore candidates should have good left ventricular function and be free from coronary arterial disease. Right ventricular dysfunction is not necessarily a contraindication, since even chronically dilated and hypertrophied right ventricles usually show rapid improvement in function after lung transplantation because the ventricle is now ejecting into a low resistance pulmonary vascular bed [38]. Although the right ventricular function quickly returns towards normal there can be temporary problems related to right ventricular outflow tract obstruction [11]. The mechanism for this is thought to be diminution in size of the right ventricular chamber leading to the hypertrophied walls of infundibulum coapting during systole [13]. The gradient in the right ventricular outflow will disappear once the hypertrophy regresses. There can also be problems if a severely hypertrophied right ventricle compromises left ventricular filling during diastole by the thickened and distorted interventricular septum compressing the left ventricle [39,40]. This effect, coupled with the improved systolic function of the right ventricle, creates a haemodynamic situation that can easily lead to pulmonary oedema when there has been ischaemia–reperfusion injury in the transplanted lungs.

If there is to be simultaneous repair of congenital heart disease, the defects should be 'simple', such as an atrial septal defect, perimembranous ventricular septal defect or a persistent ductus arteriosus. Some centres have repaired complex lesions, particularly in children, but the initial mortality was higher, the cardiac prognosis after repair is uncertain and complications such as endocarditis have occurred [41].

All forms of lung transplantation have the potential for airways complications both because the vascular supply to the native bronchi is less good than that to the trachea and because both the bronchial arteries and the coronary-bronchial collaterals to the transplanted lung have been divided. However, improvement in surgical techniques has reduced the frequency of such problems significantly [19,21,22] and methods have been developed for treating bronchial stenoses by stenting or cryotherapy [42–44].

Bilateral lung transplantation

This removes all the diseased lung tissue, which is of importance when one is dealing with chronically infected lungs in patients with cystic fibrosis or bronchiectasis. This operation can be performed either on or off cardiopulmonary bypass (except in patients with severe pulmonary hypertension); an operation done without bypass can help to reduce the risks of excessive bleeding during surgery but this technique subjects the first lung to be transplanted to a further insult while it is used for single lung ventilation as the second lung is implanted. Bilateral transplants can be performed through a clam-shell incision, which gives much better access to both pleural cavities with better control of bleeding from adhesions, etc.

Single lung transplantation

This can often be carried out without bypass. The posterolateral incision allows a good view of the entire pleural space. Alternative incisions (median sternotomy or clam-shell) may be useful when additional procedures are required such as contralateral lung volume reduction surgery. The single lung procedure technique allows choice of which side is to be operated upon, which can be an important advantage if there has been previous thoracic surgery. The heart and contralateral lung remain innervated. This operation allows the most efficient use of donor organ by allowing for up to three recipients to receive organs from one donor [10].

The most important disadvantage of this operation is the ventilation–perfusion mismatch that can occur both early after the operation from ischaemia–reperfusion injury at the time of surgery or later due to lung rejection [45,46]. Ventilation–perfusion mismatch is a particular problem in patients receiving transplants for pulmonary hypertension. In these patients the transplanted lung, which has a normal pulmonary vascular resistance, functions in parallel with the native lung, which has a very high resistance but normal airways resistance and compliance. This leads to the great majority of the blood flow going to the transplanted lung while ventilation remains evenly divided between the two lungs. During rejection, most of the pulmonary blood flow will still go to the transplanted lung but, because of increased airways resistance and reduced compliance of this lung, the majority of the ventilation will be diverted to the native lung. This can lead to a marked reduction in oxygen saturation and profound symptoms. Such an adverse response during a rejection episode will not be seen in patients receiving transplants for restrictive or obstructive lung disease where both ventilation and perfusion tend to favour the transplanted lung. However, in patients with chronic obstructive pulmonary disease, postoperative problems with air trapping in the native lung causing mediastinal shift may occur, particularly when there is early dysfunction of the transplanted lung due to ischaemia–reperfusion injury (see Chapter 15).

Bilateral lung transplantation can be used in nearly all situations where single lung transplantation can be applied and may have advantages for the recipient at the cost of performing one transplantation rather than two; there is evidence that bilateral lung transplantation can produce better short- and long-term results than single lung transplantation in both patients with parenchymal lung disease [47,48] and those with pulmonary hypertension [49]. The improved long-term results seen with bilateral lung transplantation (50) may partly reflect the higher number of normally functioning bronchoalveolar units in such patients, which can make them more resistant to the effect of bronchiolitis obliterans syndrome.

During the early years of thoracic transplantation, heart–lung transplantation was the only option for patients requiring other than an isolated heart transplant and the operation was used for patients with both parenchymal lung disease and pulmonary vascular disease [51,52]. During the last decade the number of heart–lung transplantations worldwide has fallen, concurrently with a dramatic rise in the numbers of single and bilateral lung transplantations for all indications including pulmonary vascular disease [50]. A major reason for this has been the rapid increase in the number of patients awaiting lung transplantation, while the availability of lungs suitable for transplantation has remained static or even fallen. Organ allocation rules have also played a role so that very few combined heart–lung transplantations are performed in North America whereas the operation is used more frequently in Europe [53].

Current practice

Many centres, particularly in North America, now perform bilateral lung transplantation for both parenchymal lung disease and pulmonary hypertension even in the presence of structural heart disease [49]. However in the UK and Europe, where heart–lung blocks have been more easily available, there is a tendency to perform heart–lung transplantation for primary and secondary hypertension [53] and for some types of parenchymal lung disease such as cystic fibrosis [54]. The heart from certain recipients of heart–lung transplants can be suitable for subsequent heart transplantation [29], although this concept has never been applied widely in North America. Worldwide only about 100 heart–lung transplantations are now performed annually [50], with the majority of these operations being performed in Europe [53].

The management of patients with Eisenmenger's syndrome (severe pulmonary hypertension associated with congenital heart disease and hypoxaemia due to a right to left or a bidirectional shunt) [55] varies between cen-

tres. If lung transplantation with simultaneous repair is to be performed, most units prefer to undertake a bilateral lung transplantation to avoid the ventilation–perfusion mismatch that may occur after single lung transplantation for pulmonary hypertension. Given the availability of a heart–lung block, however, many centres (including our own) would prefer to perform a combined heart and lung transplantation for all but the very simplest of congenital heart disease [56].

Indications and contraindications

The indications for, and contraindications to, lung transplantation in general have been described elsewhere [57,58] and are reviewed in Chapter 12. There have been no randomized trials to compare the use of different types of lung transplantation in specific conditions. Hence, the practice of each transplant centre is determined by historical and organizational factors as well as by the published information that is available and by the clinical experience and opinions of the transplant team.

During the development of our transplant programme, we applied heart–lung transplantation to the full range of pulmonary vascular and parenchymal lung diseases [51]; however, we currently restrict the use of heart–lung transplantation to patients requiring surgery because of primary pulmonary hypertension and its variants, cystic fibrosis or congenital heart disease with Eisenmenger's syndrome.

Contraindications

The general contraindications to heart–lung transplantation are similar to those for other types of lung transplantation (see Chapter 12). The absolute need for cardiopulmonary bypass during this procedure, combined with the extensive nature of the surgery, results in an increased risk of haemorrhagic complications; this makes previous surgery via a lateral thoracotomy or the presence of major aortopulmonary collaterals specific contraindications to heart–lung transplantation [28,30,31]. In our experience of patients with congenital heart disease who had undergone prior surgery, only 3/17 (18%) patients who had undergone median sternotomy died during the perioperative period as opposed to 22/34 (65%) who had had previous lateral thoracotomy ($p < 0.001$). Early death was even more frequent in the patients with complex pulmonary atresia and major aortopulmonary collaterals (16/20; 80%). Death was usually due to multiorgan failure secondary to bleeding and multiple transfusions [59]. We now regard these conditions as contraindications to combined heart–lung transplantation. The problem of previous surgery is not restricted to those who have undergone cardiac procedures, since similar problems can be caused by some of the types of pleurodesis that have been used in patients with cystic fibrosis or other parenchymal lung disease and by the sites of previous open lung biopsies. For this reason surgical pleurodesis and operative lung biopsies are best avoided in patients who may need transplant surgery subsequently.

The timing of surgery is critical for success; an operation on a patient with advanced secondary organ dysfunction, poor nutritional status or refractory infection is unlikely to be successful. Unfortunately, some patients are referred at too late a stage for transplantation and, because of the scarcity of suitable donor organs, some patients may deteriorate while awaiting surgery to a point where transplantation is no longer likely to be successful.

There is no lower age limit to heart–lung transplantation but the results in young children are not as good as in older children and adults [59,60]. A supportive family is extremely important when a child is to receive a transplant. Patient adherence to follow-up protocols and drug therapy can be a particular issue in adolescents and young adults. Most centres would set an upper age limit of 50 years for heart–lung transplantation [50]. We found that older patients with congenital heart disease did less well than younger patients; this was possibly due to long-term damage to other organs such as the kidneys and liver from longstanding cyanosis; because of these very poor results, we now try to avoid transplantation in this group of patients.

A group of patients about which there has been some controversy are young adults with Eisenmenger's syndrome related to Down's syndrome. Only the occasional patient in this situation has received a transplant because of the medical complications to which these patients are prone [61,62].

Indications

The decision to recommend transplantation must be based on a comparison of the expected outcome, with continued medical therapy, with that of transplantation both in terms of survival and quality of life. The criteria for transplantation are continuing to evolve with improvements in the medical management of each condition.

Primary pulmonary hypertension

Primary pulmonary hypertension is a rare condition which often has a genetic basis [63]. The initial symptoms are nonspecific and so diagnosis is often delayed. When untreated, the condition follows a progressive downhill course and eventually the patient will die from right ventricular failure; in a Registry study, the median survival

time from diagnosis was 2.8 years [64]. However, significant progress has been made in the treatment of this condition using anticoagulation [65] and vasodilator agents [66,67]. Patients who have a good functional capacity (New York Heart Association (NYHA) class I or II) and who have no evidence of right heart failure at right heart catheterization (cardiac index >2.1 L/min per m^2, mixed venous oxygen saturation >63% and right atrial pressure <10 mmHg (1.3 kpa)) should be tested for responsiveness to pulmonary vasodilators; those who respond can benefit from long-term treatment with a calcium channel blocking agent [66]. Patients in NYHA class III or IV who have right heart failure can benefit from long-term treatment with intravenous epoprostenol (prostacyclin) regardless of whether they show any acute response to pulmonary vasodilators [68]. Patients receiving such treatment have an improved short-term survival as compared with those receiving conventional therapy and this benefit appears to persist in the longer term [67,69]. Some patients will have a marked improvement in their symptoms and functional capacity during epoprostenol therapy. By stabilizing their condition and preventing progressive right heart failure with hepatic and renal dysfunction, such treatment can improve the outcome after transplantation [56]. However, intravenous therapy with epoprostenol carries a significant risk of serious complications including catheter-related sepsis and thromboembolism. In addition, an interruption in the supply of epoprostenol, due to pump failure or operator error, may lead to a rapid deterioration in the clinical condition of some patients. Therefore, patients undergoing this treatment need to be under the care of a physician with a specific interest in pulmonary hypertension and to be supported by a multidisciplinary team [70]. The substantial and sustained response to prostacyclin that occurs in many primary pulmonary hypertension patients has led to a change in practice so that patients are usually not listed for transplantation until they have had a trial of epoprostenol therapy. However, we currently feel that patients who meet the criteria for this treatment should undergo an initial assessment to clarify whether transplantation is a therapeutic option if medical therapy does not produce a satisfactory therapeutic response. Unless there is an early response, suitable patients should be listed for transplantation with the option of removing them from the list if there is improvement subsequently. This is because of the risk of further deterioration during the waiting time for transplantation and the poor results of transplantation in patients with end-stage disease causing renal and liver dysfunction with ascites, jaundice and coagulation abnormalities.

Thromboembolic pulmonary hypertension must be distinguished from primary pulmonary hypertension because

this disease is best treated by pulmonary thromboendarterectomy rather than by transplantation [71, 72].

Cystic fibrosis

Patients with cystic fibrosis (CF) require transplantation of both lungs to allow the removal of the severely
bronchiectatic and chronically infected native lungs. This
can be achieved either by heart–lung transplantation or by
bilateral sequential lung transplantation [22]. Historically,
our preference has been to use the combined heart–lung
transplant in these patients because of the excellent healing of the tracheal anastomosis that is usually achieved with
this operation. This is a particular advantage in CF, where
infection of a poorly healing anastomosis can lead to serious complications. Currently, the increasing scarcity of
donor organs for all forms of thoracic organ transplantation and the falling incidence of airway complications after
bilateral lung transplantation has influenced us to also use
bilateral lung transplantation for this group of patients.

The indications for transplantation in CF and specific
issues for the post-transplantation management of CF
patients are reviewed in Chapter 8. A problem of special concern in selecting CF patients for transplantation
is that of antibiotic-resistant bacterial infection and of
fungal infections. The issue of when to exclude patients
with multiple-resistant or pan-resistant organisms [57]
from transplantation had been controversial [73]. It is not
clear that all such patients are at high risk after transplantation perhaps because sensitivity profiles of *Pseudomonas*
species in CF patients frequently change under antibiotic pressure and resistance during in vitro testing does
not always equate with clinical resistance [57]. In addition, patients with resistant organisms often have advanced
disease and so have a particularly bad prognosis without
transplantation. However, some strains of *Burkholderia* are
highly virulent and pose a special threat; patients with these
should be excluded [74,75]. In other cases resistant infection should be regarded as a risk factor that may lead to
exclusion when other adverse factors are present such as
poor nutritional state (see also Chapters 12 and 20).

Coexistent disease of the heart and the lungs

In principle, heart–lung transplantation could be used to
treat patients with coexistent diseases affecting both the
heart and the lungs, for example a patient with severe
chronic obstructive pulmonary disease and heart failure
due to coronary heart disease. In practice, heart–lung transplantation is rarely used in this way because most of the
potential candidates are above the age limit for transplantation or have other contraindications to surgery.

Congenital heart disease

This indication for transplantation is not covered in detail
elsewhere in this volume and so it will be reviewed here;
many patients with complex congenital heart disease cannot be treated by other forms of lung transplantation.

There are four groups of patients with congenital heart
disease who might benefit from heart–lung transplantation. By far the largest group are those with unrepaired
congenital heart disease and pulmonary hypertension –
so-called Eisenmenger's syndrome [14,55]. The second
group are those patients with previously repaired defects
who have progressive pulmonary hypertension; because
these patients have already had their defect corrected, they
may be suitable for bilateral lung transplantation and the
medical management of their pulmonary hypertension
should be similar to that for patients with primary pulmonary hypertension. The third group are those with a con-
genitally inadequate pulmonary vascular bed (pulmonary
atresia, a ventricular septal defect and major aortopulmonary collateral arteries or 'complex pulmonary atresia')
[76]. Currently, we do not recommend heart–lung transplantation to this group of patients because of the poor
clinical results. Finally, there are a small number of patients
with uncorrectable congenital lung abnormalities such as
peripheral pulmonary arterial or venous stenoses. These
abnormalities may be a part of syndromes such as Alagille
syndrome [77], in which the patient may require simultaneous transplantation of the liver. In the absence of intra-
cardiac defects, these children may also be suitable for
single or double lung transplantation.

Assessment

The assessment should be performed by a multidisciplinary team including physicians and surgeons experienced in the management of patients before and after
transplantation as well as in the management of congenital heart disease. The objectives of the assessment process
are to confirm the diagnosis, ensure that optimum medical treatment has been applied, assess the severity of the
patient's condition and thereby determine whether transplantation is indicated at that stage. Contraindications to
transplantation should be identified and an assessment of
whether a patient has a realistic chance of receiving a transplant if he/she is added to the waiting list at that centre.
Due to the scarcity of organs suitable for transplantation,
there is no benefit from adding patients who are developing
secondary organ failure to the list since they are unlikely
to remain suitable for transplantation during the waiting
period.

Patients with congenital heart disease should undergo a range of investigations similar to those performed in other candidates for lung transplantation (see Chapter 12) In addition, patients with congenital heart disease must have a complete anatomical diagnosis, which can usually be obtained by a combination of echocardiography, cardiac magnetic resonance imaging and, when necessary, by ultrafast computed tomography. The positions of the great vessels and the anatomy of the systemic venous system must be defined to allow the surgical approach to be planned. Abnormalities of atrial situs and pulmonary venous return should be noted but are not barriers to surgery since complete cardiac and pulmonary replacement will occur. In patients considered to have Eisenmenger's syndrome, the haemodynamic situation should be carefully documented to detect occasional patients who have been previously misdiagnosed and who have relatively normal pulmonary pressures that may make them eligible for isolated heart transplantation. Many of the patients will have already undergone cardiac catheterization and angiography to see whether conventional cardiac surgery is possible but, in the small group of older patients who have already undergone repair and might be suitable for bilateral lung transplantation, coronary angiography should be performed. Exercise performance as measured by a six minute walk test can be useful in assessing the exact level of the patient's limitation and to assess changes with time. Respiratory function tests are generally unhelpful since they do not reflect the severity of the pulmonary vascular disease or the patient's disability. A 24 hour creatinine clearance test and liver function tests should be undertaken. As many patients with congenital heart disease and pulmonary hypertension have chronic liver congestion or polycythaemia and these may be associated with coagulation abnormalities, full haematological investigations should be performed.

Medical management of patients with congenital heart disease and pulmonary hypertension tends to be supportive, with treatment of the complications rather than of the disease itself. Contrary to previous practice, it is not now thought beneficial to haemodilute these patients, unless they have symptoms of hyperviscosity [78].

Measures to lower the pulmonary vascular resistance (PVR) are singularly ineffective and the use of calcium channel blockers may actually be harmful by acutely lowering systemic pressure and thereby increasing the right-to-left shunt, which may lead to syncope and death. Long-term oxygen therapy has been shown to be beneficial in children [79]; although its value is unproven in adults, it may provide symptomatic benefit.

In patients with Eisenmenger's syndrome, closure of the systemic-to-pulmonary connection will only hasten death.

Patients with complex pulmonary atresia are unsuitable for heart–lung transplantation because of the surgical risks of haemorrhage and death [59] but palliative surgery may be possible to enhance the pulmonary blood supply with the aim of ultimate biventricular repair [76].

Timing of transplantation

The clinical decision about when to recommend placing a patient on the waiting list is difficult because of the appreciable early risks of transplantation, which must be weighed against the patient's expected prognosis with medical therapy and their quality of life. In addition, the waiting time for heart–lung transplantation can be prolonged and the patient must be able to survive this period. Listing should be considered when the patient's condition is deteriorating and their life expectancy is about two years. Unfortunately, in patients with Eisenmenger's syndrome, there are no clear-cut guides to prognosis and the recommendation for transplantation remains one of clinical judgement.

Patients with Eisenmenger's syndrome generally have a substantially better prognosis than those with other types of pulmonary hypertension; for example, the 25 year survival after the diagnosis of an Eisenmenger ventricular septal defect is 42% [80]. This is possibly due to the 'protective' nature of the right-to-left shunt and because the pulmonary hypertension is present early and is only slowly progressive, giving the right ventricle more time to adapt [81,82]. Patients with congenital heart disease and pulmonary hypertension therefore behave differently from those with primary pulmonary hypertension and similar pulmonary artery pressures; right heart function is better and right atrial pressure lower in the former group than in the latter [81].

In view of the good overall prognosis of Eisenmenger's syndrome, selection of patients for transplantation must be based on a process of risk stratification and it must take into account the patients' quality of life as well as their anticipated survival. The published guidelines for this group of patients merely specify that they should be in NYHA functional class III or IV, with severe and progressive symptoms despite optimal medical management [58]. Features that have been found to be associated with a poor prognosis are listed in Table 14.1 [83–85].

The exception to the more benign prognosis of pulmonary hypertension associated with congenital heart disease is the group of patients who have already had an intracardiac repair but have gone on to progressive pulmonary hypertension despite this; these patients behave similarly to those with primary pulmonary hypertension and may deteriorate rapidly. This is probably because they

Table 14.1. Adverse prognostic factors in adult patients with Eisenmenger's syndrome

NYHA class III or IV
Deteriorating functional capacity
Syncope
Refractory right heart failure
Severe hypoxaemia
Presentation at a younger age
Complex cardiac defect[a]
Supraventricular arrhythmia
Degree of electrocardiographic right ventricular hypertrophy
Right ventricular dysfunction (echocardiographic dilatation and hypokinesis)
Raised serum creatinine

Note: NYHA, New York Heart Association.
[a]Simple defects are atrial septal defect, ventricular septal defect and persistent ductus arteriosus.
Source: Data from refs. 55, 83 and 84

no longer have a shunt to prevent the pulmonary artery pressure from becoming suprasystemic. This group should be regarded in the same way as those with primary pulmonary hypertension.

The guidelines for paediatric transplantation are similar to those for adults, but because the diagnoses are more varied and the disease spectrum more diverse, prognostic features have been more difficult to develop and most patients are selected empirically. Because of the relatively poor post-transplant prognosis in younger children, it is vital to exclude other correctable cardiac defects and no heart–lung transplantation should be undertaken unless it is considered a life-saving procedure.

Surgical techniques

Donor selection and management

A key problem in heart–lung transplantation is the necessity for an organ donor where all three organs are suitable for transplantation and can be allocated to the heart–lung recipient. Heart–lung blocks are rarely available in the USA because of a policy of preferentially offering all transplantable hearts first for the most urgent (United Network for Organ Sharing (UNOS) status 1) heart transplant candidates. The criteria for donor selection vary between centres; our own include age of less than 55 years, no history of significant cardiopulmonary disease and preferably, no history of smoking. Cardiac assessment and management is similar to that for transplantation of the heart alone [86]. Cardiac function should be satisfactory with either no or

minimal inotropic support being provided. The electrocardiogram should show sinus rhythm and no pathological Q-waves or unequivocal evidence of left ventricular hypertrophy. Repolarization changes are common after brain death and do not preclude organ donation. Fluid management requires careful attention, since hypovolaemia in the donor may result in an excessive use of inotropes but injudicious fluid administration can promote pulmonary oedema, which can occur after brain death. Hormone replacement therapy and the use of data obtained by placing a pulmonary artery flotation catheter to direct both fluid administration and the use of inotropic agents can significantly improve donor management [87]. Further assessment of ventricular function can be made by transthoracic echo or by transoesophageal echocardiography, which can be performed at the start of the operation for organ retrieval.

Lung function, as assessed by arterial gases, should be adequate; an arterial oxygen pressure (PaO_2 > 12 kPa (90 mmHg) on an F_1O_2 (fraction of oxygen in inspired gas) $\leq$ 35%, or $PaO_2 \geq$ 40 kPa (300 mmHg) on 100% oxygen, are considered satisfactory. Pulmonary compliance, as assessed by the inspiratory pressures required for mechanical ventilation, must be close to normal. Donor sputum is cultured to identify any pathogens that may require specific treatment in the recipient during the post-transplantation period; because of the shortage of potential donors, lung atelectasis and positive sputum cultures are not regarded, in themselves, as contraindications to organ harvesting. However, a heavy bacterial or fungal growth must exclude the donor. There should be, however, no evidence of consolidation within the lung parenchyma. Initially unsuitable lungs may sometimes be improved by a therapeutic fiberoptic bronchoscopy and physiotherapy. Although the length of mechanical ventilation is an important factor influencing the incidence of pulmonary infection, we do not use a specific time limit. The donor is given a 'cocktail' of intravenous antibiotics (cefuroxime, gentamicin, metronidazole and sodium fusidate) prior to organ harvesting.

Overall, only about 20% of solid organ donors have lungs that are considered suitable for transplantation. The common causes of exclusion are: chest trauma with severe lung contusion or laceration bronchial aspiration during resuscitation, severe neurogenic pulmonary oedema with a poor gas exchange and infection, which is usually related to prolonged positive pressure ventilation.

The donor must be screened for other transmissible diseases, particularly for hepatitis B-specific antigen and for antibodies against both hepatitis C virus and human immunodeficiency virus. The donor and recipient cytomegalovirus (CMV) status are determined serologically.

Donor–recipient matching

For heart–lung transplantation, the donor's and recipient's lung sizes should be matched to avoid problems of pulmonary atelectasis or persistent pleural effusions or pneumothorax postoperatively. The donor chest size should be slightly smaller than those of the recipient. Size matching may be based on either external measurements of the thoracic cage or the chest X-ray film [51]. The patient's original lung pathology must also be considered because patients with emphysema will have a large thoracic cavity, relative to their body size, whereas those with restrictive disease will have a small pleural space.

ABO blood group compatibility is essential but we have allowed 'minor' ABO mismatches (e.g. placing a group O organ into a group B patient) [88]. We do not match for rhesus (Rh) blood group; whenever organs from an Rh-positive donor are transplanted into a female Rh-negative recipient with child-bearing potential anti-D immunoglobulin is administered to prevent the formation of Rh antibodies (see Chapter 24).

Ideally we aim to use CMV-negative donors for CMV-negative recipients. This is because patients who are immunologically naive to CMV and who develop a primary infection after transplantation are at the greatest risk of serious tissue-invasive disease and of infection that relapses after treatment (see Chapter 21). However, the current shortage of donor organs frequently makes CMV matching impractical.

Organ preservation

For heart–lung transplantation, the heart and both lungs must be preserved simultaneously. Two general approaches have become established in clinical practice. The first is to preserve the lungs by a flush cooling technique while separately administering a cardioplegia solution to the heart [89]; the second is to systemically cool the donor using cardiopulmonary bypass to preserve the lungs, combined with cardioplegia to preserve the heart [30].

In the pulmonary flush technique a pulmonary vasodilator such as alprostadil (prostaglandin E₁) [90] or epoprostenol (prostacyclin) [91] is usually administered via the pulmonary artery to reduce pulmonary vasoconstriction during the cooling process and thereby promote uniform cooling. A variety of preservation solutions have been used with both 'intracellular' [92] and 'extracellular' [91] characteristics; both types of solution have produced satisfactory clinical results and it appears that adequate cooling of the lungs is the essential feature of all these methods.

Our approach has been to use donor cooling with cardiopulmonary bypass and this approach has been described in detail elsewhere [30,51]. This technique requires a portable cardiopulmonary bypass machine that can be transported to the donor's hospital and used to produce systemic cooling of the donor to a core temperature of 10 °C. The circulation is then arrested and cardioplegia is administered. The lungs are cooled mainly by flow through the bronchial circulation. The method does have the drawback of needing to take a cardiopulmonary bypass system to the donor hospital. It has been criticized because of the potential adverse effects of cardiopulmonary bypass on donor lung; however, in our experience this method has provided satisfactory lung preservation.

The various preservation methods available have never been compared directly in a randomized clinical trial. Practice has evolved on the basis of individual centres' experience. The pulmonary flush technique has become the method used by most centres but this seems to be on the basis of simplicity and practicality rather than any clear evidence for its superiority; the optimum method for pulmonary preservation has not been determined.

Excision of the donor organs

Once donor cooling has been accomplished and cardioplegia administered, the pleural cavities are opened and the pericardium excised. The heart and lung block can then be dissected under ideal conditions. The trachea is clamped as high as possible and the organs immersed in cold blood (obtained from the pump reservoir or pulmonary venous flow), wrapped in several sterile polythene bags and loosely packed with crushed ice in an insulated container for transportation.

Surgery in the recipient

The surgical technique is based on that originally described by Reitz and colleagues [93] and has been described elsewhere [51]. The management of anaesthesia is described in Chapter 15. Originally the operation was always performed through a median sternotomy but more recently the transverse thoracosternotomy (clam-shell) incision has also been used in cases where bleeding from pleural adhesions or collateral vessels has been anticipated to be a problem. The clam-shell incision was introduced for bilateral lung transplantation [22]; it offers excellent access to the pleural spaces and posterior mediastinal structures but its use is associated with more postoperative pain and usually it requires the use of epidural analgesia during the early postoperative phase; in addition it has occasionally caused late complications and so is not used routinely at our centre [94].

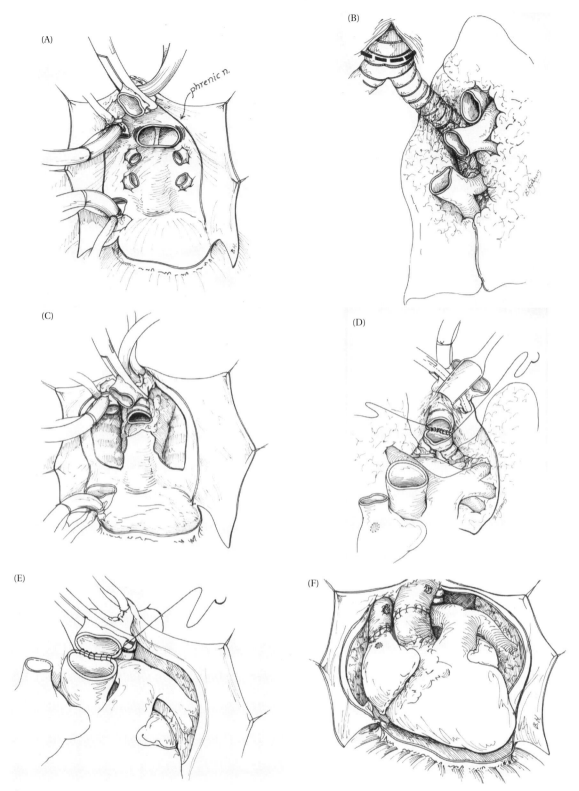

Figure 14.2 Surgical technique for heart–lung transplantation. (Reproduced with permission from ref. 51). (A) The recipient has been cannulated for cardiopulmonary bypass in preparation for a domino transplant with separate cannulae in the superior vena cava and inferior vena cava. The recipient's heart has been removed intact by dividing the great vessels, the superior vena cava, inferior vena cava/right atrial junction and the pulmonary veins. (B) The recipient's diseased lungs are removed en bloc by dividing the trachea at a point just above the carina. (C) The empty pericardial cavity following removal of the recipient's heart and lungs. (D) The donor heart–lung block is inserted through the pericardial cavity, passing each lung into its corresponding pleural cavity through limited incisions in the pericardium. The donor and recipient trachea then are anastomosed. (E) The aortic anastomosis is completed. (F) Finally the right atrial or superior vena cava and inferior vena cava anastomoses are completed.

After establishing cardiopulmonary bypass, the recipient's heart is excised (Figure 14.2). If the heart is to be used for cardiac transplantation into another patient [29], the atria are kept intact by direct cannulation of the superior vena cava and the junction of the inferior vena cava and the right atrium. In other cases the method of cannulation and excision of the heart is similar to that used for the conventional orthotopic cardiac transplantation. The pleural cavities are then opened widely; the posterior pericardium is kept intact with only limited incisions being made around the hila. Preserving the pericardium helps to prevent prolapse of the donor heart into the pleural cavity and reduces the risk of bleeding or of injury to the phrenic nerves. Dissection of the hilum is conducted by staying as near as possible to the main bronchus, particularly posteriorly, to avoid injury to the vagus nerves. The bronchial arteries must be identified and secured. The lungs are then removed en bloc by dividing the trachea just above its bifurcation.

The donor organs are prepared by trimming the ascending aorta to a level about 2.5 cm above the aortic valve. The right atrium is prepared for anastomosis. In the conventional technique, the superior vena cava is ligated and an incision is made from the orifice of the inferior vena cava towards the right atrial appendage, curving anteriorly to avoid the area of the sino-atrial node. In the 'domino' technique the right atrium is left intact. The bronchial tree is cleared by suction through the trachea.

The trachea is trimmed just above the bifurcation taking care to preserve the peritracheal tissue so as to avoid injury to the coronary-bronchial collaterals which are present within the heart–lung block (Figure 14.1). Donor and recipient aorta are then anastomosed and the atrial anastomosis performed. In the conventional technique donor and recipient right atria are joined in a manner similar to orthotopic cardiac transplantation. In the domino technique, separate anastomoses are made between donor and recipient superior vena cavae and between donor and recipient inferior venae cavae.

Postoperative care

Postoperative care is considered in detail in Chapter 15. After a routine transplantation, the heart–lung recipient typically has good initial cardiac and respiratory function. Cardiac function is rarely problematic in this situation although inotropic support may be required in the early postoperative period. Cardiac management is normally more straightforward than that required after heart transplantation [86] and this is partly because the transplanted heart and lungs are a matched physiological system. A period of lung dysfunction may occur due to ischaemia–reperfusion injury; this can usually be managed by the use of controlled mechanical ventilation, inhaled nitric oxide, fluid restriction and diuresis. Ventilation can be delivered via a conventional single lumen endotracheal tube. Weaning from ventilation may have to be delayed until the effect of any ischaemia–reperfusion injury has subsided but otherwise follows conventional lines. However, some patients with CF who have had severe carbon dioxide retention prior to transplantation will need a longer period of ventilation while their acid–base balance and respiratory centre become 'reset' to normal CO_2 levels. Those patients whose operation has been performed through a clam-shell technique will require epidural analgesia during the early postoperative phase. All patients should receive antibiotic prophylaxis against infection and in CF patients this must be selected to provide cover for the organisms present preoperatively; CF patients also require prophylaxis against gastrointestinal complication (Chapter 8).

Excessive intraoperative or postoperative blood loss can be a serious complication of heart–lung transplantation. Postoperative bleeding must be tackled vigorously by correction of coagulation abnormalities (Chapter 24) and early reoperation to prevent haemodynamic instability and the use of large volumes of blood products that may combine to produce renal, hepatic and pulmonary dysfunction.

Subsequent clinical management and results

Once discharged from the intensive care unit, the management of heart–lung transplant recipients is similar to that for other recipients of lung transplants. Immunosuppression protocols vary between units and are discussed in Chapter 18. Careful attention should be paid to physiotherapy and prophylaxis against infection. The transplanted lungs are denervated and so postural drainage techniques are required to promote the expectoration of any sputum that may be present. Subsequent rehabilitation is similar to that used for other types of thoracic surgery.

Acute rejection usually affects the transplanted lung before the transplanted heart [34,35], so monitoring is focused on signs of pulmonary rejection. Respiratory symptoms and the plain chest X-ray are useful in the early postoperative period; serial spirometric measurements should be started as soon as possible as these are the best guide to the onset of pulmonary rejection. The diagnosis of rejection should be confirmed by bronchoscopy and transbronchial biopsy (Chapter 23). Isolated heart rejection can occasionally occur but the frequency is too low to justify routine surveillance endomyocardial biopsies. We monitor the cardiac allograft clinically, electrocardiographically and by echocardiography. Endomyocardial biopsies are performed when clinically indicated but in practice they are rarely required.

Both the transplanted heart and the transplanted lung are denervated. This does not cause major physiological problems, however, and breathing patterns are normal at rest [95] and the cardiopulmonary response to exercise is similar to that seen in recipients of orthotopic heart transplants [96]. Heart–lung transplantation improves the quality of life of patients with end-stage cardiopulmonary disease [97].

Most of the long-term problems encountered after heart–lung transplantation are those common to all forms of lung transplantation including complications of immunosuppression (opportunistic infection, malignancy and drug-specific toxicity such as nephrotoxicity) together with obliterative bronchiolitis/bronchiolitis obliterans syndrome, which is currently the problem that limits the long-term benefits of all types of lung transplant. These issues are addressed elsewhere in this volume.

Primary pulmonary hypertension was found to be a risk factor for obliterative bronchiolitis in one study [98]. However, in our patients, the incidence has been similar in all patient groups. Children operated on under the age of nine years had a higher incidence of obliterative bronchiolitis and therefore a poorer long-term survival than older children and adults [60]. This was irrespective of whether they were operated on for congenital heart disease and pulmonary hypertension or for other lung disease. Factors that might contribute to this finding could include the small size of airways in young children, difficulty in cooperating with physiotherapy, late reporting of symptoms and difficulty in obtaining meaningful respiratory function tests in very small children, which could all delay the diagnosis of acute rejection or infection – risk factors for subsequent obliterative bronchiolitis. However, another study in children operated on for CF has failed to confirm that patient age was a risk factor for obliterative bronchiolitis [99].

Chronic cardiac rejection (cardiac allograft vasculopathy or transplant-associated coronary arterial disease) is an important complication of cardiac transplantation [100]. This may also affect the heart within a heart–lung transplant; however, in practice, the incidence of this disease is much lower than that seen with isolated heart transplantation [101–104] and, when it does occur, it is usually in patients who already have advanced obliterative bronchiolitis [37].

Survival after heart–lung transplantations that was reported to the International Registry was 62% at one year, 40% at five years and 26% at 10 years [50,105]. The half-life for survival was 2.8 years while the conditional half-life in those patients who survived the first year was 8.2 years. The one year survival for both single and bilateral lung transplants was somewhat higher at one year (71% and 72%, respectively); survival rates at five years were 40% for single lungs and 47% for bilateral lungs and those at 10 years were 17% and 31%, respectively. The overall half-lives after these two operations are 3.6 and 4.5 years, respectively, and the conditional half-lives of those that survive for more than one year are 5.7 and 7.9 years, respectively. Thus heart–lung transplantation has a higher short-term mortality rate than either single or double lung transplantation, while the long-term survival (reflected in the conditional half times) is better than that seen after single lung transplantation and similar to that seen after bilateral lung transplantation. Thus, in the Registry data, heart–lung transplantation was associated with a higher early mortality rate than bilateral lung transplantation but a similar long-term outcome.

In our own series of 465 heart lung transplantations, survival at one year was 63%, at five years 47% and 10 years 34%. One year survival has increased from 61% for those operated on before 1993 to 69% for those undergoing surgery between 1993 and 2001. The survival rate in all patients given a transplant for CF was 70% at one year and 51% at five years.

Patients who have undergone heart–lung transplantation are a heterogeneous group and the crude survival rates after the different lung transplant procedures should not be compared uncritically. Unfortunately, the Registry report did not break down the results of heart–lung transplantation by diagnosis or by other risks factors. Multivariate analysis of the larger lung transplant data set has revealed that a preoperative diagnosis of either congenital heart disease or primary pulmonary hypertension (two of the commonest indications for heart–lung transplantation) are both important risk factors after isolated lung transplantation (with odds ratios for death of 2.04 and 1.5, respectively). Thus case-mix and preoperative diagnosis may be factors influencing the higher initial mortality reported after heart–lung transplantation.

Retransplantation

Obliterative bronchiolitis is the commonest serious long-term complication of all types of lung transplantation. It often fails to respond to medical therapy and causes both morbidity and mortality. When the condition has progressed to the point that a patient is once again in respiratory failure, retransplantation is the only possible therapeutic option, although the results of second transplantations are inferior to those of first operations [106]. Early in our experience of heart–lung transplantation we offered selected patients with obliterative bronchiolitis a second heart–lung procedure, but this approach was associated with a high perioperative mortality. Since the majority of heart–lung recipients with advanced obliterative bronchiolitis are free from angiographic coronary disease, we have subsequently used single lung transplantation to treat selected patients with obliterative bronchiolitis. In this setting, the single lung transplantation has a lower perioperative mortality than the combined procedure and it can result in a satisfactory clinical outcome with good physical rehabilitation of the patient. However, this approach is not suitable for those patients who have developed bilateral pulmonary sepsis as a complication of obliterative bronchiolitis or for those with chronic cardiac rejection. In addition many patients must be excluded for other reasons such as ciclosporin nephrotoxicity. Our general approach is to apply the same selection criteria as are used for first transplantations; however, risk factors and relative contraindications must be given greater weight because of the lower overall survival rate after second transplantations. Pulmonary retransplantation remains a controversial practice because of the inferior results compared with those of first transplantations and the shortage of lungs suitable for transplantation [107]. In practice, because of the scarcity of donor lungs very few second transplantations are performed.

Domino heart transplantation

One of the criticisms of the combined heart–lung transplant is that it requires the use of three donor organs, while the main factor that limits all form of organ transplantation is the supply of suitable organs. However, heart–lung transplantation is applied mainly in circumstances (CF and primary pulmonary hypertension) where the most satisfactory alternative operation would be bilateral lung transplantation and the heart of the heart–lung transplantation recipient can sometimes be used for a transplant in a patient who requires heart transplantation alone: a 'domino' heart transplant [108]. In cases of complex congenital heart disease, where the heart is unsuitable for the domino procedure, the heart–lung transplantation is frequently the only satisfactory operation for the recipient.

Domino heart transplantation has several potential advantages over standard cadaveric heart transplantation, including an opportunity for a thorough evaluation of the donor, more controlled donor retrieval and the possibility for prospective donor–recipient matching, including prospective human leukocyte antigen (HLA) matching. This may be particularly useful when dealing with heart transplant candidates who have preformed cytotoxic anti-HLA antibodies and who require a prospective cross-match against donor cells before a transplant can be safely performed.

Where both the heart–lung transplantation and the domino transplantation are performed in the same centre, a short ischaemia time for the heart transplantation is possible. In addition, the domino heart has not been exposed to the adverse effects of brain death [109–111] and so may have very good initial function; thus it may be better able to cope with a moderately elevated pulmonary vascular resistance in the heart transplant recipient. In our experience, recipient pulmonary vascular resistance has not been a factor that influenced the outcome after domino transplantation [108]. We have not experienced any problems with recipient infection with hearts obtained from CF donors.

Nevertheless, domino heart transplantation does have limitations. The early mortality rate has not been lower than that seen in cadaveric transplantation, which is surprising considering the potential benefits of using a graft from a living donor with a short ischaemic time. One factor contributing to this may be the issue of sex and size matching between donor and recipient. Heart–lung transplantation in CF patients yields a high proportion of hearts from small female donors that are relatively small for most heart transplant recipients, who are typically male. In addition, we have noticed a trend towards a worse survival in patients who have received hearts from pulmonary hypertensive donors.

Importantly, we have observed a very low long-term attrition rate in recipients of domino heart transplants and a low incidence of angiographic coronary disease [112]. The 10 year actuarial survival after domino heart transplantation at our centre is 58% [108], which is higher than that generally observed after cadaveric heart transplantation [50].

Conclusion

Heart–lung transplantation was the first clinically successful form of lung transplantation. It was initially used to treat patients with primary or secondary hypertension but was subsequently applied to those with respiratory failure due to parenchymal lung disease. Alternative procedures (single and bilateral lung transplants) have subsequently been developed and have replaced the heart–lung transplantation for the treatment of most parenchymal lung diseases. Bilateral lung transplantation is essential for those with septic lung disease due to CF. In addition, the Registry data suggest that bilateral lung replacement is associated with a better long-term survival than that seen after single lung transplantation. Replacement of both lungs can be achieved by either heart–lung or bilateral sequential lung transplantation.

Comparisons of data between centres can be biased by factors other than the operative procedure used. The Registry data must be used with care because treatments have not been allocated in a randomized way. Therefore the optimum strategy for lung transplantation in each disease remains uncertain. Heart–lung transplantation is the only procedure that can be used in cases of complex congenital heart disease and Eisenmenger's syndrome. Many European centres, including our own, prefer this operation for all cases of Eisenmenger's syndrome and for cases of primary pulmonary hypertension but such patients are often treated in other centres, especially in North America, by bilateral lung transplantation. Both heart–lung and bilateral lung transplantation can be used in CF, with many centres favouring the latter approach. The criticism of an 'unnecessary' heart transplantation as part of the combined procedure can be countered to some extent by the low incidence of cardiac allograft vasculopathy after heart–lung transplantation and the potential for recycling of the recipient's heart in a domino heart transplantation. Heart–lung transplantation is no longer used for conditions such as chronic obstructive pulmonary disease or diffuse lung disease.

Heart–lung transplantation produces an excellent degree of rehabilitation and quality of life with acceptable long-term survival rates. Currently, its application is limited by the scarcity of suitable donor organs and the long-term outcome is limited by the problem of obliterative bronchiolitis.

REFERENCES

1 Demikhov V. *Experimental transplantation of vital organs*, transl. B. Haigh. Consultants Bureau, New York, 1962.

2 Castaneda AR, Zamora R, Schmidt-Habelmann P, et al. Cardiopulmonary autotransplantation in primates (baboons): late functional results. *Surgery* 1972; **72**: 1064–1070.

3 Cooley DA, Bloodwell RD, Hallman GL, Nora JJ, Harrison GM, Leachman RD. Organ transplantation for advanced cardiopulmonary disease. *Ann Thorac Surg* 1969; **8**: 30–46.

4 Lillehei CW. Discussion of Wildevuur C R, Benfield J R. A review of 23 human lung transplantations by 20 surgeons. *Ann Thorac Surg* 1970; **9**: 489–515.

5 Barnard CN, Cooper DK. Clinical transplantation of the heart: a review of 13 years' personal experience. *J R Soc Med* 1981; **74**: 670–674.

6 Reitz BA, Wallwork JL, Hunt SA, et al. Heart–lung transplantation: successful therapy for patients with pulmonary vascular disease. *N Engl J Med* 1982; **306**: 557–564.

7 Radley-Smith R, Yacoub MH. Heart and heart–lung transplantation in children [Abstract]. *Circulation* 1986; **76**(Suppl IV): 24.

8 Modry DL, Kaye MP. Heart and heart–lung transplantation: the Canadian and world experience from December 1967 to September 1985. *Can J Surg* 1986; **29**: 275–279.

9 Hardy J, Webb W, Dalton M, Walker G. Lung homotransplantation in man. *JAMA* 1963; **186**: 1065–1074.

10 Unilateral lung transplantation for pulmonary fibrosis. Toronto Lung Transplant Group. *N Engl J Med* 1986; **314**: 1140–1145.

11 Fremes SE, Patterson GA, Williams WG, Goldman BS, Todd TR, Maurer J. Single lung transplantation and closure of patent ductus arteriosus for Eisenmenger's syndrome. Toronto Lung Transplant Group. *J Thorac Cardiovasc Surg* 1990; **100**: 1–5.

12 Starnes VA, Stinson EB, Oyer PE, et al. Single lung transplantation: a new therapeutic option for patients with pulmonary hypertension. *Transplant Proc* 1991; **23**: 1209–1210.

13 Aeba R, Griffith BP, Hardesty RL, Kormos RL, Armitage JM. Isolated lung transplantation for patients with Eisenmenger's syndrome. *Circulation* 1993; **88**: II452–II455.

14 Wood P. The Eisenmenger syndrome or pulmonary hypertension with reversed central shunt. *Br Med J* 1958; **2**: 701–709.

15 Pigula FA, Gandhi SK, Ristich J, et al. Cardiopulmonary transplantation for congenital heart disease in the adult. *J Heart Lung Transplant* 2001; **20**: 297–303.

16 Lupinetti FM, Bolling SF, Bove EL, et al. Selective lung or heart–lung transplantation for pulmonary hypertension associated with congenital cardiac anomalies. *Ann Thorac Surg* 1994; **57**: 1545–1548; discussion 1549.

17 Spray TL, Mallory GB, Canter CE, Huddleston CB, Kaiser LR. Pediatric lung transplantation for pulmonary hypertension and congenital heart disease. *Ann Thorac Surg* 1992; **54**: 216–225.

18 Patterson GA, Cooper JD, Dark JH, Jones MT. Experimental and clinical double lung transplantation. *J Thorac Cardiovasc Surg* 1988; **95**: 70–74.

19 Daly RC, Tadjkarimi S, Khaghani A, Banner NR, Yacoub MH. Successful double-lung transplantation with direct bronchial artery revascularization. *Ann Thorac Surg* 1993; **56**: 885–892.

20 Patterson GA, Todd TR, Cooper JD, Pearson FG, Winton TL, Maurer J. Airway complications after double lung transplantation. Toronto Lung Transplant Group. *J Thorac Cardiovasc Surg* 1990; **99**: 14–21.

21 Calhoon JH, Grover FL, Gibbons WJ, et al. Single lung transplantation. Alternative indications and technique. *J Thorac Cardiovasc Surg* 1991; **101**: 816–825.

22 Pasque MK, Cooper JD, Kaiser LR, Haydock DA, Triantafillou A, Trulock EP. Improved technique for bilateral lung

transplantation: rationale and initial clinical experience. *Ann Thorac Surg* 1990; **49**: 785–791.

23 Ueno T, Smith JA, Snell GI, et al. Bilateral sequential single lung transplantation for pulmonary hypertension and Eisenmenger's syndrome. *Ann Thorac Surg* 2000; **69**: 381–387.

24 Starnes VA, Barr ML, Cohen RG. Lobar transplantation. Indications, technique, and outcome. *J Thorac Cardiovasc Surg* 1994; **108**: 403–411.

25 Starnes VA, Barr ML, Cohen RG, et al. Living-donor lobar lung transplantation experience: intermediate results. *J Thorac Cardiovasc Surg* 1996; **112**: 1284–1291.

26 Jones J, Payne WD, Matas AJ. The living donor – risks, benefits and related concerns. *Transplant Rev* 1993; **7**: 115–128.

27 Jamieson SW, Stinson EB, Oyer PE, et al. Heart–lung transplantation for irreversible pulmonary hypertension. *Ann Thorac Surg* 1984; **38**: 554–562.

28 Griffith BP, Hardesty RL, Trento A, et al. Heart–lung transplantation: lessons learned and future hopes. *Ann Thorac Surg* 1987; **43**: 6–16.

29 Yacoub MH, Banner NR, Khaghani A, et al. Heart–lung transplantation for cystic fibrosis and subsequent domino heart transplantation. *J Heart Transplant* 1990; **9**: 459–467.

30 Yacoub MH, Khaghani A, Banner N, Tajkarimi S, Fitzgerald M. Distant organ procurement for heart and lung transplantation. *Transplant Proc* 1989; **21**: 2548–2550.

31 Copeland JG. Heart–lung transplantation: current status. *Ann Thorac Surg* 1987; **43**: 2–3.

32 Royston D. Aprotinin therapy in heart and heart–lung transplantation. *J Heart Lung Transplant* 1993; **12**: S19–S25.

33 Banner NR, Yacoub MH. Physiology of the orthotopic cardiac transplant recipient. *Semin Thorac Cardiovasc Surg* 1990; **2**: 259–270.

34 McGregor CG, Baldwin JC, Jamieson SW, et al. Isolated pulmonary rejection after combined heart–lung transplantation. *J Thorac Cardiovasc Surg* 1985; **90**: 623–626.

35 Wahlers T, Khaghani A, Martin M, Banner N, Yacoub M. Frequency of acute heart and lung rejection after heart–lung transplantation. *Transplant Proc* 1987; **19**: 3537–3538.

36 Dawkins KD, Jamieson SW, Hunt SA, et al. Long-term results, hemodynamics, and complications after combined heart and lung transplantation. *Circulation* 1985; **71**: 919–926.

37 Smith JA, Stewart S, Roberts M, et al. Significance of graft coronary artery disease in heart–lung transplant recipients. *Transplant Proc* 1995; **27**: 2019–2020.

38 Kramer MR, Valantine HA, Marshall SE, Starnes VA, Theodore J. Recovery of the right ventricle after single-lung transplantation in pulmonary hypertension. *Am J Cardiol* 1994; **73**: 494–500.

39 Yacoub MH. Two hearts that beat as one. *Circulation* 1995; **92**: 156–157.

40 Yacoub MH. Hemodynamics of 'domino' heart transplantation. The role of ventriculo-ventricular interaction and after load mismatch. *G Ital Cardiol* 1997; **27**: 540–543.

41 Spray TL. Lung transplantation in children with pulmonary hypertension and congenital heart disease. *Semin Thorac Cardiovasc Surg* 1996; **8**: 286–295.

42 Spatenka J, Khaghani A, Irving JD, Theodoropoulos S, Slavik Z, Yacoub MH. Gianturco self-expanding metallic stents in treatment of tracheobronchial stenosis after single lung and heart and lung transplantation. *Eur J Cardiothorac Surg* 1991; **5**: 648–652.

43 Maiwand MO, Zehr KJ, Dyke CM, et al. The role of cryotherapy for airway complications after lung and heart–lung transplantation. *Eur J Cardiothorac Surg* 1997; **12**: 549–554.

44 Gaer JA, Tsang V, Khaghani A, et al. Use of endotracheal silicone stents for relief of tracheobronchial obstruction. *Ann Thorac Surg* 1992; **54**: 512–516.

45 Kramer MR, Marshall SE, McDougall IR, et al. The distribution of ventilation and perfusion after single-lung transplantation in patients with pulmonary fibrosis and pulmonary hypertension. *Transplant Proc* 1991; **23**: 1215–1216.

46 Levine SM, Jenkinson SG, Bryan CL, et al. Ventilation–perfusion inequalities during graft rejection in patients undergoing single lung transplantation for primary pulmonary hypertension. *Chest* 1992; **101**: 401–405.

47 Sundaresan RS, Shiraishi Y, Trulock EP, et al. Single or bilateral lung transplantation for emphysema? *J Thorac Cardiovasc Surg* 1996; **112**: 1485–1495.

48 Bavaria JE, Kotloff R, Palevsky H, et al. Bilateral versus single lung transplantation for chronic obstructive pulmonary disease. *J Thorac Cardiovasc Surg* 1997; **113**: 520–528.

49 Conte JV, Borja MJ, Patel CB, Yang SC, Jhaveri RM, Orens JB. Lung transplantation for primary and secondary pulmonary hypertension. *Ann Thorac Surg* 2001; **72**: 1673–1680.

50 Hosenpud JD, Bennett LE, Keck BM, Boucek MM, Novick RJ. The Registry of the International Society for Heart and Lung Transplantation: 18th official report – 2001. *J Heart Lung Transplant* 2001; **20**: 805–815.

51 Yacoub M, Banner N. Recent developments in lung and heart–lung transplantation. In: Morris P, Tilney N, eds. *Transplantation reviews*, vol. 3. WB Saunders, Philadelphia, 1989: 1–29.

52 Khaghani A, Banner N, Ozdogan E, et al. Medium-term results of combined heart and lung transplantation for emphysema. *J Heart Lung Transplant* 1991; **10**: 15–21.

53 Pielsticker EJ, Martínez FJ, Rubenfire M. Lung and heart–lung transplant practice patterns in pulmonary hypertension centers. *J Heart Lung Transplant* 2001; **20**: 1297–1304.

54 Yacoub MH, Gyi K, Khaghani A, et al. Analysis of 10-year experience with heart–lung transplantation for cystic fibrosis. *Transplant Proc* 1997; **29**: 632.

55 Vongpatanasin W, Brickner ME, Hillis LD, Lange RA. The Eisenmenger syndrome in adults. *Ann Intern Med* 1998; **128**: 745–755.

56 Conte JV, Robbins RC, Reichenspurner H, Valentine VG, Theodore J, Reitz BA. Pediatric heart–lung transplantation: intermediate-term results. *J Heart Lung Transplant* 1996; **15**: 692–699.

57 International guidelines for the selection of lung transplant candidates. The American Society for Transplant Physicians (ASTP)/American Thoracic Society (ATS)/European Respiratory Society (ERS)/International Society for Heart and Lung Transplantation (ISHLT). *Am J Respir Crit Care Med* 1998; **158**: 335–339.

58 Maurer JR, Frost AE, Estenne M, Higenbottam T, Glanville AR. International guidelines for the selection of lung transplant candidates. The International Society for Heart and Lung Transplantation, the American Thoracic Society, the American Society of Transplant Physicians, the European Respiratory Society. *J Heart Lung Transplant* 1998; **17**: 703–709.

59 Radley-Smith R, Banner N, Khaghani A, Yacoub MH. Cardiothoracic transplantation for congenital heart disease in teenagers and adults [Abstract]. *Heart* 2001; **85**: 62–63.

60 Radley-Smith R, Yacoub M, Pomerance A. OB is commoner after heart–lung transplantation in younger children [Abstract]. *J Heart lung Transplant* 1993; **12**(1 Part 2): S69.

61 Leonard H, Eastham K, Dark J. Heart and heart–lung transplantation in Down's syndrome. The lack of supportive evidence means each case must be carefully assessed. *Br Med J* 2000; **320**: 816–817.

62 Bridges ND, Mallory GB Jr, Huddleston CB, Canter CE, Sweet SC, Spray TL. Lung transplantation in children and young adults with cardiovascular disease. *Ann Thorac Surg* 1995; **59**: 813–821.

63 Thomas AQ, Gaddipati R, Newman JH, Loyd JE. Genetics of primary pulmonary hypertension. *Clin Chest Med* 2001; **22**: 477–491.

64 D'Alonzo GE, Barst RJ, Ayres SM, et al. Survival in patients with primary pulmonary hypertension. Results from a national prospective registry. *Ann Intern Med* 1991; **115**: 343–349.

65 Fuster V, Steele PM, Edwards WD, Gersh BJ, McGoon MD, Frye RL. Primary pulmonary hypertension: natural history and the importance of thrombosis. *Circulation* 1984; **70**: 580–587.

66 Rich S, Kaufmann E, Levy PS. The effect of high doses of calcium-channel blockers on survival in primary pulmonary hypertension. *N Engl J Med* 1992; **327**: 76–81.

67 Higenbottam TW, Spiegelhalter D, Scott JP, et al. Prostacyclin (epoprostenol) and heart–lung transplantation as treatments for severe pulmonary hypertension. *Br Heart J* 1993; **70**: 366–370.

68 Barst RJ, Rubin LJ, Long WA, et al. A comparison of continuous intravenous epoprostenol (prostacyclin) with conventional therapy for primary pulmonary hypertension. The Primary Pulmonary Hypertension Study Group. *N Engl J Med* 1996; **334**: 296–302.

69 Rubin LJ, Mendoza J, Hood M, et al. Treatment of primary pulmonary hypertension with continuous intravenous prostacyclin (epoprostenol). Results of a randomized trial. *Ann Intern Med* 1990; **112**: 485–491.

70 Recommendations on the management of pulmonary hypertension in clinical practice. *Heart* 2001; **86**(Suppl 1): I1–I13.

71 Jamieson SW. Pulmonary thromboendarterectomy. *Heart* 1998; **79**: 118–120.

72 Jamieson SW, Nomura K. Indications for and the results of pulmonary thromboendarterectomy for thromboembolic pulmonary hypertension. *Semin Vasc Surg* 2000; **13**: 236–244.

73 Webb AK, Egan J. Should patients with cystic fibrosis infected with *Burkholderia cepacia* undergo lung transplantation? *Thorax* 1997; **52**: 671–673.

74 Aris RM, Routh JC, LiPuma JJ, Heath DG, Gilligan PH. Lung transplantation for cystic fibrosis patients with *Burkholderia cepacia* complex. Survival linked to genomovar type. *Am J Respir Crit Care Med* 2001; **164**: 2102–2106.

75 De Soyza A, McDowell A, Archer L, et al. *Burkholderia cepacia* complex genomovars and pulmonary transplantation outcomes in patients with cystic fibrosis. *Lancet* 2001; **358**: 1780–1781.

76 Castaneda AR, Mayer JE, Lock JE. Tetralogy of Fallot, pulmonary atresia and diminutive pulmonary arteries. *Progr Pediatr Cardiol* 1992; **1**: 50–60.

77 Crosnier C, Lykavieris P, Meunier-Rotival M, Hadchouel M. Alagille syndrome. The widening spectrum of arteriohepatic dysplasia. *Clin Liver Dis* 2000; **4**: 765–778.

78 Thorne SA. Management of polycythaemia in adults with cyanotic congenital heart disease. *Heart* 1998; **79**: 315–316.

79 Bowyer JJ, Busst CM, Denison DM, Shinebourne EA. Effect of long term oxygen treatment at home in children with pulmonary vascular disease. *Br Heart J* 1986; **55**: 385–390.

80 Kidd L, Driscoll DJ, Gersony WM, et al. Second natural history study of congenital heart defects. Results of treatment of patients with ventricular septal defects. *Circulation* 1993; **87**(2 Suppl): I38–I51.

81 Hopkins WE, Ochoa LL, Richardson GW, Trulock EP. Comparison of the hemodynamics and survival of adults with severe primary pulmonary hypertension or Eisenmenger syndrome. *J Heart Lung Transplant* 1996; **15**: 100–105.

82 McCurry KR, Keenan RJ. Controlling perioperative morbidity and mortality after lung transplantation for pulmonary hypertension. *Semin Thorac Cardiovasc Surg* 1998; **10**: 139–143.

83 Cantor WJ, Harrison DA, Moussadji JS, et al. Determinants of survival and length of survival in adults with Eisenmenger syndrome. *Am J Cardiol* 1999; **84**: 677–681.

84 Daliento L, Somerville J, Presbitero P, et al. Eisenmenger syndrome. Factors relating to deterioration and death. *Eur Heart J* 1998; **19**: 1845–1855.

85 Saha A, Balakrishnan KG, Jaiswal PK, et al. Prognosis for patients with Eisenmenger syndrome of various aetiology. *Int J Cardiol* 1994; **45**: 199–207.

86 Banner N, Boscoe M, Khaghani A. Postoperative care of the heart transplant patient. In: O'Donnell J, Nacul F, eds. *Surgical intensive care medicine*. Kluwer Academic Publishers, Boston, 2001: 741–760.

87 Wheeldon DR, Potter CD, Oduro A, Wallwork J, Large SR. Transforming the 'unacceptable' donor: outcomes from the adoption of a standardized donor management technique. *J Heart Lung Transplant* 1995; **14**: 734–742.

88 Hunt BJ, Yacoub M, Amin S, Devenish A, Contreras M. Induction of red blood cell destruction by graft-derived antibodies

after minor ABO-mismatched heart and lung transplantation. *Transplantation* 1988; **46**: 246–249.

89 Baldwin JC, Frist WH, Starkey TD, et al. Distant graft procurement for combined heart and lung transplantation using pulmonary artery flush and simple topical hypothermia for graft preservation. *Ann Thorac Surg* 1987; **43**: 670–673.

90 Mayer E, Puskas JD, Cardoso PF, Shi S, Slutsky AS, Patterson GA. Reliable eighteen-hour lung preservation at 4 degrees and 10 degrees C by pulmonary artery flush after high-dose prostaglandin E1 administration. *J Thorac Cardiovasc Surg* 1992; **103**: 1136–1142.

91 Wallwork J, Jones K, Cavarocchi N, Hakim M, Higenbottam T. Distant procurement of organs for clinical heart–lung transplantation using a single flush technique. *Transplantation* 1987; **44**: 654–658.

92 Jamieson SW, Baldwin J, Stinson EB, et al. Clinical heart–lung transplantation. *Transplantation* 1984; **37**: 81–84.

93 Reitz BA, Pennock JL, Shumway NE. Simplified operative method for heart and lung transplantation. *J Surg Res* 1981; **31**: 1–5.

94 Macchiarini P, Ladurie FL, Cerrina J, Fadel E, Chapelier A, Dartevelle P. Clamshell or sternotomy for double lung or heart–lung transplantation? *Eur J Cardiothorac Surg* 1999; **15**: 333–339.

95 Shea SA, Horner RL, Banner NR, et al. The effect of human heart–lung transplantation upon breathing at rest and during sleep. *Respir Physiol* 1988; **72**: 131–149.

96 Banner NR, Lloyd MH, Hamilton RD, Innes JA, Guz A, Yacoub MH. Cardiopulmonary response to dynamic exercise after heart and combined heart–lung transplantation. *Br Heart J* 1989; **61**: 215–223.

97 O'Brien BJ, Banner NR, Gibson S, Yacoub MH. The Nottingham Health Profile as a measure of quality of life following combined heart and lung transplantation. *J Epidemiol Community Health* 1988; **42**: 232–234.

98 Kshettry VR, Kroshus TJ, Savik K, Hertz MI, Bolman RM. Primary pulmonary hypertension as a risk factor for the development of obliterative bronchiolitis in lung allograft recipients. *Chest* 1996; **110**: 704–709.

99 Balfour-Lynn IM, Martin I, Whitehead BF, Rees PG, Elliott MJ, de Leval MR. Heart–lung transplantation for patients under 10 with cystic fibrosis. *Arch Dis Child* 1997; **76**: 38–40.

100 Banner N. Coronary arterial disease in the cardiac allograft. In: Rose ML, ed. *Transplant associated cornary artery vasculopathy.* Landes Bioscience, Georgetown, TX, 2001: 1–25.

101 McCarthy PM, Starnes VA, Theodore J, Stinson EB, Oyer PE, Shumway NE. Improved survival after heart–lung transplantation. *J Thorac Cardiovasc Surg* 1990; **99**: 54–59; discussion 59–60.

102 Madden BP, Hodson ME, Tsang V, Radley-Smith R, Khaghani A, Yacoub MY. Intermediate-term results of heart–lung transplantation for cystic fibrosis. *Lancet* 1992; **339**: 1583–1587.

103 Richardson M, Pomerance A, Mitchell AG, Banner NR, Yacoub M. Coronary artery disease in heart–lung transplant recipients: angiographic and histological findings [Abstract]. *J Heart Lung Transplant* 1994; **13**: S40.

104 Radley-Smith RC, Burke M, Pomerance A, Yacoub MH. Graft vessel disease and obliterative bronchiolitis after heart/lung transplantation in children. *Transplant Proc* 1995; **27**: 2017–2018.

105 Hertz MI, Taylor DO, Trulock EP, et al. The Registry of the International Society for Heart and Lung Transplantation: 19th official report – 2002. *J Heart Lung Transplant* 2002; **21**: 950–970 (and online: www.ISHLT.org).

106 Adams DH, Cochrane AD, Khaghani A, Smith JD, Yacoub MH. Retransplantation in heart–lung recipients with obliterative bronchiolitis. *J Thorac Cardiovasc Surg* 1994; **107**: 450–459.

107 Novick RJ. Heart and lung retransplantation; should it be done? *J Heart Lung Transplant* 1998; **17**: 635–642.

108 Anyanwu AC, Banner NR, Radley-Smith R, Khaghani A, Yacoub MH. Long-term results of cardiac transplantation from live donors: the domino heart transplant. *J Heart Lung Transplant* 2002; *in press.*

109 Novitzky D, Rose AG, Cooper DK. Injury of myocardial conduction tissue and coronary artery smooth muscle following brain death in the baboon. *Transplantation* 1988; **45**: 964–966.

110 Novitzky D, Rhodin J, Cooper DK, Ye Y, Min KW, DeBault L. Ultrastructure changes associated with brain death in the human donor heart. *Transpl Int* 1997; **10**: 24–32.

111 Bittner HB, Chen EP, Biswas SS, Van Trigt P III, Davis RD. Right ventricular dysfunction after cardiac transplantation: primarily related to status of donor heart. *Ann Thorac Surg* 1999; **68**: 1605–1611.

112 Anyanwu A, Banner N, Mitchell A, Khaghani A, Yacoub M. Low incidence and severity of transplant coronary artery disease after domino heart transplantation. *J Heart Lung Transplant* 2000; **19**: Abstract 81.

Anaesthesia and intensive care

Michael J. Boscoe and Shane J. George

Harefield Hospital, Harefield, Middlesex, UK

Introduction

The anaesthetist has several roles in a cardiothoracic transplant programme. These include preoperative assessment of candidates for transplantation, management of the organ donor, intraoperative management and postoperative care of the recipient. Details of the general anaesthetic approach to patients undergoing pulmonary and cardiac surgery are outside the scope of this chapter, which will focus on the issues specific to lung and heart–lung transplantation.

Pretransplant assessment

Case selection criteria are well established (see Chapter 12) and most units use some type of proforma to collect data during the process of assessment for transplantation. This collates essential data including blood type and lymphocytotoxic antibody screen, body size measurements, findings from the physical examination, data from haematological, biochemical and microbiological screening, together with radiological reports and the results of lung function and cardiac catheterization data.

The anaesthetic appraisal will be influenced by the type of lung transplant that is required (single lung, double lung, or heart and lung). This will be affected by the nature of the underlying cardiopulmonary disease as well as the approach of the individual transplant programme (see Chapters 13 and 14).

Previous thoracic surgery or vascular collaterals associated with Eisenmenger's syndrome increase the risk of a prolonged operation and of needing to transfuse large volumes of blood products with consequent haemodynamic instability and risk of renal complications. In the case of live-related donor lobe of lung transplantation, detailed

case conferences are typical to discuss the implications for both the donors and recipient. The team may recommend delaying putting the patient on the active waiting list if the preoperative status can be optimized by further treatment.

Active infection should not be present but bacterial colonization may be present in patients with conditions such as cystic fibrosis (CF). This situation must be carefully monitored whilst the patient is on the waiting list. Surgery is contraindicated at the time if an active infection is present with pyrexia. Very low body weight in CF patients can be managed during the waiting period with a percutaneous enteral gastrotomy tube to allow overnight supplemental enteral feeding.

An important consideration is whether early extubation is likely to be possible after surgery. Failure to wean from mechanical ventilation in a reasonable time predisposes to pulmonary problems including infections and sepsis. Risk factors include poor nutritional status, especially in patients with CF, or in those with musculoskeletal problems, for example scoliosis or excessive obesity.

A small number of transplant candidates will already be ventilated for end-stage respiratory disease. Prior intubation and ventilation has been found to be indicative of a poor outcome [1]. CF patients in this category are particularly high risk in this situation, because they usually develop active infection that can progress to a sepsis syndrome. However, other groups may be considered on an individual basis, particularly if the respiratory system is an isolated problem. Washington University (USA) recently reported a 40% five year survival in 'stable' patients receiving transplants while ventilated versus 0% in the unstable group [2]. Although CF patients do not fare well when intubated and ventilated, we have found that they can often be successfully bridged to transplantation with noninvasive nasal ventilation (Hodson, Chapter 8).

Retransplantation, normally because of bronchiolitis obliterans, is uncommon because of the scarcity of suitable donor organs; rarely, a patient who has already had a lung transplant operation may be considered suitable for a second operation usually as a redo single lung transplantation (SLT) after bilateral lung or combined heart–lung transplantation or as a new SLT on the contralateral side in the case of a previous SLT. The decision whether to proceed with such a high risk case must be made by the transplant team as a whole, bearing in mind the population of the patients on the waiting list and the scarcity of donor organs suitable for transplantation.

Donor management

Brain death

The determination of brain death is pivotal in setting in motion the events leading to organ transplantation. Since the concept was first described in 1959 [3], various attempts have been made to update the medical definition, particularly taking into account modern imaging techniques, as well as responding to concerns from the public. In the USA, the Harvard Medical School criteria [4] are generally accepted, whereas in the UK the report from the Conference of the Medical Royal Colleges [5] is referred to. Clinical neurological examination remains the mainstay of diagnosis. Scientific knowledge about the process of brain death is constantly evolving, resulting in updated guidelines [6,7] and in reviews [8,9]. The clinical criteria for brain death are listed in Table 15.1 [8]. The fundamental prerequisites for diagnosis are accepted as: a known and irreversible cause for the patient's coma, the absence of complex medical conditions that may confound the clinical assessment (including severe biochemical or endocrine disturbances and hypothermia with a core temperature $<32\ ^\circ$C or severe hypotension), and the absence of drug intoxication, poisoning or neuromuscular blocking agents. The use of confirmatory tests are optional in adults (Table 15.2) [10].

Management of the potential organ donor

Thoracic organs suitable for transplantation are scarce and it is particularly difficult to find donors where the heart and both lungs are suitable for combined heart and lung transplantation. The donor management should be based on an understanding of the patient's previous clinical condition and the pathophysiology of brain death. The aim is to prevent further organ injury and to optimize medical treatment before assessing whether the organs are suitable for

Table 15.1. General clinical criteria for brain death in adults and children. Doctors must comply with the legislation and guidelines applicable in their country when making a diagnosis of brain death (brain-stem death)

Coma of known cause
Absence of motor responses
Absence of pupillary response to light and pupils at mid-position
    with respect to dilatation (4–6 mm)
Absence of corneal reflexes
Absence of caloric responses
Absence of gag reflex
Absence of coughing in response to tracheal suctioning
Absence of sucking and rooting reflexes
Absence of a respiratory drive at a $PaCO_2$ that is 60 mmHg (8 kPa)
    or 20 mmHg (2.7 kPa) above normal baseline values
Interval between two evaluations, according to patient's age
    term to 2 months old, 48 hours
    2 months to 1 year old, 24 hours
    >1 year to <18 years old, 12 hour
    > 18 years old, interval optional
Confirmatory tests
    Term to 2 months old, 2 confirmatory tests
    2 months old to 1 year old, 1 confirmatory test
    1 year old to <18 years old, optional
    >18 years old, optional

Table 15.2. Confirmatory tests sometimes used in the diagnosis of brain death

Test	Limitations
Cerebral angiography	May damage renal function
MRI scan	Blood flow in posterior fossa not imaged
EEG	A measure of whole brain death
Evoked potentials	Only tests auditory and visual pathways
Transcranial doppler	Needs experienced operator
Repeat tests at 6 hours	Donor may deteriorate in this time
Cerebral scintigraphy (^{99m}Tc)	Needs specialist equipment and operator

Note: MRI, magnetic resonance imaging; EEG, electroencephalogram.

lung or heart transplantation [10,11]. Steps must be taken to counteract the inevitable deterioration in autonomic stability after brain-stem death and to avoid the common situation where the donor is unnecessarily supported by large doses of inotropes whilst remaining severely hypovolaemic [10]. Table 15.3 summarizes the management of brain death in the potential donor. The intensivist should identify any reversible causes of poor gas exchange, including

Table 15.3. Management of the potential organ donor after brain death

Problem	Sign	Treatment
Loss of temperature control	Hypothermia or hyperpyrexia	Warming or cooling blankets (keep temperature 33–37 °C)
Haemodynamic instability	Hypertension	Short acting beta- and alpha-blocking agents and vasodilators
	Hypotension	Fluids, replacement vasopressin
Diabetes insipidus	Polyuria, dehydration	Vasopressin (avoid high dose) or desmopressin
	Hypernatraemia	Hypotonic fluids
Dehydration	Oliguria	Treat hypotension and provide adequate fluid replacement
Acute lung injury	Low compliance, hypoxia	Control fluid balance
		Avoid barotrauma during ventilation
Brain PAF release	Coagulopathy	Keep temperature > 33 °C?
Cardiac arrhythmias		?Beta blockade
Endocrine dysfunction	Diabetes mellitus	Insulin to maintain sugar 5–8 mmol/L
	Decrease TSH, T3, T4	T3 infusion (4 μg/hr followed by 3 μg/hr)
	Diabetes insipidus	Vasopressin 1 U followed by 1–4 U/hour

Note: PAF, platelet-activating factor; TSH, thyroid-stimulating hormone; T3 and T4, triiodothyronine, thyroxine; DDAVP, synthetic vasopressin.

right main bronchus intubation, excessive secretions obstructing the airways and alveolar hypoventilation. Regular bronchial suction, avoidance of an excessive use of crystalloid solutions, and the use of positive end-expiratory pressure are the mainstays of management.

Brainstem compression due to tentorial hernia hole results in systemic hypertension from a transient phase of sympathetic overactivity together with bradycardia due to vagal stimulation (Cushing's reflex). This catecholamine storm is associated with subendocardial haemorrhage and myocardial necrosis. Protection of the heart is difficult, yet appropriate use of a short-acting beta-blocker (esmolol), vasodilatation and fluid replacement will be sufficient in most cases. The lungs are vulnerable to pulmonary oedema due to acute left ventricular failure and mitral regurgitation during this period. Barotrauma from ventilation of the noncompliant lungs and super-added infection may contribute to the pulmonary insult. Endocrine disturbances can contribute to the cardiac deterioration, which may be reversed by thyroid replacement using triiodothyronine [12]. The instability of these patients requires time-consuming attention of the intensivist.

Transoesophageal echocardiography (TOE), using a portable device, is increasingly being used by transplant retrieval teams to assess donor heart function and optimize therapy [13]. The TOE will highlight hypovolaemia and help to avoid excessive use of vasoconstrictors, which can reduce organ perfusion. Anatomical defects including atrial septal defects can be readily identified. Interpretation of left ventricular function requires special care because of the frequently altered loading conditions; systemic hypotension is common in this situation [13–15]. Regional

wall abnormalities can provide evidence of coronary artery disease. Criteria for donor acceptance and management have been reviewed in detail elsewhere [11,16].

Gore et al. showed that 65% of potential donors have potentially usable hearts and 31% have usable lungs [17], yet 23% of organs offered were inappropriately turned down. The shortage of potential donors and the enthusiasm of the transplant team to harvest the organs has to be tempered with the need to ensure the best outcomes for both the patient and the transplant unit as a whole. Shumway et al. have highlighted the need for widening these criteria to include previously excluded groups to combat the donor shortage [18]. There is also a need to persuade emergency room (accident and emergency) physicians to ventilate otherwise unsalvageable patients as potential donors. Table 15.4 lists the current donor criteria for lung transplantation at our centre.

Anaesthetic management of the lung transplant recipient

Preparation

In general, these patients are not premedicated as we aim to control pulmonary vascular resistance from the outset and sedation will tend to increase this by virtue of hypercarbia. Those patients who are not hypercarbic should be sent to the operating room sitting up while receiving oxygen; those with chronic obstructive pulmonary disease and carbon dioxide retention may require controlled oxygen therapy. Therapy specific to the underlying lung condition must be

Table 15.4. Typical donor criteria for lung transplantation

Donors younger than 60 years (55 for HLT)

No history of primary pulmonary disease or cardiac disease in heart
and lung donors

Serial chest X-ray films normal

Adequate gas exchange $PaO_2 > 300$ mmHg on 100% oxygen and
PEEP ≤ 5 cmH$_2$O

Normal lung compliance (peak pressure < 30 cmH$_2$O at 15 mL/kg
tidal volume

Bronchoscopic examination normal, no evidence of aspiration or
inflammation in airways

No previous surgery on donor lung or hemithorax

Recipient matching for ABO group and size

No malignancy (except primary intracranial tumour)

Negative screening tests for HIV and hepatitis

Note: HIV, human immunodeficiency virus; PEEP, positive
end-expiratory pressure; HLT, heart–lung transplant.

continued, for example epoprostenol (prostacyclin) infusion in primary pulmonary hypertension or noninvasive ventilation in CF patients and others with end-stage respiratory failure. Abstinence from food for six hours and fluid for three hours is ideal because fear and apprehension may delay gastric emptying. Polycythaemic patients, including those with Eisenmenger's syndrome, should be given intravenous fluids, as dehydration may precipitate thrombotic complications. Nonnephrotoxic broad spectrum antibiotics are given prophylactically and the precise choice will depend on local factors; CF patients need appropriate antipseudomonal drug therapy guided by the results of the most recent sputum culture. No other special measures are required to prevent infection above those considered good anaesthetic practice, as these have not been shown to improve survival [19].

Patient monitoring, vascular access and induction of anaesthesia

Patients undergoing lung or heart–lung transplantation have very little cardiopulmonary reserve and induction is a potentially dangerous phase of the operation. In general, the appropriate level of monitoring is that required for any sick cardiothoracic patient (Table 15.5).

A 20 G radial arterial cannula is inserted under local anaesthesia. If perioperative complications are predicted, including massive blood transfusion, we may also insert a femoral arterial line after the patient is anaesthetized, because peripheral vasoconstriction may become a problem, making monitoring difficult. Intra-arterial continuous blood gas monitoring is an emerging technology that may have a role in selected cases [20].

A 14 G peripheral venous cannula is also inserted prior to induction of anaesthesia. Sufficient time should be allowed for vascular access, particularly when previous venous thrombosis is common, as in patients with CF or congenital heart disease. If peripheral venous access is impossible, a subclavian line may have to be inserted, with the patient in a semisupine position, as many patients cannot tolerate a Trendelenburg position for internal jugular line placement, although a subclavian approach carries a higher risk of pneumothorax.

The patient may resist lying flat for induction. Rapid sequence induction to prevent regurgitation of gastric contents is usually unnecessary if the patient has been fasted since being called by the transplant coordinator; the technique is best avoided, since it may be dangerous in this situation. Once the patient is anaesthetized, a quadruple or quintuple lumen central venous cannula is inserted into the right internal jugular vein and this is accompanied by an introducer for a pulmonary artery flotation catheter with side arm to enable rapid infusion of warmed fluids through its wide bore lumen. We prefer to use sulfadiazine- and chlorhexidine-coated catheters for transplant patients [21], although a potential risk of anaphylaxis has recently been reported [22]. An efficient blood warmer, for example Hotline $^®$, is used routinely. A sterile warm air blanket (Bair Hugger $^®$) is placed over the lower torso by the scrub nurse, when positioning of the patient allows this. Table 15.5 outlines the anaesthetic preparation for lung transplantation.

The choice of anaesthetic drug regimen is not as important as the experience of the anaesthetist. We use either etomidate or propofol with fentanyl as induction agents with pancuronium as muscle relaxant, followed by either sevoflurane or isoflurane to produce a balanced anaesthetic. A number of animal studies have demonstrated the benefit of free radical scavengers, including *N*-acetylcysteine and allopurinol on organ preservation but the optimum dose in humans has not been established [23,24].

The pulmonary artery (PA) flow-directed catheter and TOE have complementary roles in monitoring. The TOE probe can be placed easily and provides images at every stage of the operation without affecting the surgical field. Problems with right ventricular function can be rapidly identified and an estimate of the volume status of the heart can also be made by observation of the left ventricle. The PA catheter can be placed preinduction and can give early warning of cardiovascular decompensation, although this is not done routinely in our practice. The PA catheter may be difficult to place in the presence of poor right ventricular function and tricuspid regurgitation due to pulmonary hypertension, which commonly exist in this group of patients. It is also less reliable in determining the left

Table 15.5. Anaesthetic checklist (with comments) prior to induction

ECG	6 lead
Venous access	14 G, quad rt int jug, pulmonary art
Arterial access	20 G radial (19 G femoral in selected cases)
Fiberoptic bronchoscope	Check double lumen tube, bronchial toilet for CF patients
Omniplane TOE	To monitor right heart function and pulmonary venous anastomoses
Warm air blanket (Bair Hugger®)	To prevent cooling during nonbypass cases and during closure
Blood warmer	Temperature maintenance
Resuscitation drugs	Vasoconstrictors and adrenaline
Inhaled nitric oxide	To optimize right heart function and minimize effects of ischaemia–reperfusion injury
External defibrillator pads	To defibrillate in redo operations
Prepare for insertion of PA catheter	Timing depends on operation
Check availability of surgeon and preparation for insertion of chest drains	Preparation for airway and cardiovascular emergencies during induction

Note: ECG, electrocardiogram; quad rt int jug, quadruple lumen catheter inserted into right internal jugular vein or alternatively multilumen central venous catheter; Art, artery; CF, cystic fibrosis; TOE, transoesophageal echo; PA, pulmonary artery.

ventricular filling, particularly in the presence of severe pulmonary hypertension. However, the ability to measure both the PA pressure and the cardiac output directly offers an advantage over the TOE. Knowledge of these parameters can be a help to guide the decision about whether it is necessary to go on to cardiopulmonary bypass (CPB). The problem of placing the catheter in the pulmonary artery can be solved by temporarily pulling the catheter back, and the surgeon repositioning it after the arterial anastomosis has been completed.

In the case of combined heart and lung transplantation, injury to either left or right ventricle due to preservation or ischaemia–reperfusion injury can be problematic and in this case information from the TOE will invaluable. If left ventricular dysfunction is suspected, a left atrial line can usually be inserted surgically. Similarly, a PA catheter may be inserted directly if the passage of a pulmonary artery flotation catheter proves problematical.

Although collapse during induction is rare, particular risks are associated with specific lung pathologies. Patients with obstructive lung disease with bullae can suffer circulatory collapse following positive pressure ventilation due to either respiratory tamponade of the heart or rupture of a bulla causing a tension pneumothorax. Prior fluid loading reduces the risk of hypotension, and correction with a vasoconstrictor such as metaraminol or neosynephrine may be necessary. Diagnosis of a pneumothorax can usually be made by auscultation and observation of chest movement; however, breath sounds may be quiet in patients with chronic obstructive pulmonary disease (COPD), and end-tidal CO_2 is useful at this stage as this monitor can provide rapid evidence of both effective ventilation and cardiac output. Immediate chest drainage or even sternotomy may be

Table 15.6. Airway management according to the type of lung transplant

Heart and lung transplant	Single lumen tube
Single lung transplant	Double lumen tube, usually left sided, but check for preference of surgeon
Sequential double lung	Double lumen tube, usually left sided but check for preference of surgeon
Double lung using CPB	Single lumen tube

Note: CPB, cardiopulmonary bypass.

life saving and the surgical team should be available during induction to assist as necessary. Pulmonary hypertensive crisis during induction of a patient with primary pulmonary hypertension can be troublesome. We find that adrenaline is a most useful drug in the acute situation, since traditional pulmonary vasodilators are ineffective at this stage.

Following discussion with the surgeon about the likely operative approach the anaesthetist will plan to ventilate the lungs separately for a SLT or a double lung transplant (DLT) that is to be performed off bypass. Occasionally the planned operation will change, for example if the heart in a heart–lung bloc is found to be inadequate heart–lung transplant (HLT) may be converted to a DLT. The methods of airway management and lung separation are described in Table 15.6.

Although most centres use disposable double lumen tubes, for example Bronchocath®, some prefer to use a Carlen's pattern tube with carinal hook. This tube has a short bronchial extension and is placed in the left main bronchus. It is usually suitable for either left or right lung isolation. It has the advantage of being easily positioned and is not prone to displacement. However, it does not easily allow the passage of a fibreoptic bronchoscope or a large suction catheter and therefore is not suitable for use in infective lung disease. In addition, it must be replaced by a conventional plastic tube at the end of the operation. Similarly, the Univent tube, which is a single lumen tube with an integral small lumen bronchus blocker, does not allow effective suction in these patients with thick secretions; but it does offer the theoretical advantage of the surgeon being able to collapse either side with full access to almost the entire length of the bronchus [25]. Like other plastic tubes it suffers from slippage and the risk of loss of lung isolation.

It is important that the surgical team recognize that placement of double lumen tubes is a relatively blind technique. Success can be improved with the aid of the flexible fibreoptic bronchoscope, but abnormal anatomy in the trachea or mediastinal displacement can affect outcome. Failure to isolate the lungs at a crucial part of an operation can become a life-threatening emergency, sometimes forcing the rapid institution of cardiopulmonary bypass.

Following intubation of the patient, the anaesthetist can be faced with three types of emergency that demand a quick diagnosis and appropriate management; low compliance, hypotension and hypoxaemia (see Table 15.7). A fall in oxygen saturation may be caused by a number of factors including tube malplacement, excessive bronchial secretions, hypotension and air trapping. Low compliance in the absence of reversible complications may have to be

Table 15.7. Emergencies that may occur during induction of anaesthesia

Low compliance
Tube occluding upper lobe bronchus
Overinflated bronchial or tracheal cuff
Tension pneumothorax
Bronchospasm
Sputum plug

Hypotension
Tamponade of heart due to air trapping, e.g. in emphysema and CF
Hypovolaemia and IPPV
Drug reaction
Pulmonary hypertensive crisis

Hypoxaemia
Failure to ventilate
Low blood pressure
Pulmonary hypertensive crisis

Note: CF, cystic fibrosis; IPPV, intermittent positive pressure ventilation.

managed by permissive hypercapnia. This means using low tidal volumes and peak pressures and has been successfully applied in other situations such as in the management of acute lung injury [26]. Complications of this technique include those of hypercarbia and a fall in blood pH, a rise in pulmonary artery pressure and further hypoxaemia due to decreased alveolar ventilation. A sophisticated ventilator should be available which allows a choice of inspiratory:expiratory (I:E) ratios. Reversed I:E or prolonged I:E ratios are each occasionally helpful depending on the underlying lung pathology. Salient points for the preparation of these patients are listed in Table 15.8.

Special considerations apply to the use of pulmonary lobe transplants from live donors. The technique uses a lower lobe from each of two volunteer donors instead of cadaveric whole lungs [27]. The main indication has been for CF patients. Besides the ethical problems of this procedure, there is frequently a risk of morbidity for the donor and a prolonged recovery phase for the recipient. Both Pittsburgh [28] and Harefield groups have described their experience [29]. Table 15.9 gives an outline of the current anaesthetic management of patients in the live donor programme at our hospital.

Planning for postoperative analgesia

Combined heart and lung transplantation is usually performed via a median sternotomy, which does not produce particular problems with postoperative pain. In contrast, a lateral thoracotomy for SLT or a clam-shell incision for DLT are far more painful and require a carefully planned approach to pain control. For those patients undergoing HLT, a fentanyl or remifentanil infusion during anaesthesia, followed by a morphine infusion in intensive care is appropriate. Epidural anaesthesia has been shown to facilitate early extubation and improve oxygenation as well as providing excellent pain relief following lung resection [30]. The same considerations apply during lung transplantation. In the case of SLT for emphysema it is very desirable to extubate in the operating room to minimize mediastinal shift. Some centres will place an epidural just prior to induction when a thoracotomy or clam-shell incision is used [31]. We place an epidural in non-CPB cases at the end of surgery and prior to extubation. In cases where CPB has been used, there are concerns regarding the risks of an epidural haematoma in the presence of coagulopathy due to heparin effect or bleeding diathesis [32]. Nonsteroidal analgesics should be avoided because of their nephrotoxicity, which is synergistic with immunosuppressive agents such as ciclosporin and tacrolimus.

Table 15.8. Anaesthetic considerations for lung transplantation

Pulmonary vascular disease	
Usual operations: HLT or DLT	Pre-op i.v. if polycythaemic
Blood available	In theatre for all
Anticoagulation: coumarin	? Vitamin K in selected cases
Heparin infusion	Expect heparin resistance
Prior surgery using aprotinin	Care with test dose
Plan for reversal of intracardiac shunt	Have vasoconstrictor ready
Plan for pulmonary hypertensive crisis	Have weak (1:100 000) adrenaline ready
Patient may be small	Care to avoid nerve injuries
Obstructive lung disease	
Usual operation SLT or DLT	
Check plain CXR and CT for bullae	Chest drain ready; ?emergency sternotomy
History of bronchospasm	Bronchodilators pre-op, expect quiet breath sounds
Plan for hypotension with tamponade	Preload and have vasoconstrictor ready
All patients receiving double lumen tubes	Have fiberoptic bronchoscopic ready
Cystic fibrosis	
Thick copious secretions	May need fiberoptic bronchoscopy through single lumen tube first. Will need 14 F gauge catheters
	May have indwelling vascular device (Portacath® or Vascport®)
Thrombosed veins due to multiple previous courses of antibiotics	May need central venous line placement for anaesthetic induction (prefer subclavian in lying position to int jugular head down)
May be small and cachectic, diabetic	Care to avoid nerve injuries
Pulmonary fibrosis	
Usual operation SLT	
Expect low compliance	May need sophisticated ventilator
? Pulmonary hypertension	
Low functional residual capacity	May become hypoxic quickly if delay in establishing airway
Laboratory studies	
Haemoglobin	Guide to early blood transfusion
Serum creatinine	Guide to renal management
Serology	Hepatitis, CMV sero-status
	? Need to use CMV-negative blood products

Note: HLT, heart–lung transplant; DLT, double lung transplant; SLT, single lung transplant; CXR, chest X-ray film; CT, computed tomography scan; CMV, cytomegalovirus; i.v., intravenous.

Intraoperative care

The anaesthetist will plan to use single lung ventilation using a double lumen tube for SLT or DLT operations. CPB is necessary for HLT but is optional for other lung transplant operations and should be available in case of an emergency situation where cardiovascular or pulmonary decompensation necessitates its use to complete the procedure.

Role of transoesophageal echocardiography

Suriani has recently reviewed TOE during organ transplantation [33] and a summary of its applications in lung transplantation appears in Table 15.10. Following lung transplantation TOE is used to assess the pulmonary venous anastomosis, PA anastomoses and the presence of thrombus and intra-cardiac shunts (a patent foramen ovale is present in up to 25% of the general population). Both TOE and a PA catheter may be helpful in assessing ventricular filling [33]. Finally, TOE guidance is helpful to monitor de-airing of the heart after HLT (Table 15.10).

Fluid management

Appropriate fluid management is critical. Excessive crystalloid infusions should be avoided and 4.5% human albumin solution may be used in those with polycythaemia or after a low haemoglobin has been corrected with blood.

Table 15.9. The anaesthetic management of donors and recipients for live donor pulmonary lobe transplants

Donor	Arterial and central venous lines
	Epoprostenol (prostacyclin) infusions to keep systolic pressure at 90 mmHg (12 kPa) to dilate PAs
	Epidural anaesthesia
	Blood pulmoplegia recipient compatible (from blood bank) to lobe
Recipient	Temperature < 37.5 °C
	No *B. cepacia*, no active fungal infection
	Not on full ventilation
	No excessive risk (ethically unsound)
	Art and peripheral veins under local
	Beware air trapping during induction
	Continuous cardiac output, MvO$_2$ PA catheter
	Aprotinin
	Noradrenaline infusion on bypass if low perfusion pressure, ? shunts, bacteraemia
Postbypass	Keep lungs dry with frusemide, allow oliguria
	Avoid starch: ventilate 48 hours, control PA pressure
	Ventilate new lungs with minimum F_1O_2
	Minimum barotrauma
	Epidural inserted on day 2 with normal clotting

Note: PA, pulmonary artery; MvO$_2$, maximum oxygen uptake; F_1O_2, fraction of inspired oxygen.

The use of mannitol remains controversial. We routinely administer 20 g in the CPB machine, although its free radical scavenging effect is limited at this dose.

Oliguria can be treated with loop diuretics or with ultrafiltration on CPB or by hemodiafiltration or even extracorporeal membrane oxygenation (ECMO) with ultrafiltration. Controversy surrounds the routine use of dopaminergic agonist drugs such as dopamine, dopexamine and fenoldopam, though the latter has recently been suggested as prophylaxis against ciclosporin toxicity [34]. The natriuretic peptide, urodilatin [35], has been used, particularly for resistant cases following furosemide (frusemide) infusion, but data are not yet available that this improves outcome.

Use of blood products

Heart–lung and lung transplants may require large volumes of blood products. Patients with complex congenital heart disease (Eisenmenger's syndrome) may have collaterals involving the pleura. Those with parenchymal disease, such as CF, will have multiple vascularized pleural adhesions and enlarged mediastinal lymph nodes with enhanced blood supply. In both groups various coagulopathies may coexist. The volume of blood transfusion required has decreased considerably over the past 10 years. This has been due to better selection of recipients, better surgical techniques including use of topical fibrin and aprotinin glues, and the routine use of systemic aprotinin. We use high dose aprotinin for all lung transplants [36]. Although it has been argued that similar results can be obtained with cheaper alternatives such as epsilon-aminocaproic acid [37] and tranexamic acid, recent data suggest that aprotinin has additional benefits in modifying the inflammatory response and reducing some of the effects of ischaemia–reperfusion injury on the lung, both during the retrieval procedure and in the patient [38,39]. A cell saver may be used in those patients undergoing CPB to reduce the need for red cell transfusion though this may sometimes lead to increased use of clotting factors. Although, a range of laboratory clotting tests are available, the thromboelastogram is widely used by transplantation anaesthetists [40], partly because of its ability to produce rapid results through near-patient testing. The test has not been completely validated and, as a consequence, haematology laboratories have been reluctant to adopt it and it remains a near-patient monitoring technique. However, data have shown that its use in monitoring platelet function, fibrinolysis and the hypercoaguable state have led to reduced use of blood products [41]. Lung transplant recipients who are seronegative for cytomegalovirus (CMV) are particularly susceptible to CMV pneumonitis and we use only CMV-negative white blood cell-depleted blood for this group of patients.

Management of right heart dysfunction including the use of inhaled nitric oxide

The management of the right heart is critical to successful anaesthesia for lung transplantation. Table 15.11 shows the causes of right heart failure following lung transplantation that are frequently due to increased pulmonary vascular resistance. Thus pulmonary allograft dysfunction is often associated with right ventricular (RV) dysfunction.

RV distension is usually apparent when the heart is exposed. TOE can be used to detect any bowing of the intraventricular septum. Typically, the left ventricle appears underfilled on TOE and the right ventricle is distended with diminished contractility, sometimes with severe tricuspid regurgitation (which will allow an estimate of PA pressure to be made). Paradoxically a sudden fall in pulmonary vascular resistance can result in right heart failure due to RV outflow tract obstruction in patients with severe RV

Table 15.10. Applications of TOE in lung transplantation

Stage of operation	Recognition of:
Induction of anaesthesia	Acute pulmonary hypertension
Sequential double lung transplantation	Decompensation of right ventricle when each pulmonary artery clamped
Following reperfusion of lung	Monitoring filling of both ventricles
Check venous anastomoses	Left atrium, pulmonary veins, thrombus
Weaning from CPB	Monitoring ventricular function
	Diastolic performance
De-airing of heart	Particularly following heart–lung transplant
Identification of intracardiac shunts	Atrial septal defects, PFO

Note: CPB, cardiopulmonary bypass; PFO, patent foramen ovale.

Table 15.11. Causes of right heart dysfunction during lung transplantation

Underlying lung pathology	PPH
	Emphysema
	Cystic fibrosis
	Pulmonary fibrosis
Poor myocardial preservation (ischaemia–reperfusion injury)	Following HLT only
	RV often disproportionately affected
Lung preservation injury	Increased RV afterload
Poor myocardial protection during CPB	SLT or DLT done with CPB
	RV often disproportionately affected
Protamine reaction	Rise in pulmonary vascular resistance

Note: PPH, primary pulmonary hypertension; HLT, heart–lung transplant; RV, right ventricle; CPB, coronary pulmonary bypass; SLT, single lung transplant; DLT, double lung transplant.

hypertrophy [42]. Options for the treatment of right heart failure are listed in Table 15.12.

The decision to electively use CPB for single or double lung transplantation will depend on the surgical preference and remains controversial in some situations [43,44]. It is generally accepted that cases of primary pulmonary hypertension will require the use of CPB for SLT or DLT. In other pathologies, clamping of the contralateral pulmonary artery following implantation of the first lung will divert all the cardiac output into the new lung, which may be vulnerable to pulmonary oedema because of the effects of the preservation process. Elective CPB may be protective in this situation but carries its own risks of increased surgical bleeding and promotion of a systemic inflammatory state. Proponents of CPB argue that there are few data from its use in cardiac surgery that bypass per se damages the lungs [44]. The contrary view is that the postischaemic lung

is particularly sensitive to injury and the added insult of CPB and so bypass should be reserved for those patients with severe pulmonary hypertension [43].

Emergency CPB may be required when a patient cannot tolerate single lung ventilation. CPB is easier to institute via the right chest than through the left and this may influence the choice of which of the two lungs should be operated upon first. Alternatively the femoral vessels can be prepared for CPB if it should be required. Two studies have produced inconsistent conclusions regarding risk factors for emergency institution of CPB [45,46].

Management during the postimplant phase of surgery

Pulmonary gas exchange may not be optimal in the immediate postimplantation period. This can be due to a number of reasons including inadequate cardiac output, problems with vascular anastomoses, inadequate ventilation (tube position, secretions or lobar collapse) or parenchymal lung injury (ischaemia–reperfusion injury, fluid overload), and very rarely hyperacute rejection.

The newly implanted lung has recently undergone a period of ischaemia and the integrity of the alveolar capillary membrane is under threat. Ischaemia–reperfusion injury will be manifest by a fall in lung compliance, deterioration in gas exchange, rise in pulmonary vascular resistance and pulmonary oedema. The choice and volume of intravenous fluids administered may exacerbate pulmonary dysfunction. Ventilation–perfusion inequality must be initially treated with a high fraction of inspired oxygen (F_1O_2). We prefer to reduce the F_1O_2 as quickly as possible to a level that produces an arterial oxygen saturation of 95% because of the risk of oxygen toxicity in the presence of free radicals [47]. A number of interventions may positively influence graft viability

Table 15.12. Options for the management of right heart failure

Phosphodiesterase inhibitors	Lusotropic activity on left and right ventricles
	Pulmonary vasodilators, bronchodilators
	Drop SVR, need noradrenaline in 30% of cases to maintain SBP
Epoprostenol (prostacyclin) infusion	Drops SVR and PVR, may increase shunt
Intra-aortic balloon pump	May help LV function
Inhaled nitric oxide	Lowers pulmonary vascular resistance, ?helps ischaemia–reperfusion injury
ECMO	Aortic IVC may rest LV and lungs

Note: SVR, systemic vascular resistance; SBP, systemic blood pressure; PVR, pulmonary vascular resistance; ECMO, extracorporeal membrane oxygenation; IVC, intravenous catheter; LV, left ventricle.

including the use of antioxidants [48], protease inhibitors (e.g. aprotinin) [49] and the use of neutrophil-depleted blood [50].

A phosphodiesterase (PDE) inhibitor is given routinely during rewarming after CPB and also non-CPB cases. In our institution, either the type 3 PDE inhibitor enoximone (not licensed in the USA) or milrinone is used. Milrinone has the advantage of being miscible with many other drugs and also with dextrose. PDE inhibitors cause a significant fall in systemic vascular resistance, which in about a third of cases will need to be corrected with noradrenaline. The PDE inhibitors are pulmonary vasodilators [51]. The mechanism of action of PDE inhibitors is complex. There is evidence from animal studies that drugs of this class, including zaprinast [52], theophylline [53] and rolipram [54] may reduce lung ischaemia–reperfusion injury and there are ongoing trials using a type 5 PDE inhibitor, sildenafil, as a pulmonary vasodilator [55].

Inhaled nitric oxide (NO) is now used widely in cardiothoracic surgery [56] and may be of help in the management of acute pulmonary allograft failure due to ischaemia–reperfusion injury, as well as in reducing pulmonary vascular resistance. Inhaled NO has been used to avoid the necessity for CPB while implanting the second lung in sequential bilateral lung transplantation [57]. The role of universal prophylactic NO has not been established [58]. We use a dedicated NO administration system that uses feedback mechanisms to maintain constant concentrations of NO despite varying ventilatory parameters (INOvent®, Ohmeda) [59]. Initial NO concentrations of 40 ppm can usually be rapidly reduced to 20 ppm or less. Since the introduction of inhaled NO, epoprostenol (prostacyclin) infusions are rarely used following lung implantation because NO produces selective pulmonary vasodilatation whereas prostacyclin can also produce a fall in systemic vascular resistance.

In cases that are refractory to pharmacological therapy, additional support for the lungs and the heart may become necessary [60]. A recent study reported a 60% survival to discharge in selected cases receiving ECMO after lung transplantation [61].

Termination of cardiopulmonary bypass

Particular care should be taken not to overload the heart, in particular the right ventricle at the termination of bypass. TOE is especially useful for monitoring at this stage. Protamine, which is used to reverse the effect of heparin following CPB, may increase the pulmonary vascular resistance and cause RV dysfunction. Inhaled NO should be available to counteract this effect. Clotting factors should also be to hand for administration in the light of information gained from the thromboelastogram or other clotting tests.

Termination of anaesthesia

A double lumen tube will now be exchanged for a single lumen tube. Bronchial anastomoses may now be checked bronchoscopically. Chest drains are inserted surgically and connected to a controlled suction system. Atrial and ventricular pacing wires are attached in the case of an HLT and these should be tested prior to transfer. A pacing box should accompany the heart–lung patient to the intensive care unit. Particular care should be taken to avoid fluid overload. Catastrophic cardiac distension can result in bradycardia that is resistant to pacing.

Early extubation

There has been a vogue in recent times for early extubation across a range of cardiothoracic surgical procedures from paediatric to open heart surgery. Traditional views including the need to reduce the work of breathing have given way to new arguments that take into account new and better techniques of analgesia, better haemostasis and better methods of maintaining body temperature in the presence of reasonable cardiac output and oxygenation. It is logical to review the management of lung transplants [62] and compare them with patients undergoing lung resection. However, we feel that the only group that clearly benefit from very early extubation, (in the operating room) are COPD patients who have received an SLT where mediastinal shift during positive pressure ventilation due to the compliant native lung may produce a problem and necessitate independent ventilation of each lung [63]. There are few data to confirm that early extubation in other types of lung transplant improves the outcome. However, it is logical to suggest that obtunded ciliary function will be aided by active and early coughing and that the negative aspects of mechanical ventilation (barotrauma, transfer of infection, influence on the circulation) can be avoided by early extubation. It is possible, however, that the transient pulmonary edema and reduced pulmonary compliance that may occur due to ischaemia–reperfusion injury may be helped by ventilation. In a recent uncontrolled study, Westerlind combined continuous positive airway pressure (CPAP) with an epidural using bupivacaine and sufentanil and was able to reduce length of ventilation after lung transplantation from two days to four hours [64].

Intensive care management

The role of the intensive care unit (ICU) in a lung transplant programme can be considered under three headings: before transplantation, immediate post-transplantation care, and readmission to the ICU (Figures 15.1 and 15.2). The diagnosis and management of infection and rejection are discussed elsewhere and will not be addressed in this chapter (see Chapters 16 and 20).

Pretransplant ICU management

Respiratory units are now capable of managing extremely compromised patients with advanced respiratory techniques including noninvasive ventilation. However ICU admission and invasive positive pressure ventilation may be required because of acute respiratory complications or because of progression of the underlying pulmonary disease. A careful search should be made for any reversible factor such as infection. The results of ICU management of chronic respiratory failure can be encouraging [65]. Many transplant programmes consider mechanical ventilation as a reason to remove patients from the active transplant list. However, if the patient's condition has stabilized, and the

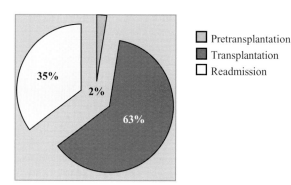

Figure 15.1 Relative length of stay of lung transplant patients in intensive care in Harefield Hospital 1999–2001.

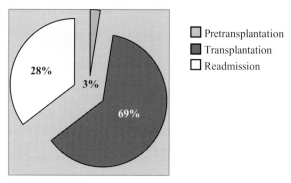

Figure 15.2 Relative proportion of patients admitted to intensive care in Harefield Hospital 1999–2001.

function of other organ systems is satisfactory, the results of transplantation can be acceptable in carefully selected cases [2,66,67]. The goal of management is to reattain the predeterioration state, so transplantation can be accomplished in a stable situation. In addition to intensive physiotherapy, treatment of infection and supportive therapy to other organ systems, procedures that can make transplantation difficult must be avoided, for example talc pleurodesis and pleural abrasions for pneumothorax.

Management immediately after transplantation

Immediate postoperative progress can be rapid, with discharge from the ICU the day after surgery being common. Perioperative, operative and graft–host interactions, however, can lead to a prolonged ICU stay for some patients. The chronic shortage of organs and the severity of illness of the recipient may lead to acceptance of suboptimal organs. Similarly preservation strategies may not be successful and the function of the transplanted lungs may become compromised as a result. In addition, the lung disease may be only a part of the underlying disorder and other organ systems may fail.

Respiratory management

Standard ventilation parameters are generally set for the uncomplicated postoperative case with tidal volume of 7–10 mL/kg, a ventilation mode that allows a peak airway pressure of < 40 cm H_2O and a small amount (5 cm H_2O) of positive end-expiratory pressure (PEEP). F_iO_2 is maintained as low as possible to allow a saturation of 95%, to minimize oxygen toxicity to the new lung and allow early detection of deteriorating gas exchange. PCO_2 is kept low to decrease pulmonary artery pressure [68]. Ventilation strategies need to be modified for single lung transplantation (see below).

Graft function

The newly transplanted lung is required to be functional immediately at least sufficiently well to allow time for further recovery. A number of factors may affect early graft function. These include donor–recipient size matching, immunology factors (such as preformed anti-human leukocyte antigen (HLA) antibodies, which can cause hyperacute rejection) and preservation injury. Technical problems with pulmonary venous or other anastomoses may first become apparent in the postoperative period. Post-transplantation injury may occur during reperfusion or because of barotrauma or fluid overload.

Monitoring trends with pulse oximetry, tidal volume (with pressure control ventilation) or peak airway pressures (with volume controlled ventilation), inspection of bronchial secretions (for pink-stained pulmonary oedema) and early chest X-ray films will give warning of developing graft failure. The oxygenation index [69] is a commonly used parameter to assess graft function (mean airway pressure × percentage inspired oxygen/partial pressure of arterial oxygen); normal < 25. Graft failure leads to an increase in this index. The possibility of technical problems with vascular anastomoses can be investigated by TOE [33,70]. Hypoxia is initially managed by increasing F_iO_2, increased PEEP, and the use of inhaled pulmonary vasodilators (NO, epoprostenol, etc.). Pulmonary oedema is managed with increased PEEP, aggressive fluid restriction and decreased pulmonary artery pressures [69,71–73].

Where graft function remains poor despite the above measures, ECMO support may be used while the lung recovers. The early use of ECMO may lead to better outcomes [61,69,74,75], and an oxygenation index value greater than 30 is used as an indicator for its institution. In the ICU,

ECMO lines may be inserted percutaneously via the femoral vessels or the patient may be returned to the operating theatre for cannulation of the ascending aorta and right atrium. Weaning from ECMO is determined by improvement in the graft function.

Mechanical airway problems (stricture or dehiscence of the anastomosis) or phrenic nerve injury can significantly delay the process of weaning from ventilation [76–78]. Later, graft complications of infection, rejection, and anastomotic problems can dominate ICU stay, with frequent need for mobile x-rays and ultrasound examinations, bronchoscopies, transbronchial biopsies and transfers to the imaging department for procedures such as computed tomography (CT) scans.

For patients with a slow recovery from surgery, discharge from the ICU is often dependent on the facilities of the stepdown support unit available. Where single organ support can be managed in a high dependency environment, discharge can be earlier with the resultant psychological benefit for the patient.

Ventilation issues specific to single lung transplants

With single lung transplantation, the different compliances of the transplanted and native lung mean that if both lungs are ventilated with the same pressure (single lumen endotracheal tube), one lung will be overinflated and the other underinflated. In this situation carefully regulated pressure controlled ventilation can ensure inflation of the less compliant lung and this is the ventilation mode of choice. PEEP and inverse ratio ventilation that augments auto PEEP must be avoided and long expiratory times are used to allow adequate deflation of the more compliant lung.

Emphysema and alpha-1-trypsin deficiency

In emphysema the native lung is very compliant and adequate ventilation of the transplanted lung to allow good gas exchange may result in hyperinflation of the native lung. This can lead to mediastinal shift with haemodynamic compromise [79–82]. Predictors of hyperinflation include very low pretransplantation FEV_1 (< 15% predicted), a high residual volume (> twice predicted), pulmonary hypertension and prolonged postoperative ventilation. Where the function of the pulmonary graft is adequate, extubation with the return to spontaneous breathing and the consequent negative intrathoracic pressure will decrease the propensity to mediastinal shift. Therefore most patients are rapidly weaned to allow early extubation [62,68].

Where mediastinal shift is a persistent problem, two main strategies may be used. Lung volume reduction surgery on the emphysematous lung will usually resolve the

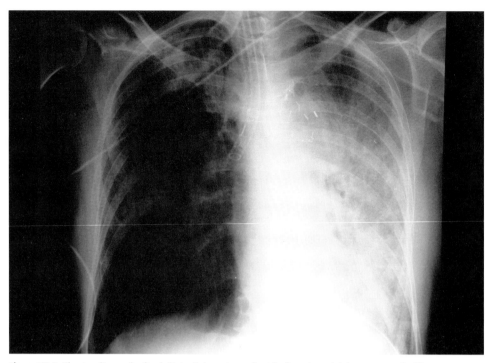

Figure 15.3 Chest radiograph after left single lung transplant for lymphangioleiomyomatosis. The transplanted lung has suffered preservation injury. Double lumen ventilation has been used to treat mediastinal shift due to air trapping in the native right lung during positive pressure ventilation.

problem and, where the lungs are known to be grossly hyperinflated, this can be combined with the initial transplant as a prophylactic procedure. Alternatively, where there is poor compliance of the transplanted lung due to preservation injury, which may improve with time, a conservative strategy of ventilatory management may be used. This usually necessitates ventilation using a double lumen tube with differential ventilation of the two lungs using separate ventilators with appropriate parameters set for each (Figure 15.3). The duration of double lumen ventilation should be minimized, as the smaller lumen makes bronchial suction less effective and leads to more lobar collapse, in addition the technique requires a greater depth of sedation than that required for ventilation via a single lumen endotracheal tube. Weaning can be effected by allowing a patient trigger to synchronize the two ventilators and gradual equalization of pressures before changing the tube back to a single lumen tube.

Diffuse (interstitial) lung disease

In patients with advanced pulmonary fibrosis, the transplanted lung is more compliant and therefore receives most of the ventilation. In addition, most of the perfusion is directed away from the pulmonary hypertensive native lung [83]. Therefore, the transplanted lung has to cope with the

bulk of the cardiac output, which makes it prone to pulmonary oedema.

Again, differential lung ventilation may be required, in this case to protect the newly transplanted lung from hyperinflation and barotrauma. In our unit, we aim for aggressive weaning with early extubation and intermittent noninvasive support if necessary. Others have opted for 48–72 hours of elective ventilation [84].

Weaning from mechanical ventilation

Early weaning can occur provided there is adequate lung function and complications such as severe preoperative CO_2 retention and surgical injury of the phrenic nerve are absent. As respiratory function improves, conventional weaning strategies can be employed. Early extubation is facilitated by effective pain management and epidural analgesia plays a major role in this. One advantage of having patients who are already well versed in respiratory technology is that compliance with noninvasive ventilation techniques is good. Therefore earlier extubation with reliance on noninvasive techniques may be a successful strategy. Where tracheal intubation is likely to be prolonged we favour early tracheostomy, to allow a reduction in sedation and more purposeful physiotherapy.

The tracheostomy should be large enough to allow entry of a normal bronchoscope that allows both diagnostic and therapeutic suction and the ability to obtain transbronchial biopsies. Where a percutaneous technique is used, care must be taken to avoid inserting the dilator too far and so void the tracheal or bronchial anastomosis.

Modern ventilators are powerful and sophisticated enough to maintain adequate gas exchange in the face of severely abnormal lung function. This may mean that, although weaning is repeatedly unsuccessful in a patient with poor graft function, ventilation can maintain adequate oxygenation. This may condemn a patient to a prolonged stay on ICU with no realistic hope of weaning. The results of early retransplantation in this group of patients are poor [85].

Mechanical airway problems of phrenic nerve injury, diaphragm damage and anastomotic leaks can significantly impair the weaning process and delay extubation [76–78].

Cardiovascular management

Significant haemodynamic changes may occur after lung transplantation; their management is based on identification of the underlying cause. This must be done quickly; the investigation must begin with an evaluation of trends in the patient's observations and other data including drain losses and current haematology and biochemistry results. Following a careful examination of the patient, information may be obtained from an up-to-date chest X-ray film, measurement of cardiac output and pulmonary pressures via the PA catheter and the findings of a TOE examination. These techniques, in combination, will reveal the mechanisms underlying the problem and guide therapy.

Excessive blood loss usually occurs in cases where there has been previous lung surgery or pleural infections, or in patients with Eisenmenger's syndrome and extensive collateral vessels, and particularly when one of these factors is present and CPB has been used [86]. The management is surgical, with simultaneous measures to correct any coagulation abnormality that may be present. The need to administer a large volume of blood components is associated with significant fluid shifts, haemodynamic instability and a proinflammatory state that gives rise to an increased risk of renal and pulmonary failure.

CPB, the need for large volumes of blood and blood products, or release of toxic components from abscesses or the infected native lung can lead to a prolonged period of vasoplegia after surgery, with pronounced vasodilatation. Management includes the use of a noradrenaline infusion and, where this is unsuccessful, an infusion of vasopressin [87].

The above changes can increase pulmonary vascular resistance substantially and the native right ventricle may

fail in the face of this. The management of right ventricular dysfunction has been discussed above, and includes the use of optimal ventilation strategies combined with inotropes, PDE inhibitors, inhaled pulmonary vasodilators (NO, epoprostenol) and, if these measures fail, the use of ECMO or an RV assist device.

Mechanical compression of the heart with blood (tamponade), air (pneumopericardium, pneumothoraces), or the lungs (hyperinflation/auto PEEP, mediastinal shift) can severely compromise cardiac output. The management is surgical drainage of air or correction of the ventilatory problem as discussed above.

In contrast, in patients with good cardiovascular function, hypertension can be a significant problem, but can be managed by a combination of either an angiotensin converting enzyme (ACE) inhibitor or an angiotensin AII receptor antagonist together with diuretics [88]. In severe and refractory cases the intravenous alpha- and beta-adrenergic blocking agent labetalol may be used.

Renal management

The use of nephrotoxic agents, either antibiotics or immunosuppressants, in patients with haemodynamic instability will increase the risk of renal failure. The newly transplanted lungs are intolerant to minor volume overload. The aim of management is to keep the patient slightly hypovolaemic to protect the transplanted lung while maintaining adequate cardiac and renal function. Diuretics, including loop diuretics and osmotic agents are used early to achieve this. Our unit in common with others has found urodilatin to be of some benefit [89]. Should these measures fail, the propensity for infection in the immunocompromised patient means that haemofiltration is used rather than peritoneal dialysis. Further advantages to haemofiltration are the ability to control temperature and the newer ability to manage liver failure as well.

Gastrointestinal system

Systemic manifestations of the primary disorder persist despite lung transplantation [65,90]. In particular, vigorous gastrointestinal tract management is essential in CF patients, with the use of N-acetylcysteine and pancreatic enzyme supplements, to prevent gastrointestinal obstruction due to the meconium ileus equivalent syndrome. Abdominal distension secondary to ileus can impair respiratory function. General surgical causes of an acute abdomen should always be considered especially, as high dose steroids and broad spectrum antibiotics can distort normal signs and symptoms [91].

Neurological/psychological complications

Most patients undergoing lung transplantation have lived with their respiratory disease for a long time. They are frequently knowledgeable, with strong likes and dislikes, and keen to participate in decisions about their care. In addition, their carers are similarly well versed in both the primary disease and transplantation, and have a support system in place already. Despite this, major depressive episodes or panic/anxiety episodes are common in the ICU [92]. Organic brain syndromes can occur in up to 50% of cases in the early postoperative phase [93]. Immunosuppressive therapy (ciclosporin) can give rise to convulsions and high dose steroids can induce a psychosis. A brain CT scan is usually necessary to rule out an organic/mass lesion and a lumbar puncture may be necessary to exclude central nervous system infection. Management consists of reducing the dose of ciclosporin/steroids if possible and the use of sedative agents (benzodiazepines, haloperidol) if necessary. The long-term psychological outcome after transplantation is discussed in detail elsewhere (see Hallas and Wray, Chapter 25).

Readmission to ICU

Readmission is usually precipitated by acute respiratory deterioration most commonly due to infection or rejection. Other reasons for readmission include acute or chronic renal failure leading to respiratory compromise, central nervous system events and the need for ICU management of incidental conditions. Where the underlying lung function has deteriorated over time due to the bronchiolitis obliterans syndrome ('chronic rejection'), and there is no prospect of retransplantation, ICU treatment may be inappropriate and a more conservative approach should be considered, with emphasis on supportive and palliative treatment.

Anaesthesia for patients with transplanted hearts and lungs

The procedures regularly performed on lung transplant patients are bronchoscopy and bronchoalveolar lavage with or without transbronchial lung biopsy. This may be carried out under local anaesthesia or a short general anaesthetic, with the choice depending on the patient's functional status. The indications are discussed elsewhere (see Corris, Chapter 16). It is important to avoid excessive administration of intravenous fluids as the patients are likely to have low pulmonary compliance with few functioning

lymphatics. Some of these patients will be electively ventilated after the procedure until treatment of the underlying condition (rejection or infection) has had time to act.

An increasing number of patients undergo general surgical procedures in noncardiothoracic centres. The overall mortality is higher than in a nontransplant population. Anaesthetists should be aware of the potential problems and these have been reviewed [94]. In general, anaesthetic drug interactions with immunosuppressants are rarely problematical, but special attention should be paid to the commonly found problems of hypertension and impaired renal function. Intensive care facilities should be available.

The team should keep in contact with the transplant centre to obtain details of the patient's clinical background and treatment. Immunosuppression should be maintained, if necessary by the intravenous routine, and access to assays for blood levels of agents such as ciclosporin and tacrolimus are essential. Occasionally, the local hospital team will wish to refer the patient back to the transplant centre.

Conclusion

Anaesthesia and intensive care forms an important component of the multidisciplinary care of the lung transplant patient. Careful planning of each procedure and good communications with surgeons, physicians and transplant coordinators is essential to achieve the optimum outcome in each case. Perioperative mortality has fallen from 15% in the period 1988–1992 to 10% in the period 1997–2000 [1].

REFERENCES

1 Hertz MI, Taylor DO, Trulock EP, et al. The Registry of the International Society for Heart and Lung Transplantation: 19th official report – 2002. *J Heart Lung Transplant* 2002; **21**: 950–970.

2 Meyers BF, Lynch JP, Battafarano RJ, et al. Lung transplantation is warranted for stable, ventilator-dependent recipients. *Ann Thorac Surg* 2000; **70**: 1675–1678.

3 Mollaret P, Gouon M. Le coma dépassé (mémoire préliminaire). *Rev Neurol* (Paris) 1959; **101**: 3–5.

4 A definition of irreversible coma: report of the Ad Hoc Committee of the Harvard Medical School to examine the definition of brain death. *JAMA* 1968; **205**: 337–340.

5 Diagnosis of brain death: statement issued by the honorary secretary of the Conference of Medical Royal Colleges and their Faculties in the United Kingdom on 11 October 1976. *Br Med J* 1976; **2**: 1187–1188.

6 President's Commission for the Study of Ethical Problems in Medicine and Biomedical and Behavioural Research. *Defining death. A report on the medical, legal and ethical issues in the*

determination of death. Government Printing Office, Washington, DC, 1981.

7 The Quality Standards Subcommittee of the American Academy of Neurology. Practice parameters for determining brain death in adults (summary statement). *Neurology* 1995; **45**: 1012–1014.

8 Wijdicks EFM. The diagnosis of brain death. *N Engl J Med* 2001; **344**: 1215–1221.

9 Van Norman GA. A matter of life and death: what every anesthesiologist should know about the medical, legal and ethical issues of declaring brain death. *Anesthesiology* 1999; **91**: 275–287.

10 Booij LHDJ. Brain death and the care of the brain death patient. *Curr Anaesth Crit Care* 1999; **10**: 312–318.

11 Perreas KG, Milano C, Tsui S, Wallwork J. Donor management tactics for cardiothoracic transplantation. *Transplant Rev* 2000; **14**: 127–130.

12 Goarin JP, Cohen S, Riou B, et al. The effects of triiodothyronine on hemodynamic status and cardiac function in potential heart donors. *Anesth Analg* 1996; **83**: 41–47.

13 Vedrinne JM, Vedrinne C, Coronel B, Mercatello A, Estanove S, Moskovtchenko JF. Transesophageal echocardiographic assessment of left ventricular function in brain-dead patients: are marginally acceptable hearts suitable for transplantation? *J Cardiothorac Vasc Anesth* 1996; **10**: 708–712.

14 Gallardo A, Anguita M, Franco M, et al. [The echocardiographic findings in patients with brain death. The implications for their selection as heart transplant donors]. *Rev Esp Cardiol* 1994; **47**: 604–608.

15 Stoddard MF, Longaker RA. The role of transesophageal echocardiography in cardiac donor screening. *Am Heart J* 1993; **125**: 1676–1681.

16 Ghosh S, Bethune DW, Hardy I, Kneeshaw J, Latimer RD, Oduro A. Management of donors for heart and heart–lung transplantation. *Anaesthesia* 1990; **45**: 672–675.

17 Gore S, Cable D, Holland A. Organ donation from intensive care units in England and Wales: two year confidential audit of deaths in intensive care. *Br Med J* 1992; **304**: 349–355.

18 Shumway SJ, Hertz MI, Petty MG, Bolman RM III. Liberalization of donor criteria in lung and heart–lung transplantation. *Ann Thorac Surg* 1994; **57**: 92–95.

19 Lange SS, Prevost S, Lewis P, Fadol A. Infection control practices in cardiac transplant recipients. The Research Committee, Houston–Gulf Coast Chapter of the American Association of Critical-Care Nurses. *Heart Lung* 1992; **21**: 101–105.

20 Myles PS, Buckland MR, Weeks AM, Bujor M, Moloney J. Continuous arterial blood gas monitoring during bilateral sequential lung transplantation. *J Cardiothorac Vasc Anesth* 1999; **13**: 253–257.

21 George SJ, Vuddamalay P, Boscoe MJ. Antiseptic-impregnated central venous catheters reduce the incidence of bacterial colonization and associated infection in immunocompromised transplant patients. *Eur J Anaesthesiol* 1997; **14**: 428–431.

22 Stephens R, Mythen M, Kallis P, Davies D, Egner W, Rickards A. Two episodes of life threatening anaphylaxis in the same patient to a chlorhexidine–sulphadiazine-coated central venous catheter. *Br J Anaesth* 2001; **87**: 306–308.

23 Weinbroum AA, Kluger Y, Abraham RB, Shapira I, Karchevski E, Rudick V. Lung preconditioning with N-acetyl-L-cysteine prevents reperfusion injury after liver no flow–reflow: a dose–response study. *Transplantation* 2001; **71**: 300–306.

24 Weinbroum AA, Rudick V, Ben-Abraham R, Karchevski E. N-acetyl-L-cysteine for preventing lung reperfusion injury after liver ischemia-reperfusion: a possible dual protective mechanism in a dose–response study. *Transplantation* 2000; **69**: 853–859.

25 Gayes JM. Pro: one-lung ventilation is best accomplished with the Univent endotracheal tube. *J Cardiothorac Vasc Anesth* 1993; **7**: 103–107.

26 Feihl F, Eckert P, Brimioulle S, et al. Permissive hypercapnia impairs pulmonary gas exchange in acute respiratory distress syndrome. *Am J Crit Care Med* 2000; **162**: 209–215.

27 Barr ML, Schenkel FA, Cohen RG, et al. Bilateral lobar transplantation utilizing living related donors. *Artif Organs* 1996; **20**: 1110–1111.

28 Quinlan JJ, Gasior T, Firestone S, Firestone LI. Anesthesia for living-related (lobar) lung transplantation. *J Cardiothorac Vasc Anesth* 1996; **10**: 391–396.

29 Farrimond JG, Boscoe MJ. Anaesthesia for lobar lung transplantation from living donors. *Curr Anaesth Crit Care* 2000; **11**: 217–223.

30 Slinger P, Shennib H, Wilson S. Postthoracotomy pulmonary function: a comparison of epidural versus intravenous meperidine infusions. *J Cardiothorac Vasc Anesth* 1995; **9**: 128–134.

31 Myles PS, Venema HR. Avoidance of cardiopulmonary bypass during bilateral sequential lung transplantation using inhaled nitric oxide. *J Cardiothorac Vasc Anesth* 1995; **9**: 565–570.

32 Chaney MA. Intrathecal and epidural anesthesia and analgesia for cardiac surgery. *Anesth Analg* 1997; **84**: 1211–1221.

33 Suriani RJ. Transesophageal echocardiography during organ transplantation. *J Cardiothorac Vasc Anesth* 1998; **12**: 686–694.

34 Jorkasky DK, Audet P, Shusterman N, et al. Fenoldopam reverses cyclosporine-induced renal vasoconstriction in kidney transplant recipients. *Am J Kidney Dis* 1992; **19**: 567–572.

35 Meyer M, Richter R, Forssmann WG. Urodilatin, a natriuretic peptide with clinical implications. *Eur J Med Res* 1998; **3**: 103–110.

36 Royston D. High-dose aprotinin therapy: a review of the first five years experience. *J Cardiothorac Vasc Anesth* 1992; **6**: 76–100.

37 Ray MJ, O'Brien MF. Comparison of epsilon aminocaproic acid and low-dose aprotinin in cardiopulmonary bypass: efficiency, safety and cost. *Ann Thorac Surg* 2001; **71**: 838–843.

38 Mathias MA, Tribble CG, Dietz JF, et al. Aprotinin improves pulmonary function during reperfusion in an isolated lung model. *Ann Thorac Surg* 2000; **70**: 1671–1674.

39 Asimakopoulos G, Lidington EA, Mason J, Haskard D, Taylor KM, Landis RC. Effect of aprotinin on endothelial function. *J Thorac Cardiovasc Surg* 2001; **122**: 123–128.

40 Samama CM. Thromboelastography: the next step. *Anesth Analg* 2001; **92**: 563–564.

41 Shore-Lesserson L, Manspeizer HE, DePerio M, Francis S, Vela-Cantos F, Ergin MA. Thromboelastography-guided transfusion algorithm reduces transfusions in complex cardiac surgery. *Anesth Analg* 1999; **88**: 312–319.

42 Gorcsan J III, Reddy SC, Armitage JM, Griffith BP. Acquired right ventricular outflow tract obstruction after lung transplantation: diagnosis by transesophageal echocardiography. *J Am Soc Echocardiogr* 1993; **6**: 324–326.

43 McRae K. Con: lung transplantation should not be routinely performed with cardiopulmonary bypass. *J Cardiothorac Vasc Anesth* 2000; **14**: 746–750.

44 Marczin N, Royston D, Yacoub M. Pro: lung transplantation should be routinely performed with cardiopulmonary bypass. *J Cardiothorac Vasc Anesth* 2000; **14**: 739–745.

45 Gammie JS, Cheul Lee J, Pham SM, et al. Cardiopulmonary bypass is associated with early allograft dysfunction but not death after double-lung transplantation. *J Thorac Cardiovasc Surg* 1998; **115**: 990–997.

46 Triantafillou AN, Pasque MK, Huddleston CB, et al. Predictors, frequency, and indications for cardiopulmonary bypass during lung transplantation in adults. *Ann Thorac Surg* 1994; **57**: 1248–1251.

47 McCord JM. Oxygen radicals and lung injury. *Chest* 1983; **83**: 355–375.

48 Shiraishi T, Kuroiwa A, Shirakusa T, et al. Free radical-mediated tissue injury in acute lung allograft rejection and the effect of superoxide dismutase. *Ann Thorac Surg* 1997; **64**: 821–825.

49 Roberts RF, Nishanian GP, Carey JN, et al. Addition of aprotinin to organ preservation solutions decreases lung reperfusion injury. *Ann Thorac Surg* 1998; **66**: 225–230.

50 Ross S, Tribble CG, Gaughen J. Reduced neutrophil infiltration protects against lung reperfusion injury after transplantation. *Ann Thorac Surg* 1999; **67**: 1428–1433.

51 Butt AY, Dinh-Xuan AT, Pepke-Zaba J, Cremona G, Clelland CA, Higenbottam TW. In vitro pulmonary vasorelaxant effect of the phosphodiesterase inhibitor enoximone. *Angiology* 1993; **44**: 289–294.

52 Schutte H, Witzenrath M, Mayer K, et al. The PDE inhibitor zaprinast enhances NO-mediated protection against vascular leakage in reperfused lungs. *Am J Physiol Lung Cell Mol Physiol* 2000; **279**: L496–L502.

53 Featherstone RL, Kelly FJ, Chambers DJ. Theophylline improves functional recovery of isolated rat lungs after hypothermic preservation. *Ann Thorac Surg* 1999; **67**: 798–803.

54 Bleiweis MS, Jones DR, Hoffmann SC, Becker RM, Egan TM. Reduced ischemia–reperfusion injury with rolipram in rat cadaver lung donors: effect of cyclic adenosine monophosphate. *Ann Thorac Surg* 1999; **67**: 194–199; discussion 199–200.

55 Abrams D, Schulze-Neick I, Magee AG. Sildenafil as a selective pulmonary vasodilator in childhood primary pulmonary hypertension. *Heart* 2000; **84**: E4.

56 Fullerton DA, McIntyre RC Jr. Inhaled nitric oxide: therapeutic applications in cardiothoracic surgery. *Ann Thorac Surg* 1996; **61**: 1856–1864.

57 Myles PS, Weeks AM, Buckland MR, Silvers A, Bujor M, Langley M. Anesthesia for bilateral sequential lung transplantation: experience of 64 cases. *J Cardiothorac Vasc Anesth* 1997; **11**: 177–183.

58 Ardehali A, Laks H, Levine M, et al. A prospective trial of inhaled nitric oxide in clinical lung transplantation. *Transplantation* 2001; **72**: 112–115.

59 Kirmse M, Hess D, Fujino Y, Kacmarek RM, Hurford WE. Delivery of inhaled nitric oxide using the Ohmeda INOvent Delivery System. *Chest* 1998; **113**: 1650–1657.

60 Miniati DN, Robbins RC. Mechanical support for acutely failed heart or lung grafts. *J Card Surg* 2000; **15**: 129–135.

61 Meyers BF, Sundt TM III, et al. Selective use of extracorporeal membrane oxygenation is warranted after lung transplantation. *J Thorac Cardiovasc Surg* 2000; **120**: 20–26.

62 Myles PS. Early extubation after lung transplantation. *J Cardiothorac Vasc Anesth* 1999; **13**: 247–248.

63 Smiley R, Navedo A. Postoperative independent lung ventilation in a single-lung patient. *Anesthesiology* 1991; **74**: 1144–1148.

64 Westerlind A, Nilsson F, Ricksten SE. The use of continuous positive airway pressure by face mask and thoracic epidural analgesia after lung transplantation. Gothenburg Lung Transplant Group. *J Cardiothorac Vasc Anesth* 1999; **13**: 249–252.

65 Sood N, Paradowski LJ, Yankaskas JR. Outcomes of intensive care unit care in adults with cystic fibrosis. *Am J Respir Crit Care Med* 2001; **163**: 335–338.

66 Baz MA, Palmer SM, Staples ED, Greer DG, Tapson VF, Davis DD. Lung transplantation after long-term mechanical ventilation: results and 1-year follow-up. *Chest* 2001; **119**: 224–227.

67 O'Brien G, Criner GJ. Mechanical ventilation as a bridge to lung transplantation. *J Heart Lung Transplant* 1999; **18**: 255–265.

68 Callegari G, Fracchia C. Modalities of ventilation in lung transplantation. *Monaldi Arch Chest Dis* 1998; **53**: 543–546.

69 Fiser SM, Kron IL, McLendon Long S, Kaza AK, Kern JA, Tribble CG. Early intervention after severe oxygenation index elevation improves survival following lung transplantation. *J Heart Lung Transplant* 2001; **20**: 631–636.

70 Huang YC, Cheng YJ, Lin YH, Wang MJ, Tsai SK. Graft failure caused by pulmonary venous obstruction diagnosed by intraoperative transesophageal echocardiography during lung transplantation. *Anesth Analg* 2000; **91**: 558–560.

71 Thabut G, Brugière O, Leseche G, et al. Preventive effect of inhaled nitric oxide and pentoxifylline on ischemia/reperfusion injury after lung transplantation. *Transplantation* 2001; **71**: 1295–1300.

72 Bittner HB, Dunitz J, Hertz M, Bolman MR III, Park SJ. Hyperacute rejection in single lung transplantation – case report of successful management by means of plasmapheresis and antithymocyte globulin treatment. *Transplantation* 2001; **71**: 649–651.

73 Haydock DA, Trulock EP, Kaiser LR, Knight SR, Pasque MK, Cooper JD. Management of dysfunction in the transplanted lung: experience with 7 clinical cases. Washington University

Lung Transplant Group. *Ann Thorac Surg* 1992; **53**: 635–641.

74 Ko WJ, Chen YS, Chou NK, Lee YC. ECMO support for single lung transplantation. *Transplant Proc* 2001; **33**: 1939–1941.

75 Nguyen DQ, Kulick DM, Bolman RM III, Dunitz JM, Hertz MI, Park SJ. Temporary ECMO support following lung and heart–lung transplantation. *J Heart Lung Transplant* 2000; **19**: 313–316.

76 Alvarez A, Algar J, Santos F, et al. Airway complications after lung transplantation: a review of 151 anastomoses. *Eur J Cardiothorac Surg* 2001; **19**: 381–387.

77 Herrera JM, McNeil KD, Higgins RS, et al. Airway complications after lung transplantation: treatment and long-term outcome. *Ann Thorac Surg* 2001; **71**: 989–993; discussion 993–994.

78 Kshettry VR, Kroshus TJ, Hertz MI, Hunter DW, Shumway SJ, Bolman RM III. Early and late airway complications after lung transplantation: incidence and management. *Ann Thorac Surg* 1997; **63**: 1576–1583.

79 Myles PS, Ryder IG, Weeks AM, Williams T, Esmore DS. Diagnosis and management of dynamic hyperinflation during lung transplantation. *J Cardiothorac Vasc Anesth* 1997; **11**: 100–104.

80 Park SJ. Acute native lung hyperinflation. *J Heart Lung Transplant* 2000; **19**: 510.

81 Weill D, Torres F, Hodges TN, Olmos JJ, Zamora MR. Acute native lung hyperinflation is not associated with poor outcomes after single lung transplant for emphysema. *J Heart Lung Transplant* 1999; **18**: 1080–1087.

82 Yonan NA, el-Gamel A, Egan J, Kakadellis J, Rahman A, Deiraniya AK. Single lung transplantation for emphysema: predictors for native lung hyperinflation. *J Heart Lung Transplant* 1998; **17**: 192–201.

83 Pasque MK, Kaiser LR, Dresler CM, Trulock E, Triantafillou AN, Cooper JD. Single lung transplantation for pulmonary hypertension. Technical aspects and immediate hemodynamic results. *J Thorac Cardiovasc Surg* 1992; **103**: 475–481; discussion 481–482.

84 Demajo WA, Winton TL. Lung transplantation: intensive care. In: Klinck JR, Lindop LM, eds. *Anaesthesia and intensive care for organ transplantation.* Chapman & Hall, London 1998: 137–146.

85 Novick RJ, Stitt L. Pulmonary retransplantation. *Semin Thorac Cardiovasc Surg* 1998; **10**: 227–236.

86 Triulzi DJ, Griffith BP. Blood usage in lung transplantation. *Transfusion* 1998; **38**: 12–15.

87 Argenziano M, Chen JM, Choudhri AF, et al. Management of vasodilatory shock after cardiac surgery: identification of predisposing factors and use of a novel pressor agent. *J Thorac Cardiovasc Surg* 1998; **116**: 973–980.

88 Midtvedt K, Neumayer HH. Management strategies for post-transplant hypertension. *Transplantation* 2000; **70**(111 Suppl): SS64–SS69.

89 Brenner P, Meyer M, Reichenspurner H, et al. Significance of prophylactic urodilatin (INN: ularitide) infusion for the prevention of acute renal failure in patients after heart transplantation. *Eur J Med Res* 1995; **1**: 137–143.

90 Semenzato G, Agostini C. Lung transplantation in sarcoidosis: lessons learned from immunology. *Sarcoidosis Vasc Diffuse Lung Dis* 1999; **16**: 21–23.

91 Hoekstra HJ, Hawkins K, de Boer WJ, Rottier K, van der Bij W. Gastrointestinal complications in lung transplant survivors that require surgical intervention. *Br J Surg* 2001; **88**: 433–438.

92 Woodman CL, Geist LJ, Vance S, Laxson C, Jones K, Kline JN. Psychiatric disorders and survival after lung transplantation. *Psychosomatics* 1999; **40**: 293–297.

93 Goldstein LS, Haug MT III, Perl J II, et al. Central nervous system complications after lung transplantation. *J Heart Lung Transplant* 1998; **17**: 185–191.

94 Boscoe M. Anesthesia for patients with transplanted lungs and heart and lungs. *Int Anesthesiol Clin* 1995; **33**: 21–44.

16

Medical management

Paul A. Corris

Freeman Hospital, Newcastle upon Tyne, UK

Introduction and general considerations

No procedure in medicine depends as much as lung transplantation does on a team approach from various disciplines including surgeons, respiratory physicians, microbiologists, physiotherapists and nurses if success is to be achieved. To minimize any confusion and optimize patient care it is essential to develop standard treatment protocols and to organize regular multidisciplinary ward rounds on a daily basis.

Although occasionally patients are extubated in the operating theatre, the majority of patients are extubated between 12 and 24 hours after surgery. They arrive in the intensive care unit mechanically ventilated and the approach to ventilation is to minimize the risk of trauma whilst ensuring adequate oxygenation on as low a fraction of inspired oxygen as possible. A low positive end-expiratory pressure of 5 cm H_2O is usually employed. A degree of lung vascular injury resulting from factors in the donor lung, method of lung preservation and ischaemia–reperfusion injury occurs in all lungs but the severity varies considerably. Brain death itself induces systemic and local cytokine responses in the donor lungs. A severe injury is manifest by parenchymal infiltrates and significant hypoxaemia. This may require careful ventilatory management, diuresis and the use of inhaled nitric oxide. When diuretics are used it is important to ensure that the circulating blood volume is not reduced to a degree that impairs tissue perfusion. It is also important to avoid electrolyte abnormalities and uraemia. Chest drains are monitored for evidence of mediastinal or pleural haemorrhage and if this is persistent or massive, re-exploration is required. The frequency of surgical re-exploration for bleeding has decreased markedly over the years. In part this is because of improved intraoperative visualization of the entire pleural surface including the posterior mediastinum. This has been achieved by the introduction of a transverse or clam-shell incision to perform bilateral lung transplantation. The increased use of aprotinin has also contributed.

One complication unique to single lung transplantation for emphysema during mechanical ventilation via a single lumen endotracheal tube is that of gas trapping within the emphysematous native lung that leads to mediastinal shift with simultaneous atelectasis of the allograft and hyperinflation of the native lung. Split lung ventilation and occasionally native lung volume reduction may be required in such cases. Another early complication of lung transplantation is that of phrenic nerve injury, which has been documented in one series to occur in up to 30% of patients. Phrenic nerve injury may significantly complicate weaning from mechanical ventilation but in the majority of patients the paralysis is transient.

Pain control is extremely important in the immediate postoperative period to aid extubation of the patient as quickly as possible. The majority of patients benefit from effective analgesia by an epidural catheter to prevent chest pain associated with physiotherapy and coughing. The importance of adequate pain control to prevent early infectious complications cannot be overemphasized. Immunosuppression (see later) is started right away and prophylactic antibiotics also given (see later).

Management post intensive care

Post intensive care

After extubation patients are usually transferred from an intensive care unit to a stepdown ward. Central venous and arterial catheters may be removed and oxygen saturation monitored continuously by an oximeter. Chest radiographs are taken twice a day during the first week and monitored for perihilar infiltrates or septal lines, which can suggest acute rejection. The development of a pleural effusion in addition to parenchymal change may indicate acute rejection or empyema. If a clinical deterioration is seen, additional chest radiographs are performed. After the first week the frequency of radiographic and other studies can be adjusted according to the patient's clinical status. Chest radiographs have been reported as being normal in 26% of cases of acute rejection during the first month and lung function testing is a vital part of graft surveillance. Spirometry can be performed as soon as practical after surgery. Many transplant units teach patients to monitor their own function using a hand-held battery spirometer. A sustained 5–10% reduction in forced expiratory volume in 1 s (FEV_1) has been reported as being a sensitive marker of either lung rejection or infection that warrants further investigation, even in the absence of clinical symptoms or chest radiographic abnormalities. All patients who undergo single lung transplantation are given a perfusion scan within the first week after transplantation. The graft should have immediate preferential perfusion compared with the native lung and any evidence of hypoperfusion of the new lung raises the probability of vascular anastamotic stricture or thrombosis. Vascular anastamotic complications are rare, but carry a high mortality. Pulmonary venous obstruction leads to increasing parenchymal infiltrates and both arterial and venous strictures or thromboses lead to persistent hypoxaemia. The diagnosis requires a high index of suspicion and confirmation via the use of transoesophageal echocardiography and pulmonary angiography. Treatment may comprise judicious use of thrombolytic agents where thrombosis is significant, balloon dilatation or surgery. The principle problem in the early management following lung transplantation is that it is impossible to differentiate between opportunist infections of the lung and lung rejection. Both complications present with identical respiratory symptoms and physical signs that include fever, cough, shortness of breath, malaise and crackles on auscultation. Chest radiography is also often unhelpful because pulmonary infiltrates and pleural effusions are common to both and in the early postoperative period may also occur as a result of lung vascular injury of the donor lung.

Bronchoscopy in the early postoperative period

Fibreoptic bronchoscopy with bronchoalveolar lavage (BAL) and transbronchial biopsy (TBB) has an essential role in the monitoring of a lung allograft in the early postoperative period. Bronchoscopy is carried out in response to the development of respiratory symptoms including a new infiltrate on chest radiograph, a drop in lung function or an unexplained fever. Although TBB may have a 15–28% false negative rate for rejection it remains the 'gold standard' in practical terms for the diagnosis of acute lung rejection [1]. It is generally believed that four to six biopsies should be taken and that serial sections should be reported by a pathologist familiar with lung transplantation pathology and graded using the guidelines established by the International Society for Heart and Lung Transplantation [2]. A deterioration in clinical condition may also be caused by lung infection and moreover a number of studies have shown that infection and rejection may be seen concurrently in the early period following transplantation. For these reasons it is important to perform BAL at the same time as TBB to provide samples for microbiological and cytological examination for bacteria, fungi and viruses.

Immunosuppression

Standard therapy is a three drug regimen based on either ciclosporin or tacrolimus. The other components are corticosteroids and either azathioprine or mycophenolate mofetil. Both tacrolimus and ciclosporin A are given orally twice a day and concentration in whole blood is measured at trough level by monoclonal assay. A trough level of 300–350 mg ciclosporin/mL or 10–15 mg tacrolimus/mL represents target levels initially but target trough levels may be adjusted on an individual basis in patients with rejection or infectious complications. Oral prednisolone is begun at 1 mg/kg per day and the dose lowered by 0.2 mg/kg per week with a target maintenance dose of 0.2 mg/kg at the time of hospital discharge. The initial dose of azathioprine is 2–3 mg/kg, the dose being adjusted according to white blood cell count. Mycophenolate mofetil is commenced at a dose of 1.5 g twice a day. Both ciclosporin A and tacrolimus are metabolized by the liver such that interactions with a number of commonly used drugs may alter the concentrations of both agents. Rapid elevations in levels because of drug interactions cause acute toxicity whereas rapid reductions allow rejection to occur (see Chapter 18).

Early infection prophylaxis

It is routine for patients to receive prophylactic antibiotics following surgery and it is common for patients to receive cover against both staphylococci and anaerobic organisms until healing of the bronchial anastamosis has

Table 16.1. Histological grading of acute cellular rejection

Grade	Normal severity	Extent of perivascular infiltrates
A0	No rejection	No significant abnormality
A1	Minimal	Infrequent perivascular mononuclear cell infiltrates mainly surrounding venules with a thickness of just a few cells
A2	Mild	More frequent infiltrates that involve veins and arteries that are more than several cells thick
A3	Moderate	More exuberant mononuclear cell infiltrates that extend from the perivascular space into the alveolar interstitium
A4	Severe	Infiltrates extend into the alveolar space with pneumonocyte damage; there may be necrosis of vessels and lung parenchyma

been identified. Flucloxacillin and metronidazole are commonly used. Patients who have septic lung conditions are often colonized with *Pseudomonas* species and they should receive appropriate antibiotic cover according to pretransplantation cultures. Recipients with airways colonized by *Aspergillus* spp. are generally given antifungal treatment to reduce the incidence of disseminated fungal infections, as well as of infections of the bronchial and anastamotic site. There is no clear consensus and units employ a variety of strategies including nebulized amphotericin 20 mg twice a day, low dose intravenous amphotericin or oral itraconazole. Some donor lung lavages show evidence of *Candida* spp., and the prophylactic use of fluconazole is usually employed. Patients with evidence of lung injury or who have required a prolonged period of mechanical ventilation often continue with nebulized colomycin to help prevent colonization of lungs with Gram-negative organisms. Patients at high risk for the subsequent development of cytomegalovirus disease will often start prophylaxis with oral ganciclovir during this early postoperative period (see Chapter 21).

Early complications

Acute rejection

Acute rejection is seen in up to 40% of recipients within the first 30 days of transplantation. Episodes that occur in the first two weeks typically cause fever, chills, malaise, increasing tightness in the chest, cough and worsening dyspnoea. Physical examination may reveal signs of pleural effusion and crackles.

Pulmonary function studies may show deteriorating lung function and hypoxaemia. Chest radiographs may demonstrate interstitial infiltrates with or without pleural effusions. The principle morphological change found in acute rejection is a perivascular lymphocytic infiltrate that may extend into alveolar septae in the later stages of rejection. In addition, airways may show a lymphocytic infiltrate. It is usual to perform TBB on each lobe from one lung, as rejection may be patchy and multiple biopsies from different lobes afford a greater chance of positive diagnosis. Many studies have tried to establish reliable, less invasive methods of diagnosing rejection on blood or BAL cells and fluid. To date, none has proved sufficiently sensitive and specific for routine clinical use, although the Pittsburgh group reported some success using the donor-specific primed lymphocyte response of BAL cells to diagnose lung allograft rejection. The grading of acute pulmonary rejection is based on the intensity of lymphocyte infiltrate as described in Table 16.1 (see Chapter 23).

Acute rejection is a complex integrated immune response stimulated by the recognition of histocompatibility antigens on the surface of donor cells. The most important histocompatability antigens are those of the major histocompatability complex (MHC). T-cell recognition of foreign MHC occurs via a complex interaction between the donor antigens, antigen presenting cells and the T-cell antigen receptor, together with accessory costimulatory molecules. Adhesion molecules such as vascular cell adhesion molecule (VCAM) 1 and intercellular adhesion molecule (ICAM) 1 facilitate the process. Following interaction, the T cell becomes 'activated', a term that refers to a cascade of events including signal transduction, gene transcription and release of cytokines (see Chapter 17). Episodes of acute vascular rejection are usually treated with pulsed methyl prednisolone at 10 mg/kg intravenously for three days followed by augmented oral prednisolone (see Chapter 18). Rejection episodes resistant to increased corticosteroids

Table 16.2. Staging of bronchiolitis
obliterans syndrome (BOS)

Stage 0	$FEV_1 > 90\%$
	$FEF_{25-75} > 75\%$
Stage 0-p	FEV_1 81–90% and/or
	$FEF_{25-75} \leq 75\%$
Stage 1	FEV_1 66–80%
Stage 2	FEV_1 51–65%
Stage 3	$FEV_1 < 50\%$

Percentages refer to baseline value.
FEV_1, forced expiratory volume in 1 s; FEF_{25-75},
forced expiratory flow at between 25% and 75%
of vital capacity.

may be treated by T-cell antibody, photophoretic therapy or total lymphoid irradiation. In general, however, the response to methylprednisolone is brisk, with symptoms improving within 24 hours. Within one week of completion of therapy, allograft function should have improved dramatically. Failure to achieve this end-point warrants immediate re-evaluation.

Infection

The principle cause of early postoperative death is infection. Bacterial pneumonia is common in the early postoperative period and affects up to 35% of patients [3]. The factors that influence the development of pneumonia include immunosuppression, alteration of the natural defence mechanisms such as a depressed cough reflex, and reduced clearance, in part because of depressed ciliary beat frequency. The initial approach to determining the cause of pneumonia in a patient who has received a lung allograft is not different from that of any other immunocompromised patient. TBB, however, is usually carried out at an earlier stage because acute rejection may present with identical clinical features. Sputum should be sent for Gram stain, and culture and blood cultures are taken. Fibreoptic bronchoscopy is carried out with lavage and protected brush specimens from the involved segments. The high incidence of pneumonia is caused by Gram-negative rod-shaped bacteria such as *Pseudomonas* species. All transplant centres have reported typical pneumonia organisms such as *Streptococcus pneumoniae, Haemophilus influenzae, Mycoplasma pneumoniae, Legionella pneumophila* and *Staphylococcus aureus*. Although patients with cystic fibrosis do not have a higher frequency of pneumonia they do have an increased frequency of *Pseudomonas* species

isolated from sputum and lavage, and such patients benefit from prophylactic nebulized colomycin to prevent the development of pneumonia. Cytomegalovirus (CMV) is the most common viral pathogen. A recipient negative for CMV antibody who receives an organ from an antibody-positive donor has the potential for the most severe disease [4]. Antibody-positive patients who receive lungs from either antibody-positive or antibody-negative donors may also develop CMV disease but the risk is not as great as in the former category. Antibody-negative patients who receive lungs from antibody-negative donors have a negligible risk provided they receive seronegative blood products. CMV disease typically presents with fever, increasing breathlessness and/or abdominal pain and is usually associated with leukopenia. Much literature has been published concerning the prophylaxis of CMV disease in lung transplant recipients. The high incidence of CMV disease in antibody-negative recipients of lungs from positive donors led to a number of strategies and practice still varies widely. The development of oral ganciclovir taken as 1 g three times per day for up to three months after transplantation has been adopted by many groups. It is virostatic rather than virocidal and so infection typically occurs when prophylaxis is discontinued. The advantage of delaying the onset of CMV disease is that the degree of immunosuppression is usually less and the patient's overall condition more robust at the later date and so the host is more able to deal with the pathogen. A second approach is to use pre-emptive therapy with ganciclovir based on weekly testing for antigenaemia in the at-risk patients. This is conceptionally more scientific, but practically challenging as it relies on repeated blood sampling and the availability of a reliable antigenaemia testing service.

Ganciclovir at 5 mg/kg intravenously twice a day for two to three weeks is the treatment of choice for established CMV infection. The dose must be adjusted for renal insufficiency and leukopenia. Herpes virus pneumonia was reported as a common problem in early heart and lung transplant recipients and for that reason aciclovir prophylaxis has traditionally been given for up to 6–12 weeks after transplantation. *Pneumocystis carinii* is one of the potential opportunist infections following lung transplantation but has been virtually eliminated by the widespread use of prophylaxis. Without prophylaxis, infection was reported in up to 88% of heart–lung transplant recipients. It is rare before six months after transplantation, but prophylaxis is usually started within the first month. Prophylactic treatment is taken twice daily for three days each week using trimethaprim 160 mg and sulphamethoxazole 800 mg in combination (co-trimoxazole). Infection with *Candida* or

Aspergillus species is a potential problem when these organisms are isolated from the airway of the donor lung at harvest or from the recipient lung following explantation. They may invade the bronchial anastamosis in the early postoperative period and infect not only devitalized tissue at the anastamosis but also ischaemic areas of the bronchus, with the potential to cause life-threatening haemorrhage. Prophylaxis for susceptible patients is as discussed above and frank infection treated with fluconazole, itraconazole or intravenous amphotericin and flucytosine as indicated previously.

Transition to out-patient management

Most lung transplant recipients remain in hospital for at least three weeks after transplantation for surveillance and physiotherapy. Patients also require a good deal of education regarding warning signs of infection or rejection and information relating to their drug therapy. Once recipients have achieved a sufficient level of independence they can be discharged to housing adjacent to the hospital, where they can continue postoperative training and rehabilitation for days or weeks prior to returning home. Highly deconditioned recipients benefit greatly from intensive rehabilitation. Patients must be trained in the use of a portable minispirometer before discharge. Daily spirometry can detect resection at an early stage.

Outpatient management

The number of lung transplant recipients continues to grow and as a consequence respiratory physicians play an increasing role in the management of these patients. They must be aware, however, of when to refer recipients back to transplant centres for specialist investigation. The major complications encountered in the first few months following transplantation are similar to those encountered early and comprise rejection and infection. Differences in the presentation of rejection and the causes of infection occur in this stage rather than in the early postoperative period. In addition a number of other disorders associated with immune suppression are seen and these require prompt management if the recipient is to realize the maximum potential from the transplantation. Although two thirds of recipients experience at least one episode of acute rejection within the first two years the incidence is greatest in the first six months and declines markedly thereafter [5]. After six months, chronic rejection, recognized histologically by bronchiolitis obliterans and functionally by the bronchiolitis obliterans syndrome (BOS), begins to emerge [6].

Bronchiolitis obliterans syndrome (BOS)

BOS has become the leading cause of death following lung transplantation and affects up to two thirds of all long-term survivors [7,8] (see Chapters 19 and 23). Prevention is complicated and remains one of the major challenges facing lung transplantation today. Histologically it is recognized by obliteration of bronchioles by organizing fibrin associated with fibroblasts and mononuclear cells. Immunohistology shows that the walls of the bronchioles are infiltrated by CD8 lymphocytes [9]. The small bronchioles are left as fibrous bands extending out to the pleura, with associated dilatation and bronchiectasis of proximal airways. Vascular sclerosis affecting both pulmonary arteries and veins may be seen in conjunction with obliterative bronchiolitis. The leading risk factor for chronic rejection is the severity and persistence of acute rejection. Those recipients affected by recurrent or persistent acute cellular rejection that fails to respond to repeated therapy with corticosteroids are at the highest risk. Other complications that also may increase the risk include infection with CMV, severe lung injury in the early post-transplantation period and mismatch of the human leukocyte antigen A locus [10]. The diagnosis of bronchiolitis obliterans syndrome is made on the basis of an irreversible decline in FEV_1 after all other causes of allograft dysfunction have been excluded [6]. It is categorized functionally into five groups, as shown in Table 16.2. Since biopsy specimens from up to one third of recipients with chronic rejection do not demonstrate bronchiolitis obliterans, histological confirmation via TBB is not necessary. Bronchiolitis obliterans usually results in a progressive loss of function due to airflow obstruction over a period; however, a few patients appear to stabilize with an attenuation in the loss of FEV_1. The most common clinical manifestations of BOS are dyspnoea on exertion, cough and sputum. Patients with BOS will commonly develop proximal bronchiectasis and become colonized with Gram-negative infections as the disease progresses. Recurrent pulmonary infection is common at this stage. Effective treatment of BOS remains difficult. The majority of centres begin therapy with a pulse of corticosteroids but this generally is ineffective. Cytolytic therapy may stabilize lung function in some patients and switching patients from ciclosporin-based immunosuppression to tacrolimus appears to stabilize lung function in others. Other approaches include total lymphoid irradiation, cyclophosphamide and sirolimus (see Chapter 18). Current research aims to identify those patients at risk prior to functional damage when more targeted immunosuppression may be successful in preventing irreversible bronchiolar obliteration.

Surveillance

Many transplant centres perform surveillance bronchoscopy, which includes TBBs at predetermined intervals, and show evidence that changes in the management take place in up 50% of patients as a result of this practice [11,12]. Other transplant centres have stopped carrying out biopsies as there is no evidence that the incidence of obliterative bronchiolitis in units carrying out surveillance biopsies is lower than in those centres who perform bronchoscopy only when required by clinical indication. The development of newer and more specific immunosuppressive drugs, however, may well mandate a return to the practice of performing regular surveillance biopsies.

Complications in intermediate and long-term survivors

Infection

Bacterial infection is common in long-term survivors, leading to both lower respiratory tract infections and pneumonia. The usual organisms leading to community-acquired pneumonias in a nontransplant population predominate. Although many fungal species have the potential to cause life-threatening infection in lung recipients, *Aspergillus* species are by far the most important. Invasive aspergillosis usually occurs in recipients who were previously colonized by *Aspergillus fumigatus* and who undergo treatment for rejection. Invasive disease requires treatment with intravenous amphotericin B, usually using a liposomal product. Amphotericin may also be inhaled if there is involvement of the bronchial mucosa. The level of immunosuppression is also lowered. Some centres elect to treat recipients who become colonized by *Aspergillus* with oral itraconazole. It is unclear whether this approach eliminates the possibility of invasive disease. Tuberculosis is a rare cause of infection, probably because of the preoperative prophylaxis in at-risk recipients with isoniazid and careful selection of donors. The few cases reported respond well to therapy. A whole gamut of opportunist infections have been reported in lung transplant recipients, including nocardiasis and, as with other immunocompromised hosts, results of treatment are best with early bacterial conformation and specific targeted therapy as soon as possible. The use of early BAL or fine-needle aspiration of nodules is recommended.

Lymphoproliferative disease

Epstein–Barr virus (EBV) is associated with post-transplantation lymphoproliferative disease (PTLD), which results from immortalization of B cells that are either monoclonal or polyclonal in origin. Most adult recipients have immunity to EBV, but when a seronegative recipient receives an organ from a seropositive donor the risk of primary infection is high and nearly 50% of such infections are associated with PTLD. Reactivation of latent EBV infection also occurs following intense immunosuppression for rejection. PTLD is usually asymptomatic until the burden of tumour interferes with lung function or leads to symptoms in other sites such as intestinal obstruction. Less commonly enlargement of peripheral lymph nodes occurs. Recipients at risk from a primary infection may be monitored for EBV antibodies to early intermediate antigens or for EBV mRNA in peripheral blood detected by the polymerase chain reaction. Evidence that links a high level of EBV mRNA in the blood with PTLD is emerging and suggests that this approach may identify recipients who have subclinical PTLD. Many patients who develop PTLD respond to a reduction in the level of systemic immunosuppression. Routine chemotherapy carries a high risk of morbidity and subsequent mortality. Newer treatment options comprise the use of monoclonal antibodies and utilizing recipients' natural killer cells obtained by venesection and activated in vitro with interleukin 2 [4] prior to subsequent reinfusion of activated cells [13]. Despite the fact that PTLD can be controlled in the majority of instances it still leads to the premature death of some lung transplant recipients and more research into novel therapeutic approaches is required.

Drug-induced complications

Most transplant recipients have impaired renal function as a result of ciclosporin- or tacrolimus-induced vasoconstriction of the afferent renal arteriole leading to a reduction in glomerular filtration rate. The cause of the vasoconstriction is multifactorial and includes increased production of vasoconstrictors such as endothelin 1 and direct effects of ciclosporin on calcium channels in vascular smooth muscle [14]. Although renal tubular abnormalities were initially thought to be the cause of ciclosporin-induced renal dysfunction, it is now believed that they are a consequence of chronic hypoperfusion. A degree of chronic nephrotoxicity occurs in virtually all patients after lung transplantation but a minority will require renal replacement therapy in the form of haemodialysis or renal transplantation as the result of severe chronic renal failure. The concurrent administration of many drugs can potentiate nephrotoxicity and particular care needs to be taken when coprescribing nonsteroidal anti-inflammatory drugs and aminoglycoside antibiotics. Drugs that block calcium channels have been shown to be at least in part protective against acute and chronic nephrotoxicity. Systemic hypertension is also a side effect of the calcineurin inhibitors and approximately two thirds of previously normotensive patients will develop hypertension.

Neuromuscular complications

Approximately 25–30% of lung transplant recipients will develop neurological problems including headache, confusion, seizures, strokes, peripheral neuropathy and myopathy. The majority of complications relate to the neurotoxic effects of both ciclosporin and tacrolimus. One important syndrome relates to posterior leukoencephalopathy, when a patient may present with a constellation of symptoms that include tremor, headache, encephalopathy, seizures, cortical blindness and confusion. Patients become hypertensive, and although the syndrome most commonly appears in the early post-transplantation period, it has been recorded much later. The diagnosis is supported by characteristic white matter changes on magnetic resonance imaging (see Chapter 22) which reflects microvascular injury. These findings are commonly reversible with initial discontinuation and then a reduction in the level of calcineurine inhibitors. Patients who develop major seizures commonly have coexistent hypomagnesaemia and general are younger recipients. Control of seizures is best managed with valproate, which does not interfere with calcineurin inhibitor levels. Myopathy is a complication of therapy with ciclosporin and corticosteroids. Ciclosporin has been implicated as the causative factor in the development of a proximal myopathy with features of mitochondrial dysfunction. The reduced maximum exercise capacity following successful lung transplantation seems to be caused by reduced peripheral muscle activity as the result of this mitochondrial dysfunction rather than any ventilatory limitation of the lungs themselves.

Osteoporosis

Bone mineral density is reduced in many patients with advanced chronic pulmonary disease and studies have demonstrated a 15% reduction in bone mineral density during the first six months of surgery. One study showed that 73% of patients following lung transplantation had spine and femoral bone mineral densities below the fracture threshold. Since the majority of bone loss appears to

occur within the first six months, prophylactic therapy with bisphosphonates and calcium supplementation should be commenced from the start.

Gastrointestinal complications

Approximately 20% of patients develop gastrointestinal complications including gastroparesis, gastritis, peptic ulcer disease, cholelithiasis and colonic perforation. Gastroparesis leads to significant morbidity and occurs as a direct result of the action of ciclosporin on gastric motility and also as a result of vagal nerve damage during surgery. Azathioprine, ciclosporin and tacrolimus can be associated with acute pancreatitis.

Nonlymphoproliferative malignancies

Patients after lung transplantation are susceptible to a number of nonlymphatic tumours [15]. Skin tumours are most common, particularly squamous cell carcinoma. As a consequence, lung transplantation recipients must avoid excessive exposure to sunlight. Other tumours seen with greater frequency in the transplant population include sarcomas and carcinomas of the cervix and hepatobiliary system.

Other drug-related complications

Ciclosporin induces gum hypertrophy, hirsuties and diabetes. Tacrolimus causes less gum hypertrophy and hirsuties but is a more potent inducer of diabetes.

Outcome and results

Provided that patients are appropriately selected, the results of heart–lung, single lung and bilateral lung transplantation are good. The International Society of Heart and Lung Transplant has demonstrated an improvement in survival over the last decade, although overall survival still lags behind that of patients receiving liver, kidney or heart transplantation. None the less, lung transplantation has become an accepted therapy for many end-stage pulmonary or pulmonary vascular diseases. The one year survival rate should now be 75–80%, with a five year survival of 50–55%. Functional results in survivors measured in terms of FEV_1 and exercise performance are good, and recipients of two lungs can expect to attain their normal predicted FEV_1 and vital capacity between six months and one year post-transplantation in the absence of complications, although the diffusing capacity usually remains reduced. All patients should expect restoration of a normal lifestyle, with little or no functional restriction during normal activities of daily living. Maximum exercise performance is limited by peripheral muscle function rather than cardiac or ventilatory limitation.

Exercise data comparing six minute walking distance and maximum oxygen consumption during an incremental symptom limited exercise test show that successful lung transplant recipients return to a normal six minute walking distance by one year, with no evidence of desaturation on exercise irrespective of the operation. In addition to prolonging life, lung transplantation also improves the quality of life as determined by standardized measures of health status [16]. There are increasing numbers of recipients surviving to 10 years and patients who have not developed BOS by five years, are free from other long-term complications and have a good potential for long-term survival.

Disease recurrence

There has been great interest in the study of lungs after successful transplantation to see whether the original lung disease will recur in the allograft. Mature granulomata have been described in the lungs of patients receiving a transplant for sarcoidosis and alveolar cell carcinoma, lymphangioleiomyomatosis and Langerhans cell granulomatosis [17] have all been demonstrated to recur in the lung allograft following transplantation for these indications. So far there is no evidence that patients with chronic obstructive pulmonary disease, including those with emphysema associated with alpha-1-antitrypsin deficiency, will develop recurrence of their original disease and presumably this is as a result of smoking cessation. There have been two case reports of recurrent giant cell interstitial pneumonitis in pulmonary allografts after transplantation for this condition [18] but to date there have been no reports of interstitial pulmonary fibrosis of the usual type recurring. There have been no reports of primary pulmonary hypertension recurring in lung transplant recipients for this condition.

Medical management of lung candidates awaiting lung transplantation

Good communication between a potential lung transplant recipient's physician and the transplant centre physician is essential. Transplant centres must be aware of changes in the condition of candidates and all must be aware that candidates may deteriorate to the point where transplantation is no longer feasible. It is important for patients to remain as mobile as possibly, emphasizing the need for

pulmonary rehabilitation, including nutritional support. Some patients who develop cachexia will require percutaneous endoscopic gastronomy feeding in order to reverse the cachexia, and exercise rehabilitation will improve muscle strength. One area relates to the decision whether to intubate a young patient awaiting lung transplantation. This clearly can be considered where there is an acute on chronic deterioration, for example due to pneumonia, where control of the acute problem may lead to successful weaning from the ventilator. Patients who develop the need for intubation as a result of progressive deterioration in the natural history of their disease, however, should not be mechnically ventilated, since this confers a significant adverse outcome as compared with nonintubated patients. The critical shortage of donor lungs therefore mitigates against intubating patients who develop progressive respiratory failure. Some patients have received chronic ventilatory support via nasal intermittent positive pressure ventilation. This does not appear to lead to an adverse outcome, as does intubation, and consideration of this form of support should be discussed on an individual basis.

Summary

Lung transplantation is an effective therapy for patients with end-stage lung disease. The major practical problems facing lung transplantation continue to be a shortfall of suitable donor organs as compared with the number of potential recipients, and the development of obliterative bronchiolitis. Patients with advanced pulmonary airway, parenchymal or vascular disease who receive lung transplantation and remain free from obliterative bronchiolitis enjoy an excellent standard of life with normal or near normal restoration of activity and good prospects of prolonged survival.

REFERENCES

1 Guilinger RA, Paradis IC, Dauber JH, et al. The importance of bronchoscopy with transbronchial biopsy and bronchoalveolar lavage in the management of lung transplant recipients. *Am J Respir Care Med* 1995; **152**: 2037–2043.

2 Yousem S, Berty G, Brunt E, et al. A working formulation for the standardisation of nomenclature on the diagnosis of heart and lung rejection: Lung Rejection Study Group. *J Heart Transplant* 1990; **9**: 593–601.

3 Kramer MR, Marshal SE, Stance CA, et al. Infectious complications in heart–lung transplantation. Analysis of 200 episodes. *Arch Intern Med* 1993; **153**: 2010–2016.

4 Wreghitt TG, Hakim M, Gray JJ, et al. Cytomegalovirus infections in heart and heart–lung transplant recipients. *J Clin Pathol* 1988; **41**: 660–667.

5 Bando K, Paradis IL, Komatsu K, et al. Analysis of time-dependent risks for infection, rejection and death after pulmonary transplantation. *J Thorac Cardiovasc Surg* 1995; **109**: 49–59.

6 Estenne M, Maurer JR, Boehler A, et al. Bronchiolitis obliterans syndrome 2001: an update of the diagnostic criteria. *J Heart Lung Transplant* 2002; **21**: 297–310.

7 Bando K, Paradis IL, Konishi H, et al. Obliterative bronchiolitis after lung and heart lung transplantation: an analysis of risk factors and management. *J Thorac Cardiovasc Surg* 1995; **110**: 4–14.

8 Sundaresan S, Trulock EP, Mohanankumar T, et al. Prevalence and outcome of bronchiolitis obliterans syndrome after lung transplantation. *Ann Thorac Surg* 1995; **60**: 1341–1347.

9 Milne DS, Gascoigne AD, Wilkes J, et al. The immunohistological features of obliterative bronchiolitis following lung transplantation. *Transplantation* 1992; **54**: 748–750.

10 Kroshus TJ, Kshettry VR, Savik K, John E, Hertz MI, Bolman RMI. Risk factors for the development of bronchiolitis obliterans syndrome after lung transplantation. *J Thorac Cardiovasc Surg* 1997; **114**: 195–202.

11 Guilinger RA, Paradis IL, Dauber JH, et al. The importance of bronchoscopy with transbronchial biopsy in the management of lung transplant recipients. *Am J Respir Care Med* 1995; **152**: 2037–2043.

12 Yousem SA, Paradis IL, Griffith BP. Can transbronchial biopsy aid in the diagnosis of bronchiolitis obliterans in lung transplant recipients? *Transplantation* 1994; **57**: 151–153.

13 Nalesnik MA, Rao AS, Furakawa H, et al. Autologous lymphokine-activated killer cell therapy of Epstein–Barr virus-positive and negative lymphoproliferative disorders arising in organ transplant recipients. *Transplantation* 1997; **63**: 1200–1205.

14 Rossi NF, Chuchill PC, McDonald FD, et al. Mechanisms of cyclosporin A-induced renal vasoconstriction in the rat. *J Pharmacol Exp Ther* 1989; **250**: 896–901.

15 Penn I. Incidence and treatment of neoplasia after transplantation. *J Heart Lung Transplant* 1993; **12**: S328–S336.

16 Gross CR, Savik SK, Bolman RM, Hertz MI. Long term health status and quality of life outcomes of lung allograft recipients. *Chest* 1995; **108**: 1587–1593.

17 Gabbay E, Corris PA. Recurrence of Langerhan's cell granulomata and its subsequent treatment following transplantation. *Thorax* 98; **53**: 326–327.

18 Frost AE, Keller CA, Brown RW et al. Giant cell interstitial pneumonitis: disease recurrence in the transplanted lung. *Annu Rev Respir Dis* 1993; **148**: 1401–1402.

17

Immunological mechanisms of graft injury

Marlene L. Rose[1] and Ian V. Hutchinson[2]

[1]Imperial College London and Harefield Hospital, Harefield, Middlesex, UK
[2]Manchester Hospital, Manchester, UK

Overview

In the clinical situation the vast majority of transplants are allografts, organs transplanted between genetically different individuals of the same species. These will be the focus of this chapter. However, the future may hold the option of xenografting where organs are transplanted from one species to another. Commercial and other considerations have dictated the choice of the pig as a potential donor for humans. Where appropriate, mention will be made of xenotransplantation.

Graft rejection is often categorized according to the tempo at which it happens. The terms hyperacute, acute and chronic rejection are used to describe graft damage that occurs in minutes to hours, days to weeks, or months to years after transplantation, respectively [1]. However, the mechanisms responsible for acute rejection may be activated late after transplantation, while the changes characteristic of chronic rejection may be seen very early after transplantation in some recipients. Hence it is generally better to think in terms of the underlying mechanisms and accept that the immune system will do its utmost, using almost every specific and nonspecific mechanism it can muster, to destroy the transplanted tissue. In general, if steps were not taken to overcome the mechanisms of rejection then the majority of grafts would be lost very quickly.

To complicate matters, the graft itself responds to the transplantation procedure and to its new and often hostile environment. The period of cold ischaemia during the transplantation procedure elicits the expression of a range of new molecules, including adhesion molecules, proinflammatory cytokines and chemokines. These serve to promote the infiltration of the graft by recipient leukocytes, first by neutrophils, followed by monocytes and macrophages then ultimately by lymphocytes. This orderly procession of cells into a wound over several days sterilizes, removes debris, initiates repair and establishes a local immune reaction. Such regulated inflammation is a beneficial process. However, in the face of a persistent source of antigen, in the normal case an infection, immune lymphocytes drive the inflammatory response of monocytes and granulocytes, leading to tissue damage in an attempt to eliminate the infection. In the case of a transplant, the grafted tissue itself is the source of persistent antigen and, without immunosuppression, would be severely damaged. Even when the infiltration and inflammatory process is greatly dampened with immunosuppression the local release of inflammatory cytokines such as tumour necrosis factor alpha (TNF-α) and interferon gamma (IFN-γ) changes the expression of histocompatibility and adhesion molecules within the transplant, making the graft a better target for the immune response. Finally, in an extension of the repair process, both the graft and the infiltrating leukocytes release an array of growth factors, but the chronicity of this process leads to fibrosis and arteriosclerosis.

Hyperacute rejection

Introduction

If the recipient already has circulating antibodies against the graft, these will bind in the transplant as soon as the blood supply is restored to the organ. The endothelial cells lining the blood vessels of the new organ are the principal targets. The preformed antibodies may be directed at either human leukocyte antigens (HLA) or at an endothelial antigen. Their binding may either kill or activate the endothelium, leading to intravascular thrombosis and coagulation, occluding the graft vessels (2,3). This blockage of the blood supply to the graft is dramatic. A newly anastomosed graft turns pink as the blood flow is restored, but then the graft rapidly darkens in colour and begins to swell in a matter of minutes.

Preformed antibodies in allotransplantation

How do these preformed antibodies arise? There are three possibilities: blood transfusions, previous transplants and pregnancy. Patients awaiting a transplant may have received blood transfusions. This exposure to foreign cells, from another individual, induces the appearance of anti-HLA antibodies in perhaps 20% of transfused patients. As an aside, paradoxically those who do not become sensitized by blood transfusion may accept a (kidney) transplant more readily, a phenomenon known as the blood transfusion effect. This will be discussed later. Other patients may already have had a transplant against which they have made antibodies. Women who have been pregnant, particularly multiparous women, may have very high levels of antibodies directed at the paternal antigens of foetal origin. Indeed, histocompatibility laboratories use pregnancy sera as tissue typing reagents. Finally, antibodies against blood group antigens can cause hyperacute rejection. For most organs it is not possible to transplant across an ABO incompatibility, and grafts have to be performed according to the rules of blood transfusion. An interesting exception to these rules appears to be transplantation of ABO mismatched hearts into neonatal human recipients [4].

Preformed antibodies in xenotransplantation

In pig-to-human xenotransplantation, natural antibodies in human serum specific for porcine carbohydrate blood group-like antigens, in particular an epitope called 'gal-alpha-1,3-gal' containing two linked galactose molecules, bring about the immediate demise of pig xenografts (5,6). This applies, too, to donors other than pigs because the same carbohydrate antigens exist in all potential donor species apart from primates.

Avoidance of hyperacute rejection of allografts

Nowadays, clinical hyperacute rejection is exceedingly rare. The majority of surgeons will never see a case of hyperacute rejection because tissue typing laboratories devote an enormous amount of effort to identifying and characterizing antibodies in potential transplant recipients that could bind to donor antigens. The basic test is known as the 'leukocyte cross-match test'. At the time of harvesting of the donor organs, recipient serum is mixed with donor blood leukocytes in the presence of complement (serum enzymes that can be triggered to lyse cell membranes). If the recipient serum contains antidonor antibodies and kills the donor cells then the cross-match test is positive and the transplant cannot go ahead. One limitation of the test performed this way is that it uses leukocytes rather than endothelial cells, so that rare positive reactions against endothelium may be missed.

Variations in the cross-match test are used in the period before transplantation. One of these is the panel reactivity antibody (PRA) test. A panel of, say, 60–100 different leukocyte samples that express a wide range of antigens is tested with the recipient serum. The serum may kill 40%, 60% or even 100% of the cell samples in the panel. A 100% reactivity virtually excludes the possibility of transplantation, while lesser degrees of reactivity on the panel can be analysed to identify the specificity of antibodies present to improve the chances of finding a cross-match-negative donor. Usually antibodies to major histocompatibility complex (MHC) class II antigens are less problematic than those against MHC class I antigens, for example. Nowadays this search for antibodies is carried out in some laboratories using more sensitive methodology, for example using a flow cytometer (the so-called flow cross-match test) and beads coated with purified MHC antigens rather than cells. However, greater sensitivity detects more cross-match-positive patients and may exclude them from transplantation, so the appropriate level of sensitivity has to be determined.

Avoidance of hyperacute rejection of xenografts

For xenotransplantation there are four possible options to avoid hyperacute rejection: remove the antibody from the recipient, remove the complement from the recipient, remove the antigen from the donor organ or protect the endothelium of the donor blood vessels from complement-mediated damage. The first requires plasmapheresis of the recipient followed by the administration of potent (and toxic) immunosuppressive agents such as cyclophosphamide or methotrexate to prevent the reappearance of the antibodies [7]. This has been done with only limited success in animal models. Decomplementation of the recipient is an experimental procedure using a factor isolated from cobra venom that activates and therefore removes all of the third component of complement (C3), thereby inhibiting complement-mediated cell killing [8–10]. This is a short-term treatment that can be repeated only until antibodies appear to neutralize the cobra venom factor. In any case, complement is an important and valuable part of the innate immune system.

Removing the carbohydrate antigen from pig tissues has been achieved by inactivating an enzyme, galactosyl transferase, which is important in making the carbohydrate antigen. This technology may provide animal organs lacking the blood group antigens against which humans have natural antibodies [11]. Finally, some endothelial cell surface proteins break down complement very quickly. One is called decay accelerating factor (DAF), but pig DAF is not very efficient at breaking down human complement. Thus pigs have been given the gene for human DAF and there is some evidence that organs from these human DAF transgenic pigs are more resistant to hyperacute rejection (12–14). A good review of these and other approaches has been published [15]. The effect of such manipulations on xenograft acceptance in humans is, as yet, unknown.

Acute rejection

Introduction

It is remarkable that, of the 5×10^{11} T cells present in the average human, up to 1 in 1000 can directly recognize a transplanted organ [16]. Furthermore, each cell has the capacity to divide very rapidly, doubling in numbers every 8 to 18 hours so that each T can (in theory) produce between a thousand and a million daughter cells specific for graft antigens. The principal points here are the large numbers of T cells that can recognize and respond to a transplant, and the enormous capacity the immune system has for expansion.

Major histocompatibility complex molecules and their normal function

MHC molecules are central to the normal physiology and function of T cells. The T cells have receptors that bind to peptide fragments of foreign antigens held in a binding groove of MHC molecules. T-cell receptors bind strongly to the combined peptide and MHC molecule, but very weakly indeed to either peptide or MHC molecule alone.

The peptide-binding grooves of the MHC molecules on normal tissues are occupied by peptides derived from the proteins of the cells on which the MHC molecules are expressed (Figure 17.1). Recognition of self peptide antigens presented by MHC molecules is usually avoided because potentially self-reactive T cells have been deleted in the thymus, a process called negative selection. At the same time the thymus positively selects T cells that do bind weakly to MHC molecules so that they can recognize self MHC presenting foreign peptide complexes [17]. In the course of a virus infection, the self peptides in self MHC

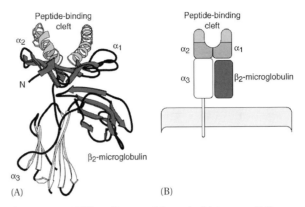

Figure 17.1 (a) Ribbon diagram of the major histocompatibilty complex (MHC) class I molecule showing the peptide-binding cleft in a groove formed by the alpha helix conformation of the α_1 and α_2 domains. (b) Shown schematically, the MHC class I molecule is a heterodimer of a membrane-spanning α-chain (43 000 kDa) noncovalently linked to β_2-microglobulin (12 000 kDa). (Reproduced with permission from *Immunobiology, the immune system in health and disease*, fourth edition, ed. Janeway CA, Travers P, Walport M, Capra JD. Elsevier Science Ltd, Amsterdam 1999.)

molecules are replaced by peptides from the virus. The T cells 'see' the self MHC–foreign peptide complexes and respond to destroy the virus-infected cells [18].

Antigen presenting cells

Recognition of MHC molecules is not itself sufficient to activate T cells for graft destruction. The antigen (MHC–peptide complex) must be presented on the surface of leukocytes or endothelial cells. One set of leukocytes in the body is especially good at activating T cells. These cells are known as 'professional antigen presenting cells' [19]. In a sense virtually all nucleated cells in the body are antigen presenting cells (APCs) because they express MHC class I antigens and, if they become infected with a virus, are capable of displaying arrays of MHC class I–virus peptide complexes. However, professional APCs have the distinction of being able to acquire foreign antigens, process them (into peptide fragments) and create MHC–peptide complexes that are displayed on the cell surface. In addition, professional APCs carry other cell surface molecules called 'costimulation molecules' that interact with corresponding molecules on the T-cell surface and are necessary for the proper activation of T cells [20,21] (Figure 17.2). Such costimulatory interactions involve B7.1 and B7.2 (CD80 and CD86) molecules on the APCs and CD28 and CTLA-4 on T cells [22], or CD40 on

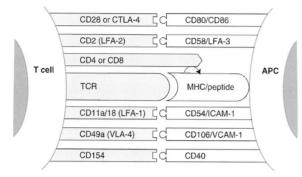

Figure 17.2 Costimulatory molecules are needed for T-cell activation. Diagrammatic representation to demonstrate interactions between APCs (such as a dendritic cell or B cell) and T cells that result in T-cell activation. TCR, T-cell receptor; MHC, major histocompatibility complex; APC, antigen presenting cell; ICAM, intracellular adhesion molecule; VCAM, vascular cell adhesion molecule; LFA, lymphocyte function-associated antigen; VLA, very late antigen.

APCs and its ligand CD40L (CD154) on T cells [23]. The most potent professional APCs are the dendritic cells, but macrophages and B cells have professional APC activity too.

Of particular importance in transplantation is the fact that the most potently immunogenic cell in an organ transplant, the cell that stimulates the rejection response the most, is the so-called 'passenger leukocyte' (24,25). All tissues have within them bone marrow-derived dendritic cells that are temporarily resident. There is a turnover of these cells, whose function is to detect antigen exposure in the tissues and to activate the protective immune response. Inevitably these cells are part of the transplant. It was shown that removal of passenger dendritic cells from rat transplants [24,26,27] could reduce the immune response so much that the organs were not rejected acutely, although they do undergo chronic rejection at later times. Clinical attempts to remove passenger dendritic cells from human organs by perfusion with monoclonal antibodies to leukocytes during the period of storage, alas, did not have a measurable outcome on graft rejection [28].

Direct and indirect allorecognition

Direct allorecognition

We can distinguish two ways in which transplanted tissues are recognized by T cells. These are known as direct and indirect allorecognition [29–31].

The phenomenon of direct allorecognition, the inherent capacity of the immune system to recognize and respond to transplanted tissues, has been studied in great detail.

Why should there be so many cells in a person capable of recognizing the antigens of someone else [16]?

When a transplant is introduced, unmatched MHC molecules on the graft are recognized by the T cells of the recipient because of the following:

(a) All T cells are programmed in the thymus to recognize MHC antigens and it is only those that have receptors for self MHC–self peptide complexes that are eliminated. Thus the vast numbers remaining will contain T cells capable of binding with sufficient affinity to the foreign MHC–foreign peptide complexes to respond. Furthermore, the MHC antigens are expressed densely on most cells, providing plenty of antigen for avid binding and recognition. This has been described as the 'high determinant density' concept of allorecognition.

(b) The peptide-binding grooves of the unmatched MHC molecules of the donor and the recipient will differ and will therefore display a different array of normal tissue peptides. To the T cells of the recipient such foreign MHC–foreign peptide complexes resemble self MHC molecules presenting, say, virally derived foreign peptides. Indeed, it has been shown that T cells recognizing virus-infected self cells will respond to foreign MHC antigens. Hence, this is the 'cross-reactivity' concept of allorecognition. It has also been described as the 'multiple binary complex' hypothesis because there are many possible donor-derived peptides so, again, many T cells may respond.

These two possibilities to explain the high numbers of alloreactive cells are not mutually exclusive, and to a large extent overlap anyway. Regardless of the details, the important feature of allorecognition is the very large numbers of T cells that can be activated by a transplant.

Minor histocompatibility antigens

Incidentally, so far only major histocompatibility differences have been described. Minor histocompatibility antigens have been identified too. However, these still involve the MHC molecules. Simply put, minor histocompatibility antigens are peptides (albeit presented by MHC molecules) [32,33]. As outlined above, normal cells bear on their surface MHC molecules complexed with peptides derived from normal cellular proteins. Some normal proteins vary from one person to another (allelic variants, say allele 1 and allele 2). Thus the same MHC molecule on cells from two people having different alleles of a normal protein express MHC–peptide complexes that can be distinguished by T cells, namely MHC plus peptide from allele 1 or MHC plus peptide from allele 2. These minor histocompatibility antigens (MHC molecules with allelic peptides) can contribute to allorecognition so that, even when the donor and recipient are very closely matched for their MHC antigens, minor histocompatibility differences can trigger rejection responses.

Indirect allorecognition

So far only direct allorecognition has been discussed. Direct allorecognition is relevant only in the nonphysiological context of transplantation (or, perhaps, in pregnancy if the maternal immune system is exposed to paternal antigens of the fetus). In contrast, indirect allorecognition occurs according to the normal physiological pathways of antigen recognition by T cells [34–37]. As alluded to before, peptides from a pathogen (such as virus peptides described above) are taken up and presented in the grooves of MHC molecules to the receptors of T cells. In this case the T cells and the APCs presenting the MHC–peptide complex are the same, so the T cells see *self MHC* plus *foreign (viral) peptides*. Essentially the same thing happens when donor antigens are shed from a graft and are taken up and presented by recipient APCs, so the recipient T cells see *self MHC* plus *foreign (donor) peptide* (Figure 17.3). Hence, indirect allorecognition is the same as the physiologically normal recognition of foreign antigens by T cells.

The relative capacity for direct and indirect allorecognition

One of the major differences between direct and indirect allorecognition is the number of T cells with receptors that can recognize the graft. In the case of direct allorecognition, the frequency of reactive cells is 1 in 1000 to 1 in 10 000. In contrast, the frequency of indirectly alloreactive T cells is 1 in 100 000 to 1 in a million, two or three orders of magnitude fewer cells.

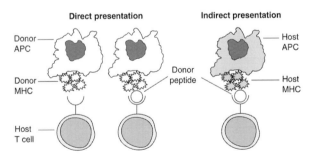

Figure 17.3 Pathways of antigen presentation. Diagrammatic representation of mechanisms whereby recipient T cells recognize allo-class II determinants. Recipient T cells recognize donor MHC determinants on donor APC (direct presentation) or they recognize donor MHC peptides, which have been released from donor cells and processed and presented by host APC within self MHC molecules (indirect presentation). APC, antigen presenting cell; MHC, major histocompatibility complex.

Effector responses in acute rejection

The response to clinical organ transplants is dependent on T cells. Experimentally it has been shown that rodents depleted or deficient of T cells are unable to reject allografts. These T cells recognize the graft as foreign because they have antigen-specific receptors, but the mechanism by which they destroy the graft may be specific (antibodies or cytotoxic T cells) or nonspecific (inflammation or delayed-type hypersensitivity). Any or all of the mechanisms may contribute to acute graft damage, depending on the type of graft and the degree of histoincompatibility between the donor and the recipient [38–41].

Role of CD4+ T cells

Various studies have been conducted in which subpopulations of T cells have been transferred into animals devoid of any T cells, to determine which are capable of rejecting a transplant. It is very clear that CD4+ T cells play a central role in graft destruction [42] (Figure 17.4). CD4+ T cells may bring about damage to the graft in four ways. First, they could act as cytotoxic (killer) T cells. CD4+ T cells can be cytotoxic. However, because they directly recognize MHC class II antigens that are present on activated endothelium but virtually nowhere else in transplanted organs, such cells

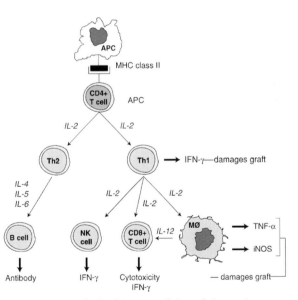

Figure 17.4 Central role of CD4+ T cells in graft destruction. Diagram shows that activation of CD4+ T cells results in Th1 or Th2 cells, production of their characteristic cytokine profiles and maturation of effector mechanisms. APC, antigen presenting cell; MHC, major histocompatibility complex; IFN, interferon; TNF, tumour necrosis factor; iNOS, inducible nitricoxide synthase; Mφ, macrophase; IL, interleukin.

may be responsible for endothelialitis but are unlikely to be a major mechanism of parenchymal cell damage.

Alternatively, the CD4+ T cells may act as 'helper' T cells in the activation of B cells and their differentiation into plasma cells making antibodies against the graft. They can act in this manner only if they have been activated by the indirect allorecognition pathway because they must interact with MHC class II molecules on recipient B cells. Help for B-cell activation is provided by cytokines released by the T helper (Th) cells. CD4+ Th cells are divided into two subsets according to the cytokines they produce. It is the Th2 subset of cells that make the cytokines necessary to promote antibody production. These cytokines include interleukin IL-4, IL-5 and IL-6, formerly known as B-cell growth factor (BCGF) 1, BCGF-2, and B-cell differentiation factor (BCDF).

In contrast, the CD4+ Th cells may be of the Th1 subset that makes IFN-γ and IL-2. Such cells may be activated by the direct or the indirect pathways of allorecognition. IFN-γ has many effects in the transplant situation. It increases the expression of adhesion molecules of the graft endothelium, facilitating the adhesion of circulating leukocytes to the blood vessel walls and their transmigration into the graft. Graft infiltration is one of the hallmarks of acute rejection. IFN-γ activates macrophages and induces them to release enzymes, free radicals and other noxious agents (intended to clear an infection) as well as inflammatory cytokines such as IL-1 and tumour necrosis factor alpha (TNF-α). This pathway (graft-specific T cells activating macrophages in a manner analogous to type IV or delayed-type hypersensitivity) seems to be very important in graft damage. In particular, recipients of kidney, heart or liver transplants who have either been shown to be high producers of TNF-α in vitro or who have a TNF-α genotype associated with higher TNF-α production are more likely to lose their graft to acute rejection. IFN-γ also increases the expression of MHC class II molecules on the graft parenchyma and endothelial cells and increases the ability of APCs to activate T cells by increasing their ability to process and present antigen and to express costimulatory molecules.

In xenografts, the role of the Th1 cell is partly replaced by that of the natural killer cell that responds to the lack of self MHC antigens on the xenograft by producing IFN-γ. Initial immune recognition by T cells, presumably by the indirect allorecognition pathway, is still necessary so that xenograft rejection does not occur in recipients entirely lacking T cells. Otherwise, histologically, acute xenograft rejection resembles that of allograft rejection.

Finally, the other Th1 cytokine, IL-2, mentioned above has a major influence on graft rejection too. It is a growth factor for T and B cells, dramatically increasing their proliferation and survival. Blocking IL-2 production with the calcineurin inhibitors ciclosporin [43] or tacrolimus [44], blocking uptake of IL-2 by IL-2 receptors using monoclonal antibodies to CD25 (one of the chains of the IL-2 receptor) [45] or blocking the intracellular signalling through the IL-2 receptor with sirolimus [46,47] all suppress graft rejection. One of the cell types dependent on IL-2 for activation is the CD8+ cytotoxic T lymphocyte (CTL), which will be discussed below.

Role of CD8+ T cells

The part played by the CTL in graft rejection is still a matter of debate amongst immunologists [42]. To damage the graft these CTL must be activated by the direct pathway of allorecognition, otherwise they would not recognize and kill the donor tissue. Highly activated CTL can be recovered from grafts undergoing rejection [48], and activated CTLs injected into tissues cause cell death and necrosis at the injection site [49]. On that basis, the presence of CTLs in rejection and their potential to damage tissues, CTLs probably do play a role in acute graft rejection. However, rejection can occur in the absence of histological evidence of graft cell lysis. When naive CD8+ T cells are transferred into a transplant recipient with no other T cells they do not become activated and bring about graft rejection [50–52]. However, this merely suggests that, in the absence of Th1 cells making IL-2, they are not able to grow and differentiate. The intravenous transfer of preactivated CD8+ T cells into graft recipients does not cause graft damage either. This may be because they do not home into the graft or they die very quickly. The latter is supported by an experiment in which activated CD8+ T cells were transferred into recipients given regular doses of IL-2 to maintain the viability of the CD8+ CTL, a protocol that did lead to organ graft rejection. Thus it seems that CD8+ CTL, recognizing the MHC class I molecules expressed on the majority of nucleated cells, can and probably do contribute to graft damage.

CTLs cause damage to target cells by inducing lytic or apoptotic cell death [53,54]. The lytic death is caused by the directed release onto the target cell surface of two molecules: perforin, which permeates the target cell membrane; and granzyme, which enters the cell and initiates the lytic programme. The cell bursts and releases its contents into the environment, and this may promote a local inflammatory response, in the case of a viral infection to clear remaining virus particles. The expression of perforin and granzyme in transplant biopsies [55] and in peripheral blood cells [56] is being studied as a molecular marker of acute rejection.

Lytic cell death is a pathological process and is not part of the turnover of cells in normal tissues. The alternative route of cell death is apoptosis, in which the nucleus fragments, the chromatin is degraded and the cell is broken up into small pieces that are rapidly phagocytosed by macrophages and destroyed without the release of any of the target cell contents. This is a physiologically normal process that regulates the overall size of cell populations, and is important in the remodelling of tissues, for example in embryogenesis. The cytotoxic T cell induces apoptosis, otherwise known as programmed cell death, in target cells by interaction with the target cell using Fas–Fas ligand (FasL) interaction [53,54]. Both types of killing are thought to play a role in graft rejection and, indeed, the apoptotic pathway may explain how CTL can damage grafts without histological evidence of tissue cell lysis.

Role of antibody

In experimental models, acute rejection is usually accompanied by production of alloantibody, but this antibody may not be damaging. Recent studies using gentically modified mice that have no antibodies but an otherwise intact immune system demonstrate that T cells are the main effectors of acute graft rejection. However, when T cells are compromised, antibodies become important as an effector of graft rejection [57]. Consistent with a role for antibodies in acute rejection, experimental studies have shown that treatment to suppress rejection reduces the binding of antibodies in the graft. In addition, there is evidence that some types of Th cell bring about graft rejection in adoptive transfer models by helping B cells to make antibodies [58,59].

There is another line of evidence that antibodies can protect allografts, both organs and tumours, from acute rejection [60]. Against expectation, the passive transfer of antidonor antibodies into rats given organ grafts protected them from rejection, an effect called passive immunological enhancement, and caused damage only when rabbit complement was injected too [61]. Thus, until recently, there was no clear evidence that antibody plays a role in acute rejection and, indeed, on the basis of the assumption that it does not, ciclosporin was vaunted as special because it prevented graft rejection but did not suppress the antibody responses that protect the recipient against infection. Now the sparing of antibody production is not considered a desirable feature of immunosuppression, particularly in view of the evidence that antibodies play a role in chronic rejection.

In human recipients post-transplant monitoring of antibody production is done in only a few centres, and it is likely that antibody-mediated rejection is underestimated. Antibody-mediated rejection is a diagnosis made after the exclusion of other possibilities. For example, a heart graft may begin to fail in the absence of histological evidence of cell-mediated acute rejection. In such cases plasmapheresis and additional immunosuppression with cyclophosphamide or methotrexate have been attempted, but with little success. Thus the consensus on the role of antibodies in acute rejection is much as it is with the role of CTL. They may be present, they can cause damage and, in some patients, probably do contribute to acute graft rejection.

Overcoming acute rejection

Introduction

Given the various mechanisms of acute rejection one might expect to have to use a variety of approaches to prevent acute graft loss. The major strategies are to minimize immune activation, to reduce the number of T cells in the recipient, to prevent T-cell activation and proliferation and to suppress inflammation. The aim is to induce long-term graft acceptance with minimal immunosuppression. Indeed, the ultimate achievement would be long-term graft acceptance without the need for continued immunosuppression, in other words immunological tolerance of the graft.

HLA matching

Immune activation of the recipient can be minimized by matching of the MHC antigens of the donor with those of the recipient. Of the MHC class I and class II loci, it is considered most important to match for HLA-A, HLA-B and HLA-DR antigens. That is not to say that HLA-C, HLA-DP and HLA-DQ antigens are unimportant in transplantation but analyses have shown that they have a lesser effect on graft outcome than HLA-A, -B and -DR. In any case, because HLA antigens are all located quite close together in the MHC gene complex on the short arm of chromosome 6 (6p21.1) and are therefore inherited as haplotypes, matching for some HLA antigens may lead to fortuitous matching for other HLA antigens. Since an individual is diploid, having one set of genes from his or her mother and the other from the father, there are two HLA-A antigens that need to be matched, two HLA-B antigens and two HLA-DR antigens. Hence a full match is a 'six antigen match' according to standard tissue typing practices. This is the optimal situation, when a donor and recipient share all six antigens. A 'zero match' or 'six antigen mismatch' is the worst possible situation. In between, the statistics of graft survival according to HLA mismatch show that graft outcome gets worse as the degree of mismatch increases. However, it is most important to match for the HLA-DR antigens, with acute rejection being minimal in recipients of fully HLA-DR matched kidneys [62] and hearts [63,64]. Other organs may not benefit as much from HLA-DR matching. The beneficial effect of HLA-DR matching is explained by the fact that the CD4+ T helper cells recognize and respond to MHC class II antigens of the graft, so that matching for the human MHC class II antigens HLA-DR minimizes the activation of alloreactive CD4+ T cells.

Great progress has been made in tissue typing methodology. Perhaps the greatest advance is the replacement of serological HLA typing methods with rapid molecular genetic approaches based on the polymerase chain reaction to amplify DNA from the donor and the recipient. For serological typing a panel of antibodies is required that is specific for each HLA antigen. Because monoclonal tissue typing reagents proved exceptionally difficult to make, most laboratories relied on pregnancy sera, containing complex mixtures of antibody specificities that required immense experience in interpretation and, in any case, were available in only limited quantities. In contrast, the polymerase chain reaction is performed with cheap and easily made primers specific for each HLA allele and the results are straightforward to interpret. Most laboratories now use molecular methods for the typing of class II antigens and some class I antigens.

Many cardiothoracic transplant centres do not routinely consider HLA matching for two reasons. Historically it took too long to perform the HLA typing (no longer a consideration) and clinical imperatives often overrode any potential benefit of HLA matching. After all, a poor mismatch can be compensated for by greater immunosuppression, but this increases the risk of toxic side effects, infections and malignancies. Despite the need for increased immunosuppression, HLA matching is still beneficial [63,64].

Immunosuppressive agents

The first immunosuppressive agents to be used clinically were steroids. Steroids have two major uses: as low maintenance doses given over a long period after transplantation or as large bolus doses given as a very short course. With reference to the description above, low dose steroids in effect mainly counteract the immune changes associated with the release of proinflammatory cytokines in the graft. Low dose steroids suppress the activation of macrophages, reduce the expression of adhesion molecules on endothelium, suppress the expression of MHC antigens on the graft and interfere with the antigen presenting function of dendritic cells. Low dose steroids also inhibit the proliferation of lymphocytes by interrupting the intracellular signalling pathways necessary for cell activation. In contrast,

high dose bolus steroids are used to treat rejection episodes because activated lymphocytes are susceptible to steroid-induced apoptosis. Hence bolus steroids are used to eliminate large numbers of activated B and T cells from patients experiencing rejection episodes.

Steroids alone do not completely prevent T-cell activation, partly because they are too toxic to be given at sufficient doses. Thus the next sort of immunosuppressive agent introduced was antiproliferative, acting to prevent the vast expansion in the numbers of activated lymphocytes of which the immune system is capable (see above). The agent that achieved clinical acceptance as an antiproliferative agent was azathioprine, and for many years the standard immunosuppressive protocol was dual immunosuppression with these two agents.

In the 1980s a new agent was discovered, one that worked because it inhibited the synthesis of IL-2 (and other cytokines such as TNF-α and IFN-γ). This agent was ciclosporin [43]. It was discovered serendipitously and was found to prevent graft rejection before its mode of action was known [65]. Once the mode of action of ciclosporin was known another agent, originally known as FK506 but now called tacrolimus, with the same properties, namely inhibition of IL-2, production was identified through a search for agents with this activity [44]. It turned out that both ciclosporin and tacrolimus inhibit an enzyme called calcineurin, a phosphatase important in activating the IL-2 gene [66]. The clinical introduction of ciclosporin [67] revolutionized the practice of transplantation, improving results dramatically and widening the applicability of transplantation to patients, including children, who had not previously received a transplant. For 15 years the 'gold standard' for immunosuppression was triple therapy with steroids, ciclosporin and azathioprine. However, the calcineurin inhibitors have toxic side effects. It was hoped that tacrolimus might have a different and less toxic profile, but this has proved to be only partially so.

Antibodies have been used widely too, especially in cardiothoracic transplantation, either as pretreatment of transplant patients (induction therapy) or to treat rejection episodes. In the late 1970s these agents were sera or the globulin fraction (containing the antibodies) of sera raised in horses, goats or rabbits against human lymphocytes or thymocytes, variously antilymphocyte serum (ALS), antilymphocyte globulin (ALG) and antithymocyte globulin (ATG). Their quality and potency were difficult to control, although such preparations are still manufactured and used today. The advent of the monoclonal antibody era led to attempts to make monoclonal antilymphocyte preparations. The virtue of monoclonal antibodies is that endless supplies of a reliably active product could be made.

The difficulty was that we did not know which antibodies in a crude ALS were active. Indeed, it turned out that most of the antibodies in ATG are not immunosuppressive. Those antibodies directed at molecules associated with the T-cell receptor, in particular the CD3 molecules, were found to be immunosuppressive and a monoclonal agent OKT3 (specific for CD3) achieved widespread use [68]. However, it is too effective in some respects, causing overimmunosuppression in some patients, leading especially to viral infections and, in some cases, to post-transplantation lymphoproliferative disorders (PTLD). Other monoclonal agents have been prepared and tested, and will be described below.

Another approach to achieve selectivity for lymphocytes was to inhibit biochemical pathways upon which lymphocytes rely for their proliferation and activation. One such agent is mycophenolate, which inhibits an enzyme, inosine monophosphate dehydrogenase (IMPDH), involved in the de novo pathway of DNA synthesis [69]. Proliferating lymphocytes are almost uniquely dependent on the de novo pathway of DNA synthesis, so mycophenolate has a remarkably lymphocyte-specific effect. It inhibits the expansion of both T- and B-cell numbers, thereby preventing antibody production, as well as the cellular mechanisms of graft rejection. Another advantage of mycophenolate over azathioprine is that it is a noncompetitive inhibitor of DNA synthesis (in fact, it inhibits a cofactor necessary for IMPDH activity) unlike azathioprine, which is incorporated as a purine analogue into the DNA of dividing cells, causing DNA damage and therefore having mutagenic activity.

The most recent drug to be approved for clinical use is sirolimus (rapamycin) [47]. This agent inhibits the activating signals into lymphocytes delivered by the IL-2 receptor. Its action is still being elucidated, but it is known to interfere with progression of lymphocytes through the cell cycle in response to IL-2. Thus it is an antiproliferative agent that works by interfering with the IL-2 pathway of lymphocyte activation. It can be seen that immunosuppressive drugs act on different pathways of the immune activation cascade (Figure 17.5). It is disappointing that, once effector mechanisms come into play, we know of no drugs that inhibit their actions.

Induction of graft acceptance and tolerance

The use of immunosuppressive agents is fraught with potential side effects, and it would be better to manage the patients without them. How, though, might this be achieved? In animals, particularly in rodents, it is quite easy to induce long-term graft acceptance by some manipulation either before or after transplantation. (Note that-long term graft

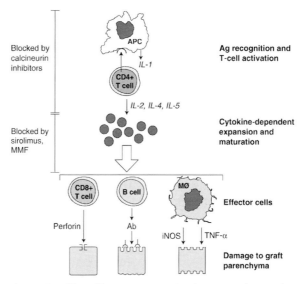

Figure 17.5 Effect of immunosuppressive drugs on pathways of immune activation. The diagram shows that early T-cell activation, resulting in IL-2 production, is inhibited by the calcineurin inhibitors. Calcineurin inhibitors have no effect on cytokine-dependent T-cell proliferation and maturation, but this stage is blocked by sirolimus and mycophenolate (MMF). None of the existing drugs inhibits damage mediated directly by effector cells. Ab, antibody; Ag, antigen; for other abbreviations see Figure 17.4.

survival in this context means 100 days, hardly an acceptable clinical definition.) There are some human transplant recipients who have stopped taking their immunosuppression for one reason or another, or who are on very low maintenance doses of drugs. Given that graft acceptance and, perhaps, immunological tolerance of the graft is possible, the mechanisms thought to underlie this acceptance have been studied extensively. Obviously the aim is to understand these mechanisms so that we can deliberately induce unresponsiveness to the graft. Some think that we know enough already and ought to be applying this knowledge now. In fact there is a huge programme in the USA, the Immune Tolerance Network, funded by the US government, with the stated aim of inducing transplantation tolerance in patients.

Manipulation of the graft

In the first place one could think about manipulating the graft. At least it is accessible at the time of transplantation. There are several things that could be done. The first and so far unsuccessful approach would be to deplete the graft of passenger leukocytes, either by perfusion of antibodies [28] or storage in a way that does not favour leukocyte survival [70]. Instead of antibodies, the graft might be perfused with cytokines to change the characteristics of the dendritic cells into those necessary for the induction of tolerance.

Grafts from donors that have been stressed (and have increased expression of heat shock proteins in the tissues) appear to survive relatively well as compared with unstressed tissues [71,72]. Xenografts placed into animals depleted of natural antibodies are not rejected when the antibody levels return, because of a process called graft accommodation [73]. We do not know the mechanism of graft protection, but one idea is that 'protective genes' are activated [74–76]. This may be related to the stress response. A better understanding of graft accommodation may enable this state to be induced in both allografts and xenografts at the time of transplantation.

Finally, because the graft is accessible it can be transfected before transplantation with various genes that may influence the immune response. Attempts have been made to transfer the genes for regulatory cytokines and other molecules such as CTLA4-Ig, in the hope that local production of these cytokines will protect the graft [77,78].

Manipulation of the recipient

The recipient, rather than the graft, may be manipulated by treatment with antigens, antibodies or drugs. The aim is to induce a state of immunological unresponsiveness against donor tissue. It is now clear that such unresponsiveness is largely due to active immune responses against donor antigens but, instead of damaging the graft, they modify or suppress the rejection responses. Indeed, there is one school of thought that clinical transplant recipients do not usually become tolerant of their transplants, an outcome readily achieved in many animal models, because the clinically used immunosuppressive agents interfere with the immune responses of graft acceptance.

Bearing in mind that specific unresponsiveness implies that only the T cells able to recognize the graft are affected, the mechanisms of graft acceptance could be deletion, anergy or suppression of donor-specific T cells.

Deletion of self-reactive T cells occurs during the natural maturation of T-cell precursors in the thymus. Any self-reactive T cells escaping that process are inactivated in the periphery, after they have left the thymus, hence the terms thymic and peripheral tolerance. One approach to tolerance induction is to introduce donor antigen into the thymus to delete the donor-reactive T cells as they are undergoing maturation. Direct injection of donor antigen into the thymus has been shown to induce graft acceptance [79], especially when this protocol is combined with a treatment to reduce the number of mature T cells in the circulation [80]. This is likely to be the mechanism of neonatal

tolerance in rats and mice, too. Rodents are born before there is any escape of T cells from the thymus into the periphery. Injection of donor bone marrow in the neonatal period introduces antigen into the thymus that deletes donor-reactive T cells and skin grafts are accepted [81]. If the bone marrow injection is delayed until seeding from the thymus occurs then skin graft tolerance is not induced. However, other nondeletional mechanisms may play a role [82] and such treatment may suppress acute rejection without affecting chronic rejection [83].

Acceptance of organ transplants can be induced in adult rodents by antigen pretreatment. An intravenous injection of donor cells a minimum of five to seven days before kidney or heart transplantation induces long-term (100 days) graft acceptance [84,85]. The requirement for pretreatment is to allow time for the active development of unresponsiveness, as discussed above, and graft acceptance can be undermined by drug treatment with, for example, steroids [86]. The same effect has been observed clinically. Individuals who have had many blood transfusions from random donors (to expose them by chance to the antigens of their organ donor), or fewer transfusions from their prospective donor, are less likely to reject their grafts [87,88]. This is known as the blood transfusion effect, and is quite paradoxical because one might have anticipated that prior antigen exposure would sensitize rather than suppress [87,89]. In fact, in rodent models, while intravenous antigen prolongs graft survival, subcutaneous antigen accelerates rejection. Thus the route of immunization, directing antigen to the APCs (macrophages) of the liver and the spleen, is important for the induction of unresponsiveness. In contrast, antigen injected into a subcutaneous site drains to the local lymph node, where the major APC is the dendritic cell, which, as outlined before, is very good at activating rejection responses. To maximize the uptake of donor antigen by the APCs in the liver, antigen can be introduced by the portal vein (or the dorsal penile vein that drains into the portal system), and this route is especially efficient in inducing unresponsiveness [90].

The whole business of arranging pretreatment with donor antigens is fraught with difficulties, even in renal transplantation, and is impracticable for cardiothoracic transplantation. However, the graft itself can be seen as a source of donor antigen capable of inducing graft acceptance. In animal models of organ transplantation, a short course (7–10 days postoperatively) of ciclosporin or tacrolimus induces long-term unresponsiveness. This probably works by delaying the activation of the graft rejection response without inhibiting the mechanisms of unresponsiveness. For example, we know that IL-2 is important in the activation of graft-damaging cells. IL-2 deprivation of T cells during the activation process causes them to undergo apoptosis or to become anergic [91], not dying but unable to respond to antigen. Antibodies to the IL-2 receptor, CD25 [45], and the new agent, sirolimus, that inhibits signalling through the IL-2 receptor [46,47] should work in this manner, too, and in fact all of the early protocols proposed to induce clinical transplantation tolerance under the auspices of the Immune Tolerance Network were based on the administration of sirolimus. However, we must be clear that the administration of other drugs may inhibit tolerance induction, although it will take some courage initially to abandon some of the mainstays of clinical immunosuppression!

Other approaches have been tried, for example blocking the interaction between APCs and T cells during the initial stages of activation. As told above, T cells require both antigen and costimulation to become activated. Without costimulation the T cells undergo apoptosis or become anergic [92–94]. The use of agents such as antibodies to CD40 or to CTLA4-Ig that block the interactions between CD40 and CD40L or between B7 (CD80 and CD86) and CD29, respectively (see above), has been shown to inhibit graft rejection in rodents [20,95–99] and monkeys [100,101]. Alas, the early clinical trials have run into some unforeseen problems.

One common feature of all these treatments is that the frequency of donor-reactive T cells in the recipient is diminished and cells capable of suppressing the activation of the rejection responses appear [102,103]. We used to call the latter cells 'suppressor T cells' but this term fell out of vogue and they are now called 'regulatory T cells'. Recent evidence suggests that anergic cells have the properties of regulatory cells [104], so that agents suppressing the IL-2 pathway or costimulation favour the induction of unresponsiveness [95,105,106]. The regulatory cells probably act on the APCs, bathing them in cytokines such as transforming growth factor beta (TGF–β) and incapacitating them in terms of their ability to activate rejection and changing them so that they activate only more regulatory cells, an effect called infectious tolerance [107,108]. This leads to an accumulation of regulatory cells and increasingly solid acceptance of the graft.

The recognition that dendritic cells can be divided into two functional subsets [109], one of which activates the cells involved in rejection while the other activates the cells involved in graft acceptance, has led to attempts to manipulate dendritic cell maturation [110]. For example, dendritic cells exposed to TGF-β activate regulatory cells (note that the production of TGF-β regulatory cells could explain infectious tolerance [111,112] and favour the induction of graft acceptance). The transfer of genes into dendritic cells

to alter their function is under investigation in several laboratories [113].

Chronic rejection

Introduction

Currently used immunosuppressive drugs prevent or limit parenchymal damage caused by infiltrating mononuclear cells in the first few months after transplantation. However, as time progresses, grafts become damaged by an insidious process resulting in obliteration of the main conduits of the graft. In the cases of heart transplantation this presents as a gradual occlusion of the coronary arteries and small blood vessels of graft origin, called transplant-associated coronary artery disease (TxCAD) or graft vasculopathy. Following lung transplantation, the main pathology is occlusion of the small and large airways by proliferating myofibroblasts and deposition of collagen and extracellular matrix. This is known as obliterative bronchiolitis or bronchiolitis obliterans syndrome (BOS) (for clinical features and histopathology, see Chapters 19 and 23).

Immunologists have to explain such disease progression in the face of strong immunosuppressive agents that strongly inhibit a type 1 response. First, it is clear that chronic rejection has antigen-dependent and antigen-independent components. The endothelial response to injury hypothesis, proposed by Ross in 1993 to explain nontransplant atherosclerosis [114] is equally applicable to transplant atherosclerosis (TxCAD) and indeed BOS. Ross proposed that an initial insult results in endothelial cell activation and upregulation of cytokines, chemokines and adhesion molecules. This leads to transendothelial migration of monocytes, which may be further modified in the vessel wall by modified low density lipoprotein (LDL), where they subsequently release cytokines and growth factors, leading to smooth muscle cell proliferation and migration.

In the case of lung transplantation, we would propose that an initial insult leads to damaged epithelial cells resulting in upregulation of cytokines, chemokines and adhesion molecules. Damaged lungs contain many neutrophils as well as macrophages and T cells [115]. Indeed, one can consider three phases of the disease process (Figure 17.6), the first being an antigen-independent phase consisting primarily of damage by neutrophils and free radicals [116]. This is followed by an alloimmune phase with lymphocytic infiltration of bronchiolar structures, then finally a chronic fibroproliferative phase leading to partial or total occlusion of the airway lumen.

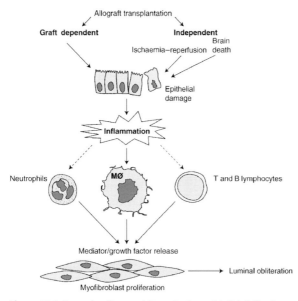

Figure 17.6 Stages leading to obliterative bronchiolitis following lung transplantation. The diagram illustrates three stages of damage following lung transplantation. First, there is antigen-independent damage to epithelial cells accompanied by neutrophil infiltration; second, there is an antigen-dependent infiltration of effector lymphocytes; and finally a chronic fibroproliferative phase leading to obliteration of the airways. Mϕ, macrophage. (Reprinted with permission from ref. 159.)

The alloimmune response in chronic rejection

Role of CD4+ T cells

CD4+ T cells have been widely implicated in experimental parenchymal and vascular rejection episodes. As in acute rejection, they can contribute to chronic rejection in three ways: (1) by provision of signals that promote the generation of CD8+ CTLs, (2) by provision of signals that promote differentiation and activation of alloantibody-producing B cells; and (3) by activating antigen-independent effector leukocytes, which damage the tissue. The best known of these effector leukocytes are activated macrophages, which damage tissue through release of mediators such as reactive oxygen intermediates, nitric oxide and degradative enzymes. In addition, cytokines released by macrophages (e.g. TNF-α) or T cells (IFN-γ) can be directly damaging to graft parenchymal cells [117,118]. IFN-γ is of particular interest as an effector mechanism of chronic rejection. Injection of human IFN-γ into severe combined immunodeficiency (SCID) mice bearing human aortic grafts caused proliferation of aortic smooth muscle cells and vessel remodelling [118].

It has to be remembered that in a nontransplant setting, these host responses serve a protective function by eradicating foreign microbes. When the same effector mechanism is activated by an effector mechanism that is not associated with a pathogenic microbe, the resultant tissue injury is known as delayed-type hypersensitivity (DTH) [119]. Acute DTH has been invoked as a possible effector mechanism in acute allograft rejection. When the antigen that evokes DTH is not eliminated one can hypothesize that the CD4+ T cells and macrophages remain persistently activated and release cytokines and growth factors that act on mesenchymal cells to promote stromal cell growth and fibrosis. It is likely therefore that chronic DTH is one of the contributing factors to chronic rejection.

Pathways of antigen presentation

The term 'antigen presenting cell' has a specific meaning; it means a cell that is able to present antigen and cause activation of resting T cells (see above for various molecules that are required for T-cell activation). Only specialized cells can cause activation of resting T cells (e.g. dendritic cells). In a nontransplant setting, T cells recognize nominal antigen in the context of self MHC. An important step in the understanding of alloreactivity came with the discovery that T cells can engage and respond to allogeneic molecules directly (Figure 17.3) [37]. This form of antigen recognition known as the direct pathway is responsible for the strong proliferative response of alloreactive CD4+ T cells seen in vitro (the mixed lymphocyte response) and quite possibly for the vigorous acute rejection seen in certain experimental strain combinations. However, it is now known that T cells can also recognize allogeneic peptides that have been processed and presented within self MHC molecules by host APCs in the same manner that T cells recognize nominal antigen (Figure 17.3). It is likely that the earliest antigraft response involves direct activation of memory CD4+ T cells by MHC class II-expressing endothelial cells [120] and donor-derived passenger leukocytes present within the graft. At later times after transplantation, naive CD4+ T cells become activated, but the activation requirements of naive T cells differ from those of memory T cells. Naive T cells can be activated either directly by donor-derived dendritic cells in the graft or indirectly by host-derived dendritic cells presenting donor-derived alloantigens. However, naive T cells can be activated only by dendritic cells in the microenvironment of secondary lymphoid tissue [121], and for this to take place alloantigens from the graft have to travel to draining lymph nodes.

There is much experimental and clinical support for the hypothesis that chronic rejection is driven by indirect presentation. We must therefore assume that, as time progresses, donor-derived parenchymal cells shed antigens that are captured by dendritic cells in secondary lymphoid tissues. Thus studies of kidney [122] and heart transplant recipients have shown that T cells from long-term patients are hyporesponsive to donor HLA presented directly, even though the patients may have chronic rejection [123]. In contrast, a study of seven cardiac transplant patients with chronic rejection showed that five of them were hyperresponsive to donor antigens presented via the indirect pathway; none of the four patients without chronic rejection were hyperresponsive to indirectly presented donor antigens [124]. There have been two small studies of lung transplant patients to date [125,126]. The studies investigated frequency of CD4+ T cells to indirectly presented peptides from the hypervariable region of mismatched MHC class I [125] or class II antigens [126]. The results showed a significantly higher precursor frequency in BOS recipients (3–24-fold higher) than recipients without BOS.

Our own studies have assessed frequency of CD4+ T cells to indirectly presented donor or third party antigen using freeze–thawed splenocytes as the source of antigen and IL-2 production as the read out (R. Stanford and M.L. Rose, unpublished data). We can confirm that in patients with BOS the frequency of T cells recognizing donor antigens via the indirect pathway was significantly higher than T cells recognizing third party antigen. This was not the case for patients without BOS (Figure 17.7).

However, one of the most interesting aspects of our study was to compare T-cell frequencies between lung and heart transplant patients. Using both historical controls [123] and controls done at the same time, the frequency of donor

reactive CD4+ T cells (in the indirect pathway) was 10 times higher in the lung than in the heart patients. Thus, after cardiac transplantation, the indirect frequency, even in patients with chronic rejection, is quite low at 1 in 100 000. In contrast, we can detect frequencies of 1 in 10 000 in patients after lung transplantation. Whether this reflects the sheer volume of tissue transplanted, lymphoid tissues in the transplanted lung, more MHC class II presenting cells in lungs than heart, or better lymphatic drainage and subsequent drainage of antigens to recipient secondary lymphoid tissues is unknown. It would seem that the immunological stimulus is greater from lungs than from heart.

Role of CD8+ T cells

The measurement of T-cell responses described above relates to CD4+ T-cell responses. Activation of CD4+ T cells leads to maturation of other effector mechanisms of immune damage (see section above) including maturation of antigen-specific cytotoxic CD8+ T cells. One would therefore predict that if frequencies of CD4+ Th cells were reduced during chronic rejection, this would also apply to frequencies of cytotoxic T cells as well. This is certainly the case after heart and kidney transplantation, where long-term patients become hyporesponsive for direct recognition of target cells by cytotoxic CD8+ lymphocytes [123]. This would confirm that patients become tolerant or anergic in the direct pathway but that the indirect pathway of antigen recognition is not inhibited by long-term immunosuppressive agents. No one has yet investigated whether the direct pathway of antigen recognition is rendered hyporesponsive after lung transplantation; this could be done measuring the extent of donor specific CD4+ Th responses as compared to third party. Alternatively cytotoxic CD8+ T cell responses could be measured. In view of the heightened indirect response in lung transplant patients mentioned above, it would be unjustifiable to assume that lung recipients become hyporesponsive in the direct pathway, as do recipients of heart and kidneys allografts.

There may be an argument for tissue-specific damage mediated by cytotoxic T cells following lung transplantation. A study of mucosal epithelia including those of the gut and lungs has identified the presence of a characteristic population of CD8+ T cells that express the adhesion molecule $\alpha_E\beta_7$ – only 2% of peripheral lymphocytes express this integrin. The integrin is identified by monoclonal antibodies to the CD103 antigen present on the α_E subunit. Significantly, the only known molecule to which the $\alpha_E\beta_7$ integrin binds with high affinity is E-cadherin, a molecule constitutively expressed by most epithelial cells [127,128]. Recently, it has been shown that CD103+ CD8+ T cells accumulate within the tubular epithelial layer of renal

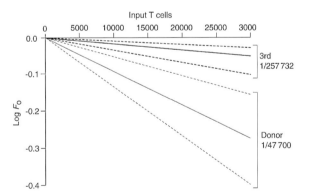

Figure 17.7 Bronchiolitis obliterans syndrome (BOS) is characterized by recognition of donor antigens presented via the indirect pathway of allorecognition. This figure shows the frequencey (F_0) of CD4+ T cells that recognize donor or third party alloantigens in patients with BOS. The steeper the curve, the higher the frequency of T cells recognizing the stimulator population. The frequency of cells to donor antigen (1/47 000) was significantly higher than the frequency of cells recognizing unrelated third party antigens (1/257 732).

biopsies showing acute rejection [129]. The same authors have suggested that TGF-β_1, expressed in renal tubules during acute rejection, promotes differentiation of local infiltrating CD8+ T cells to become CD103 positive.

The precise functional significance of interaction between E-cadherin and $\alpha_E\beta_7$-positive T cells is unclear. However, it is known that cytotoxic T cells can modulate the physiological function of intra-TEC (tubular epithelial cells) tight junctions [130] and that blockade of the $\alpha_E\beta_7$ integrin can prevent cell-mediated lysis of E-cadherin-expressing target cells in vitro [131]. This raises the possibility of tissue-specific T-cell damage to epithelial cells, which may well to apply epithelial cells lining the bronchi. It is well established that donor epithelial cells are destroyed early on after experimental tracheal transplantation and become replaced by recipient cells [132]. Adams et al. have demonstrated the importance of the epithelium in the development of BOS [133]. Using a rat tracheal syngeneic graft transplanted into the omentum, they removed the epithelium by protease digestion before grafting. The syngeneic grafts developed luminal occlusion, an effect that was inhibited by reseeding with epithelial cells. The same group has also compared different immunosuppressive drugs on BOS development and shown a direct relationship between drugs that preserve epithelial cell integrity and those that prevent airway obliteration [134]. This group has suggested that an intact epithelium somehow discourages or inhibits mesenchymal proliferation. How epithelial cells exert such an inhibitory effect is not known.

Role of antibody

There are many clinical and experimental studies showing an association between chronic production of antibody and development of chronic rejection or transplant vasculopathy following cardiac transplantation [135]. It has to be remembered that the calcineurin inhibitors (ciclosporin and tacrolimus), are able to inhibit T cell-dependent antibody responses but will have no effect on a secondary immune response involving production of antibody. After cardiac transplantation chronic production of antibodies to HLA class I antigens is associated with transplant vasculopathy [136,137]. Similarly, after lung transplantation, a multivariate analysis of risk factors associated with BOS has shown HLA mismatches at the class I locus (in this case, the HLA-A locus) and antibodies to HLA-A antigens were significantly independent predictors of development of disease [138].

Antibodies to MHC class I antigens probably contribute to chronic rejection by their ability to cause activation of parenchymal cells within the graft. Thus it has been shown that monoclonal and anti-HLA class I antibodies derived from patients cause activation of nuclear factor kappa B (NF-κB) in human macrovascular and microvascular endothelial cells [139]. In addition, ligation of MHC class I antigens causes human endothelial cells to express fibroblast growth factor receptors and to proliferate in vitro [140]. Similarly, ligation of MHC class I antigens on smooth muscle cells induces tyrosine phosphorylation, fibroblast growth factor production and cell proliferation [141]. Of direct relevance to lung transplantation, activation of an airway epithelial cell line with anti-MHC class I antibodies results in production of fibrogenic factors, allowing proliferation of adjacent fibroblasts [142]. It is likely, therefore, that chronic production of antibodies exacerbates the fibroproliferative lesions of BOS.

The role of complement activation in the development of BOS has been investigated in the rat by Kallio et al. [143]. They demonstrated an increase within the graft of complement components C3 and C5b–9, the membrane attack complex, and also increases in immunoglobulin (Ig)M and IgG during the loss of epithelium and the development of airway occlusion in the allografts. Whether complement activation is also involved in the signal transduction events described above is not known. It is also known that patients who have IgG antibodies to MHC class I antigens of donor origin prior to their transplant lose their lung allografts within six weeks of transplantation [144], again demonstrating the deleterious effect of anti-class I antibodies on lung function.

Breakdown of tolerance to self antigens

The currently accepted paradigm of chronic rejection is that it is driven by indirect recognition of HLA antigens released from the graft and processed by recipient dendritic cells in secondary lymphoid tissues. A variety of antigens are involved in this process and the phenomenon of epitope spreading has been described after transplantation (145) as in autoimmune disease. That antigens are constantly being released from the graft, and the antigen (i.e. the graft) is never cleared, contributes to the chronic immune response.

It is now clear that patients make antibodies to non-HLA antibodies after transplantation. Thus we have found that production of antibodies to the intermediate filament protein vimentin is a significant independent risk factor for the development of graft vasculopathy following cardiac transplantation [146]. Such antibodies react with both donor and recipient vimentin, and are therefore autoantibodies. Other autoantibodies have been described after solid organ transplantation; heart transplant recipients make antimyosin [147] and antiphospholipid antibodies [148], and antibodies and T-cell responses to epithelial cells have been described in renal transplant patients [149]. Endothelial cell antibodies have also been described after cardiac and renal transplantation [150–153].

It is likely that such antibodies are produced in an organ-specific manner, as a response to autoantigens being exposed or released from the damaged graft. Thus we would predict that antimyosin antibodies would not be found after renal or lung transplantation. Relatively few studies have investigated whether autoantibodies are made after lung transplantation. Our own studies showed that some lung patients had cytotoxic antibodies to an epithelial cell line (A549) prior to transplantation, and such patients had a significantly worse graft survival at one year (78% for antiepithelial cell antibody (AECA) negative compared to 56% for AECA positive, $p = 0.01$) (154). This study suggested that an organ- or cell-specific response contributes to rejection, but it did not investigate de novo antibody formation after transplantation. De novo production of antibodies to non-HLA antigens in 30% of patients with BOS has recently been described [155]. In some cases these antibodies bound to a 60 kDa antigen on epithelial cells, causing cell activation (142).

Recently, collagen V has been detected in bronchiole alveolar lavage specimens of lung transplant patients, and a small number of these patients were shown to have a DTH response against collagen V (156). The same group demonstrated that feeding collagen V to rats (inducing oral tolerance) downregulated the cellular response to lung allografts (157). Collagen V is a major component of the extracellular matrix in fibrotic lungs and the above results suggest that it is a candidate autoantigen in the pathogenesis of BOS.

It has recently been demonstrated in experimental models that allotransplantation breaks tolerance to self antigens [158]. Thus, after cardiac allotransplantation in mice, de novo T- and B-cell responses to cardiac myosin were elicited, but this response was not elicited after syngeneic heart transplantation. The same peptide of cardiac myosin that causes autoimmune myocarditis in mice was found to be the target of the autoimmune response following cardiac transplantation. The question arises whether such autoantibody responses are damaging. It was shown that preimmunization of mice with cardiac myosin caused accelerated rejection of allogeneic hearts and also caused rejection of syngeneic hearts, demonstrating the relevance of the autoimmune response to graft rejection.

Acknowledgement

The authors thank the British Heart Foundation for continued support.

REFERENCES

1 Hutchinson IV. Cardiac allograft vasculopathy – the cellular attack. *Cardiology* 2000; **89**: 16–20.
2 Kissmeyer-Nielson F, Olsen S, Petersen VP, Fjeldborg O. Hyperacute rejection of kidney allografts associated with pre-existing humoral antibodies against donor cells. *Lancet* 1966; **2**: 662–665.
3 Williams G, Hulme D, Hudson R, Morris P, Kano K, Milgrom F. Hyperacute renal homograft rejection in man. *New Engl J Med* 1968; **279**: 611–618.
4 West L, Pollock-Barziv SM, Dipchand AI, et al. ABO-incompatible heart transplantation in infants. *N Engl J Med* 2001; **344**: 793–800.
5 Oriole R, Ye Y, Koren E, Cooper DKC. Carbohydrate antigens of pig tissues reacting with human natural antibodies as potential targets for hyperacute rejection in pig-to-man organ xenotransplantation. *Transplantation* 1993; **56**: 1433–1442.
6 Oriole R, Barthod F, Berenger A-M, Ye Y, Koren E, Cooper DKC. Monomorphic and polymorphic carbohydrate antigens on pig tissues: implications for organ xenotransplantation in the pig-to-human model. *Transplant Int* 1994; **7**: 405–413.
7 Besse T, Duck L, Latinne D et al. Effect of plasmapheresis and splenectomy on parameters involved in vascular rejection of discordant xenografts in the swine to baboon model. *Transplant Proc* 1994; **26**: 1042–1044.
8 Leventhal JR, Dalmasso AP, Cromwell JW et al. Prolongation of cardiac allograft survival by depletion of complement. *Transplantation* 1993; **55**: 857–866.
9 Leventhal JR, Dalmasso AP, Cromwell JW, Manivel CJ, Bolman RM, Matas AJ. Complement depletion prolongs discordant cardiac xenograft survival in rodents and in non-human primates. *Transplant Proc* 1993; **25**: 398–399.
10 Leventhal JR, Sakiyalak P, Witson J et al. The synergistic effect of combined antibody and complement depletion on discordant cardiac xenograft survival in non-human primates. *Transplantation* 1994; **57**: 974–978.
11 Tearle RG, Tange MJ, Zannettino ZL et al. The α 1,3-galactosyl transferase knockout mouse: implications for xenotransplantation. *Transplantation* 1996; **61**: 13–19.
12 Bhatti FN, Schmoeckel M, Zaidi A, et al. Three month survival of hDAF transgenic pig hearts transplanted into primates. *Transplant Proc* 1999; **31**: 958.
13 Schmoeckel M, Bhatti FN, Zaidi A, et al. Splenectomy improves survival of hDAF transgenic pig kidneys in primates. *Transplant Proc* 1999; **31**: 961.

14 Loss M, Prezemeck M, Schidtko J, et al. Long-term survival of cyanomologous monkeys following pig-to-primate kidney xenotransplantation using hDAF transgenic donor organs. *Transplant Proc* 2000; **32**: 1095–1096.

15 D'Apice AJ, Pearse MJ. Xenotransplantation. In: Tilney NL, Strom TB, Paul LC, eds. *Transplantation biology*. Lippincott-Raven Publishers, Philadelphia, 1996: 701–716.

16 Matzinger P, Bevan M. Why do so many lymphocytes respond to major histocompatibility complex antigens? *Cell Immunol* 1997; **29**: 1–5.

17 Benoist C, Mathis D. Positive selection of the T cell repertoire: where and when does it occur? *Cell* 1989; **58**: 1027–1033.

18 Benichou G, Fedoseyeva EV. The contribution of peptide to T cell allorecognition and allograft rejection. *Int Rev Immunol* 1996; **13**: 231–243.

19 Sprent J. Antigen-presenting cells. Professionals and amateurs. *Curr Biol* 1995; **5**: 1095–1097.

20 Sayegh MH, Turka LA. The role of T cell costimulatory activation in transplant rejection. *N Engl J Med* 1998; **338**: 1813–1821.

21 Chai J-G, Vendetti S, Bartok I et al. Critical role of costimulation in the activation of naïve antigen-specific TCR-transgenic CD8⁺ T cells in vitro. *J Immunol* 1999; **165**: 1298–1305.

22 Lenschow DJ, Walunas TL, Bluestone JA. CD28/B7 system of T cell costimulation. *Ann Rev Immunol* 1996; **14**: 233–258.

23 Yamada A, Sayegh MH. The CD154–CD40 costimulatory pathway in transplantation. *Transplantation* 2002; **73** (S1): S36–S39.

24 Lechler RL, Batchelor JR. Restoration of immunogenicity to passenger cell depleted kidney allografts by the addition of donor strain dendritic cells. *J Exp Med* 1982; **155**: 31–41.

25 Krasinkas AM, Eiref SD, McLean AD, et al. Replacement of graft-resident donor-type antigen presenting cells alters the tempo and pathogenesis of murine cardiac allograft rejection. *Transplantation* 2000; **70**: 514–521.

26 McKenzie JL, Beard ME, Hart DN. The effect of donor pretreatment on interstitial dendritic cell content and rat cardiac allograft survival. *Transplantation* 1984; **38**: 371–376.

27 Prop J, Nieuwenhuis P, Wildevuur CR. Lung allograft rejection in the rat. I. Accelerated rejection caused by graft lymphocytes. *Transplantation* 1985; **40**: 25–30.

28 Goldberg LC. Pretreatment of kidney allografts with monoclonal antibodies to CD45: results of a multicentre study. CD45 Study Group. *Transplant Int* 1994; **7** (S1): S252–S254.

29 Lechler RI, Lombardi G, Batchelor JR, et al. The molecular basis of allorecognition. *Immunol Today* 1990; **11**: 83–88.

30 Sherman LA, Chattopadhyay S. The molecular basis of allorecognition. *Ann Rev Immunol* 1993; **11**: 385–402.

31 Auchincloss H, Sultan H. Antigen processing and presentation in transplantation. *Curr Opin Immunol* 1996; **8**: 681–687.

32 Goulmy E. Minor histocompatibility antigens: from T cell recognition to peptide identification. *Hum Immunol* 1997; **54**: 8–14.

33 Simpson E, Roopenian D, Goulmy E. Much ado about minor histocompatibility antigens. *Immunol Today* 1998; **19**: 108–112.

34 Shoskes DA, Wood KJ. Indirect presentation of MHC antigens in transplantation. *Immunol Today* 1994; **15**: 32–38.

35 Benham AM, Sawyer GJ, Fabre JW. Indirect T cell recognition of donor antigens contributes to the rejection of vascularized kidney allografts. *Transplantation* 1995; **59**: 1028–1032.

36 Sayegh MH, Carpenter CB. Role of indirect allorecognition in allograft rejection. *Int Rev Immunol* 1996; **13**: 221–229.

37 Hornick P, Lechler RI. Direct and indirect pathways of allorecognition: relevance to acute and chronic allograft rejection. *Nephrol Dial Transplant* 1997; **12**: 1806–1810.

38 Hall BM, Dorsch S, Roser B. The cellular basis of allograft rejection in vivo. I. The cellular requirements for first-set rejection of heart grafts. *J Exp Med* 1978; **148**: 878–889.

39 Ascher NL, Hoffmann RA, Hanto DW, Simmons RL. Cellular basis of allograft rejection. *Immunol Rev* 1984; **77**: 217–232.

40 Hutchinson IV. Cellular mechanisms of allograft rejection. *Curr Opin Immunol* 1991; **3**: 722–728.

41 Strom TB, Roy-Chaudhury P, Manfro R, et al. The Th1/Th2 paradigm and the allograft response. *Curr Opinion Immunol* 1996; **8**: 688–693.

42 Rosenberg AS, Mizuochi T, Sharrow SO, Singer A. Phenotype, specificity and function of T cell subsets and T cell interactions involved in skin graft rejection. *J Exp Med* 1987; **165**: 1296–1315.

43 Borel JF, Feurer C, Gubler HU, Stahelin H. Biological effects of cyclosporin A: a new immunosuppressive agent. *Agent Actions* 1976; **6**: 468–475.

44 Goto T. Discovery, immunopharmacology and rationale for the development of tacrolimus: a novel immunosuppressant of microbial origin. In: Lieberman R, Mukherjee A, eds. *Principles of drug development in transplantation and autoimmunity*. RG Landes Company, Austin, TX, 1996: 159–163.

45 Pascual J, Marcen R, Ortuno J. Anti-interleukin-2 receptor antibodies: basiliximab and dacluzimab. *Nephrol Dial Transplant* 2001; **16**: 1756–1760.

46 Dumont FJ, Staruch MJ, Koprak SL, Melino MM, Sigal NH. Distinct mechanisms of suppression of murine T cell activation by the related macrolides FK-506 and rapamycin. *J Immunol* 1990; **144**: 251–258.

47 Seghal SN. Immunosuppressive profile of rapamycin. *Ann NY Acad Sci* 1993; **696**: 1–8.

48 Snider ME, Armstrong L, Hudson JL, Steinmuller D. In vitro and in vivo cytotoxicity of T cells cloned from rejecting allografts. *Transplantation* 1986; **42**: 171–177.

49 Steinmuller D, Tyler JD, Snider ME, et al. Tissue destruction resulting from the interaction of cytotoxic T cells and their targets. *Ann NY Acad Sci* 1988; **532**: 106–118.

50 Bolton EM, Gracie JA, Briggs JD, Kampinga J, Bradley JA. Cellular requirements for renal allograft rejection in the athymic nude rat. *J Exp Med* 1989; **169**: 1931–1946.

51 Bradley JA, Sarawar SR, Porteous C, et al. Allograft rejection in CD4+ T cell-reconstituted athymic nude rats – the

non-essential role of host derived CD8+ T cells. *Transplantation* 1992; **53**: 477–482.

52 Hall BM. Cells mediating allograft rejection. *Transplantation* 1991; **52**: 936–946.

53 Dennert G. Molecular mechanism of target lysis by cytotoxic T cells. *Int Rev Immunol* 1997; **14**: 133–152.

54 Shresta S, Pham CT, Thomas DA, Graubert TA, Ley TJ. How do cytotoxic lymphocytes kill their targets? *Curr Opin Immunol* 1998; **10**: 581–587.

55 Vasconcellos LM, Schachter AD, Zheng XX, et al. Cytotoxic lymphocyte gene expression in peripheral blood leukocytes correlates with rejecting renal allografts. *Transplantation* 1998; **66**: 562–566.

56 Shulzhenko N, Morgun A, Zheng XX, et al. Intragraft activation of genes encoding cytotoxic T lymphocyte effector molecules precedes the histological evidence of rejection in human cardiac transplantation. *Transplantation* 2001; **72**: 1705–1708.

57 Brandle D, Joergensen J, Zenke G, Burki K, Hof RP. Contribution of donor specific antibodies to acute allograft rejection: evidence from B cell deficient mice. *Transplantation* 1998; **65**: 1489–1493.

58 Morton AL, Bell EB, Bolton EM, et al. CD4+ T cell-mediated rejection of major histocompatibility complex class I-disparate grafts: a role for antibody. *Eur J Immunol* 1993; **23**: 2078–2084.

59 VanBuskirk AM, Wakely ME, Orosz CG. Transfusion of polarised Th2-like cell populations into SCID mouse cardiac allograft recipients results in acute allograft rejection. *Transplantation* 1996; **62**: 229–238.

60 Carpenter CB, d'Apice AJF, Abbas AK. The role of antibodies in rejection and enhancement of organ allografts. *Adv Immunol* 1976; **22**: 1–65.

61 French ME, Batchelor JR. Enhancement of renal allografts in rats and man. *Transplant Rev* 1972; **13**: 115–141.

62 Morris PJ, Ting A. HLA-DR and renal transplantation. *Contemp Top Mol Immunol* 1983; **9**: 65–88.

63 Sheldon S, Hasleton PS, Yonan N, et al. Rejection in heart transplantation strongly correlates with HLA-DR antigen mismatch. *Transplantation* 1994; **58**: 719–722.

64 Smith JD, Rose ML, Pomerance A, Burke M, Yacoub MH. Reduction of cellular rejection and increase in longer term survival after heart transplantation after HLA-DR matching. *Lancet* 1995; **346**: 1318–1322.

65 Cohen DJ, Loertscher R, Rubin MF, Tilney NL, Carpenter CB, Strom TB. Cyclosporine: a new immunosuppressive agent for organ transplantation. *Ann Intern Med* 1984; **101**: 667–682.

66 Peters DH, Fitton A, Plosker GL, Faulds D. Tacrolimus: a review of its pharmacology and therapeutic potential in hepatic and renal transplantation. *Drugs* 1993; **46**: 746–794.

67 Calne RY, Rolles K, White DJG, et al. Cyclosporin A initially as the only immunosuppressant in 34 recipients of cadaveric organs: 32 kidneys, 2 pancreases and 2 livers. *Lancet* 1979; **2**: 1033–1010.

68 Cosimi AB, Burton RC, Colvin RB, et al. Treatment of acute rejection with OKT3 monoclonal antibody. *Transplantation* 1981; **32**: 535–539.

69 Allison AC, Kowalski W, Muller CD, Eugui EM. Mechanisms of action of mycophenolic acid. *Ann NY Acad Sci* 1993; **696**: 63–87.

70 Taylor MJ, Bank HL, Benton MJ. Selective killing of leucocytes by freezing: potential for reducing the immunogenicity of pancreatic islets. *Diabetes Res* 1987; **5**: 99–103.

71 Hiratsuka M, Yano M, Mora BN, Nagahiro I, Cooper JD, Patterson GA. Heat shock pretreatment protects pulmonary isografts from subsequent ischaemia–reperfusion injury. *J Heart Lung Transplant* 1998; **17**: 1238–1246.

72 Matsumoto K, Honda K, Kobayashi N. Protective effect of heat preconditioning of rat liver grafts resulting in improved transplant survival. *Transplantation* 2001; **15**: 862–868.

73 Bach FH, Turman MA, Vercellotti GM, Platt JL, Dalmasso AP. Accommodation: a working paradigm for progressing toward clinical discordant xenografting. *Transplant Proc* 1991; **23**: 205–207.

74 Bach FH, Ferran C, Candinas D, et al. Accommodation of xenografts: expression of 'protective genes' in endothelial and smooth muscle cells. *Transplant Proc* 1997; **29**: 56–58.

75 Bach FH, Hancock WW, Ferran C. Protective genes expressed in endothelial cells: a regulatory response to injury. *Immunol Today* 1997; **18**: 483–486.

76 Hancock WW. Basic science aspects of chronic rejection: induction of protective genes to prevent development of transplant arteriosclerosis. *Transplant Proc* 1998; **30**: 1585–1589.

77 Ardehali A, Reddy R, Laks H. Gene therapy and heart transplantation. *Expert Opin Investig Drugs* 2000; **9**: 1021–1027.

78 Wood KJ, Prior TG. Gene therapy and transplantation. *Curr Opin Mol Ther* 2001; **3**: 390–398.

79 Chen W, Sayegh MH, Khoury SJ. Mechanisms of acquired thymic tolerance in vivo: intrathymic injection of antigen induces apoptosis of thymocytes and peripheral T cell anergy. *J Immunol* 1998; **160**: 1504–1508.

80 Hara Y, Matsuura T, Imanishi M, Tahara H, Kurita T. Unresponsiveness to rat cardiac allografts induced by intrathymic injection of donor bone marrow cells and a short course of immunosuppression. *Transplant Proc* 1994; **26**: 3226–3228.

81 Billingham RE, Brent L, Medawar PB. Actively acquired tolerance of foreign cells. *Nature* 1953; **172**: 603–606.

82 Niimi M, Jones ND, Morris PJ, Wood KJ. Evidence that nondeletional mechanisms are responsible for inducing and maintaining unresponsiveness after intrathymic injection of non-professional antigen presenting cells. *J Heart Lung Transplant* 2000; **19**: 576–583.

83 Hillebrands JL, Raue HP, Klatter FA, et al. Intrathymic immune modulation prevents acute rejection but not the development of graft arteriosclerosis (chronic rejection). *Transplantation* 2001; **71**: 914–924.

84 Marquet RL, Heystek GA, Tinbergen WJ. Specific inhibition of organ allograft rejection by donor blood. *Transplant Proc* 1971; **3**: 708–710.

85 Fabre JW, Morris PJ. The effect of donor strain blood pretreatment on renal allograft rejection in rats. *Transplantation* 1972; **14**: 608–617.

86 Lim SM, Kogure K, White DJ. Cyclosporin A-induced tolerance is not amplified by the addition of steroid therapy. *Transpl Int* 1990; **3**: 70–72.

87 Morris PJ, Ting A, Stocker J. Leukocyte antigens in renal transplantation. I. The paradox of blood transfusions in renal transplantation. *Med J Aust* 1968; **2**: 1088–1090.

88 Salvatierra OJ, Melzer J, Potter D, et al. A seven year experience with donor-specific blood transfusions. Results and considerations for maximum efficiency. *Transplantation* 1985; **40**: 654–659.

89 Opelz G, Terasaki PI (1974). Poor kidney transplant survival with frozen blood transfusions or no transfusions. *Lancet* 1974; **ii**: 696–698.

90 Wrenshall LE, Ansite JD, Eckman PM, Heilman MJ, Stevens RB, Sutherland DE. Modulation of immune responses after portal venous injection of antigen. *Transplantation* 2001; **71**: 841–850.

91 De Silva DR, Urhdal KB, Jenkins MK. Clonal anergy is induced in vitro by T cell receptor occupancy in the absence of proliferation. *J Immunol* 1991; **147**: 3261–3267.

92 Schwartz RH. The acquisition of immunologic self-tolerance. *Cell* 1989; **57**: 1073–1081.

93 Schwartz RH. A cell culture model for T-lymphocyte clonal anergy. *Science* 1990; **248**: 1349–1356.

94 Schwartz RH. Models of T cell anergy: is there a common molecular mechanism? *J Exp Med* 1996; **184**: 1–8.

95 Alegre ML. Costimulatory molecules as targets for the induction of transplantation tolerance. *Nephrol Dial Transplant* 1999; **14**: 322–332.

96 Azuma H, Chandraker A, Nadeau K, et al. Blockade of T-cell costimulation prevents development of experimental chronic renal allograft rejection. *Proc Natl Acad Sci USA* 1996; **93**: 12439–12444.

97 Fauwrith KA, Alegre ML, Thompson CB. Induction of T cell anergy in the absence of CTLA-4/B7 interaction. *J Immunol* 2000; **164**: 2987–2993.

98 Judge TA, Zihou W, Zheng X-G, Sharpe AH, Sayegh MH, Turka LA. The role of CD80, CD86 and CTLA-4 in alloimmune responses and the induction of long-term allograft survival. *J Immunol* 1999; **162**: 1947–1951.

99 Larsen C, Elwood E, Alexander D, et al. Long-term acceptance of skin and cardiac allografts after blocking CD40 and CD28 pathways. *Nature* 1996; **381**: 434–438.

100 Kirk AD, Harlan DM, Armstrong NN, et al. CTLA4-Ig and anti-CD40 ligand prevent renal allograft rejection in primates. *Proc Natl Acad Sci USA* 1997; **94**: 8789–8794.

101 Kirk AD, Burkly LC, Batty DS, et al. Treatment with humanised monoclonal antibody to CD154 prevents acute renal allograft rejection in nonhuman primates. *Nat Med* 1999; **5**: 686–693.

102 Hutchinson IV. Suppressor T cells in allogeneic models. *Transplantation* 1986; **41**: 547–555.

103 Holan V, Mitchison NA. Haplotype specific suppressor T cells mediating linked suppression of immune responses elicited by third-party alloantigens. *Eur J Immunol* 1983; **13**: 652–657.

104 Lechler RL, Chai JG, Marelli-Berg F, Lombardi G. T-cell anergy and peripheral T-cell tolerance. *Phil Trans R Soc Lond B Biol Sci* 2001; **356**: 625–637.

105 Qin S, Cobbold S, Pope H, et al. 'Infectious' transplantation tolerance. *Science* 1993; **259**: 974–976.

106 Waldmann H, Cobbold S. How do monoclonal antibodies induce tolerance? A role for infectious tolerance? *Annu Rev Immunol* 1998; **16**: 619–644.

107 Chen ZK, Cobbold SP, Waldmann H, Metcalfe S. Amplification of a natural regulatory immune mechanism for transplantation tolerance. *Transplantation* 1996; **62**: 1200–1206.

108 Cobbold SP, Waldmann H. Infectious tolerance. *Curr Opin Immunol* 1998; **10**: 518–524.

109 Kapsenberg ML, Kalinski P. The concept of type 1 and type 2 antigen-presenting cells. *Immunol Lett* 1999; **69**: 5–6.

110 Lu L, Thomson AW. Manipulation of dendritic cells for tolerance induction in transplantation and autoimmune disease. *Transplantation* 2002; **73** (Suppl 1): S19–S22.

111 Kehral JH, Wakefield LM, Roberts AB, et al. Production of transforming growth factor beta by human T lymphocytes and its potential role in regulation of T cell growth. *J Exp Med* 1986; **163**: 1037–1050.

112 Ahuja SS, Paliogianni F, Yamada H, Balow JE, Boumpas DT. Effect of transforming growth factor beta on early and late activation events in human T cells. *J Immunol* 1993; **150**: 3109–3118.

113 Lu L, Lee WC, Takayama T, et al. Genetic engineering of dendritic cells to express immunosuppressive molecules (viral IL-10, TGF-beta and CTLA4Ig). *J Leukoc Biol* 1999; **66**: 293–296.

114 Ross R. The pathogenesis of atherosclerosis: a perspective for the 1990s. *Nature* 1993; **362**: 801–809.

115 Elssner A, Vogelmeier C. The role of neutrophils in the pathogenesis of obliterative bronchiolitis after lung transplantation. *Transpl Infect Dis* 2001; **3**: 168–176.

116 Meyer KC, Nunley DR, Dauber JH, et al. Neutrophils, unopposed neutrophil elastase, and alpha-1 anti-protease defenses following human lung transplantation. *Am J Respir Crit Care Med* 2001; **164**: 97–102.

117 Schulz R, Panas DL, Catena R, Moncada S, Olley PM, Lopachuk GD. The role of nitric oxide in cardiac depression induced by interleukin-1 beta and tumor necrosis factor alpha. *Br J Pharmacol* 1995; **114**: 27–34.

118 Tellides G, Tereb DA, Kirkles-Smith NC, et al. Interferon-γ elicits graft arteriosclerosis in the absence of leukocytes. *Nature* 2000; **403**: 207–211.

119 Libby P, Pober JS. Chronic rejection. *Immunity* 2001; **14**: 387–397.

120 Pober JS, Orosz CG, Rose ML, Savage COS. Overview: can graft endothelial cells initiate a host anti-graft immune response? *Transplantation* 1996; **61**: 343–349.

121 Laakis FG, Arekelov A, Konieczny BT, Inoue Y. Immunologic 'ignorance' of vascularised organ transplants in the absence of secondary lymphoid tissue. *Nature Med* 2000; **6**: 686–688.

122 Mason P, Robinson C, Lechler R. Detection of donor-specific hyporesponsiveness following late failure of human renal allografts. *Kidney Int* 1996; **50**: 1019–1025.

123 Hornick PI, Mason P, Yacoub MH, Rose ML, Batchelor JI, Lechler RI. Assessment of the contribution that direct allorecognition makes to the progression of transplant rejection in humans. *Circulation* 1998; **97**: 1257–1263.

124 Hornick PI, Mason PD, Baker RJ, et al. Significant frequencies of T cells with indirect anti-donor specificity in heart graft recipients with chronic rejection. *Circulation* 2000; **101**: 2405–2410.

125 SivaSai KSR, Smith MA, Poindexter NJ, et al. Indirect recognition of donor HLA class I peptides in lung transplant recipients with bronchiolitis obliterans syndrome. *Transplantation* 1999; **67**: 1094–1098.

126 Reznik SI, Jaramaillo A, SivaSai KSR, et al. Indirect allorecognition of mismatched donor HLA class II peptides in lung transplant recipients with bronchiolitis obliterans syndrome. *Am J Transplant* 2001; **1**: 228–235.

127 Cepak KL, Shaw SK, Parker SM, et al. Adhesion between epithelial cells and T lymphocytes mediated by E-cadherin and the alpha E beta 7 integrin. *Nature* 1994; **372**: 190–194.

128 Kilshaw PJ. Alpha E beta 7. *Mol Pathol* 1999; **52**: 203–207.

129 Robertson H, Wong WK, Talbot D, Burt AD, Kirby JA. Tubulitis after renal transplantation: demonstration of an association between CD103+ T cells, transforming growth factor β1 expression and rejection grade. *Transplantation* 2001; **71**: 306–313.

130 Kirby JA, Morgan JC, Shenton BK, Lennard TWJ, Proud G, Taylor RMR. Renal allograft rejection: functional impairment of kidney epithelial cell monolayers mediated by lymphokine activated killer cells and by antibody. *Transplantation* 1991; **51**: 891–895.

131 Karecla PI, Bowden SJ, Green SJ, Kilshaw PJ. Recognition of E-cadherin on epithelial cells by the mucosal T cell integrin alpha M290 beta 7 (alpha E beta 7). *Eur J Immunol* 1995; **25**: 852–856.

132 Brazelton TR, Shorthouse H, Huang X, Morris RE. Infiltrating recipient mesenchymal cells form the obliterative airway disease lesion and dramatically remodel graft tissue in a model of chronic lung rejection. *Transplant Proc* 1997; **29**: 2614

133 Adams BF, Brazelton T, Berry GR, Morris RE. The role of respiratory epithelium in a rat model of obliterative airway disease. *Transplantation* 2000; **69**: 661–693.

134 Huang X, Reichenspurner H, Shorthouse R, Cao W, Berry G, Morris ME. Heterotopic tracheal allograft transplantation: a new model to study the molecular events causing obliterative airway disease (OAD) in rats. *J Heart Lung Transplant* 1995; **14**: S49–S55.

135 Rose ML. Role of antibodies in rejection. *Curr Opin Organ Transplant* 1999; **4**: 227–233.

136 Suci-Foca N, Reed E, Marboe C, et al. The role of anti-HLA antibodies in heart transplantation. *Transplantation* 1991; **51**: 716–724.

137 Reed EF, Hong B, Ho E, Harris PE, Weinberger J, Suci-Foca N. Monitoring of soluble HLA alloantigens and anti-HLA antibodies identifies heart allograft recipients at risk of transplant-associated coronary artery disease. *Transplantation* 1996; **61**: 566–572.

138 Sundaresan S, Mohanakumar T, Smith MA, et al. HLA-A locus mismatches and development of antibodies to HLA antigens after lung transplantation correlates with development of bronchiolitis obliterans syndrome. *Transplantation* 1998; **65**: 648–653.

139 Smith JD, Lawson C, Yacoub MH, Rose ML. Activation of NF-κB in human endothelial cells induced by monoclonal and specific HLA antibodies. *Int Immunol* 2000; **12**: 563–571.

140 Harris PE, Bian H, Reed EF. Induction of high affinity fibroblast growth factor receptor expression and proliferation in human endothelial cells by anti-HLA antibodies. A possible mechanism of transplant atherosclerosis. *J Immunol* 1997; **159**: 5697–5704.

141 Bian H, Harris PE, Reed EF. Ligation of HLA class I molecules on smooth muscle cells with anti-HLA antibodies induces tyrosine phosphorylation, fibroblast growth factor receptor expression and cell proliferation. *Int Immunol* 1998; **10**: 1315–1323.

142 Jaramillo A, Zhang T, Mohanakumar T. Binding of anti-HLA class I antibodies to airway epithelial cells induces activation and growth factor production and indirectly upregulates lung fibroblast proliferation (Abstract). *J Heart Lung Transplant* 2001; **20**: 166.

143 Kallio EA, Koskinen PK, Aavik E, Vaali K, Lemstrom KB. Role of platelet derived growth factor in obliterative bronchiolitis (chronic rejection) in the rat. *Am J Respir Crit Care Med* 1999; **160**: 1324–1332.

144 Smith JD, Danskine AJ, Laylor RM, et al. The effect of panel reactive antibodies and the donor specific cross match on graft survival after heart and lung transplantation. *Transplant Immunol* 1993; **1**: 60–68.

145 Ciubotario R, Liu Z, Colavai AI, et al. Persistent allopeptide reactivity and epitope spreading in chronic rejection of organ allografts. *J Clin Invest* 1998; **101**: 398–405.

146 Jurcevic S, Ainsworth ME, Pomerance A, et al. Antivimetin antibodies are an independent predictor of transplant-associated coronary artery disease after cardiac transplantation. *Transplantation* 2001; **71**: 886–892.

147 Dunn MJ, Rose ML, Latif N, et al. Demonstration by western blotting of anti-heart antibodies before and after cardiac transplantation. *Transplantation* 1991; **51**: 806–812.

148 Laguens RP, Argel MI, Chambo JG, et al. Anti-skeletal muscle glycolipid antibodies in human heart transplantation as markers of acute rejection. *Transplantation* 1996; **62**: 211–216.

149 Deckers JG, Daha MR, Van der Kooj SW, Van der Woude FJ. Epithelial and endothelial specificity of renal graft infiltrating cells. *Clin Transplant* 1998; **12**: 285–291.

150 Dunn MJ, Crisp S, Rose ML, Taylor P, Yacoub MH. Anti-endothelial antibodies and coronary artery disease after cardiac transplantation. *Lancet* 1992; **339**: 1566–1570.

151 Ferry BL, Welsh KI, Dunn MJ, et al. Anti-cell surface endothelial antibodies in sera from cardiac and kidney transplant recipients: association with chronic rejection. *Transplant Immunol* 1997; **5**: 17–24.

152 Perrey C, Brenchley PEC, Johnson RWG, Martin S. An association between antibodies specific for endothelial cells and renal transplant failure. *Transplant Immunol* 1998; **6**: 101–106.

153 Fredrich R, Toyoda M, Czer LS, et al. The clinical significance of antibodies to human vascular endothelial cells after cardiac transplantation. *Transplantation* 1999; **67**: 385–391.

154 Smith JD, Crisp SJ, Dunn MJ, Pomerance A, Yacoub MH, Rose ML. Pre-transplant anti-epithelial antibodies and graft failure after single lung transplantation. *Transplant Immunol* 1995; **3**: 68–73.

155 Jaramillo A, Naziruddin B, Zhang L, et al. Activation of human airway epithelial cells by non-HLA antigens developed after lung transplantation: a potential etiological bronchiolitis obliterans syndrome. *Transplantation* 2001; **71**: 966–976.

156 Wilkes DS, Heidler KM, Yasufuku K, et al. Cell mediated immunity to collagen V in lung transplant recipients: correlation with collagen V release into BAL fluid (Abstract). *J Heart Lung Transplant* 2001; **20**: 167.

157 Yasufuku K, Heidler KM, O'Donnell PW, et al. Oral tolerance induced by type V collagen downregulates allograft rejection. *Am J Respir Cell Mol Biol* 2001; **25**: 26–34.

158 Fedoseyeva EV, Zhang F, Orr PL, Levin D, Buncke HJ, Benichou G. De novo autimmunity to cardiac myosin after heart transplantation and its contribution to the rejection process. *J Immunol* 1999; **162**: 6836–6842.

159 Hele DJ, Yacoub MH, Belvisi MG. The heterotopic tracheal allograft as an animal model of obliterative bronchiolitis. *Respir Res* 2001; **2**: 169–183.

18

Pharmacological immunosuppression

Nicholas R. Banner and Haifa Lyster

Harefield Hospital, Harefield, Middlesex, UK

Introduction

Pharmacological immunosuppression is required after all types of organ transplantation to prevent rejection of the allograft. Immunosuppressive drugs have a potential for serious toxicity. Due to the strength of the alloimmune response [1,2], the drugs that are currently available cannot be used as single agents to prevent rejection without unacceptable toxicity. Current practice is therefore to use combinations of agents with complementary immunosuppressive actions but differing adverse effects to achieve synergistic immunosuppression with the lowest possible toxicity [3–5].

However, this approach does not overcome the other main problem associated with the use of these drugs, which is that their effect is not specific for the immune response to the allograft. Nonspecific immunosuppression increases the risk of both infection and certain types of malignancy in the transplant recipient [6,7]. Although progress has been made through the introduction of potent immunosuppressive agents that affect predominantly those aspects of the immune response central to allograft rejection [8–10], the fundamental limitation of nonspecific immunosuppression remains.

The variety and complexity of clinical immunosuppression protocols has increased with the number of agents that are available and with the use of multiple-drug combinations; in addition, there are differing strategies for both the administration and the monitoring of individual drugs. The evidence base for treatment protocols in lung transplantation is limited. The number of lung transplantations that are performed in individual centres is usually too few to allow studies that can achieve a statistically robust conclusion. Many of the studies that have been published also have other methodological limitations that prevent unambiguous interpretation. Almost no large, multi-centre, randomized clinical trials have been conducted in the field of lung transplantation. Such studies are expensive and require financial backing that can usually be obtained only from the pharmaceutical industry. For understandable commercial reasons, drug companies have tended to concentrate their efforts on renal transplantation, which has the highest level of clinical activity and therefore market potential. Thus much of our knowledge about the use of immunosuppression for lung transplantation has been extrapolated from preclinical studies and clinical studies performed in other types of organ transplantation. While such information is clearly of value, there are specific features of lung transplantation that may limit the validity of such extrapolations; these include the greater susceptibility of lung allografts to infection and the nature of chronic pulmonary allograft dysfunction (obliterative bronchiolitis) [11], which differs from the 'chronic rejection' seen in renal and cardiac allografts that is predominately an obliterative vascular process [12,13]. Information about lung transplantation itself has to be synthesized from the results of single centre studies, Registry data and the collective experience of physicians working in the field of thoracic organ transplantation.

This chapter provides a selective overview of the information available about the use of pharmacological immunosuppression in adult transplant patients, with an emphasis on the drugs most commonly used in clinical practice.

The development of clinical immunosuppression

An increased understanding of the phenomenon of allograft rejection during the 1940s and 1950s paved the way for clinical attempts to transplant human organs. Following successful kidney transplants between genetically identical twins [14], attempts were made to transplant kidneys between genetically different individuals. Initially, the intended recipient's immune system was prepared by using total body irradiation but this did not produce an acceptable rate of success and an alternative approach was required [15,16]. Schwartz and colleagues discovered that 6-mercaptopurine has a suppressive effect on the immune response and subsequently demonstrated the drug's ability to prolong skin allograft survival [17,18]. Calne then used 6-mercaptopurine to prevent rejection of renal allografts in dogs [19]. Following this, azathioprine, the prodrug of 6-mercaptopurine, was found to be an easier agent to administer and control, leading to further successful renal transplants [20].

Medawar and colleagues had noted the effect of corticosteroids on the mononuclear cell infiltrate seen during experimental allograft rejection [21,22]. Starzl and colleagues found that large doses of corticosteroids could be used to reverse acute rejection of renal allografts in dogs who were being treated with azathioprine [23]. Thus it became apparent that combinations of drugs were required to control the alloimmune response. The combination of azathioprine and corticosteroids became established as a standard treatment for human renal allografts. Although this combination increased the chance of a successful transplant, rejection remained a frequent problem and acute rejection crises were sometimes difficult to reverse with increased doses of corticosteroids. In addition, the use of high dose corticosteroids was associated with frequent complications, including infections.

Further experimental studies confirmed the key role played by lymphocytes in acute rejection and demonstrated that lymphocyte depletion (by drainage of the thoracic duct and the use of antilymphocyte antibodies) could reduce the risk of acute rejection and so prolong allograft survival [24,25]. In certain animal models these treatments appeared to promote tolerance to the allograft. These observations led to the clinical use of antilymphocyte antibody preparations [26]. These proved to be useful in both the prophylaxis and treatment of acute rejection, but unfortunately their use did not induce long-term tolerance to allografts in humans. Such preparations continue to have a role in many immunosuppression protocols and the term 'induction therapy' has persisted to describe the use of biological anti-T-cell agents in the early post-transplantation period.

The discovery of a method to produce monoclonal antibodies in unlimited quantities [27], enabled studies to be performed to investigate the function of specific molecules (antigenic determinants) on the surface of cells during the alloimmune response and to evaluate the potential therapeutic actions of antibodies directed against

them [28,29]. The first monoclonal antibody to be used therapeutically in humans was muromonab-CD3 (OKT3) [30].

Although immunosuppression protocols based on azathioprine, corticosteroids and antilymphocyte globulin enabled the clinical development of renal and hepatic transplantation, the initial results of cardiac, and especially of pulmonary transplantation, were poor. Two specific problems in lung transplantation were the continuing risk that infection could be introduced into the allograft through the respiratory tract and problems with healing of the bronchial anastomosis, which were partly due to the need to use large doses of corticosteroids [31].

The next major advance in immunosuppressive therapy came with the discovery of ciclosporin [8,32]. Ciclosporin proved to be an effective and specific inhibitor of T-cell activation and did not have unwanted effects on the bone marrow or on the innate immune system [33]. However, early clinical studies rapidly revealed that it had serious dose-limiting nephrotoxicity in humans [34,35]. Nevertheless, immunosuppressive protocols based on ciclosporin proved to be more effective than those that had previously been available and its use was associated with a marked improvement in the results of both renal and cardiac transplantation [36,37]. The introduction of ciclosporin was one of the factors that led to clinically successful lung transplantation [38].

The discovery of tacrolimus [39], another potent inhibitor of T-cell activation, which had a molecular structure completely different from that of ciclosporin but which proved to have an identical primary mechanism of action, contributed to research into the molecular mechanisms underlying activation of T cells [40]. Understanding of the mechanisms involved in T-cell activation has grown in parallel with the discovery of new immunosuppressive agents [41]. This knowledge provided a rational basis for the use of combinations of immunosuppressive agents to control rejection and it led to the idea that agents could be developed to specifically target different stages in this process. Such an approach led to the re-evaluation of a previously abandoned compound, mycophenolic acid, as an immunosuppressive agent [42]. In the future, a knowledge of the three-dimensional structure of key enzymes and receptors within the lymphocyte may allow the de novo design of new immunosuppressive agents.

The alloimmune response

Allograft rejection is conventionally divided into three categories according to the time at which it occurs after transplantation; each of these syndromes has a different pathogenesis.

Hyperacute rejection

Hyperacute rejection was first described in renal transplantation [43–45] and it has subsequently been recognized to occur after both cardiac [46] and pulmonary transplants [47,48], although it has not been reported after liver transplantation. In hyperacute rejection, preformed antibodies against antigens of the ABO blood group system, or human leukocyte antigens (HLA)/major histocompatability complex (MHC) antigens bind to the endothelium of the allograft; this causes endothelial activation, complement binding, and intravascular coagulation, which leads to the rapid destruction of the graft. Damage begins to occur immediately following the surgical vascularization of the transplanted organ. This type of rejection is now rarely seen because it can be prevented by ABO matching between the recipient and donor and by screening transplant candidates for anti-HLA antibodies; those who have such antibodies must also undergo a lymphocytotoxic cross-match against the donor before transplantation can be safely performed. When hyperacute rejection does occur, it does not respond to conventional immunosuppressive therapy and requires specific treatment aimed at both the removal of the preformed antibodies and prevention of the production of further antibody [49].

Acute rejection

Typically this first occurs within the first three months of transplantation but may occur later. Some patients will experience persistent or recurrent episodes of acute rejection. Acute rejection sometimes occurs years after transplantation because of changes in the patient's immunosuppressive therapy or poor adherence to the treatment protocol.

Acute rejection is predominantly a cellular process [50,51]. It is initiated by helper T cells (Th) that recognize either foreign HLA on the surface of cells within the graft (direct recognition) or antigens from the allograft that have been processed by antigen presenting cells of the host (indirect recognition) [52]. Direct recognition appears to be the most important mechanism in acute rejection. Binding of the receptor of a helper T cell to allogeneic HLA will, if coupled to a secondary signal caused by binding between adhesion molecules on the surface of the T cell and the antigen presenting cell, lead to activation of the T cell via a cascade of intracellular signals [53]. The activated T cell will generate cytokines including interleukin 2 (IL-2), which has an autocrine effect on the T cell itself as well as recruiting and stimulating effector cells including cytotoxic T cells, monocytes and eosinophils and helping to activate alloreactive B cells leading to antibody production. The helper T cell itself is stimulated to progress through the cell cycle leading to cell division and a clonal expansion of cells with the same alloreactivity. Thus acute rejection is initiated by alloreactive helper T cells that act as a cytokine-producing 'engine', which leads to amplification of the immune response through cell division and the recruitment of other cells. The effector mechanisms that subsequently lead to the destruction of the graft include: the action of cytotoxic T cells, which induce target cell necrosis in an MHC-restricted manner via molecules such as granzyme and perforin as well as by inducing apoptosis through the binding of Fas to Fas-ligand [54]; less specific (non-MHC restricted) cell killing will also occur by the recruitment of activated macrophages, natural killer cells and eosinophils [55,56].

Acute rejection is susceptible to immunosuppressive drugs that can be used both to prevent it and to reverse breakthrough episodes of rejection. The action of immunosuppressive agents can be largely understood by their effects on the intracellular signals that lead to T-cell activation.

Chronic rejection

Both donor antigen-dependent and independent processes contribute to the development of chronic allograft dysfunction or 'chronic rejection'. The manifestations of this process vary with the organ transplanted; renal [12] and cardiac allografts [13] are prone to an obliterive vascular process whereas the lung is subject to a fibroproliferative obliteration of the bronchioles. The pathogenesis of this bronchiolitis obliterans syndrome (BOS) is multifactorial and our knowledge of the mechanisms involved is far from complete. The risk factors that have been identified include both nonimmunological factors such as the organ ischaemia time during the transplantation [57] and immunological factors including acute rejection [58]. The link with acute rejection raises the possibility that more effective immunosuppression may lead to a reduction in the incidence of BOS.

Immunosuppressive agents

The T-cell activation cascade

A simplified model of the sequence of events that leads to activation of a helper T cell is shown in Figure 18.1. The

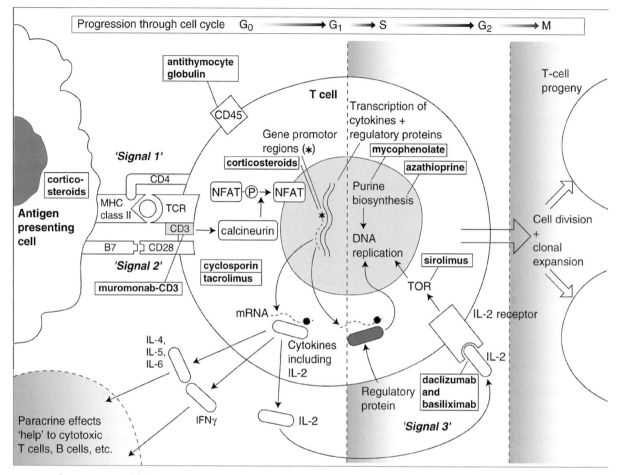

Figure 18.1 Simplified model of the events that occur during T-cell activation. The sites of action of each of the immunosuppressive agents discussed in this chapter are shown. Polyclonal antithymocyte globulin is shown as binding to the common leukocyte antigen but, in reality, contains antibodies which bind to many different T-cell antigens. NFAT, nuclear factor of activated T-cells; TCR, T-cell receptor; MHC, major histocompatibility complex; P, phosphate; CD, cluster of differentiation antigen; TOR, target of rapamycin; IL, interleukin; IFN-γ, interferon gamma. For further details, see the text.

early, calcium-dependent, phase of activation begins when the T-cell receptor (TCR) binds to a complementary MHC class II molecule with an associated peptide in its antigen presentation groove 'Signal 1'. Full activation also requires a second event or 'Signal 2', which is caused by binding between complementary adhesion molecules on the surface of the antigen presenting cell and the T cell [53,59]. Signal transduction from the TCR occurs via the CD3 complex [60–62]. Subsequent intracellular signalling involves the inositol triphosphate/diacyglycerol pathway and mobilization of intracellular calcium [63]. This leads to activation of the protein phosphatase calcineurin [40]. Calcineurin dephosphorylates the nuclear factor of activated T cells (NFAT) allowing its active moiety to translocate to the nucleus and

so bind to the promoter regions of various genes encoding cytokines such as IL-2, regulatory proteins and the IL-2 receptor [64]. The pattern of cytokine expression depends on the nature of the helper T cell (Th1 or Th2) and can lead to either recruitment of cytotoxic T cells and other effector cells or to the provision of help to B cells for antibody production [65]. The expression of IL-2 leads to autocrine, stimulation of the T cell [66]. Binding of IL-2 to its receptor initiates a second sequence of intracellular signals involving the mammalian target of rapamycin (sirolimus) (TOR), which leds to DNA synthesis and replication and culminates in cell division [67]. The sites of action of the various immunosuppressive agents are indicated in Figure 18.1.

The calcineurin inhibitors

Mechanism of action of ciclosporin and tacrolimus

Although ciclosporin and tacrolimus have very different molecular structures and physicochemical properties, the principal mechanism of their immunosuppressive action is the same, inhibition of the phosphatase calcineurin. They thereby interrupt the early phase of T-cell activation and the production of IL-2 [40,68].

Neither drug acts directly on calcineurin. Both bind initially to intracellular proteins known as immunophilins (cyclophilins for ciclosporin and the FK-506 binding proteins (FKBP) for tacrolimus) to form a drug–immunophilin complex [69,70]. It is this complex that inhibits calcineurin (a calcium- and calmodulin-dependent phosphatase) and thereby prevents the dephosphorylation of the cytoplasmic form of NFAT [40,64]. In vitro, tacrolimus is 10–100 times more potent than ciclosporin [71,72]; one explanation for this difference is that tacrolimus binds far more strongly to FKBP than ciclosporin does to cyclophilin.

Although the main action is identical, there are a number of differences between the two drugs that may be of clinical importance. Some studies have indicated that the expression of active transforming growth factor beta (TGF-β) is increased by ciclosporin but not by tacrolimus [73]. Enhanced expression of TGF-β is associated with fibrosis and so could play a role in long-term failure of the transplanted organ [74]. However, other studies have failed to confirm this difference between the drugs [75].

Production of antibodies against both HLA and non-HLA antigens has been associated with chronic rejection. In one study, the use of tacrolimus was associated with a reduction in the production of antibodies against vimentin (which are associated with cardiac allograft vasculopathy) [76]. This finding needs confirmation and further studies are required to determine whether important differences in antibody production occur after lung transplantation.

P-glycoprotein is a member of the ATP-binding cassette proteins and it actively transports a variety of substrates across biological membranes [77]. Both tacrolimus and ciclosporin are P-glycoprotein substrates but ciclosporin has a significantly higher affinity for it. Ciclosporin can induce overexpression of P-glycoprotein [78], but this phenomenon has not been seen with therapeutic concentrations of tacrolimus [79]. It has been speculated that in some circumstances ciclosporin-related overexpression of P-glycoprotein may be linked with episodes of transplant rejection [80,81].

Pharmacokinetics and administration of ciclosporin

Oral and intravenous forms are available. Ciclosporin is no longer subject to patent control and a number of oral formulations are available; because of the drug's lipophilic nature and relatively high molecular weight, its absorption after oral administration is influenced by the formulation used. Absorption of the original oral formulation (Sandimmun or Sandimmune made by Sandoz/Novartis pharmaceuticals) was heavily influenced by dietary intake and other factors so that absorption varied within individuals over time. Neoral (Novartis) is a newer, microemulsion formulation, of ciclosporin that has a more rapid and consistent pattern of absorption [82]. Oral bioavailability of Neoral is generally better than that of Sandimmun [82]. Food decreases the rate and extent of absorption. Absorption of Neoral may be altered by changes in gastrointestinal function and, for example, is poor during the first few days after heart transplantation, probably because of the effects of cardiopulmonary bypass used during surgery [83]; it seems likely that similar abnormalities may occur after lung transplant operations performed using cardiopulmonary bypass to support the recipient during surgery. A number of other formulations of ciclosporin are now available in different countries. Owing to their lack of bioequivalence, patients should not be switched between preparations without careful monitoring and adjustment of the dose required.

Ciclosporin is a highly lipophilic compound and it binds to a variety of intracellular proteins. This results in a large volume of distribution. Only a small fraction of ciclosporin in blood is unbound while the majority is bound to lipoproteins or protein bound within erythrocytes [84,85]. Thus measurement of ciclosporin concentration in whole blood can be influenced by factors such as haematocrit; furthermore, there is no direct relationship between this concentration and that present at the site of action.

Ciclosporin is eliminated by the liver; in common with many immunosuppressive agents and other drugs, it is subject to metabolism by the cytochrome P450 system, mainly by P450-3A. More than 30 metabolites have been identified, some of which possess a degree of immunosuppressant activity and contribute to toxicity [86]. This metabolism is the cause of important pharmacokinetic interactions between ciclosporin and other drugs. The elimination half-life of ciclosporin after oral or intravenous administration varies between 10 and 27 hours. Ciclosporin is normally administered at 12-hourly intervals.

Orally administered ciclosporin is subject to considerable first pass metabolism by cytochrome P450 in the intestinal mucosa, as well as in liver, which reduces its systemic bioavailability. Bioavailability of Neoral averages 43% but has a reported range of 17–68% [82]. Therefore, when ciclosporin is administered intravenously, a lower dose is required to achieve the same blood concentration. The optimum protocol for intravenous administration is uncertain. If steady-state infusions are used, the blood concentration will not vary and exposure to the drug will be much lower than that which would occur with the same pre-dose (trough) concentration during oral administration. Therefore it may be more appropriate to administer it by intermittent infusions over two or three hours and to measure the resulting trough level before the next infusion.

Ciclosporin has a variety of toxicities that can occur at concentrations within the therapeutic range. This, coupled with the marked variations in absorption and metabolism between individuals, as well as the possibility of interactions with other drugs and dietary substances, necessitates careful monitoring of blood levels during therapy.

Pharmacokinetics and administration of tacrolimus

Tacrolimus is available as one proprietary product (Prograf); it is often referred to by its premarketing designation FK-506. Both oral and intravenous formulations are available. The oral bioavailability of tacrolimus is 20–25% [87], so that the intravenous dose is lower than that needed orally. Food reduces the rate and extent of absorption; however, the magnitude of this effect is unlikely to be clinically important [88]. Tacrolimus binds extensively to red blood cells and plasma proteins [89], hence its clearance is influenced by haematocrit and plasma albumin levels in the transplant recipient [90].

Tacrolimus is almost completely metabolized prior to elimination via cytochrome P450-3A; this occurs primarily in the liver but also in the intestinal mucosa [91–93]. Up to 15 metabolites have been identified and at least one appears to have immunosuppressive properties [87]. The main route of elimination is in the bile, with less than 1% excreted unchanged in the urine. The elimination half-life of tacrolimus has been found to vary between 12 and 35 hours depending on clinical circumstances, being longest in normal subjects and shortest in recipients of liver transplants [87]. Tacrolimus is normally administered twice daily. The drug is highly bound to cells and proteins and it is hypothesized that it is the free fraction of drug that is available for hepatic elimination. This is supported by the observation that factors that reduce drug binding such as low plasma protein levels or low haematocrit are associated with more rapid clearance of the drug [90].

As with ciclosporin, metabolism of tacrolimus via the cytochrome P450 system forms the basis of a number of important pharmacokinetic drug interactions. Tacrolimus

Table 18.1. Drug-specific side effects of the calcineurin inhibitors. The relative frequency of each side effect is indicated. The complications that are common to all types of pharmacological immunosuppression (infection and malignancy) are not included in this or later tables unless there are particular issues related to a specific drug

	Ciclosporin	Tacrolimus
Nephrotoxicity	++	++
Hypertension	++	+
Neurotoxicity	+	++
Headache, including migraine, tremor, occasionally seizures, cortical blindness, paraesthesia, burning sensation in hands and feet		
Glucose intolerance and diabetes mellitus	+	++
Hyperlipidaemia	++	+
Gingival hypertrophy	++	−
Hypertrichosis	+	−
Alopecia	−	+
Hyperuricaemia and gout	+	+
Hyperkalaemia and hypomagnesaemia	+	+
Liver dysfunction	+/−	+/−
Gastrointestinal symptoms	+	+
Pancreatitis	+	+
Haemolytic-uraemic syndrome/TTP	+	+
Gynaecomastia	+	+

Note: TTP, thrombocytopenic purpura; plus and minus signs indicate relative frequency of side effects.

also has a low therapeutic index and so requires monitoring of drug levels during therapy.

Adverse effects

As would be expected from their identical primary mechanism of action, there are great similarities between the adverse effects caused by ciclosporin and by tacrolimus. Both cause nephrotoxicity, which limits the dose that can be used clinically. However there are some important differences between the toxicity of the two agents and these are summarized in Table 18.1.

Nephrotoxicity is the most common serious side effect of treatment with either drug [35,94]. It can be categorized into acute and chronic forms [95]. Acute toxicity is dose and blood level related and is potentially reversible, i.e. renal function usually improves following a reduction in dose. The mechanism of acute toxicity is predominantly an effect on renal haemodynamics; calcineurin inhibitors cause vasoconstriction of the afferent arteriole, resulting in reduced renal blood flow, decreased glomerular filtration rate and increased sodium retention. Chronic nephrotoxicity is associated with irreversible structural changes in the kidney that appear to result both from chronic ischaemic damage and from direct toxicity to the renal parenchyma [95]. Management involves reducing the dose of the calcineurin inhibitor as far as possible (often by introducing alternative immunosuppressive agents) [96], careful control of hypertension (perhaps using calcium antagonists) [97,98] and the use of angiotensin converting enzyme inhibitors if there is proteinuria.

There are differences in the cosmetic side effects of the two drugs that may necessitate a switch from one calcineurin inhibitor to the other in some patients (Table 18.1). It has been suggested that, from this perspective, tacrolimus may be more suitable for use by children and female patients because it does not stimulate excessive hair growth. However, the choice of calcineurin inhibitor must be made in the light of all their effects and there have been reports of an increased incidence of lymphoproliferative disease [99] and case reports of drug-induced cardiomyopathy in paediatric patients treated with tacrolimus [100].

Hypertension is a common problem after organ transplantation and occurs in about 60% of lung transplant recipients by five years after surgery [57]. Drug treatments with calcineurin inhibitors and corticosteroids are important contributory factors [101]. There is evidence from clinical trials in heart transplantation that hypertension may be less frequent in patients treated with tacrolimus than in those treated with ciclosporin [102,103].

Hyperlipidaemia is also frequent after transplantation. Like hypertension, it is a multifactorial problem and is related to the use of both corticosteroids [104] and calcineurin inhibitors [105,106]. However, tacrolimus therapy appears to be associated with a lower incidence of hyperlipidaemia than is ciclosporin [103,106].

New onset diabetes mellitus is another serious complication of organ transplantation. It is related both to treatment with corticosteroids and to the use of calcineurin inhibitors [107–109]. The incidence of post-transplantation diabetes is greater in patients treated with tacrolimus than in those receiving ciclosporin [109].

Clinical use

The introduction of ciclosporin was an important step forward in the development of pharmacological immunosuppression because of its powerful and specific action in preventing T-cell activation. Randomized trials demonstrated the efficacy of the original Sandimmun formulation of ciclosporin after renal transplantation [36,110–112]. Its

use was not tested so rigorously in other settings but its value in heart transplantation rapidly became apparent [37,113]. The availability of ciclosporin was one of the factors that led to lung transplants being performed successfully [38].

Subsequently, it became apparent that the variable absorption of the Sandimmun formulation could influence its effectiveness as an immunosuppressant [114,115] and this led to the introduction of the microemulsion formulation of ciclosporin with its better absorption characteristics [82,116]. In lung transplant recipients with cystic fibrosis, the Neoral formulation results in better drug absorption [117]. Clinical trials demonstrated a reduction in the incidence of acute rejection after renal transplantation compared with that seen using the Sandimmun formulation [118,119]. Patient and graft survival as well as side effects were comparable with the two formulations. Neoral also reduced the incidence of corticosteroid resistant rejection after heart transplantation [120]. The microemulsion formulation also allowed the early use of oral therapy in patients after liver transplantation where the Sandimmun formulation was not absorbed well because of a lack of normal bile flow [121,122]; use of the microemulsion formulation was associated with a lower incidence of acute rejection after liver transplants [123]. Overall, the use of the Neoral microemulsion formulation has been associated with a reduction in the incidence of acute rejection in kidney, heart and liver transplants [124]. However, there has been no change in graft and patient survival and in some studies the use of Neoral has been associated with an increased incidence of side effects [124]. Overall, the microemulsion formulation is more effective than the original formulation; however, the differences are not dramatic, which is as might be expected, since the active agent is unchanged and, in clinical practice, the dose is normally adjusted in the light of both the clinical response and the measurements of the drug concentration in blood.

Tacrolimus was introduced after ciclosporin. It has been compared with ciclosporin in a number of randomized clinical trials that have been performed mainly in liver and renal transplants. In general, these studies were conducted using the Sandimmun formulation of ciclosporin in the control group; this may be particularly relevant to the outcome of the liver studies, where Sandimmun is very poorly absorbed in the immediate period after surgery. In addition these were 'open label' because of the need to adjust the dose of both tacrolimus and ciclosporin in the light of their blood concentration. Furthermore, the protocol-specified dose and target levels of tacrolimus were adjusted during some of the trials. This, combined with the very different potency of the two drugs, has obscured whether the comparisons were made using the optimum dose of each agent.

In renal transplantation, the use of tacrolimus was associated with a reduction in the incidence of acute rejection, with similar graft function, graft survival and adverse events [109,125]. Similarly, acute rejection rates and steroid-resistant acute rejection were reduced after liver transplantation [126,127]. Only small-scale studies have been performed after heart transplantation; the efficacy of tacrolimus and ciclosporin appeared similar but with some differences in the incidence of specific adverse effects [103]. No multicentre trials have been completed in lung transplantation, although there are data from individual centres to support the view that tacrolimus may be somewhat more effective than ciclosporin in preventing acute and chronic rejection after lung transplantation [128–130].

Many studies have examined the role of transferring patients from ciclosporin to tacrolimus in cases of acute rejection that is refractory to conventional therapy. Unfortunately, the nature of the study populations and the clinical situation usually precludes the use of randomized studies. Therefore the data from such studies are generally anecdotal and uncontrolled. Nevertheless the data do support the view that switching from ciclosporin to tacrolimus as part of the treatment for refractory rejection may be beneficial [131,132].

In summary, there is reasonable evidence that both the microemulsion formulation of ciclosporin (Neoral) and tacrolimus provide more effective immunosuppression than the original Sandimmun formulation of ciclosporin. There is some evidence that tacrolimus may be more effective than Neoral ciclosporin in certain circumstances but the data are not conclusive. Since the primary mechanism of action is the same for the two drugs, any advantage must be related either to pharmacokinetic differences or to the differences in their chemical structure and binding proteins.

Corticosteroids

These are chemically modified derivatives of the naturally occurring adrenal hormone cortisol. The agents in this group differ in their pharmacokinetics as well as in their glucocorticoid and mineralocorticoid activity (Table 18.2).

Mechanism of action

Corticosteroids (glucocorticosteroids) have multiple effects on both innate and acquired immunity as well as having nonspecific anti-inflammatory effects [133]. They act by crossing the cell membrane, binding to specific glucocorticoid receptors in the cytoplasm, and then trans-

Table 18.2. Relative potency of the corticosteroids

Compound	A Relative anti-inflammatory potency	B Relative sodium-retaining potency	Ratio A/B
Cortisone	0.8	0.8	1
Hydrocortisone (cortisol)	1	1	1
Prednisone	4	0.8	5
Prednisolone	4	0.8	5
Methylprednisolone	5	0.5	10

locate to the nucleus and, by binding to glucocorticoid response elements, either increase or decrease gene expression [134,135]. Corticosteroids inhibit macrophage function and antigen processing [136,137], reduce cytokine gene transcription (including IL-1, IL-2, interferon gamma) [138–141], as well as inhibiting the synthesis of protein, RNA and DNA in lymphocytes; they thereby prevent T-cell proliferation. Corticosteroids can also induce apoptosis (programmed cell death) in lymphocytes [142].

Corticosteroids exhibit anti-inflammatory effects. One mechanism involves an increase in the production of lipocortin, which inhibits phospholipase A_2 [143], an enzyme involved in arachidonic acid metabolism, affecting both the cyclo-oxygenase and 5-lipoxygenase pathways. However, other mechanisms are also involved, including inhibition of gene transcription regulated by the nuclear factor kappa B (NF-κB) [144,145]. The correlation between the immunosuppressive effect of these drugs and their anti-inflammatory action is poor [143] and while dexamethasone is a potent anti-inflammatory drug it is not effective as an immunosuppressive agent [146].

Pharmacokinetics and administration

A variety of preparations are available with differing pharmacokinetic properties. Prednisone, prednisolone and methylprednisolone are the agents most commonly used in transplantation because they are potent glucocorticoids with low mineralocorticoid effects and they have proved to be effective immunosuppressants. Prednisolone and prednisone are the corticosteroids used most commonly for oral administration whereas methylprednisolone is usually used for intravenous administration. Prednisone is metabolized in the liver to prednisolone (a reversible transformation) [147]. Prednisolone is completely bioavailable after oral administration [148]. The pharmacokinetics of these agents is complex because of variable binding to plasma proteins, which, in the case of prednisolone, is dose

Table 18.3. Side effects of the corticosteroids

- Increased appetite and weight gain
- Cushing's syndrome (moon face, obesity, buffalo hump, skin striae, hirsutism)
- Diabetes mellitus
- Hypertension
- Hyperlipidaemia
- Corticosteroid-related bone disease (osteoporosis and avascular osteonecrosis)
- Poor wound healing
- Dermatological problems: skin thinning and striae; acne (in the young), bruising and ecchymosis (older patients)
- Peptic ulceration (including increased risk of perforation)
- Ophthalmological problems including glaucoma, cataracts and risk of ophthalmic infection
- Pancreatitis
- Proximal myopathy
- Tendon rupture
- Neuropsychiatric effects including sleep disturbance, euphoria, depression, de novo psychosis (or risk of aggravating schizophrenia), convulsions (and aggravation of epilepsy)
- Fluid retention
- Hypokalaemia
- Leukocytosis
- Suppression of the adrenal cortex, leading to dependence on exogenous corticosteroids
- Menstrual irregularity and amenorrhea
- Growth retardation in children

dependent [149,150] and the reversible conversion of each agent into the other [151,152].

Glucocorticoids are metabolized via the cytochrome P450 system in the liver and the resulting metabolites are excreted in the urine. The elimination half-life of methylprednisolone is 2–3 hours [153,154] and that of prednisolone 2.5–4.5 hours [150].

Adverse effects

Table 18.3 lists the adverse effects of corticosteroids. The multiple immunosuppressive actions of these potent drugs means that their use is associated with a significant risk of infection, particularly when they are used at high dose. Their metabolic effects are also important [155], particularly the risk of new onset diabetes and their ability to exacerbate pre-existing diabetes that is dose-related [107,156].

Corticosteroid-related bone disease

Corticosteroid-related bone disease (osteopenia, osteoporosis and avascular osteonecrosis) have become an increasing problem in patients receiving long-term treatment. Osteoporosis is a multifactorial disease and its incidence is related not only to the dose and duration of corticosteroid therapy but also to the patient's age, sex and mobility. Patients who have been in respiratory failure with limited mobility for a long time before transplantation and those who have been treated with corticosteroids before transplantation are at increased risk. Fortunately prophylactic measures are available against this problem and these will be reviewed here.

Osteopenia is defined as a bone mineral density (BMD) between 1 and 2.5 standard deviations below the young adult mean and osteoporosis as a BMD more than 2.5 standard deviations below this [157]. Lung transplant recipients are at increased risk of osteoporosis both before and after transplantation. Risk factors before transplantation include decreased mobility, hypoxaemia, malnutrition, vitamin D deficiency, tobacco use and corticosteroid use [158,159]. Cystic fibrosis is associated with osteopenia due to pancreatic insufficiency, vitamin D deficiency, calcium malabsorption and hypogonadism [160].

The immunosuppressive regimens used to prevent allograft rejection include glucocorticosteroid and calcineurin inhibitors (ciclosporin and tacrolimus), which are associated with rapid bone loss. The incidence of osteoporotic fractures ranges from 8% to 65% during the first year after transplantation [161]. Bone loss is related to dose and length of glucocorticoid exposure, with doses greater than 10 mg prednisolone daily resulting in substantial bone loss. In corticosteroid-induced osteoporosis the trabecular bones (ribs, vertebrae and distal ends of long bones) are especially affected and prone to fractures [161].

Rapid bone loss and fractures tend to occur in the first year after transplantation [161–165], hence prophylaxis management should be started as early as possible. A number of prophylactic approaches have been used. Elemental calcium supplementation with at least 1000 mg daily (1500 mg daily in postmenopausal women) may be of benefit [157]. Calcitriol can enhance the intestinal absorption of calcium [157,166]. In postmenopausal women, hormone replacement therapy (HRT) prevents bone loss related to oestrogen deficiency. Oestrogens improve BMD in women treated with glucocorticoids and animal studies suggest that they also prevent ciclosporin-induced bone loss [161]. Hence, it is recommended that postmenopausal women and premenopausal women with amenorrhea receive HRT both before and after transplantation unless there are definite contraindications. Progesterone must also be given in those women with an intact uterus to prevent endometrial hyperplasia.

Bisphosphonates (etidronate, alendronate, pamidronate) are pyrophosphate analogues that bind strongly to the bone mineral hydroxyapatite. They thereby inhibit osteoclast activity and bone resorption. Cyclical etidronate therapy (14 days of etidronate followed by 76 days of calcium supplements) can prevent glucocorticoid-induced osteoporosis [167–169]. Alendronate has also been shown to prevent bone loss in patients receiving therapy with corticosteroids [170].

Calcitonin can also inhibit bone reabsorption but its effect wanes after two years of use, perhaps because of the development of blocking antibodies or receptor downregulation [171,172].

Clinical use

Corticosteroids comprised the first drugs to be used for clinical immunosuppression and were found to be highly effective immunosuppressive agents; however, their use has not been assessed using randomized clinical trials. They remain of central importance in many current protocols for maintenance immunosuppression as well as being the agent of first choice for treating acute cellular rejection [23,173–175].

The main corticosteroids used clinically are methylprednisolone, prednisolone and prednisone. Methylprednisolone is administered intravenously in high doses early after surgery as prophylaxis against rejection and to ameliorate the effects of ischaemia–reperfusion injury. It is also administered intravenously as the first-line treatment for acute (cellular) rejection. Prednisolone and prednisone are given orally as part of many maintenance immunosuppression protocols as prophylaxis against rejection; they are also given in higher doses as part of the consolidation phase of treatment for more severe episodes of acute rejection [174].

Patients undoubtedly differ in their response to corticosteroids, perhaps due partly to differences in cytochrome P450 activity between individuals. However, no method of pharmacokinetic or pharmacodynamic monitoring has become established and the adjustment of the dose used for maintenance therapy is a matter of clinical judgement. Due to the side effects of corticosteroids, which are related to dose and duration of therapy as well as individual factors, the dose used is usually tapered down during the long-term maintenance phase and, in some centres, corticosteroids are actively withdrawn [175–177].

Inhibitors of DNA synthesis

Azathioprine

Azathioprine is a synthetic imidazole derivative of 6-mercaptopurine that acts as an antimetabolite and inhibits purine synthesis. It was used in combination with corticosteroids as prophylaxis against rejection during the pioneering period of clinical allogeneic renal transplantation with pharmacological immunosuppression [20]. Like corticosteroids, its use as an immunosuppressive agent was never subjected to assessment in randomized clinical trials. It has now been partially replaced by mycophenolate, which has been found to be a more effective immunosuppressant at least in renal and heart transplantation.

Mechanism of action

Azathioprine is a prodrug that is converted in the liver to 6-mercaptopurine; this readily crosses cell membranes and is converted intracellularly into a number of purine thio-analogues including thioinosinic acid (6-thioinosine monophosphate) [178].

Azathioprine acts at a late stage in the process of lymphocyte activation. Thioinosinic acid inhibits the synthesis of both guanylic and adenylic acids from inosinic acid by inhibiting several enzymes including adenylsuccinate synthetase, adenylsuccinate lyase, and inosine monophosphate dehydrogenase. In addition, thioinsinic acid is converted into thioguanylic acid and thence thiodexoguanosine triphosphate, which interferes with DNA synthesis and can also be incorporated into DNA. A build up of thiopurine ribonucleotides also produces feeback inhibition of de novo purine biosynthesis. By inhibiting DNA synthesis, azathioprine inhibits the S phase of the lymphocyte cell cycle and thereby inhibits the proliferation of both T and B lymphocytes [179,180]. It is potentially mutagenic and may induce chromosomal breaks. Azathioprine also interferes with the synthesis of polyadenylate-containing RNA [181].

Pharmacokinetics and administration

Azathioprine is well absorbed after oral administration, with peak serum levels occuring at one to two hours, the elimination half-life is four to six hours. It is normally administered once daily [182]. The recommended initial oral dose is 4–5 mg/kg followed by a maintenance dose of 1–4 mg/kg per day although doses above 2 mg/kg per day frequently produce leukopenia with continued treatment and the dose must be adjusted in the light of changes in the white blood cell count. Oral bioavailability is about 50%, suggesting that the dose should be reduced during intravenous administration. Azathioprine is metabolized to 6-mercaptopurine in the liver; 6-mercaptopurine is metabolized via the thiopurine methyltransferase and the xanthine oxidase pathways and the resulting metabolites (predominantly inactive 6-thiouric acid) are excreted in the urine. No dose adjustment is required in renal failure because only 10% of a dose is eliminated as unchanged drug. Metabolism

Table 18.4. Side effects of azathioprine

- Dose-related bone marrow suppression
- Nausea
- Hepatotoxicity including cholestatic jaundice and rarely Budd–Chiari syndrome
- Hair loss
- Hypersensitivity reactions, which are uncommon in transplant patients (fever, malaise, arthralgia, myalgia, rash, diarrhoea, hypotension, interstitial nephritis)
- Pancreatitis (rare)
- Pneumonitis (rare)
- Thrombophlebitis (after intravenous administration)

via xanthine oxidase is the basis for an important drug interaction with allopurinol [183–185]. Polymorphism in the thiopurine methyltransferase gene contributes to variation between individuals in their response to azathioprine [186–188].

Adverse effects

Table 18.4 describes the adverse effects of azathioprine. In clinical practice dose-related bone marrow suppression is the most common problem to be encountered [189]. Leukopenia is usually the first manifestation but thrombocytopenia and anaemia will follow if the dose is not reduced. A macrocytic anaemia without leukopenia [190,191] is sometimes seen with long-term therapy. Some patients are intolerant of azathioprine because of nausea but this usually responds to a reduction in the dose. Liver dysfunction is not uncommon in the early postoperative phase of thoracic organ transplantation; azathioprine must be considered as a potential cause and it may be necessary to switch patients to an alternative therapy such as mycophenolate. Severe obstructive jaundice is uncommon and the Budd–Chiari syndrome is a rare late complication of azathioprine therapy [192–195]. Hypersensitivity reactions have been reported but are uncommon in the post-transplantation population [196].

Skin cancer is more common in immunosuppressed individuals and is probably related largely to the immunosuppressed state itself; however, there is some evidence that azathioprine therapy may be a particular risk factor [197–199].

Clinical use

Azathioprine is used as part of many maintenance immunosuppression protocols for prophylaxis against rejection; it is normally used in combination with a calcineurin inhibitor and corticosteroids. However, mycophenolate has been demonstrated to be more effective than azathio-

prine after both renal and heart transplantation and it has gradually replaced azathioprine in these conditions, although its superiority for liver and lung transplant patients has not yet been demonstrated by a randomized clinical trial.

Mycophenolate mofetil and mycophenolic acid

Mycophenolic acid, a natural fermentation product of several *Penicillium* species, is an uncompetitive inhibitor of the rate-limiting enzyme in the pathway of de novo purine synthesis, inosine monophosphate dehydrogenase [200]. Mycophenolate mofetil is the synthetic morpholinoethyl ester prodrug of mycophenolic acid. Mycophenolate has become established as an alternative immunosuppressive agent to azathioprine and has been shown to be more effective than azathioprine in renal and cardiac transplantation [201–204].

Mechanism of action

Purine synthesis is accomplished by two separate pathways: the de novo pathway and the salvage pathway. Most cells can utilize both pathways but proliferating lymphocytes are dependent on the de novo pathway. Since mycophenolic acid inhibits only de novo synthesis, it has a selective effect on proliferating B and T lymphocytes that are unable to recycle purine bases. Furthermore, it selectively inhibits the type II isoform of inosine monophosphate dehydrogenase, which predominates in proliferating lymphocytes [205]. As a result, mycophenolic acid has a specific action on proliferating lymphocytes while having less effect on other proliferating cells [206]. Hence it has a high therapeutic ratio as an immunosuppressant [200]. In contrast azathioprine inhibits multiple steps in purine metabolism and has more widespread effects on proliferating cells. Unlike azathioprine, mycophenolic acid does not become incorporated into DNA.

Inhibition of purine synthesis leads to depletion of guanosine nucleotides; depletion of deoxyguanosine triphosphate inhibits DNA synthesis while depletion of guanosine triphosphate inhibits the formation of glycoproteins including cell surface molecules that play a role in cell adhesion, intercellular communication and lymphocyte traffic through the vascular epithelium [207–209].

Mycophenolic acid inhibits both cellular and humoral immune responses [206,210,211]. Early events in T-lymphocyte activation, including IL-2 production, are not affected and the cell is arrested in the S phase of the cell cycle. Mycophenolic acid can also inhibit the proliferation of human smooth muscle cells, which could be of value in the management of chronic rejection [212].

Pharmacokinetics and administration

Mycophenolate mofetil is available in oral and intravenous formulations. The recommended starting dose for renal transplant patients is 1 g twice daily and for heart transplant recipients 1.5 g twice daily. Mycophenolate is rapidly absorbed after oral administration and converted to the active drug mycophenolic acid. The mean bioavailability after oral administration is 94% [213]; consequently oral and intravenous doses are the same. The maximum plasma concentration (C_{max}) occurs approximately two hours after oral administration. Food lowers the C_{max} of mycophenolic acid; however, systemic exposure (area under the curve, AUC) is not affected. Mycophenolic acid undergoes enterohepatic recirculation, which causes a secondary peak in plasma concentration between 6 and 12 hours after administration [214, 215].

Mycophenolic acid is strongly bound to plasma albumin in a concentration-dependent manner. Binding is not altered by ciclosporin, tacrolimus and prednisolone, or by warfarin, digoxin and phenytoin. As with many highly protein bound drugs, the pharmacological activity of mycophenolate is a function of the free mycophenolic acid concentration in the plasma [216]. Renal dysfunction is associated with decreased binding and an increase in the free fraction of mycophenolic acid [217].

The half-life of mycophenolic acid is approximately 18 hours [213]. It is metabolized in the liver mainly to mycophenolic acid glucuronide, which is pharmacologically inactive [218]. The glucuronide is excreted predominantly via the kidneys. However it is also excreted into bile and subsequently deconjugated by gut bacteria and reabsorbed, producing an enterohepatic recirculation [216].

Adverse effects

The adverse effects of mycophenolate are shown in Table 18.5. It is generally well tolerated and is free from renal, metabolic and cardiovascular toxicity. The main dose-related side effects are bone marrow suppression (usually leukopenia) and gastrointestinal symptoms (particularly nausea and diarrhoea). Bone marrow suppression is less common than that seen with azathioprine whereas gastrointestinal symptoms are more common [201–203].

Table 18.5. Side effects of mycophenolate mofetil

- Gastrointestinal symptoms; particularly nausea and diarrhoea (less commonly dyspepsia, vomiting, abdominal pain, oesophagitis, pancreatitis, gastrointestinal bleeding or perforation)
- Bone marrow suppression, most commonly leukopenia (less frequently anaemia, thrombocytopenia)
- Dizziness, headache

The incidence of some opportunistic infections may be increased by the use of mycophenolate, although this appears to reflect its more effective immunosuppressive action rather than being a specific effect of the drug. Side effects may be increased in patients with substantially impaired renal function [217,219].

Clinical use

Mycophenolate mofetil has been evaluated as an immunosuppressive agent used in combination with ciclosporin and corticosteroids for prophylaxis against rejection after renal and cardiac transplantation [201–204]. In renal transplantation, mycophenolate proved to be superior to either placebo [201] or azathioprine [202,203] in preventing rejection. In general the risk:benefit ratio was most favourable using a dose of 2 g daily [220]. A flaw in the study design of the heart transplant trial prevented a clear cut result from being obtained from analysis of the intention to treat data. However, analysis of patients according to the treatment received confirmed the finding of the renal studies that mycophenolate (3 g per day) was superior to azathioprine as a prophylaxis against acute rejection [204].

Mycophenolate has also been found to be a useful component in the treatment of acute rejection [221] and acute refractory rejection [222].

In small nonrandomized studies after lung transplantation, acute rejection episodes were less frequent in those patients receiving mycophenolate as compared with those treated with azathioprine [223–225]. Currently there is a multicentre trial comparing mycophenolate with azathioprine each used together with ciclosporin and corticosteroids in de novo lung transplants. The primary end-point of this study is the incidence of bronchiolitis obliterans syndrome.

Sirolimus and its analogues

Sirolimus (rapamycin) has recently been approved for use as a component of maintenance immunosuppression after renal transplantation. It can be combined with ciclosporin to produce an increased level of immunosuppression but, although it is not nephrotoxic itself, it potentiates the nephrotoxicity of ciclosporin. Everolimus (SDZ-RAD), an analogue of sirolimus, is undergoing clinical investigation. Most of the information available about the clinical use of sirolimus comes from the field of renal transplantation. In these studies sirolimus has been administered either with ciclosporin or without a calcineurin inhibitor. There is currently little clinical information available about the use of sirolimus and tacrolimus in combination. Although both drugs bind to FKBP and can antagonize each other's action in vitro when either is present in excess, it is unlikely that such effects will occur at concentrations that are used clinically.

Mechanism of action

Sirolimus is structurally similar to tacrolimus and binds intracellularly to FKBP [226]; but, unlike tacrolimus, it does not affect the early calcium-dependent phase of T-cell activation [227]. The sirolimus–FKBP complex inhibits signal transduction from the IL-2 receptor by binding to TOR proteins and it thereby inhibits progression of the T cell from the G_1 to the S phase of the cell cycle [227–229].

Sirolimus has similar inhibitory effects on the proliferation of vascular smooth muscle cells [230], which could be important in preventing or treating chronic vascular rejection. In animal models of airway transplantation, sirolimus inhibits the fibroproliferative response to transplantation [231, 232], raising the possibility that sirolimus may be of value in the prevention and treatment of obliterative bronchiolitis.

Pharmacokinetics and administration

Sirolimus is currently only available as an oral formulation. After oral administration, sirolimus is rapidly absorbed, producing a peak in blood concentration after one to three hours. However, bioavailability is low due to first pass metabolism mediated by cytochrome P450 in both the intestinal mucosa and the liver, as well as counter-transport by intestinal P-glycoprotein [91,233,234]. Systemic exposure is linearly related to dose [234]. Absorption is influenced by food, which may lead to variations in pharmacokinetics within subjects. A consistent relationship between administration and both meals and ciclosporin administration is recommended to reduce pharmacokinetic variability [235]. It is suggested that the administration of ciclosporin and sirolimus should be separated by at least four hours.

Sirolimus is extensively bound to red blood cells. Hepatic metabolism is via cytochrome P450-3A to form demethylated and hydroxylated metabolites that do not have significant immunosuppressive effects; these are eliminated mainly in the faeces. The elimination half-life was 62 hours in renal transplant patients who were also receiving ciclosporin [236].

This long half-life permits the drug to be administered once daily. At a fixed daily dose, it takes approximately six days for sirolimus levels to reach a steady state, which is a shorter period than would be expected from the elimination half-life. A loading dose of three times maintenance dose can be used to achieve therapeutic concentrations more quickly.

Table 18.6. Side effects of sirolimus

- Thrombocytopenia
- Leukopenia
- Anaemia
- Hypercholesterolaemia
- Hypertriglyceriaemia
- Abnormal liver function
- Hypokalaemia
- Diarrhoea
- Arthralgia
- Abdominal pain
- Tachycardia
- Pancreatitis
- Pneumonitis
- Potentiation of ciclosporin nephrotoxicity
- Thrombotic thrombocytopenic purpura (with ciclosporin)

Sirolimus was used at fixed doses in the pivotal studies of its use in combination with ciclosporin after renal transplantation [237,238]. However, concentration-controlled administration is now recommended, with the target blood level being adjusted depending on whether ciclosporin is also being coadministered (8 ng/mL (range 4–12) with ciclosporin and 16 ng/mL (range 12–20) without ciclosporin).

A lower dose of sirolimus is needed to achieve the same blood level when it is coadministered with ciclosporin because of the pharmacokinetic interaction between the two drugs involving both cytochrome P450 and P-glycoprotein. Although no formulation is available for intravenous administration, it would be expected that the intravenous dose would be lower than that needed orally because of the significant first pass metabolism that occurs.

Adverse effects

The agent-specific side effects of sirolimus are shown in Table 18.6. Some adverse effects, including thrombocytopenia, leukopenia and hyperlipidaemia are dose related [239]. Sirolimus is not intrinsically nephrotoxic [240,241]. But it potentiates the nephrotoxicity of ciclosporin [237, 238,242]. This effect is dose related and becomes apparent once the drugs have been coadministered for several months; it is reversible if ciclosporin is withdrawn after three months [243].

Clinical use

Most of the data that are currently available have been obtained in the field of renal transplantation. In clinical trials performed in recipients of renal transplants, sirolimus was more effective in preventing acute rejection than either placebo [238] or azathioprine [237] when administered in combination with ciclosporin and corticosteroids.

In both these studies sirolimus was administered at a single fixed dose of either 2 mg or 5 mg per day; the 2 mg regimen appeared to be as effective as 5 mg. Unfortunately, the improved control of rejection did not translate into improved renal (graft) function. These studies confirmed that sirolimus potentiates the nephrotoxicity of ciclosporin [237,238,242].

Studies have been performed to investigate whether sirolimus can be used as an alternative to ciclosporin immediately after renal transplantation [240,241] or whether sirolimus-based immunosuppression can allow ciclosporin to be withdrawn safely early after transplantation [243]. The use of sirolimus instead of ciclosporin in combination with corticosteroids and either azathioprine [240] or mycophenolate [241] resulted in similar acute rejection rates and graft survival rates with the ciclosporin-based regimens (although the size of these studies was relatively small, which limited their ability to detect such differences), and the elimination of ciclosporin was associated with improved renal function. In the study where ciclosporin was withdrawn at three months, although withdrawal was associated with a trend towards a higher rate of acute rejection, graft survival was similar and renal function was better at one year in those in whom ciclosporin had been withdrawn [243].

At present the approved indication for sirolimus is for use in combination with ciclosporin and corticosteroids for maintenance immunosuppression during the early phase after renal transplantation. The long-term use of the combination of sirolimus and ciclosporin is not recommended because of the risk of nephrotoxicity.

Biological anti-T-cell agents

This group of agents consists of a variety of antibodies (both natural and engineered) directed against antigenic determinants on the surface of T cells. They all must be administered parenterally and all are capable, in varying degrees, of stimulating an antibody response directed against themselves that can modify their activity.

Antithymocyte globulin antilymphocyte globulin

These polyclonal antibodies were introduced into clinical practice in the 1960s [26]. A number of products are currently available either commercially or from specific transplant centres. They are produced by immunizing either rabbits (e.g. Thymoglobulin, Sangstat) or horses (e.g. Lymphoglobuline, Sangstat, or ATGAM, Upjohn) with human lymphocytes or thymocytes. The antibodies produced by a group of animals are collected and pooled before being processed and assayed for clinical activity. The spectrum of

antibodies present and the potency of the product may vary with the immunogen used, the species immunized, and procedures used to adsorb unwanted antibodies, as well as assays used to assess potency during the manufacturing process. These products are complex biological preparations that have broadly similar actions but they are not bioequivalent. Historically, there was considerable batch to batch variability but this problem has been minimized by modern techniques of production and quality control.

Mechanism of action

Due to the presence of multiple antibodies in these preparations, their mechanism of action is complex and is not completely understood. Thymoglobulin (Sangstat) is a typical antithymocyte globulin (ATG) in current clinical use. It is a pasteurized preparation of rabbit immunoglobulin (Ig) G from animals that were immunized with human thymocytes (rabbit antithymocyte globulin or RATG). It contains antibodies directed against a wide range of molecules present on T cells including CD3, CD4, CD8, CD28, CD45, and CD80/CD86 (B7-1 and B7-2) as well as antibodies against non-T-cell antigens present on erythrocytes, monocytes, platelets and neutrophils [244,245]. It also contains antibodies directed against B lymphocytes [246].

Immediately after the administration of RATG, transient lymphocyte activation can occur, leading to the release of tumour necrosis factor (TNF) and other cytokines that produce symptoms such as chills, fever, rigors, headache and hypotension (the 'first dose' or 'cytokine release' syndrome) [244].

The main immunosuppressive effect of ATG is related to its ability to deplete circulating T lymphocytes [247]. A number of mechanisms may contribute to this, including opsonization of antibody-coated cells, complement-mediated cell lysis and apoptosis [247–249]. In addition the function of antibody-coated cells may be modulated, making them hyporesponsive, although the mechanisms underlying this effect are not completely understood [249,250].

Pharmacokinetics and administration

RATG is administered by an intravenous infusion (via a central venous catheter to prevent thrombophlebitis). Infusions are typically given over four to eight hours. ATG has a low volume of distribution (0.12 L/kg per min) [251]. Serum levels fall rapidly due to antibody binding to circulating lymphocytes and other cells [252], and is cleared from the serum with a half-life of two to three days. However, bound ATG can persist for a much longer period and the mean elimination half-life is approximately 30 days [251]. Rabbit-derived ATGs are generally more potent than equine

Table 18.7. Side effects of antithymocyte globulin

- Leucopenia, anaemia, thrombocytopenia
- Local reactions at administration site, including pain and phlebitis (usually avoided by central venous administration)
- Systemic reaction including fever, chills, tachycardia, hypotension, dyspnoea, vomiting (most frequent with the first dose – minimized by premedication with corticosteroids and an antihistamine)
- Anaphylactoid reactions
- Serum sickness (delayed fever, rash, joint pain and muscle pain); usually only after repeated administration
- Increased incidence of infection, particularly viral infections, such as CMV
- Increased incidence of PTLD

Note: CMV, cytomegalovirus; PTLD, post-transplantation lymphoproliferative disease.

ATGs and the latter are usually administered at higher doses (e.g. Thymoglobulin, a rabbit ATG, 1.25–2.5 mg/kg per day for prophylaxis and 2.5–5 mg/kg per day for treatment of rejection compared with Lymphoglobuline, an equine ATG, 10 mg/kg per day for prophylaxis and 10–20 mg/kg per day for treatment).

Adverse effects

Table 18.7 describes the side effects associated with the use of antilymphocyte globulin. The symptoms that accompany the first dose appear to be related to the release of cytokines but are generally less intense than those seen after the administration of muromonab-CD3. They can be ameliorated by premedication with paracetamol (acetaminophen), an antihistamine and a corticosteroid. The release of cytokines may be related to the increased incidence of cytomegalovirus infection that is seen after the administration of ATG [253]. Post-transplant lymphoproliferative disease is also more common after the use of ATG [254]. However, the risk appears lower than seen after treatment with muromonab-CD3 [254], perhaps because of the intrinsic anti-B-cell effects of ATG [255].

Clinical use

Antilymphocyte globulins have been used for induction therapy [256] as part of treatment for hyperacute or antibody-mediated rejection (where its activity against B cells as well as T cells is important), and to treat acute (cellular) rejection [257].

Muromonab-CD3

Muromonab-CD3 (Orthoclone OKT3, Cilag Biotech) is a murine monoclonal antibody which is specific to the ϵ-chain of the TCR–CD3 complex expressed on the surface of T cells. It was the first monoclonal antibody to become commercially available for clinical use. Its monoclonal nature results in a uniform product and it has a well-defined mechanism of action.

Mechanism of action

Muromonab-CD3 is directed specifically against the CD3 antigen, which is present on mature circulating T cells and on medullary thymocytes [258]. Because the CD3 complex plays a role in signal transduction, antibody binding leads to transient T-cell activation and the release of cytokines, which are responsible for the acute side effects of the drug and which may contribute to the risk of subsequent viral infections and of post-transplantation lymphoproliferative disease [259–263]. CD3-positive cells are rapidly cleared from the circulation after the first dose due to both modulation of expression of the TCR–CD3 complex and opsonization of T cells, leading to their subsequent removal by the reticuloendothelial system [264]. Modulation is probably the most important mechanism because CD3-positive cells rapidly reappear at the end of treatment. Loss of the TCR–CD3 complex renders the T cell temporarily unable to recognize and respond to alloantigen.

As a murine antibody, muromonab-CD3 can elicit a xenogeneic antibody response in the patient. Both anti-idiotypic and anti-isotypic antibodies may develop [265]. These antibodies may block the therapeutic effect of muromonab-CD3 and necessitate the use of immunological monitoring during treatment.

Pharmacokinetics and administration

Muromonab-CD3 is administered by intravenous injection; the recommended dose for adult patients is 5 mg per day. Serum levels decrease rapidly after the administration of a single dose, falling to 10% of the peak level by 24 hours after the injection [266]. Plasma concentrations increase gradually during a course of treatment but decrease rapidly thereafter [267]. The route of elimination appears to be via binding to CD3 on lymphocytes and its subsequent removal [268]. Higher concentrations are observed during prophylactic administration than during the treatment of rejection, perhaps because of the increased number of CD3-positive cells present during rejection.

The elimination half-life is approximately 36 hours during prophylactic administration and 18 hours during the treatment of rejection [269,270]. Once daily administration is recommended. Elimination may be accelerated by the development of human anti-mouse antibody and so therapy must be monitored.

Table 18.8. Side effects of muromonab-CD3

- Cytokine-release syndrome, especially with the first two doses (fever, chills, malaise, rigors, headache, nausea and vomiting, diarrhoea and abdominal pain; less commonly chest pain, dyspnoea, wheezing, acute pulmonary oedema, hyper- or hypotension, cardiovascular collapse)
- Neurological complications are less common but may be serious.

  Seizures

  Aseptic meningitis (meningeal symptoms, CSF pleocytosis with normal or reduced glucose level and negative microbiological and virological studies)

  Encephalopathy and cerebral oedema
- Cytokine-mediated renal dysfunction
- Anaphylactic and other hypersensitivity reactions
- Intravascular thrombosis in allograft or elsewhere
- Risk of infection related to the intensity of immunosuppression and to the cytokine release phenomenon; particularly CMV
- Increased incidence of PTLD

Note: CSF, cerebrospinal fluid; CMV, cytomegalovirus; PTLD post-transplantation lymphoproliferative disease.

Adverse effects

The side effects of muromonab-CD3 are described in Table 18.8. Antibody binding to the CD3 complex results in 'cytokine-release syndrome' causing fever, malaise, chills and rigors; in addition serious cardiovascular, respiratory and neurological complications may occur [271–276]. This reaction is common with the first two doses when the number of CD3-positive circulating T cells is highest. This can be minimized by the use of methylprednisolone as part of the premedication prior to the first two doses of the course. Corticosteroids can attenuate the acute side effects associated with the cytokine release phenomenon [277]; the administration of paracetamol and an antihistamine may also help to minimize symptoms. Muromonab-CD3 can less frequently cause pulmonary oedema, cardiovascular collapse, seizures and renal failure [276,278–280]. The risk of infectious complications and malignancy is related to the overall level of immunosuppression and to the influence of cytokines on viral activation [253,262, 281].

Clinical use

Muromonab-CD3 has been used for induction therapy immediately after transplantation and for the treatment of acute rejection including 'steroid-resistant' rejection [30,264,282–284].

Antibodies directed against the interleukin-2 receptor

IL-2 and its receptor play a key role in T-cell activation [285–287]. The IL-2 receptor (IL-2R) complex consists of three subunits denoted as α, β and γ. The β- and γ- subunits are constitutively expressed on resting lymphocytes, have signal transduction properties, and together form a low affinity receptor for IL-2; the early phase of lymphocyte activation leads to upregulation of these subunits and de novo expression of the α-subunit to form the high affinity receptor [288–290]. The α-subunit (CD25) has no role in signal transduction but it stabilizes the interaction between IL-2 and the $\beta\gamma$-subunit [287]. Rodent monoclonal antibodies directed against the IL-2R (also known as the T-cell activation complex or Tac) were found to prevent acute rejection [285,291,292] and subsequently two biologically engineered antibodies against IL-2Rα (CD25) have been developed for clinical use.

Mechanism of action of daclizumab and basiliximab

Both antibodies have been genetically engineered [293] from mouse anti-Tac antibodies to replace most of murine protein content and thus reduce their immunogenicity. Basiliximab [294] is a chimeric human–mouse antibody and daclizumab [295] is a fully 'humanized' antibody where only the antigen-binding site is of murine origin; only about 10% of the protein mass of daclizumab is of murine origin [296]. Basiliximab retains the antigen-binding affinity of the original antibody whereas the humanization process has resulted in some reduction in the affinity of daclizumab [10,296].

Both agents bind to IL-2Rα and thereby inhibit IL-2-driven proliferation [10,296–298]; they are therefore specific for activated lymphocytes. Their constant regions are composed of human IgG. Neither antibody causes lymphocyte activation or depletion of the total number of circulating T cells [299]. In addition, the antibodies can downregulate the expression of IL-2R and trigger antibody-dependent cell-mediated cytotoxicity [297,299].

Pharmacokinetics and administration

Daclizumab and basiliximab are both administered by intravenous infusion. The recommended treatment schedules for renal transplantation are: basiliximab 20 mg by infusion two hours before surgery and 20 mg again on post-operative day 4 [294]; daclizumab 1 mg/kg prior to surgery and again every two weeks thereafter for a total of five doses [295]. These agents can be administered via a peripheral vein. Both have small volumes of distribution (5.3 L for daclizumab [299] and 4.9 L for basiliximab [300]). The antibodies have a longer half-life and therefore duration of action than unmodified murine monoclonal antibodies; the chimeric antibody, basiliximab, has an elimination half-life of approximately 6.5 days [300] whereas the humanized daclizumab has a half-life of approximately 20 days [299].

Adverse effects

Since neither antibody causes lymphocyte activation, these agents are not associated with the acute cytokine release syndrome that is associated with the administration of muromonab-CD3 or polyclonal ATG. The absence of lymphocyte activation may have other advantages such as avoidance of an increased risk of some opportunistic infections such as cytomegalovirus (CMV) [301]. These antibodies have remarkably few side effects, with no increase in adverse reactions above those seen in the control groups of several clinical trials [298,302–304], although severe hypersensitivity reactions have been observed occasionally.

Clinical use

The mechanism of action of these two antibodies is identical and the differences between them are their affinity for CD25 (higher for basiliximab), their elimination half-life (longer for dalizumab) and their recommended schedule of administration. Placebo-controlled clinical trials have demonstrated that basiliximab and daclizumab are effective in reducing the incidence of acute rejection after renal transplantation when combined with ciclosporin and corticosteroids (with [298] or without [302–304] azathioprine). Smaller studies have also indicated efficacy in other circumstances such as heart transplantation [305].

An early study with an unmodified rat anti-Tac antibody demonstrated that anti-IL2R therapy could be as effective as induction therapy with polyclonal ATG in preventing acute rejection while producing fewer side effects [292]. However, no large-scale clinical trials have been conducted to determine whether the daclizumab and basiliximab are as effective as polyclonal ATG.

Theoretically, once rejection has become established (with amplification of alloreactive T cells, the expression of multiple cytokines, and the recruitment of a variety of other cells), an antagonist of a single cytokine would not be expected to reverse the response. Although one study with an unmodified anti-Tac antibody indicated that anti-IL-2R therapy may be effective in reversing acute rejection [306] this finding was not confirmed in another study [307]. The potential of basiliximab or daclizumab to potentiate the effect of other antirejection therapies has not been investigated.

Drug interactions

Pharmacokinetic interactions

Most immunosuppressive agents have a low therapeutic index with serious toxicity occurring close to the dose and blood concentration that produces an immunosuppressive effect, for example nephrotoxicity in the case of ciclosporin and tacrolimus. There are two main mechanisms by which the coadministration of other drugs can alter the pharmacokinetics of immunosuppressive agents and thereby cause toxicity or loss of efficacy; these are effects on drug-metabolizing enzymes (particularly cytochrome P450) and effects on P-glycoprotein.

Cytochrome P450

The calcineurin inhibitors (ciclosporin and tacrolimus) and the TOR inhibitor, sirolimus, are metabolized by the cytochrome P450-3A enzyme system [308]. There are a number of other drugs that affect the activity of this enzyme system; these drugs can be divided into enzyme inducers and enzyme inhibitors (Table 18.9). Enzyme inducers increase cytochrome P450 activity, resulting in increased metabolism and clearance of drugs such as ciclosporin. If the dose of the drug is not adjusted to compensate for this, such an interaction can lead to rejection of the transplant.

Enzyme inhibitors cause decreased metabolism and, without adjustment of the dose administered, will produce an increased risk of toxicity, for example ciclosporin-related nephrotoxicity. Enzyme inhibitors have also been deliberately used to reduce the dose of immunosuppressant required and thus the cost of treatment. Both ketoconazole and diltiazem have been combined with ciclosporin in this way [309–313]; itraconazole reduces the metabolism of tacrolimus [314].

Table 18.9. Some important examples of drugs that either inhibit or induce cytochrome P450-3A and thereby alter the metabolism of ciclosporin, tacrolimus and sirolimus

Enzyme inhibitors	Enzyme inducers
Macrolide antibiotics: erythromycin, clarithromycin	Rifampicin
Imidazole antifungals: itraconazole, fluconazole, ketoconazole	Anticonvulsants: phenytoin, phenobarbital, carbamazepine
Calcium channel blockers, especially diltiazem and verapamil	

Table 18.10. Mechanisms of pharmacokinetic interactions between immunosuppressive agents

	Tacrolimus	Corticosteroids	Azathioprine	Mycophenolate	Sirolimus
Ciclosporin	Cytochrome P450, P-glycoprotein	Cytochrome P450		?	Cytochrome P450, P-glycoprotein
Tacrolimus		Cytochrome P450		?	Cytochrome P450, FKBP
Corticosteroids					Cytochrome P450

Note: FKBP, FK-506-binding protein.

P-glycoprotein

P-glycoprotein actively transports a variety of substrates across biological membranes. It is found in a number of normal human tissues including intestinal epithelial cells, biliary canalicular membranes, proximal kidney cells, the blood–brain barrier and in the haematological compartment [315]. As a result it can influence the absorption of drugs from the gut, their distribution between body compartments, as well as their metabolism and excretion [77]. The P-glycoprotein pump, located in the intestinal wall, transports many cytochrome P450 substrates and prevents the entry of a variety of foreign compounds into the systemic circulation.

A number of drugs compete as substrates for P-glycoprotein and thereby inhibit each other's transport across cell membranes; these include ciclosporin, calcium channel blockers and antiarrhythmic agents. P-glycoprotein antagonists can be divided into two groups: those that are substrates and are transported themselves (e.g. ciclosporin) and those that are not [315]. It has been speculated that P-glycoprotein may play a role in the interaction of cyclosporin and mycophenolate mofetil [77].

Foods and herbal remedies

Grapefruit juice increases the oral bioavailability of ciclosporin but it has no effect after intravenous ciclosporin administration [316,317]. Grapefruit is an inhibitor of intestinal cytochrome P450, which is responsible for the first pass metabolism of many medications, but it does not alter liver cytochrome P450 activity. The P-glycoprotein pump may also be inhibited by grapefruit juice, resulting in increased bioavailability of ciclosporin [316,317].

Information regarding possible interactions with herbal remedies is often lacking. This is in part due to the fact that dietary supplements and herbal remedies are not regulated as rigorously as conventional medicines. Reports of such interactions are on the increase [318,319]. Many patients do not consider herbal supplements to be medications and hence do not include them in any drug history requested by health professionals.

St John's Wort (Hypericum perforatum) contains a variety of phytochemicals that contribute to its pharmacological activity. These result in the induction of the cytochrome P450 enzyme system and intestinal P-glycoprotein, causing a decrease in ciclosporin bioavailability and thereby increasing the risk of cellular rejection [320,321].

Interactions between immunosuppressive agents

With the increasing number of immunosuppressive agents that are available, and the use of complex multidrug regimens, drug interactions between the immunosuppressive agents themselves are becoming increasingly important (Table 18.10). Ciclosporin and tacrolimus will inhibit each other's metabolism but there is no clinical indication to administer them together because they have the same mechanism of action [322].

High dose corticosteroids may decrease ciclosporin metabolism by inhibiting cytochrome P450 [323]. Ciclosporin, in turn, can inhibit the metabolism of prednisolone [324]. A study in renal transplant patients found that tacrolimus dose requirements fell with time as corticosteroids were weaned; this finding suggested that corticosteroids may increase the metabolism of tacrolimus [90].

Mycophenolate does not alter the metabolism of ciclosporin or tacrolimus but systemic exposure to mycophenolate is greater in patients being treated with tacrolimus than in those receiving ciclosporin [325]. This may be partly because tacrolimus inhibits the glucuronidation of mycophenolate [326] but is probably largely because ciclosporin increases the metabolism of mycophenolate [327,328].

The mechanisms of the interactions between sirolimus and ciclosporin are not fully understood. Pharmacokinetic interactions involve P-glycoprotein and cytochrome P450 in the intestine and cytochrome P450 in the liver. However, the mechanism by which sirolimus potentiates ciclosporin nephrotoxicity despite control of ciclosporin blood concentrations is currently unknown.

Interaction with antimicrobial agents

Infection is a frequent complication in transplant patients. A number of antimicrobial agents are metabolized through the cytochrome P450 system and can alter the metabolism of immunosuppressive agents. Rifampicin is a powerful inducer of cytochrome P450, can cause a considerable reduction in ciclosporin or tacrolimus levels [329,330] and would probably have a similar effect on sirolimus. It also increases the metabolism of prednisolone and may halve the effective dose received; this interaction can easily be overlooked, since corticosteroid levels are not routinely monitored [331,332].

Many other antimicrobials are known to inhibit the metabolism of ciclosporin, tacrolimus and, probably, sirolimus. The interactions encountered most frequently are those with imidazole antifungal agents (ketoconazole [313,333], fluconazole [334] and itraconazole [314,335] and the macrolide antibiotics (erythromycin [336–338] and clarithromycin [339,340]).

Interactions with anticovulsants
Postoperative convulsions may occur after thoracic organ transplantation and are probably related to drug therapy, particularly ciclosprin and corticosteroids [341], together with electrolyte imbalances. Young adults appear to be most at risk. Many anticonvulsants are powerful enzyme inducers of cytochrome P450 and can lower the levels of drugs including ciclosporin, tacrolimus and corticosteroids [154,342–344].

Interactions with oral contraceptive agents and hormone replacement therapy
Contraception is an important issue for younger female transplant recipients and hormone replacement therapy (HRT) is an essential component of prophylaxis against osteoporosis in older women, There have been reports that oestrogen- and progestogen-containing preparations, and also the gonadotrophin inhibitor danazol, may inhibit ciclosporin metabolism, resulting in increased blood levels [345–348]. Preparations with cyclical variations in the dose of these hormones may lead to fluctuating levels of immunosuppression. Whenever possible, preparations that provide a constant dose should be used, i.e. progesterone-only oral or depot contraceptive agents and noncyclical forms of HRT. The dose of ciclosporin may need to be adjusted when commencing and when discontinuing therapy. Danazol also increases tacrolimus levels [349]. Tacrolimus may alter the metabolism of oral contraceptives.

Interactions with statins
Many immunosuppressive agents can contribute to hyperlipidaemia, which is a common problem after organ transplantation. 3-Hydroxy-3-methylglutaryl CoA reductase inhibitors (statins) are now the most widely prescribed lipid-lowering agents and clinical trials have shown a reduction in cardiac events and mortality in hyperlipidaemic nontransplant patients [350–352]. However, many of the statins are metabolized through the cyctochrome P450 system, and pharmacokinetic interactions between statins and ciclosporin have been observed that result in an increased risk of rhabdomyolysis or myopathy [353,354]. It has been recommended that concurrent administration of statins and immunosuppressive agents metabolized by cytochrome P450 should be undertaken with caution, using low doses, and patients should be closely monitored [355]. All patients should be advised to report any side effects such as muscle pain, tenderness or weakness, particularly if accompanied by malaise or fever. Pravastatin may be safer than many of the statins because its interaction with ciclosporin is minimal [356].

Calcium channel blockers
These drugs are frequently used to treat hypertension and may have renal protective properties in transplant recipients. Both diltiazem and verapamil inhibit the metabolism of ciclosporin and tacrolimus [357,358].

Allopurinol
Renal dysfunction is common in transplant patients and ciclosporin itself can cause hyperuricaemia. Consequently, some transplant patients will develop gout. Allopurinol, which is frequently used as a prophylactic agent to prevent recurrent episodes, acts by inhibiting xanthine oxidase, so reducing the production of uric acid. However, xanthine oxidase is also involved in the metabolism of azathioprine; coadministration of the two drugs may cause serious bone marrow suppression. It is generally recommended that, if treatment with allopurinol is required, the dose of azathioprine should be reduced to 25% of the original dose and the patient's blood count must be carefully monitored [183–185,359]. However, a safer alternative may be to switch the patient from azathioprine to mycophenolate as it has no interaction with allopurinol.

Management of pharmacokinetic interactions
The information available about many interactions is based on either in vitro and animal data or clinical case reports. Since there are marked differences in pharmacokinetic parameters between individuals, the magnitude of drug interactions may also be expected to vary between patients. Strong drug interactions will have an effect in most cases (e.g. rifampicin, anticovulsants, imidazole antifungals, nondihydropyridine calcium channel blockers) whereas weaker interactions may be more apparent in

some individuals than in others. It is not possible to predict the size of an effect for a specific patient.

Management depends on an awareness of the interactions that are known to occur and others that may be expected on theoretical grounds. Where there is a choice of effective agents, the physician should choose a drug that is unlikely to cause a serious interaction, for example pravastatin to treat hypercholesterolaemia or sodium valproate to control postoperative seizures. Macrolide antibiotics should be avoided whenever possible. Occasionally, it may be appropriate to modify the immunosuppressive regimen to accommodate the new treatment, for example changing from azathioprine to mycophenolate to allow the use of allopurinol.

When a drug that may interact with the immunosuppressive therapy has to be used, plans should be made to monitor immunosuppressant drug levels, efficacy and toxicity, more frequently so that the dose administered can be adjusted. It must be appreciated that the maximum effect of an interaction may be delayed since enzyme induction will not occur immediately. Where the metabolism of a drug is reduced, its half-life will be prolonged and the time required to reach a new steady state (four to five half-lives) will be increased. Increased monitoring, therefore, may be needed for a prolonged period. Furthermore, additional monitoring and dose adjustment will be required again when the interacting drug is discontinued [314]. A useful 'rule of thumb' is that, when the interacting drug is discontinued, more frequent monitoring should continue until the dose of the immunosuppressant required and drug level have returned to those observed before commencing the interacting drug.

Pharmacodynamic interactions

Interactions between drugs with similar side effects can result in additive or even synergistic toxicity. The most common problem to arise in practice is the need to use other nephrotoxic drugs with either ciclosporin or tacrolimus; examples include nonsteroidal anti-inflammatory agents [360], aminoglycoside antibiotics [361,362], intravenously administered amphotericin [363,364], high dose co-trimoxazole [365], foscarnet [366], aciclovir [367] and fibrates [368,369]. The myelosuppressive effects of azathioprine and mycophenolate can be exacerbated by other drugs that cause bone marrow toxicity, including ganciclovir and co-trimoxazole.

Ciclosporin can sometimes cause hyperkalaemia, which can be exacerbated by angiotensin converting enzyme inhibitors [370], angiotensin receptor blockers [371] and potassium-retaining diuretics.

Whenever possible, drugs that do not potentiate the toxicity of the existing treatment regimen should be used. However, such interactions cannot always be avoided; in such cases careful monitoring is necessary and the additional treatment should be discontinued as soon as possible.

Over-the-counter medicines

In most countries, there are a number of preparations available without prescription that may cause problems to patients receiving pharmacological immunosuppression: for example, nonsteroidal anti-inflammatory drugs [360] (which are available alone and are also present in a number of proprietary products) and the herbal remedy St John's Wort [321]. To avoid problems with such drugs, all transplant patients must be educated about the possibility of drug interactions and the importance of informing the pharmacist of their ongoing treatment before purchasing 'over-the counter' drugs. Information packs for family physicians and the provision of a telephone help-line for patients and doctors can also help to prevent prescribing errors.

Therapeutic drug monitoring

Most immunosuppressive agents have dose-limiting toxicity in dose ranges used for clinical immunosuppression. There are substantial variations between individuals in the rate at which drugs are metabolized. In addition, the relationship between the dose administered and systemic exposure to the drug can be influenced by a variety of factors, including dietary intake, the coadministration of other drugs and the use of herbal remedies.

These observations have led to the use of measurements of the concentrations of several immunosuppressive agents in the blood and concentration-guided dose adjustment with the aim of maximizing efficacy while minimizing the risk of toxicity. This strategy is described as therapeutic drug monitoring (TDM).

TDM has certain general limitations. The concentration measured (usually that in whole blood) is not the concentration at the site of action and need not bear a direct relationship to it. The trough (pre-dose or minimum) level is usually determined, but this may not always be the most appropriate surrogate measure of the drug's effect. Therefore, the optimum timing and the utility of such measurements must be empirically determined for each drug. The concentrations measured in individual patients are subject to a degree of day-to-day variation that is independent of the dose ingested. The recommended therapeutic blood concentrations are broad; furthermore, the appropriate drug concentration may vary according to the clinical situation and the other immunosuppressive agents that are being administered. TDM can be of particular value in the management of the coadministration of drugs that have pharmacokinetic interactions and in investigations of cases of unexpected toxicity or lack of efficacy as well as documenting patient nonadherence with the therapy prescribed.

An alternative approach is that of pharmacodynamic drug monitoring. This approach seeks to measure the therapeutic action of the drug either directly [372] or indirectly. Indirect measurements using in vitro assays of T-cell activation following exposure to a mitogen or antigens may be used to assess the overall effect of a combination of immunosuppressive agents [373–375]. While these techniques have great potential, it has not been established whether they are predictive of clinical events; the complexity of the alloimmune response may make it difficult to model using such in vitro assays.

Ciclosporin

Whole blood is the preferred matrix for ciclosporin measurements [376]. The relation between ciclosporin trough concentration and immunosuppressive efficacy has been studied extensively. However, the 'therapeutic range' derived from a population of patients is usually wide and individuals with ciclosporin levels within range can still experience either rejection or nephrotoxicity [377].

The frequency of measurement depends on clinical factors such as the time elapsed since transplantation, intercurrent illness, evidence of rejection or toxicity and concomitant treatment with drugs that affect ciclosporin's pharmacokinetics. In the immediate post-transplantation period the recommended frequency of monitoring is once every 24 to 48 hours [378]. The frequency can be gradually reduced, once the patient has become clinically stable, to monthly for the first year and then at one- to three-monthly intervals thereafter. However, additional measurements should be performed if clinical signs or symptoms suggest that dosage adjustments may be necessary or if the patient is given another medication known to interact.

There are three immunoassays available in addition to a high performance liquid chromatography method. The immunoassays show a positive bias, probably due to cross-reactivity of ciclosporin metabolites, i.e. these assays are not completely specific for the parent drug. A survey conducted in 1994–5 showed that most centres recommend a higher range of target concentrations during the early postoperative period [378]. Doses are then tapered to a lower maintenance concentration, usually three to six months

after transplantation (although some centres taper the dose over 12 months or more). The survey also showed that the target range of ciclosporin concentration used for heart transplants is higher than that for kidney or liver transplants.

Efforts should be made to maintain stable blood ciclosporin concentrations, as fluctuations in blood level have been found to be a risk factor for acute rejection of both lung and kidney transplants [379,380]. The microemulsion formulation of ciclosporin (Neoral) has better absorption characteristics, which result in an improved correlation of trough concentration level with systemic exposure (AUC) compared with the original Sandimmun formulation ($r = 0.66$ versus 0.17) [381].

Studies of the absorption of Neoral have led to a new approach in TDM, that of absorption profiling and the use of limited sampling strategies to obtain a better estimate of systemic exposure. The greatest degree of inter- and intra-individual variability in ciclosporin blood concentrations occurs during the absorption phase (i.e. the first four hours postdose) [382]. Measurements obtained during this period provide a better measure of exposure than the conventional pre-dose 'trough' level (C_0).

In liver and kidney transplantation, the measurement of blood concentration two hours after the administration of an oral dose (C_2), which approximates to the maximum concentration (C_{max}), has been shown to be a better predictor of the clinical effect than C_0. Another approach to estimation of AUC is to obtain a limited number of blood samples during the four hour absorption phase [383–386].

Tacrolimus

Whole blood is the matrix currently recommended for the measurement of tacrolimus concentrations. There are two immunoassay kits available (IMX and Pro-Trac), both of which use the same monoclonal antibody but have different methods of detection. In addition, a highly specific liquid chromatography/tandem mass spectrometry method has been developed [387].

A number of studies have compared the immunoassays with the chromatography/spectrometry method; they have all observed a positive bias, with the immunoassays ranging from 3% to 20% [387–389]. This bias is due to cross-reactivity of several tacrolimus metabolites in the immunoassays [390].

The target range used for tacrolimus trough concentration varies with time after transplantation and the type of transplant as well as varying between transplant centres. In 1995 a preliminary target range of 5–20 μg/L was recommended [391].

A global survey was conducted in 1997 to determine the therapeutic ranges for tacrolimus currently employed in 30 selected centres [387]. The majority were using immunoassays. Most centres recommended a higher target range during the early postoperative and postrescue period and then decreased to a lower maintenance range. In liver and kidney transplants the ranges recommended were 10–15 μg/L initially and reduced to 5–10 μg/L for long-term therapy. Slightly higher target ranges were suggested for heart (10–18 μg/L followed by 8–15 μg/L). There were no major differences between the target ranges for primary or rescue treatment or when tacrolimus was used as part of 'double' or 'triple' drug immunosuppression regimens or between adult and paediatric patients.

The correlation between trough level and AUC is generally high, indicating that pharmacokinetic profiling methods are not necessary for monitoring tacrolimus therapy [392–394].

Mycophenolic acid

Mycophenolate mofetil is rapidly hydrolysed to mycophenolic acid after oral administration and the esterfied prodrug cannot be detected in plasma. More than 99% of mycophenolic acid (mycophenolate) in blood is retained in the plasma fraction and plasma is recommended as the matrix of choice for its measurement [395,396]. High performance liquid chromatography is considered to be the reference method of measurement; in addition an enzyme-multiplied immunoassay technique is available [397].

A low systemic exposure to mycophenolic acid (AUC) is a risk factor for acute rejection [398,399]. At a constant dose of mycophenolate mofetil, exposure to mycophenolate increases with time after renal transplantation [398,399].

While there is a clear relationship between systemic exposure to mycophenolate (AUC) and its therapeutic action, the value of mycophenolate trough levels or limited sampling strategies to estimate AUC remain to be established [399]. The enterohepatic circulation of mycophenolate produces a biphasic concentration curve that could limit the value of trough level monitoring [398].

The major clinical trials that studied mycophenolate mofetil as a maintenance immunosuppressant after renal or heart transplantation used fixed dose regimens, in combination with ciclosporin and corticosteroids, and did not use TDM. The more recent observations that mycophenolate levels differ between patients receiving ciclosporin or tacrolimus [325–327] have raised the possibility that concentration-controlled mycophenolate therapy may be particularly important in patients treated with tacrolimus [400].

Sirolimus

Sirolimus is extensively bound in red blood cells and whole blood is the recommended matrix for measurement of sirolimus. There is no immunoassay available and measurements are made by high performance liquid chromatography combined with detection by either ultraviolet light or by mass spectrometry. The latter method is preferable because it is specific for the parent compound [401,402].

Trough levels observed after 2 mg of sirolimus was administered to renal transplant recipients in combination with ciclosporin were 8 ± 4 ng/mL [237,238]. The probability of acute rejection was related to the trough level in individual patients, suggesting that adjustment of sirolimus dose according to trough levels may help to reduce the incidence of acute rejection [239]. Some side effects have been found to be concentration related, including thrombocytopenia, leukopenia and hyperlipidaemia [239].

The target sirolimus blood levels that have been used in studies of immunosuppression without a calcineurin inhibitor have been considerably higher (20–30 ng/mL immediately after transplantation falling to 15 ng/mL for maintenance therapy) [240,241]. Currently the recommended ranges of blood concentrations are 4–12 ng/mL when administered with ciclosporin and 12–20 ng/mL without. Systemic exposure (AUC) is strongly correlated with both the 12 and the 24 hour trough concentrations [236].

Other agents

No methods have been established for the routine monitoring of azathioprine, corticosteroids, daclizumab or basiliximab. ATG and muromonab-CD3 are not monitored directly but their effects can be monitored through changes in the number of circulating lymphocytes with specific surface markers (e.g. CD3-positive cells). The development of human anti-mouse antibody, which may block the effects of muromonab-CD3, can also be monitored [403–406].

Clinical immunosuppression

The clinical use of immunosuppressive agents will be addressed briefly since the management of acute and chronic rejection is discussed in detail elsewhere in this book.

Table 18.11. Potential advantages and disadvantages of 'induction therapy' with biological anti T-cell agents

Advantage	Disadvantage
Intensified immunosuppression early after transplantation when the risk of rejection is greatest	First dose side effects with muromonab-CD3 and with ATG
Reduced incidence of acute rejection	Increased incidence and severity of infection including CMV
Delay of rejection until graft function becomes stable	Increased risk of PTLD
Reduced reliance on drugs with difficult pharmacokinetics in the postoperative phase	Increased cost related to the drug and need for further antimicrobial prophylaxis
Ability to delay introduction of nephrotoxic drugs such as ciclosporin	Nephrotoxicity of muromonab-CD3
	No evidence of graft-specific tolerance in humans

Note: ATG, antithymocyte globulin; CMV, cytomegalovirus; PTLD, post-transplantation lymphoproliferative disease.

Immunosuppression can be considered to consist of several phases: initial or induction therapy, maintenance treatment (which may be adjusted with increasing time after transplantation) and the management of rejection.

Induction therapy

Some transplant centres use induction therapy (ATG, muromonab-CD3, daclizumab or basiliximab) immediately after lung transplantation [407]. There are both advantages and disadvantages in the use of an induction agent (Table 18.11) and the relative importance of these varies depending on the type of transplant as well as the induction agent involved.

Induction therapy can reduce the incidence of acute rejection; in one study of ATG induction in lung transplantation, this was associated with a trend towards a lower incidence of BOS [408]. However, the use of ATG and muromonab-CD3 antibody treatment is associated with an increased risk of infection [409], which is a particular concern in lung transplantation. The newer biologically engineered antibodies have improved the control of acute rejection after renal transplantation without increasing the

risk of infection [298,302–4]. However, there is currently no evidence that the use of these agents in lung transplantation will reduce the risk of bronchiolitis obliterans.

Maintenance immunosuppression

Currently most centres use a triple drug regimen for maintenance immunosuppression consisting of a calcineurin inhibitor (ciclosporin or tacrolimus), corticosteroids and an antiproliferative agent (mycophenolate mofetil or azathioprine).

Although some single centre or small multicentre studies have suggested that tacrolimus may be superior to ciclosporin for maintenance therapy after lung transplantation [128,130], there have been no large randomized multicentre controlled trials to confirm this; therefore the choice of calcineurin inhibitor is currently determined by other considerations such as the differing side effect profiles of the two drugs and by physician preference.

Mycophenolate has been found to be superior to azathioprine for controlling acute rejection after renal and heart transplantation [201–204] and may be of benefit after lung transplantation [224,225]. A multicenter trial comparing these two drugs after lung transplantation is nearing completion and this will clarify whether mycophenolate is better at preventing acute rejection or bronchiolitis obliterans.

After the period of highest risk for acute rejection (three to six months after transplantation) most physicians gradually reduce the doses of both the calcineurin inhibitor and corticosteroids to reduce the risk of side effects. Unfortunately, there is currently no laboratory test that can indicate how far immunosuppression should be reduced in an individual patient. Therefore practice in this area varies between transplant centres and even between individual physicians; weaning of drugs such as corticosteroids must be conducted on a 'trial and error' basis.

Treatment of acute rejection

Changes in the chest radiograph are frequently an indicator of rejection early after transplantation whereas functional (spirometric) changes are the commonest presenting feature thereafter. Whenever possible the diagnosis should be confirmed by bronchoscopy, bronchoalveolar lavage and transbronchial biopsy because clinical differentiation of acute rejection from pulmonary infection is frequently difficult, and sometimes the two conditions may coexist [410,411].

The choice of treatment will depend on several factors (Table 18.12). Most episodes will respond to a course of

Table 18.12. Factors that may influence the choice of treatment for an episode of acute rejection

- Background immunosuppression including adequacy of drug levels
- Histological severity as assessed by biopsy
- Clinical severity and impact on graft function
- History of previous rejection
- Response during treatment (functional and histological)

intravenous injections of methylprednisolone followed by a temporary increase in the maintenance dose of oral prednisolone [174]. The dose of the other maintenance immunosuppressive drugs should be adjusted appropriately. If the episode has occurred later after transplantation, when some of the prophylactic antimicrobial therapy has been discontinued, prophylaxis should be restarted. Some centres favour the use of a follow-up transbronchial lung biopsy after treatment because lymphocytic infiltrates may persist despite an apparently good functional response [412].

More severe episodes, and those which do not respond to corticosteroids, may require treatment with ATG or muromonab-CD3 [413]. The risk of corticosteroid resistant rejection is in part related to the efficacy of the maintenance immunosuppression protocol that is being used [120,126]. However, steroid-resistant rejection is also more common more than six months after lung transplantation [414].

Many centres will change the background immunosuppression that is being used in cases of severe or recurrent rejection, for example substituting tacrolimus for ciclosporin [131,132,415] or mycophenolate for azathioprine [221,222,224,416].

Treatment of bronchiolitis obliterans syndrome

Bronchiolitis obliterans is the most common serious long-term complication of lung transplantation. It is often regarded as 'chronic rejection' of the transplanted lung but it is a multifactorial process and is related to both immune and nonimmune factors. The disease has an active inflammatory phase that is followed by a fibroproliferative phase, which leads to a patchy obliteration of the small airways of the lung. Histological proof is often difficult to obtain in life and so the diagnosis is often made on functional criteria after excluding other causes of deteriorating lung function (bronchiolitis obliterans syndrome, BOS) [417]; computed tomography (CT) chest and pulmonary radionucleotide studies can provide supportive data. Like many chronic diseases, bronchiolitis obliterans frequently follows a variable course, with episodes of acute deterioration punctuated by periods of relative stability.

In view of its complex pathogenesis and variable clinical course, it is perhaps not surprising that it has been difficult to demonstrate unequivocally that increased immunosuppression is beneficial in this condition. Various measures have been investigated, usually in small single centre studies, including switching from ciclosporin to tacrolimus [418] or from azathioprine to mycophenolate [224,419], treatment with muromonab-CD3 or ATG [420,421] and the use of total nodal lymphoid irradiation [422].

Unfortunately many patients continue to follow a downhill course despite these measures. At this stage they may develop recurrent infections because of either their degree of immunosuppression or the development of secondary bronchiectasis. Since infection is often the terminal event in such patients, a judicious reduction in immunosuppression coupled with careful antimicrobial prophylaxis may help to extend the life of patients with advanced disease. In those few patients where retransplantation may be a realistic possibility, care should be taken to protect their renal function as far as it is possible to do so.

Adjunctive antimicrobial prophylaxis

Due to the nonspecific nature of pharmacological immunosuppression, infection remains one of the most common complications after lung transplantation [57]. The risks of infection can be reduced by antimicrobial prophylaxis such as the use of co-trimoxazole to prevent *Pneumocystis carinii* pneumonia, nebulized amphotericin to reduce the risk of pulmonary *Aspergillus* infection and prophylaxis or monitoring and pre-emptive therapy to control CMV infection

Conclusion

Steady progress has been made in the field of pharmacological immunosuppression and the incidence of acute rejection after heart, liver and kidney transplantation has fallen. Many of the immunosuppressive agents and protocols have not been rigorously tested in lung transplant patients. However, this situation is changing and randomized multicentre trials with adequate statistical power are now being conducted in lung transplantation. It remains to be determined whether improved pharmacological immunosuppression will have a substantial impact on the long-term problem of bronchiolitis obliterans.

A wider choice of immunosuppressive agents will probably help transplant physicians to minimize the burden of drug toxicity in their patients. However the problems associated with nonspecific immunosuppression (infection, lymphoproliferative disease and an increased risk of other malignancies) will remain until a method of inducing graft-specific tolerance is ready for clinical application.

REFERENCES

1 Matzinger P, Bevan MJ. Hypothesis: why do so many lymphocytes respond to major histocompatibility antigens? *Cell Immunol* 1977;**29**: 1–5.

2 Sherman LA, Chattopadhyay S. The molecular basis of allorecognition. *Annu Rev Immunol* 1993; **11**: 385–402.

3 Tilney NL, Padberg WM, Lord RH, et al. Synergy between subtherapeutic doses of cyclosporine and immunobiological manipulations in rat heart graft recipients. *Transplantation* 1988; **46**(2 Suppl): 122S–128S.

4 Ueda H, Hancock WW, Cheung YC, Diamantstein T, Tilney NL, Kupiec-Weglinski JW. The mechanism of synergistic interaction between anti-interleukin 2 receptor monoclonal antibody and cyclosporine therapy in rat recipients of organ allografts. *Transplantation* 1990; **50**: 545–550.

5 Squifflet JP, Sutherland DE, Rynasiewicz JJ, Field J, Heil J, Najarian JS. Combined immunosuppressive therapy with cyclosporin A and azathioprine. A synergistic effect in three of four experimental models. *Transplantation* 1982; **34**: 315–318.

6 Penn I. Post-transplant malignancy: the role of immunosuppression. *Drug Saf* 2000; **23**: 101–113.

7 Fishman JA, Rubin RH. Infection in organ-transplant recipients. *N Engl J Med* 1998; **338**: 1741–1751.

8 Borel JF, Feurer C, Gubler HU, Stahelin H. Biological effects of cyclosporin A: a new antilymphocytic agent. *Agents Actions* 1976; **6**: 468–475.

9 Allison AC, Almquist SJ, Muller CD, Eugui EM. In vitro immunosuppressive effects of mycophenolic acid and an ester pro-drug, RS-61443. *Transplant Proc* 1991; **23**(2 Suppl 2): 10–14.

10 Amlot PL, Rawlings E, Fernando ON, et al. Prolonged action of a chimeric interleukin-2 receptor (CD25) monoclonal antibody used in cadaveric renal transplantation. *Transplantation* 1995; **60**: 748–756.

11 Cooper JD, Billingham M, Egan T, et al. A working formulation for the standardization of nomenclature and for clinical staging of chronic dysfunction in lung allografts. International Society for Heart and Lung Transplantation. *J Heart Lung Transplant* 1993; **12**: 713–716.

12 Azuma H, Tilney NL. Immune and nonimmune mechanisms of chronic rejection of kidney allografts. *J Heart Lung Transplant* 1995; **14**: S136–S142.

13 Banner NR. Coronary arterial disease in the cardiac allograft. In: Rose ML, ed. *Transplant-associated coronary artery disease.* Landes Bioscience, Georgetown, TX, 2001; 1–25.

14 Merrill JP, Murray JE, Harrison JH, Guild WR. Successful homotransplantation of the kidney between identical twins. *JAMA* 1956; **160**: 277–282.

15 Hume DM, Jackson BT, Zukoski CF, Lee HM, Kauffman HM, Ecdahl RH. The homotransplantation of kidneys and of fetal liver and spleen after total body irradiation. *Ann Surg* 1960; **152**: 354–373.

16 Merill JP, Murray JE, Harrison JH, Freidman EA, Dealy JBJ, Dammin GJ. Successful homotransplantation of the kidney between non-identical twins. *N Engl J Med* 1960; **262**: 1251–1260.

17 Schwartz R, Dameshek W. The effect of 6-mercaptopurine on homograft reactions. *J Clin Invest* 1960; **39**: 952–958.

18 Schwartz R, Stack J, Damashek W. Effect of 6-mercaptopurine on antibody production. *Proc Soc Exp Biol Med* 1958; **99**: 164–167.

19 Calne RY. The rejection of renal homografts: inhibition in dogs by 6-mercaptopurine. *Lancet* 1960; **1**: 417–418.

20 Murray JE, Merill JP, Harrison JH, Wilson RE, Dammin GJ. Prolonged survival of human kidney homografts by immunosuppressive drug therapy. *N Engl J Med* 1963; **268**: 1315–1323.

21 Billingham RE, Krohn PL, Medawar PB. Effect of locally applied cortisone acetate on survival of skin homografts in rabbits. *Br Med J* 1951; **2**: 1049–1053.

22 Billingham RE, Krohn PL, Medawar PB. Effect of cortisone acetate on survival of skin homografts in rabbits. *Br Med J* 1951; **1**: 1157–1163.

23 Marchioro TL, Axtell HK, LaVia MF, Waddell WR, Strazl TE. The role of adrenocorticosteroids in reversing established homograft rejection. *Surgery* 1964; **55**: 412–417.

24 Woodruff MFA, Anderson NF. Effect of lymphocyte depletion by thoracic duct fistula and administration of antilymphocyte serum on the survival of skin homografts in rats. *Nature* 1963; **200**: 702.

25 Levy RH, Medawar PB. Some experiments on the action of anti-lymphoid antisera. *Ann NY Acad Sci* 1966; **129**: 164–177.

26 Starzl TE, Marchioro TL, Hutchinson DE, Porter KA, Cerilli GJ, Brettschneider L. The clinical use of antilymphocyte globulin in renal homotransplantation. *Transplantation* 1967; **5**(Suppl): 1100–1105.

27 Kohler G, Milstein C. Continuous cultures of fused cells secreting antibody of predefined specificity. *Nature* 1975; **256**: 495–497.

28 Kung P, Goldstein G, Reinherz EL, Schlossman SF. Monoclonal antibodies defining distinctive human T cell surface antigens. *Science* 1979; **206**: 347–349.

29 Reinherz EL, Kung PC, Goldstein G, Schlossman SF. Further characterization of the human inducer T cell subset defined by monoclonal antibody. *J Immunol* 1979; **123**: 2894–2896.

30 Cosimi AB, Burton RC, Colvin RB, et al. Treatment of acute renal allograft rejection with OKT3 monoclonal antibody. *Transplantation* 1981; **32**: 535–539.

31 Wildevuur CR, Benfield JR. A review of 23 human lung transplantations by 20 surgeons. *Ann Thorac Surg* 1970; **9**: 489–515.

32 Borel JF, Kis ZL. The discovery and development of cyclosporine (Sandimmune). *Transplant Proc* 1991; **23**: 1867–1874.

33 Green CJ, Allison AC. Extensive prolongation of rabbit kidney allograft survival after short-term cyclosporin-A treatment. *Lancet* 1978; **1**: 1182–1183.

34 Calne RY, Rolles K, White DJ, et al. Cyclosporin A initially as the only immunosuppressant in 34 recipients of cadaveric organs: 32 kidneys, 2 pancreases, and 2 livers. *Lancet* 1979; **2**: 1033–1036.

35 Myers BD, Ross J, Newton L, Luetscher J, Perlroth M. Cyclosporine-associated chronic nephropathy. *N Engl J Med* 1984; **311**: 699–705.

36 Canadian Multicenter Transplant Study Group. A randomized clinical trial of cyclosporine in cadaveric renal transplantation. *N Engl J Med* 1983; **309**: 809–815.

37 Sarris GE, Moore KA, Schroeder JS, et al. Cardiac transplantation: the Stanford experience in the cyclosporine era. *J Thorac Cardiovasc Surg* 1994; **108**: 240–252.

38 Reitz BA, Wallwork JL, Hunt SA, et al. Heart–lung transplantation: successful therapy for patients with pulmonary vascular disease. *N Engl J Med* 1982; **306**: 557–564.

39 Kino T, Hatanaka H, Miyata S, et al. FK-506, a novel immunosuppressant isolated from a *Streptomyces*. II. Immunosuppressive effect of FK-506 in vitro. *J Antibiot* (Tokyo) 1987; **40**: 1256–1265.

40 Schreiber SL, Crabtree GR. The mechanism of action of cyclosporin A and FK506. *Immunol Today* 1992; **13**: 136–142.

41 Sigal NH, Dumont FJ. Cyclosporin A, FK-506, and rapamycin: pharmacologic probes of lymphocyte signal transduction. *Annu Rev Immunol* 1992; **10**: 519–560.

42 Eugui EM, Almquist SJ, Muller CD, Allison AC. Lymphocyte-selective cytostatic and immunosuppressive effects of mycophenolic acid in vitro: role of deoxyguanosine nucleotide depletion. *Scand J Immunol* 1991; **33**: 161–173.

43 Williams GM, Hume DM, Hudson RP Jr, Morris PJ, Kano K, Milgrom F. 'Hyperacute' renal-homograft rejection in man. *N Engl J Med* 1968; **279**: 611–618.

44 Patel R, Terasaki PI. Significance of the positive crossmatch test in kidney transplantation. *N Engl J Med* 1969; **280**: 735–739.

45 Terasaki PI, Kreisler M, Mickey RM. Presensitization and kidney transplant failures. *Postgrad Med J* 1971; **47**: 89–100.

46 Smith JD, Danskine AJ, Laylor RM, Rose ML, Yacoub MH. The effect of panel reactive antibodies and the donor specific crossmatch on graft survival after heart and heart–lung transplantation. *Transplant Immunol* 1993; **1**: 60–65.

47 Choi JK, Kearns J, Palevsky HI, et al. Hyperacute rejection of a pulmonary allograft. Immediate clinical and pathologic findings. *Am J Respir Crit Care Med* 1999; **160**: 1015–1018.

48 Scornik JC, Zander DS, Baz MA, Donnelly WH, Staples ED. Susceptibility of lung transplants to preformed donor-specific HLA antibodies as detected by flow cytometry. *Transplantation* 1999; **68**: 1542–1546.

49 Bittner HB, Dunitz J, Hertz M, Bolman MR III, Park SJ. Hyperacute rejection in single lung transplantation – case report of successful management by means of plasmapheresis and antithymocyte globulin treatment. *Transplantation* 2001; **71**: 649–651.

50 Hall BM, Dorsch S, Roser B. The cellular basis of allograft rejection in vivo. I. The cellular requirements for first-set rejection of heart grafts. *J Exp Med* 1978; **148**: 878–889.

51 Rosenberg AS, Mizuochi T, Sharrow SO, Singer A. Phenotype, specificity, and function of T cell subsets and T cell interactions involved in skin allograft rejection. *J Exp Med* 1987; **165**: 1296–1315.

52 Hornick P, Lechler R. Direct and indirect pathways of alloantigen recognition: relevance to acute and chronic allograft rejection. *Nephrol Dial Transplant* 1997; **12**: 1806–1810.

53 Sayegh MH, Turka LA. The role of T-cell costimulatory activation pathways in transplant rejection. *N Engl J Med* 1998; **338**: 1813–1821.

54 Russell JH, Ley TJ. Lymphocyte-mediated cytotoxicity. *Annu Rev Immunol* 2002; **20**: 323–370.

55 Adams DO, Hamilton TA. The cell biology of macrophage activation. *Annu Rev Immunol* 1984; **2**: 283–318.

56 Doody DP, Stenger KS, Winn HJ. Immunologically nonspecific mechanisms of tissue destruction in the rejection of skin grafts. *J Exp Med* 1994; **179**: 1645–1652.

57 Hosenpud JD, Bennett LE, Keck BM, Boucek MM, Novick RJ. The Registry of the International Society for Heart and Lung Transplantation: 18th official report – 2001. *J Heart Lung Transplant* 2001; **20**: 805–815.

58 Heng D, Sharples LD, McNeil K, Stewart S, Wreghitt T, Wallwork J. Bronchiolitis obliterans syndrome: incidence, natural history, prognosis, and risk factors. *J Heart Lung Transplant* 1998; **17**: 1255–1263.

59 Crabtree GR. Contingent genetic regulatory events in T lymphocyte activation. *Science* 1989; **243**: 355–361.

60 Abramowicz D, Schandene L, Goldman M, et al. Release of tumor necrosis factor, interleukin-2, and gamma-interferon in serum after injection of OKT3 monoclonal antibody in kidney transplant recipients. *Transplantation* 1989; **47**: 606–608.

61 Barber EK, Dasgupta JD, Schlossman SF, Trevillyan JM, Rudd CE. The CD4 and CD8 antigens are coupled to a protein-tyrosine kinase (p56lck) that phosphorylates the CD3 complex. *Proc Natl Acad Sci USA* 1989; **86**: 3277–3281.

62 Rudd CE. CD4, CD8 and the TCR–CD3 complex: a novel class of protein-tyrosine kinase receptor. *Immunol Today* 1990; **11**: 400–406.

63 Weiss A, Imboden JB. Cell surface molecules and early events involved in human T lymphocyte activation. *Adv Immunol* 1987; **41**: 1–38.

64 Liu J. FK506 and cyclosporin, molecular probes for studying intracellular signal transduction. *Immunol Today* 1993; **14**: 290–295.

65 Mosmann TR, Cherwinski H, Bond MW, Giedlin MA, Coffman RL. Two types of murine helper T cell clone. I. Definition

according to profiles of lymphokine activities and secreted proteins. *J Immunol* 1986; **136**: 2348–2357.

66 O'Garra A. Interleukins and the immune system 1. *Lancet* 1989; **1**: 943–947.

67 Kuo CJ, Chung J, Fiorentino DF, Flanagan WM, Blenis J, Crabtree GR. Rapamycin selectively inhibits interleukin-2 activation of p70 S6 kinase. *Nature* 1992; **358**: 70–73.

68 Mathew A, Talbot D, Minford EJ, et al. Reversal of steroid-resistant rejection in renal allograft recipients using FK506. *Transplantation* 1995; **60**: 1182–1184.

69 Siekierka JJ, Staruch MJ, Hung SH, Sigal NH. FK-506, a potent novel immunosuppressive agent, binds to a cytosolic protein which is distinct from the cyclosporin A-binding protein, cyclophilin. *J Immunol* 1989; **143**: 1580–1583.

70 Walsh CT, Zydowsky LD, McKeon FD. Cyclosporin A, the cyclophilin class of peptidylprolyl isomerases, and blockade of T cell signal transduction. *J Biol Chem* 1992; **267**: 13115–13118.

71 Sawada S, Suzuki G, Kawase Y, Takaku F. Novel immunosuppressive agent, FK506. In vitro effects on the cloned T cell activation. *J Immunol* 1987; **139**: 1797–1803.

72 Wiederrecht G, Lam E, Hung S, Martin M, Sigal N. The mechanism of action of FK-506 and cyclosporin A. *Ann NY Acad Sci* 1993; **696**: 9–19.

73 Mohamed MA, Robertson H, Booth TA, Balupuri S, Kirby JA, Talbot D. TGF-beta expression in renal transplant biopsies: a comparative study between cyclosporin-A and tacrolimus. *Transplantation* 2000; **69**: 1002–1005.

74 El-Gamel A, Awad M, Sim E, et al. Transforming growth factor-beta 1 and lung allograft fibrosis. *Eur J Cardiothorac Surg* 1998; **13**: 424–430.

75 Khanna A, Cairns V, Hosenpud JD. Tacrolimus induces increased expression of transforming growth factor-beta 1 in mammalian lymphoid as well as nonlymphoid cells. *Transplantation* 1999; **67**: 614–619.

76 Jurcevic S, Dunn MJ, Crisp S, et al. A new enzyme-linked immunosorbent assay to measure anti-endothelial antibodies after cardiac transplantation demonstrates greater inhibition of antibody formation by tacrolimus compared with cyclosporine. *Transplantation* 1998; **65**: 1197–1202.

77 van Gelder T, Klupp J, Sawamoto T, Christians U, Morris RE. ATP-binding cassette transporters and calcineurin inhibitors: potential clinical implications. *Transplant Proc* 2001; **33**: 2420–2421.

78 Jette L, Beaulieu E, Leclerc JM, Beliveau R. Cyclosporin A treatment induces overexpression of P-glycoprotein in the kidney and other tissues. *Am J Physiol* 1996; **270**: F756–F765.

79 Hauser IA, Koziolek M, Hopfer U, Thevenod F. Therapeutic concentrations of cyclosporine A, but not FK506, increase P-glycoprotein expression in endothelial and renal tubule cells. *Kidney Int* 1998; **54**: 1139–1149.

80 Zanker B, Barth C, Stachowski J, Baldamus CA, Land W. Multidrug resistance gene *MDR1* expression: a gene transfection in vitro model and clinical analysis in cyclosporine-treated patients rejecting their renal grafts. *Transplant Proc* 1997; **29**: 1507–1508.

81 Vergara E, Gomez-Morales M, Ramirez C, et al. P-glycoprotein expression in acute kidney graft rejection. *Transplant Proc* 1998; **30**: 2425–2426.

82 Mueller EA, Kovarik JM, van Bree JB, Tetzloff W, Grevel J, Kutz K. Improved dose linearity of cyclosporine pharmacokinetics from a microemulsion formulation. *Pharm Res* 1994; **11**: 301–304.

83 Banner NR, David OJ, Leaver N, et al. Pharmacokinetics of oral cyclosporine (Neoral) in heart transplant recipients during the immediate period after surgery. *Transpl Int* 2002; **15**: 649–654.

84 Gurecki J, Warty V, Sanghvi A. The transport of cyclosporine in association with plasma lipoproteins in heart and liver transplant patients. *Transplant Proc* 1985; **17**: 1997–2002.

85 Lemaire M, Tillement JP. Role of lipoproteins and erythrocytes in the in vitro binding and distribution of cyclosporin A in the blood. *J Pharm Pharmacol* 1982; **34**: 715–718.

86 Christians U, Sewing KF. Cyclosporin metabolism in transplant patients. *Pharmacol Ther* 1993; **57**: 291–345.

87 Venkataramanan R, Swaminathan A, Prasad T, et al. Clinical pharmacokinetics of tacrolimus. *Clin Pharmacokinet* 1995; **29**: 404–430.

88 Christiaans M, van Duijnhoven E, Beysens T, Undre N, Schafer A, van Hooff J. Effect of breakfast on the oral bioavailability of tacrolimus and changes in pharmacokinetics at different times posttransplant in renal transplant recipients. *Transplant Proc* 1998; **30**: 1271–1273.

89 Beysens AJ, Wijnen RM, Beuman GH, van der Heyden J, Kootstra G, van As H. FK 506: monitoring in plasma or in whole blood? *Transplant Proc* 1991; **23**: 2745–2747.

90 Undre NA, Schafer A. Factors affecting the pharmacokinetics of tacrolimus in the first year after renal transplantation. European Tacrolimus Multicentre Renal Study Group. *Transplant Proc* 1998; **30**: 1261–1263.

91 Sattler M, Guengerich FP, Yun CH, Christians U, Sewing KF. Cytochrome P-450 3A enzymes are responsible for biotransformation of FK506 and rapamycin in man and rat. *Drug Metab Dispos* 1992; **20**: 753–761.

92 Lampen A, Christians U, Gonschior AK, et al. Metabolism of the macrolide immunosuppressant, tacrolimus, by the pig gut mucosa in the Ussing chamber. *Br J Pharmacol* 1996; **117**: 1730–1734.

93 Lampen A, Christians U, Guengerich FP, et al. Metabolism of the immunosuppressant tacrolimus in the small intestine: cytochrome P450, drug interactions, and interindividual variability. *Drug Metab Dispos* 1995; **23**: 1315–1324.

94 Porayko MK, Textor SC, Krom RA, et al. Nephrotoxic effects of primary immunosuppression with FK-506 and cyclosporine regimens after liver transplantation. *Mayo Clin Proc* 1994; **69**: 105–111.

95 Kopp JB, Klotman PE. Cellular and molecular mechanisms of cyclosporin nephrotoxicity. *J Am Soc Nephrol* 1990; **1**: 162–179.

96 de Mattos AM, Olyaei AJ, Bennett WM. Nephrotoxicity of immunosuppressive drugs: long-term consequences and challenges for the future. *Am J Kidney Dis* 2000; **35**: 333–346.

97 Reams GP. Do calcium channel blockers have renal protective effects? *Drugs Aging* 1994; **5**: 263–287.

98 Rodicio JL. Calcium antagonists and renal protection from cyclosporine nephrotoxicity: long-term trial in renal transplantation patients. *J Cardiovasc Pharmacol* 2000; **35**(3 Suppl 1): S7–S11.

99 Sokal EM, Antunes H, Beguin C, et al. Early signs and risk factors for the increased incidence of Epstein–Barr virus-related posttransplant lymphoproliferative diseases in pediatric liver transplant recipients treated with tacrolimus. *Transplantation* 1997; **64**: 1438–1442.

100 Atkison P, Joubert G, Barron A, et al. Hypertrophic cardiomyopathy associated with tacrolimus in paediatric transplant patients. *Lancet* 1995; **345**: 894–896.

101 Singer DR, Jenkins GH. Hypertension in transplant recipients. *J Hum Hypertens* 1996; **10**: 395–402.

102 Pham SM, Kormos RL, Hattler BG, et al. A prospective trial of tacrolimus (FK 506) in clinical heart transplantation: intermediate-term results. *J Thorac Cardiovasc Surg* 1996; **111**: 764–772.

103 Taylor DO, Barr ML, Radovancevic B, et al. A randomized, multicenter comparison of tacrolimus and cyclosporine immunosuppressive regimens in cardiac transplantation: decreased hyperlipidemia and hypertension with tacrolimus. *J Heart Lung Transplant* 1999; **18**: 336–345.

104 Keogh A, Macdonald P, Harvison A, Richens D, Mundy J, Spratt P. Initial steroid-free versus steroid-based maintenance therapy and steroid withdrawal after heart transplantation: two views of the steroid question. *J Heart Lung Transplant* 1992; **11**: 421–427.

105 Ballantyne CM, Podet EJ, Patsch WP, et al. Effects of cyclosporine therapy on plasma lipoprotein levels. *JAMA* 1989; **262**: 53–56.

106 Abouljoud MS, Levy MF, Klintmalm GB. Hyperlipidemia after liver transplantation: long-term results of the FK506/cyclosporine A US multicenter trial. US Multicenter Study Group. *Transplant Proc* 1995; **27**: 1121–1123.

107 Hjelmesaeth J, Hartmann A, Kofstad J, et al. Glucose intolerance after renal transplantation depends upon prednisolone dose and recipient age. *Transplantation* 1997; **64**: 979–983.

108 Roth D, Milgrom M, Esquenazi V, Fuller L, Burke G, Miller J. Posttransplant hyperglycemia. Increased incidence in cyclosporine-treated renal allograft recipients. *Transplantation* 1989; **47**: 278–281.

109 Pirsch JD, Miller J, Deierhoi MH, Vincenti F, Filo RS. A comparison of tacrolimus (FK506) and cyclosporine for immunosuppression after cadaveric renal transplantation. FK506 Kidney Transplant Study Group. *Transplantation* 1997; **63**: 977–983.

110 Canadian Multicentre Transplant Study Group. A randomized clinical trial of cyclosporine in cadaveric renal transplantation. Analysis at three years. *N Engl J Med* 1986; **314**: 1219–1225.

111 Gianello P, Squifflet JP, Pirson Y, Stoffel M, Dereme T, Alexandre GP. Cyclosporine-steroids versus conventional therapy in cadaver kidney transplantation: analysis of a randomized trial at two years. *Transplant Proc* 1987; **19**: 1867–1872.

112 Calne RY. Cyclosporin in cadaveric renal transplantation: 5-year follow-up of a multicentre trial. *Lancet* 1987; **2**: 506–507.

113 Hunt SA, Gamberg P, Stinson EB, Oyer PE, Shumway NE. The Stanford experience: survival and renal function in the pre-Sandimmune era compared to the Sandimmune era. *Transplant Proc* 1990; **22**(3 Suppl 1): 1–5.

114 Grevel J, Welsh MS, Kahan BD. Cyclosporine monitoring in renal transplantation: area under the curve monitoring is superior to trough-level monitoring. *Ther Drug Monit* 1989; **11**: 246–248.

115 Grevel J, Kahan BD. Area under the curve monitoring of cyclosporine therapy: the early posttransplant period. *Ther Drug Monit* 1991; **13**: 89–95.

116 Noble S, Markham A. Cyclosporin. A review of the pharmacokinetic properties, clinical efficacy and tolerability of a microemulsion-based formulation (Neoral). *Drugs* 1995; **50**: 924–941.

117 Mikhail G, Eadon H, Leaver N, et al. An investigation of the pharmacokinetics, toxicity, and clinical efficacy of Neoral cyclosporin in cystic fibrosis patients. *Transplant Proc* 1997; **29**: 599–601.

118 Pollard SG, Lear PA, Ready AR, Moore RH, Johnson RW. Comparison of microemulsion and conventional formulations of cyclosporine A in preventing acute rejection in de novo kidney transplant patients. The UK Neoral Renal Study Group. *Transplantation* 1999; **68**: 1325–1331.

119 Keown P, Niese D. Cyclosporine microemulsion increases drug exposure and reduces acute rejection without incremental toxicity in de novo renal transplantation. International Sandimmun Neoral Study Group. *Kidney Int* 1998; **54**: 938–944.

120 Eisen HJ, Hobbs RE, Davis SF, et al. Safety, tolerability, and efficacy of cyclosporine microemulsion in heart transplant recipients: a randomized, multicenter, double-blind comparison with the oil-based formulation of cyclosporine – results at 24 months after transplantation. *Transplantation* 2001; **71**: 70–78.

121 Trull AK, Tan KK, Tan L, Alexander GJ, Jamieson NV. Enhanced absorption of new oral cyclosporin microemulsion formulation, Neoral, in liver transplant recipients with external biliary diversion. *Transplant Proc* 1994; **26**: 2977–2978.

122 Hemming AW, Greig PD, Cattral MS, et al. A microemulsion of cyclosporine without intravenous cyclosporine in liver transplantation. *Transplantation* 1996; **62**: 1798–1802.

123 Otto MG, Mayer AD, Clavien PA, Cavallari A, Gunawardena KA, Mueller EA. Randomized trial of cyclosporine microemulsion (Neoral) versus conventional cyclosporine in liver transplantation: MILTON study. Multicentre International Study in Liver Transplantation of Neoral. *Transplantation* 1998; **66**: 1632–1640.

124 Shah MB, Martin JE, Schroeder TJ, First MR. The evaluation of the safety and tolerability of two formulations of cyclosporine: Neoral and Sandimmune. A meta-analysis. *Transplantation* 1999; **67**: 1411–1417.

125 Mayer AD, Dmitrewski J, Squifflet JP, et al. Multicenter randomized trial comparing tacrolimus (FK506) and cyclosporine in the prevention of renal allograft rejection: a report of the European Tacrolimus Multicenter Renal Study Group. *Transplantation* 1997; **64**: 436–443.

126 European FK506 Multicentre Liver Study Group. Randomised trial comparing tacrolimus (FK506) and cyclosporin in prevention of liver allograft rejection. *Lancet* 1994; **344**: 423–428.

127 US Multicenter FK506 Liver Study Group. A comparison of tacrolimus (FK 506) and cyclosporine for immunosuppression in liver transplantation. *N Engl J Med* 1994; **331**: 1110–1115.

128 Griffith BP, Bando K, Hardesty RL, et al. A prospective randomized trial of FK506 versus cyclosporine after human pulmonary transplantation. *Transplantation* 1994; **57**: 848–851.

129 Keenan RJ, Konishi H, Kawai A, et al. Clinical trial of tacrolimus versus cyclosporine in lung transplantation. *Ann Thorac Surg* 1995; **60**: 580–585.

130 Treede H, Klepetko W, Reichenspurner H, et al. Tacrolimus versus cyclosporine after lung transplantation: a prospective, open, randomized two-center trial comparing two different immunosuppressive protocols. *J Heart Lung Transplant* 2001; **20**: 511–517.

131 Mentzer RM Jr, Jahania MS, Lasley RD. Tacrolimus as a rescue immunosuppressant after heart and lung transplantation. The US Multicenter FK506 Study Group. *Transplantation* 1998; **65**: 109–113.

132 Woodle ES, Thistlethwaite JR, Gordon JH, et al. A multicenter trial of FK506 (tacrolimus) therapy in refractory acute renal allograft rejection. A report of the Tacrolimus Kidney Transplantation Rescue Study Group. *Transplantation* 1996; **62**: 594–599.

133 Cohn LA. Glucocorticosteroids as immunosuppressive agents. *Semin Vet Med Surg* (Small Anim) 1997; **12**: 150–156.

134 Cupps TR, Fauci AS. Corticosteroid-mediated immunoregulation in man. *Immunol Rev* 1982; **65**: 133–155.

135 Adcock IM. Glucocorticoid-regulated transcription factors. *Pulm Pharmacol Ther* 2001; **14**: 211–219.

136 Gerrard TL, Cupps TR, Jurgensen CH, Fauci AS. Hydrocortisone-mediated inhibition of monocyte antigen presentation: dissociation of inhibitory effect and expression of DR antigens. *Cell Immunol* 1984; **85**: 330–339.

137 Mokoena T, Gordon S. Human macrophage activation. Modulation of mannosyl, fucosyl receptor activity in vitro by lymphokines, gamma and alpha interferons, and dexamethasone. *J Clin Invest* 1985; **75**: 624–631.

138 Snyder DS, Unanue ER. Corticosteroids inhibit murine macrophage Ia expression and interleukin 1 production. *J Immunol* 1982; **129**: 1803–1805.

139 Dinarello CA, Mier JW. Lymphokines. *N Engl J Med* 1987; **317**: 940–945.

140 Zanker B, Walz G, Wieder KJ, Strom TB. Evidence that glucocorticosteroids block expression of the human interleukin-6 gene by accessory cells. *Transplantation* 1990; **49**: 183–185.

141 Refojo D, Liberman AC, Holsboer F, Arzt E. Transcription factor-mediated molecular mechanisms involved in the functional cross-talk between cytokines and glucocorticoids. *Immunol Cell Biol* 2001; **79**: 385–394.

142 Planey SL, Litwack G. Glucocorticoid-induced apoptosis in lymphocytes. *Biochem Biophys Res Commun* 2000; **279**: 307–312.

143 Gruber SA, Chan GLC, Canafax DM, Matas AJ. Immunosuppression in renal transplantation. II. Corticosteroids, antilymphocyte globulin and OKT3. *Clin Transplant* 1991; **5**: 219–232.

144 Barnes PJ, Karin M. Nuclear factor-kappaB: a pivotal transcription factor in chronic inflammatory diseases. *N Engl J Med* 1997; **336**: 1066–1071.

145 Van Laethem F, Baus E, Andris F, Urbain J, Leo O. A novel aspect of the anti-inflammatory actions of glucocorticoids: inhibition of proximal steps of signaling cascades in lymphocytes. *Cell Mol Life Sci* 2001; **58**: 1599–1606.

146 Bennett WM, Barry JM. Failure of dexamethasone to provide adequate chronic immunosuppression for renal transplantation. *Transplantation* 1979; **27**: 218–219.

147 Ferry JJ, Horvath AM, Bekersky I, Heath EC, Ryan CF, Colburn WA. Relative and absolute bioavailability of prednisone and prednisolone after separate oral and intravenous doses. *J Clin Pharmacol* 1988; **28**: 81–87.

148 Al-Habet S, Rogers HJ. Pharmacokinetics of intravenous and oral prednisolone. *Br J Clin Pharmacol* 1980; **10**: 503–508.

149 Frey BM, Frey FJ. Clinical pharmacokinetics of prednisone and prednisolone. *Clin Pharmacokinet* 1990; **19**: 126–146.

150 Bergrem H, Grottum P, Rugstad HE. Pharmacokinetics and protein binding of prednisolone after oral and intravenous administration. *Eur J Clin Pharmacol* 1983; **24**: 415–419.

151 Garg V, Jusko WJ. Bioavailability and reversible metabolism of prednisone and prednisolone in man. *Biopharm Drug Dispos* 1994; **15**: 163–172.

152 Barth J, Damoiseaux M, Mollmann H, Brandis KH, Hochhaus G, Derendorf H. Pharmacokinetics and pharmacodynamics of prednisolone after intravenous and oral administration. *Int J Clin Pharmacol Ther Toxicol* 1992; **30**: 317–324.

153 Al-Habet SM, Rogers HJ. Methylprednisolone pharmacokinetics after intravenous and oral administration. *Br J Clin Pharmacol* 1989; **27**: 285–290.

154 Stjernholm MR, Katz FH. Effects of diphenylhydantoin, phenobarbital, and diazepam on the metabolism of methylprednisolone and its sodium succinate. *J Clin Endocrinol Metab* 1975; **41**: 887–893.

155 Curtis JJ, Galla JH, Woodford SY, Lucas BA, Luke RG. Effect of alternate-day prednisone on plasma lipids in renal transplant recipients. *Kidney Int* 1982; **22**: 42–47.

156 Vesco L, Busson M, Bedrossian J, Bitker MO, Hiesse C, Lang P. Diabetes mellitus after renal transplantation: characteristics, outcome, and risk factors. *Transplantation* 1996; **61**: 1475–1478.

157 Moe SM. The treatment of steroid-induced bone loss in transplantation. *Curr Opin Nephrol Hypertens* 1997; **6**: 544–549.

158 Aris RM, Neuringer IP, Weiner MA, Egan TM, Ontjes D. Severe osteoporosis before and after lung transplantation. *Chest* 1996; **109**: 1176–1183.

159 Shane E, Silverberg SJ, Donovan D, et al. Osteoporosis in lung transplantation candidates with end-stage pulmonary disease. *Am J Med* 1996; **101**: 262–269.

160 Bachrach LK, Loutit CW, Moss RB. Osteopenia in adults with cystic fibrosis. *Am J Med* 1994; **96**: 27–34.

161 Rodino MA, Shane E. Osteoporosis after organ transplantation. *Am J Med* 1998; **104**: 459–469.

162 Julian BA, Laskow DA, Dubovsky J, Dubovsky EV, Curtis JJ, Quarles LD. Rapid loss of vertebral mineral density after renal transplantation. *N Engl J Med* 1991; **325**: 544–550.

163 Horber FF, Casez JP, Steiger U, Czerniak A, Montandon A, Jaeger P. Changes in bone mass early after kidney transplantation. *J Bone Miner Res* 1994; **9**: 1–9.

164 Grotz WH, Rump LC, Niessen A, et al. Treatment of osteopenia and osteoporosis after kidney transplantation. *Transplantation* 1998; **66**: 1004–1008.

165 Pichette V, Bonnardeaux A, Prudhomme L, Gagne M, Cardinal J, Ouimet D. Long-term bone loss in kidney transplant recipients: a cross-sectional and longitudinal study. *Am J Kidney Dis* 1996; **28**: 105–114.

166 Neuhaus R, Lohmann R, Platz KP, et al. Treatment of osteoporosis after liver transplantation. *Transplant Proc* 1995; **27**: 1226–1227.

167 Mulder H, Struys A. Intermittent cyclical etidronate in the prevention of corticosteroid-induced bone loss. *Br J Rheumatol* 1994; **33**: 348–350.

168 Diamond T, McGuigan L, Barbagallo S, Bryant C. Cyclical etidronate plus ergocalciferol prevents glucocorticoid-induced bone loss in postmenopausal women. *Am J Med* 1995; **98**: 459–463.

169 Adachi JD, Bensen WG, Brown J, et al. Intermittent etidronate therapy to prevent corticosteroid-induced osteoporosis. *N Engl J Med* 1997; **337**: 382–387.

170 Saag KG, Emkey R, Schnitzer TJ, et al. Alendronate for the prevention and treatment of glucocorticoid-induced osteoporosis. Glucocorticoid-Induced Osteoporosis Intervention Study Group. *N Engl J Med* 1998; **339**: 292–299.

171 Singer FR, Aldred JP, Neer RM, Krane SM, Potts JT Jr, Bloch KJ. An evaluation of antibodies and clinical resistance to salmon calcitonin. *J Clin Invest* 1972; **51**: 2331–2338.

172 Haddad JG Jr, Caldwell JG. Calcitonin resistance: clinical and immunologic studies in subjects with Paget's disease of bone treated with porcine and salmon calcitonins. *J Clin Invest* 1972; **51**: 3133–3141.

173 Park GD, Bartucci M, Smith MC. High- versus low-dose methylprednisolone for acute rejection episodes in renal transplantation. *Nephron* 1984; **36**: 80–83.

174 Trulock EP. Management of lung transplant rejection. *Chest* 1993; **103**: 1566–1576.

175 Citterio F. Steroid side effects and their impact on transplantation outcome. *Transplantation* 2001; **72**(12 Suppl): S75–S80.

176 Hricik DE, Almawi WY, Strom TB. Trends in the use of glucocorticoids in renal transplantation. *Transplantation* 1994; **57**: 979–989.

177 Fryer JP, Granger DK, Leventhal JR, Gillingham K, Najarian JS, Matas AJ. Steroid-related complications in the cyclosporine era. *Clin Transplant* 1994; **8**: 224–229.

178 Elion GB. Symposium on immunosuppressive drugs. Biochemistry and pharmacology of purine analogues. *Fedn Proc* 1967; **26**: 898–904.

179 Elion GB. Nobel lecture. The purine path to chemotherapy. *Biosci Rep* 1989; **9**: 509–529.

180 Halloran PF, Leung S. Approved immunosuppressants. In: Norma DJ, Suki WN, eds. *Primer on transplantation*. American Society of Transplant Physicians, Thorofare, NJ, 1998, 93–102.

181 Elion GB. The purine path to chemotherapy. *Science* 1989; 244: 41–47.

182 Chan GL, Erdmann GR, Gruber SA, Matas AJ, Canafax DM. Azathioprine metabolism: pharmacokinetics of 6-mercaptopurine, 6-thiouric acid and 6-thioguanine nucleotides in renal transplant patients. *J Clin Pharmacol* 1990; **30**: 358–363.

183 Boulieu R, Lenoir A, Bertocchi M, Mornex JF. Intracellular thiopurine nucleotides and azathioprine myelotoxicity in organ transplant patients. *Br J Clin Pharmacol* 1997; **43**: 116–118.

184 Kennedy DT, Hayney MS, Lake KD. Azathioprine and allopurinol: the price of an avoidable drug interaction. *Ann Pharmacother* 1996; **30**: 951–954.

185 Cummins D, Sekar M, Halil O, Banner N. Myelosuppression associated with azathioprine-allopurinol interaction after heart and lung transplantation. *Transplantation* 1996; **61**: 1661–1662.

186 Coulthard SA, Hall AG. Recent advances in the pharmacogenomics of thiopurine methyltransferase. *Pharmacogenomics J* 2001; **1**: 254–261.

187 Escousse A, Guedon F, Mounie J, Rifle G, Mousson C, D'Athis P. 6-Mercaptopurine pharmacokinetics after use of azathioprine in renal transplant recipients with intermediate or high thiopurine methyl transferase activity phenotype. *J Pharm Pharmacol* 1998; **50**: 1261–1266.

188 Weinshilboum R. Thiopurine pharmacogenetics: clinical and molecular studies of thiopurine methyltransferase. *Drug Metab Dispos* 2001; **29**: 601–605.

189 Pollak R, Nishikawa RA, Mozes MF, Jonasson O. Azathioprine-induced leukopenia – clinical significance in renal transplantation. *J Surg Res* 1980; **29**: 258–264.

190 DeClerck YA, Ettenger RB, Ortega JA, Pennisi AJ. Macrocytosis and pure RBC anemia caused by azathioprine. *Am J Dis Child* 1980; **134**: 377–379.

191 Old CW, Flannery EP, Grogan TM, Stone WH, San Antonio RP. Azathioprine-induced pure red blood cell aplasia. *JAMA* 1978; **240**: 552–554.

192 Romagnuolo J, Sadowski DC, Lalor E, Jewell L, Thomson AB. Cholestatic hepatocellular injury with azathioprine: a case

report and review of the mechanisms of hepatotoxicity. *Can J Gastroenterol* 1998; **12**: 479–483.

193 Sparberg M, Simon N, del Greco F. Intrahepatic cholestasis due to azathioprine. *Gastroenterology* 1969; **57**: 439–441.

194 Marubbio AT, Danielson B. Hepatic veno-occlusive disease in a renal transplant patient receiving azathioprine. *Gastroenterology* 1975; **69**: 739–743.

195 Read AE, Wiesner RH, LaBrecque DR, et al. Hepatic veno-occlusive disease associated with renal transplantation and azathioprine therapy. *Ann Intern Med* 1986; **104**: 651–655.

196 Vandepitte K, Vanrenterghem Y, Michielsen P. Azathioprine hypersensitivity in a renal transplant recipient. *Transpl Int* 1990; **3**: 47–48.

197 Walder BK, Robertson MR, Jeremy D. Skin cancer and immunosuppression. *Lancet* 1971; **2**: 1282–1283.

198 Taylor AE, Shuster S. Skin cancer after renal transplantation: the causal role of azathioprine. *Acta Derm Venereol* 1992; **72**: 115–119.

199 Lennard L, Thomas S, Harrington CI, Maddocks JL. Skin cancer in renal transplant recipients is associated with increased concentrations of 6-thioguanine nucleotide in red blood cells. *Br J Dermatol* 1985; **113**: 723–729.

200 Allison AC, Eugui EM. Immunosuppressive and other effects of mycophenolic acid and an ester prodrug, mycophenolate mofetil. *Immunol Rev* 1993; **136**: 5–28.

201 Placebo-controlled study of mycophenolate mofetil combined with cyclosporin and corticosteroids for prevention of acute rejection. European Mycophenolate Mofetil Cooperative Study Group. *Lancet* 1995; **345**: 1321–1325.

202 A blinded, randomized clinical trial of mycophenolate mofetil for the prevention of acute rejection in cadaveric renal transplantation. The Tricontinental Mycophenolate Mofetil Renal Transplantation Study Group. *Transplantation* 1996; **61**: 1029–1037.

203 Sollinger HW. Mycophenolate mofetil for the prevention of acute rejection in primary cadaveric renal allograft recipients. US Renal Transplant Mycophenolate Mofetil Study Group. *Transplantation* 1995; **60**: 225–232.

204 Kobashigawa J, Miller L, Renlund D, et al. A randomized active-controlled trial of mycophenolate mofetil in heart transplant recipients. Mycophenolate Mofetil Investigators. *Transplantation* 1998; **66**: 507–515.

205 Natsumeda Y, Carr SF. Human type I and II IMP dehydrogenases as drug targets. *Ann NY Acad Sci* 1993; **696**: 88–93.

206 Eugui EM, Mirkovich A, Allison AC. Lymphocyte-selective antiproliferative and immunosuppressive effects of mycophenolic acid in mice. *Scand J Immunol* 1991; **33**: 175–183.

207 Sokoloski JA, Sartorelli AC. Effects of the inhibitors of IMP dehydrogenase, tiazofurin and mycophenolic acid, on glycoprotein metabolism. *Mol Pharmacol* 1985; **28**: 567–573.

208 Blaheta RA, Leckel K, Wittig B, et al. Mycophenolate mofetil impairs transendothelial migration of allogeneic CD4 and CD8 T-cells. *Transplant Proc* 1999; **31**: 1250–1252.

209 Bertalanffy P, Dubsky P, Wolner E, Weigel G. Alterations of endothelial nucleotide levels by mycophenolic acid result in changes of membrane glycosylation and E-selectin expression. *Clin Chem Lab Med* 1999; **37**: 259–264.

210 Grailer A, Nichols J, Hullett D, Sollinger HW, Burlingham WJ. Inhibition of human B cell responses in vitro by RS-61443, cyclosporine A and DAB486 IL-2. *Transplant Proc* 1991; **23**: 314–315.

211 Smith KG, Isbel NM, Catton MG, Leydon JA, Becker GJ, Walker RG. Suppression of the humoral immune response by mycophenolate mofetil. *Nephrol Dial Transplant* 1998; **13**: 160–164.

212 Mohacsi PJ, Tuller D, Hulliger B, Wijngaard PL. Different inhibitory effects of immunosuppressive drugs on human and rat aortic smooth muscle and endothelial cell proliferation stimulated by platelet-derived growth factor or endothelial cell growth factor. *J Heart Lung Transplant* 1997; **16**: 484–492.

213 Bullingham R, Monroe S, Nicholls A, Hale M. Pharmacokinetics and bioavailability of mycophenolate mofetil in healthy subjects after single-dose oral and intravenous administration. *J Clin Pharmacol* 1996; **36**: 315–324.

214 Wolfe EJ, Mathur V, Tomlanovich S, et al. Pharmacokinetics of mycophenolate mofetil and intravenous ganciclovir alone and in combination in renal transplant recipients. *Pharmacotherapy* 1997; **17**: 591–598.

215 Seebacher G, Mallinger R, Laufer G, et al. Pharmacokinetics of mycophenolate mofetil in heart transplant recipients. *Adv Exp Med Biol* 1998; **431**: 801–803.

216 Simmons WD, Rayhill SC, Sollinger HW. Preliminary risk–benefit assessment of mycophenolate mofetil in transplant rejection. *Drug Saf* 1997; **17**: 75–92.

217 Shaw LM, Mick R, Nowak I, Korecka M, Brayman KL. Pharmacokinetics of mycophenolic acid in renal transplant patients with delayed graft function. *J Clin Pharmacol* 1998; **38**: 268–275.

218 Nowak I, Shaw LM. Effect of mycophenolic acid glucuronide on inosine monophosphate dehydrogenase activity. *Ther Drug Monit* 1997; **19**: 358–360.

219 Puggia R, Rizzolo M, Maresca MC, Calconi G, Vianello A. Tolerance of mycophenolate mofetil is dependent on kidney function. *Transplant Proc* 1998; **30**: 2228.

220 Halloran P, Mathew T, Tomlanovich S, Groth C, Hooftman L, Barker C. Mycophenolate mofetil in renal allograft recipients: a pooled efficacy analysis of three randomized, double-blind, clinical studies in prevention of rejection. The International Mycophenolate Mofetil Renal Transplant Study Groups. *Transplantation* 1997; **63**: 39–47.

221 Mycophenolate Mofetil Acute Renal Rejection Study Group. Mycophenolate mofetil for the treatment of a first acute renal allograft rejection. *Transplantation* 1998; **65**: 235–241.

222 Mycophenolate Mofetil Renal Refractory Rejection Study Group. Mycophenolate mofetil for the treatment of refractory, acute, cellular renal transplant rejection. *Transplantation* 1996; **61**: 722–729.

223 Zuckermann A, Birsan T, Thaghavi S, et al. Mycophenolate mofetil in lung transplantation. *Transplant Proc* 1998; **30**: 1514–1516.

224 Ross DJ, Waters PF, Levine M, Kramer M, Ruzevich S, Kass RM. Mycophenolate mofetil versus azathioprine immunosuppressive regimens after lung transplantation: preliminary experience. *J Heart Lung Transplant* 1998; **17**: 768–774.

225 Zuckermann A, Klepetko W, Birsan T, et al. Comparison between mycophenolate mofetil- and azathioprine-based immunosuppressions in clinical lung transplantation. *J Heart Lung Transplant* 1999; **18**: 432–40.

226 Vilella-Bach M, Nuzzi P, Fang Y, Chen J. The FKBP12-rapamycin-binding domain is required for FKBP12-rapamycin-associated protein kinase activity and G1 progression. *J Biol Chem* 1999; **274**: 4266–4272.

227 Sehgal SN. Rapamune (RAPA, rapamycin, sirolimus): mechanism of action of immunosuppressive effect results from blockade of signal transduction and inhibition of cell cycle progression. *Clin Biochem* 1998; **31**: 335–340.

228 Dumont FJ, Staruch MJ, Koprak SL, Melino MR, Sigal NH. Distinct mechanisms of suppression of murine T cell activation by the related macrolides FK-506 and rapamycin. *J Immunol* 1990; **144**: 251–258.

229 Bierer BE, Mattila PS, Standaert RF, et al. Two distinct signal transmission pathways in T lymphocytes are inhibited by complexes formed between an immunophilin and either FK506 or rapamycin. *Proc Natl Acad Sci USA* 1990; **87**: 9231–9235.

230 Marx SO, Jayaraman T, Go LO, Marks AR. Rapamycin–FKBP inhibits cell cycle regulators of proliferation in vascular smooth muscle cells. *Circ Res* 1995; **76**: 412–417.

231 Fahrni JA, Berry GJ, Morris RE, Rosen GD. Rapamycin inhibits development of obliterative airway disease in a murine heterotopic airway transplant model. *Transplantation* 1997; **63**: 533–537.

232 Kelly PA, Gruber SA, Behbod F, Kahan BD. Sirolimus, a new, potent immunosuppressive agent. *Pharmacotherapy* 1997; **17**: 1148–1156.

233 Lampen A, Zhang Y, Hackbarth I, Benet LZ, Sewing KF, Christians U. Metabolism and transport of the macrolide immunosuppressant sirolimus in the small intestine. *J Pharmacol Exp Ther* 1998; **285**: 1104–1112.

234 MacDonald A, Scarola J, Burke JT, Zimmerman JJ. Clinical pharmacokinetics and therapeutic drug monitoring of sirolimus. *Clin Ther* 2000; **22**(Suppl B): B101–B121.

235 Kaplan B, Meier-Kriesche HU, Napoli KL, Kahan BD. The effects of relative timing of sirolimus and cyclosporine microemulsion formulation coadminstration on the pharmacokinetics of each agent. *Clin Pharmacol Ther* 1998; **63**: 48–53.

236 Zimmerman JJ, Kahan BD. Pharmacokinetics of sirolimus in stable renal transplant patients after multiple oral dose administration. *J Clin Pharmacol* 1997; **37**: 405–415.

237 Kahan BD. Efficacy of sirolimus compared with azathioprine for reduction of acute renal allograft rejection: a randomised multicentre study. The Rapamune US Study Group. *Lancet* 2000; **356**: 194–202.

238 MacDonald AS. A worldwide, phase III, randomized, controlled, safety and efficacy study of a sirolimus/cyclosporine regimen for prevention of acute rejection in recipients of primary mismatched renal allografts. *Transplantation* 2001; **71**: 271–280.

239 Kahan BD, Napoli KL, Kelly PA, et al. Therapeutic drug monitoring of sirolimus: correlations with efficacy and toxicity. *Clin Transplant* 2000; **14**: 97–109.

240 Groth CG, Backman L, Morales JM, et al. Sirolimus (rapamycin)-based therapy in human renal transplantation: similar efficacy and different toxicity compared with cyclosporine. Sirolimus European Renal Transplant Study Group. *Transplantation* 1999; **67**: 1036–1042.

241 Kreis H, Cisterne JM, Land W, et al. Sirolimus in association with mycophenolate mofetil induction for the prevention of acute graft rejection in renal allograft recipients. *Transplantation* 2000; **69**: 1252–1260.

242 Andoh TF, Lindsley J, Franceschini N, Bennett WM. Synergistic effects of cyclosporine and rapamycin in a chronic nephrotoxicity model. *Transplantation* 1996; **62**: 311–316.

243 Johnson RW, Kreis H, Oberbauer R, Brattstrom C, Claesson K, Eris J. Sirolimus allows early cyclosporine withdrawal in renal transplantation resulting in improved renal function and lower blood pressure. *Transplantation* 2001; **72**: 777–786.

244 Bonnefoy-Berard N, Vincent C, Revillard JP. Antibodies against functional leukocyte surface molecules in polyclonal antilymphocyte and antithymocyte globulins. *Transplantation* 1991; **51**: 669–673.

245 Preville X, Nicolas L, Flacher M, Revillard J. A quantitative flow cytometry assay for the preclinical testing and pharmacological monitoring of rabbit antilymphocyte globulins (rATG). *J Immunol Methods* 2000; **245**: 45–54.

246 Bonnefoy-Berard N, Genestier L, Flacher M, et al. Apoptosis induced by polyclonal antilymphocyte globulins in human B-cell lines. *Blood* 1994; **83**: 1051–1059.

247 Preville X, Flacher M, LeMauff B, et al. Mechanisms involved in antithymocyte globulin immunosuppressive activity in a non-human primate model. *Transplantation* 2001; **71**: 460–468.

248 Genestier L, Fournel S, Flacher M, Assossou O, Revillard JP, Bonnefoy-Berard N. Induction of Fas (Apo-1, CD95)-mediated apoptosis of activated lymphocytes by polyclonal antithymocyte globulins. *Blood* 1998; **91**: 2360–2368.

249 Bonnefoy-Berard N, Fournel S, Genestier L, Flacher M, Quemeneur L, Revillard JP. In vitro functional properties of antithymocyte globulins: clues for new therapeutic applications? *Transplant Proc* 1998; **30**: 4015–4017.

250 Merion RM, Howell T, Bromberg JS. Partial T-cell activation and anergy induction by polyclonal antithymocyte globulin. *Transplantation* 1998; **65**: 1481–1489.

251 Bunn D, Lea CK, Bevan DJ, Higgins RM, Hendry BM. The pharmacokinetics of anti-thymocyte globulin (ATG) following intravenous infusion in man. *Clin Nephrol* 1996; **45**: 29–32.

252 Shenton BK, White MD, Bell AE, et al. The paradox of ATG monitoring in renal transplantation. *Transplant Proc* 1994; **26**: 3177–3180.

253 Fietze E, Prosch S, Reinke P, et al. Cytomegalovirus infection in transplant recipients. The role of tumor necrosis factor. *Transplantation* 1994; **58**: 675–680.

254 Opelz G, Henderson R. Incidence of non-Hodgkin lymphoma in kidney and heart transplant recipients. *Lancet* 1993; **342**: 1514–1516.

255 Bonnefoy-Berard N, Flacher M, Revillard JP. Antiproliferative effect of antilymphocyte globulins on B cells and B-cell lines. *Blood* 1992; **79**: 2164–2170.

256 Brennan DC, Flavin K, Lowell JA, et al. A randomized, double-blinded comparison of Thymoglobulin versus Atgam for induction of immunosuppressive therapy in adult renal transplant recipients. *Transplantation* 1999; **67**: 1011–1018.

257 Gaber AO, First MR, Tesi RJ, et al. Results of the double-blind, randomized, multicenter, phase III clinical trial of Thymoglobulin versus Atgam in the treatment of acute graft rejection episodes after renal transplantation. *Transplantation* 1998; **66**: 29–37.

258 Norman DJ. Mechanisms of action and overview of OKT3. *Ther Drug Monit* 1995; **17**: 615–620.

259 Singh N, Dummer JS, Kusne S, et al. Infections with cytomegalovirus and other herpesviruses in 121 liver transplant recipients: transmission by donated organ and the effect of OKT3 antibodies. *J Infect Dis* 1988; **158**: 124–131.

260 Gaston RS, Deierhoi MH, Patterson T, et al. OKT3 first-dose reaction: association with T cell subsets and cytokine release. *Kidney Int* 1991; **39**: 141–148.

261 Hibberd PL, Tolkoff-Rubin NE, Cosimi AB, et al. Symptomatic cytomegalovirus disease in the cytomegalovirus antibody seropositive renal transplant recipient treated with OKT3. *Transplantation* 1992; **53**: 68–72.

262 Swinnen LJ, Fisher RI. OKT3 monoclonal antibodies induce interleukin-6 and interleukin-10: a possible cause of lymphoproliferative disorders associated with transplantation. *Curr Opin Nephrol Hypertens* 1993; **2**: 670–678.

263 Portela D, Patel R, Larson-Keller JJ, et al. OKT3 treatment for allograft rejection is a risk factor for cytomegalovirus disease in liver transplantation. *J Infect Dis* 1995; **171**: 1014–1018.

264 Todd PA, Brogden RN. Muromonab CD3. A review of its pharmacology and therapeutic potential. *Drugs* 1989; **37**: 871–899.

265 Chatenoud L. Humoral immune response against OKT3. *Transplant Proc* 1993; **25**:(2 Suppl 1): 68–73.

266 Goldstein G, Fuccello AJ, Norman DJ, Shield CF III, Colvin RB, Cosimi AB. OKT3 monoclonal antibody plasma levels during therapy and the subsequent development of host antibodies to OKT3. *Transplantation* 1986; **42**: 507–511.

267 Schroeder TJ, First MR, Hurtubise PE, et al. Immunologic monitoring with Orthoclone OKT3 therapy. *J Heart Transplant* 1989; **8**: 371–380.

268 Schroeder TJ, Michael AT, First MR, et al. Variations in serum OKT3 concentration based upon age, sex, transplanted organ, treatment regimen, and anti-OKT3 antibody status. *Ther Drug Monit* 1994; **16**: 361–367.

269 Bock HA, Gallati H, Zurcher RM, et al. A randomized prospective trial of prophylactic immunosuppression with ATG-fresenius versus OKT3 after renal transplantation. *Transplantation* 1995; **59**: 830–840.

270 Goldstein G, Norman DJ, Henell KR, Smith IL. Pharmacokinetic study of orthoclone OKT3 serum levels during treatment of acute renal allograft rejection. *Transplantation* 1988; **46**: 587–589.

271 Thomas DM, Nicholls AJ, Feest TG, Riad H. OKT3 and cerebral oedema. [Letter] *Br Med J* (Clin Res Edn) 1987; **295**: 1486.

272 Coleman AE, Norman DJ. OKT3 encephalopathy. *Ann Neurol* 1990; **28**: 837–838.

273 Shihab FS, Barry JM, Norman DJ. Encephalopathy following the use of OKT3 in renal allograft transplantation. *Transplant Proc* 1993; **25**(2 Suppl 1): 31–34.

274 Costanzo-Nordin MR. Cardiopulmonary effects of OKT3: determinants of hypotension, pulmonary edema, and cardiac dysfunction. *Transplant Proc* 1993; **25**(2 Suppl 1): 21–24.

275 Radhakrishnan J, Cohen DJ. Cytokine-release syndrome: general risk-factor modification – preparation of high-risk patients for use of OKT3. *Transplant Proc* 1993; **25**(2 Suppl 1): 60–62.

276 Wilde MI, Goa KL. Muromonab CD3: a reappraisal of its pharmacology and use as prophylaxis of solid organ transplant rejection. *Drugs* 1996; **51**: 865–894.

277 Chatenoud L, Ferran C, Legendre C, et al. In vivo cell activation following OKT3 administration. Systemic cytokine release and modulation by corticosteroids. *Transplantation* 1990; **49**: 697–702.

278 Stein KL, Ladowski J, Kormos R, Armitage J. The cardiopulmonary response to OKT3 in orthotopic cardiac transplant recipients. *Chest* 1989; **95**: 817–821.

279 Breisblatt WM, Schulman DS, Stein K, et al. Hemodynamic response to OKT3 in orthotopic heart transplant recipients: evidence for reversible myocardial dysfunction. *J Heart Lung Transplant* 1991; **10**: 359–365.

280 Cronin DC II, Faust TW, Brady L, et al. Modern immunosuppression. *Clin Liver Dis* 2000; **4**: 619–655, ix.

281 Swinnen LJ, Costanzo-Nordin MR, Fisher SG, et al. Increased incidence of lymphoproliferative disorder after immunosuppression with the monoclonal antibody OKT3 in cardiac-transplant recipients. *N Engl J Med* 1990; **323**: 1723–1728.

282 A randomized clinical trial of OKT3 monoclonal antibody for acute rejection of cadaveric renal transplants. Ortho Multicenter Transplant Study Group. *N Engl J Med* 1985; **313**: 337–342.

283 Norman DJ, Kahana L, Stuart FP Jr, et al. A randomized clinical trial of induction therapy with OKT3 in kidney transplantation. *Transplantation* 1993; **55**: 44–50.

284 Carrier M, Jenicek M, Pelletier LC. Value of monoclonal antibody OKT3 in solid organ transplantation: a meta-analysis. *Transplant Proc* 1992; **24**: 2586–2591.

285 Kupiec-Weglinski JW, Diamantstein T, Tilney NL. Interleukin 2 receptor-targeted therapy – rationale and applications in organ transplantation. *Transplantation* 1988; **46**: 785–792.

286 Taniguchi T, Minami Y. The IL-2/IL-2 receptor system: a current overview. *Cell* 1993; **73**: 5–8.

287 Amlot PL. The clinical and experimental use of monoclonal antibodies to the IL-2 receptor. In: Chatenoud L, ed. *Monoclonal antibodies in transplantation*. R G Landes, Austin, TX, 1995; 53–98.

288 Soulillou JP. Relevant targets for therapy with monoclonal antibodies in allograft transplantation. *Kidney Int* 1994; **46**: 540–553.

289 Amlot PL, Tahami F, Chinn D, Rawlings E. Activation antigen expression on human T cells. I. Analysis by two-colour flow cytometry of umbilical cord blood, adult blood and lymphoid tissue. *Clin Exp Immunol* 1996; **105**: 176–182.

290 Nashan B, Schwinzer R, Schlitt HJ, Wonigeit K, Pichlmayr R. Immunological effects of the anti-IL-2 receptor monoclonal antibody BT 563 in liver allografted patients. *Transpl Immunol* 1995; **3**: 203–211.

291 Soulillou JP, Peyronnet P, Le Mauff B, et al. Prevention of rejection of kidney transplants by monoclonal antibody directed against interleukin 2. *Lancet* 1987; **1**: 1339–1342.

292 Soulillou JP, Cantarovich D, Le Mauff B, et al. Randomized controlled trial of a monoclonal antibody against the interleukin-2 receptor (33B3.1) as compared with rabbit antithymocyte globulin for prophylaxis against rejection of renal allografts. *N Engl J Med* 1990; **322**: 1175–1182.

293 Mayforth RD, Quintans J. Designer and catalytic antibodies. *N Engl J Med* 1990; **323**: 173–178.

294 Onrust SV, Wiseman LR. Basiliximab. *Drugs* 1999; **57**: 207–214.

295 Wiseman LR, Faulds D. Daclizumab: a review of its use in the prevention of acute rejection in renal transplant recipients. *Drugs* 1999; **58**: 1029–1042.

296 Queen C, Schneider WP, Selick HE, et al. A humanized antibody that binds to the interleukin 2 receptor. *Proc Natl Acad Sci USA* 1989; **86**: 10029–10033.

297 Junghans RP, Waldmann TA, Landolfi NF, Avdalovic NM, Schneider WP, Queen C. Anti-Tac-H, a humanized antibody to the interleukin 2 receptor with new features for immunotherapy in malignant and immune disorders. *Cancer Res* 1990; **50**: 1495–1502.

298 Vincenti F, Kirkman R, Light S, et al. Interleukin-2-receptor blockade with daclizumab to prevent acute rejection in renal transplantation. Daclizumab Triple Therapy Study Group. *N Engl J Med* 1998; **338**: 161–165.

299 Vincenti F, Lantz M, Birnbaum J, et al. A phase I trial of humanized anti-interleukin 2 receptor antibody in renal transplantation. *Transplantation* 1997; **63**: 33–38.

300 Kovarik J, Wolf P, Cisterne JM, et al. Disposition of basiliximab, an interleukin-2 receptor monoclonal antibody, in recipients of mismatched cadaver renal allografts. *Transplantation* 1997; **64**: 1701–1705.

301 Hengster P, Pescovitz MD, Hyatt D, Margreiter R. Cytomegalovirus infections after treatment with daclizumab, an anti IL-2 receptor antibody, for prevention of renal allograft rejection. Roche Study Group. *Transplantation* 1999; **68**: 310–313.

302 Nashan B, Moore R, Amlot P, Schmidt AG, Abeywickrama K, Soulillou JP. Randomised trial of basiliximab versus placebo for control of acute cellular rejection in renal allograft recipients. CHIB 201 International Study Group. *Lancet* 1997; **350**: 1193–1198.

303 Nashan B, Light S, Hardie IR, Lin A, Johnson JR. Reduction of acute renal allograft rejection by daclizumab. Daclizumab Double Therapy Study Group. *Transplantation* 1999; **67**: 110–115.

304 Kahan BD, Rajagopalan PR, Hall M. Reduction of the occurrence of acute cellular rejection among renal allograft recipients treated with basiliximab, a chimeric anti-interleukin-2-receptor monoclonal antibody. United States Simulect Renal Study Group. *Transplantation* 1999; **67**: 276–284.

305 Beniaminovitz A, Itescu S, Lietz K, et al. Prevention of rejection in cardiac transplantation by blockade of the interleukin-2 receptor with a monoclonal antibody. *N Engl J Med* 2000; **342**: 613–619.

306 Carl S, Wiesel M, Daniel V, Staehler G. Effect of anti-IL-2-receptor monoclonal antibody BT 563 in treatment of acute interstitial renal rejection. *Transplant Proc* 1995; **27**: 854–855.

307 Cantarovich D, Le Mauff B, Hourmant M, et al. Anti-interleukin 2 receptor monoclonal antibody in the treatment of ongoing acute rejection episodes of human kidney graft – a pilot study. *Transplantation* 1989; **47**: 454–457.

308 Tilney NL, Strom TB, Kupiec-Weglinski JW. Pharmacologic and immunologic agonists and antagonists of cyclosporine. *Transplant Proc* 1988; **20**(3 Suppl 3): 13–22.

309 Schroeder TJ, Melvin DB, Clardy CW, et al. Use of cyclosporine and ketoconazole without nephrotoxicity in two heart transplant recipients. *J Heart Transplant* 1987; **6**: 84–89.

310 Gandhi BV, Kale S, Bhowmik DM, Jain AK. Concomitant administration of cyclosporine and ketoconazole in renal transplant patients. *Transplant Proc* 1992; **24**: 1715.

311 McCauley J, Ptachcinski RJ, Shapiro R. The cyclosporine-sparing effects of diltiazem in renal transplantation. *Transplant Proc* 1989; **21**: 3955–3957.

312 Valantine H, Keogh A, McIntosh N, Hunt S, Oyer P, Schroeder J. Cost containment: coadministration of diltiazem with cyclosporine after heart transplantation. *J Heart Lung Transplant* 1992; **11**: 1–8.

313 Keogh A, Spratt P, McCosker C, Macdonald P, Mundy J, Kaan A. Ketoconazole to reduce the need for cyclosporine after cardiac transplantation. *N Engl J Med* 1995; **333**: 628–633.

314 Banerjee R, Leaver N, Lyster H, Banner NR. Coadministration of itraconazole and tacrolimus after thoracic organ transplantation. *Transplant Proc* 2001; **33**: 1600–1602.

315 Scala S, Akhmed N, Rao US, et al. P-glycoprotein substrates and antagonists cluster into two distinct groups. *Mol Pharmacol* 1997; **51**: 1024–1033.

316 Edwards DJ, Fitzsimmons ME, Schuetz EG, et al. 6′,7′-Dihydroxybergamottin in grapefruit juice and Seville orange juice: effects on cyclosporine disposition, enterocyte CYP3A4, and P-glycoprotein. *Clin Pharmacol Ther* 1999; **65**: 237–244.

317 Kane GC, Lipsky JJ. Drug–grapefruit juice interactions. *Mayo Clin Proc* 2000; **75**: 933–942.

318 Klepser TB, Klepser ME. Unsafe and potentially safe herbal therapies. *Am J Health Syst Pharm* 1999; **56**: 125–138.

319 Miller LG. Herbal medicinals: selected clinical considerations focusing on known or potential drug–herb interactions. *Arch Intern Med* 1998; **158**: 2200–2211.

320 Barone GW, Gurley BJ, Ketel BL, Lightfoot ML, Abul-Ezz SR. Drug interaction between St John's wort and cyclosporine. *Ann Pharmacother* 2000; **34**: 1013–1016.

321 Ahmed SM, Banner NR, Dubrey SW. Low cyclosporin-A level due to Saint-John's-wort in heart transplant patients. *J Heart Lung Transplant* 2001; **20**: 795.

322 Wu YM, Venkataramanan R, Suzuki M, et al. Interaction between FK 506 and cyclosporine in dogs. *Transplant Proc* 1991; **23**: 2797–2799.

323 Klintmalm G, Sawe J. High dose methylprednisolone increases plasma cyclosporin levels in renal transplant recipients. *Lancet* 1984; **1**: 731.

324 Langhoff E, Madsen S, Flachs H, Olgaard K, Ladefoged J, Hvidberg EF. Inhibition of prednisolone metabolism by cyclosporine in kidney-transplanted patients. *Transplantation* 1985; **39**: 107–109.

325 Undre NA, van Hooff J, Christiaans M, et al. Pharmacokinetics of FK 506 and mycophenolic acid after the administration of a FK 506-based regimen in combination with mycophenolate mofetil in kidney transplantation. *Transplant Proc* 1998; **30**: 1299–1302.

326 Zucker K, Tsaroucha A, Olson L, Esquenazi V, Tzakis A, Miller J. Evidence that tacrolimus augments the bioavailability of mycophenolate mofetil through the inhibition of mycophenolic acid glucuronidation. *Ther Drug Monit* 1999; **21**: 35–43.

327 Smak Gregoor PJ, van Gelder T, Hesse CJ, van der Mast BJ, van Besouw NM, Weimar W. Mycophenolic acid plasma concentrations in kidney allograft recipients with or without cyclosporin: a cross-sectional study. *Nephrol Dial Transplant* 1999; **14**: 706–708.

328 Gregoor PJ, de Sevaux RG, Hene RJ, et al. Effect of cyclosporine on mycophenolic acid trough levels in kidney transplant recipients. *Transplantation* 1999; **68**: 1603–1606.

329 Daniels NJ, Dover JS, Schachter RK. Interaction between cyclosporin and rifampicin. *Lancet* 1984; **2**: 639.

330 Furlan V, Perello L, Jacquemin E, Debray D, Taburet AM. Interactions between FK506 and rifampicin or erythromycin in pediatric liver recipients. *Transplantation* 1995; **59**: 1217–1218.

331 Buffington GA, Dominguez JH, Piering WF, Hebert LA, Kauffman HM Jr, Lemann J Jr. Interaction of rifampin and glucocorticoids. Adverse effect on renal allograft function. *JAMA* 1976; **236**: 1958–1960.

332 McAllister WA, Thompson PJ, Al-Habet SM, Rogers HJ. Rifampicin reduces effectiveness and bioavailability of prednisolone. *Br Med J* (Clin Res Edn) 1983; **286**: 923–925.

333 Floren LC, Bekersky I, Benet LZ, et al. Tacrolimus oral bioavailability doubles with coadministration of ketoconazole. *Clin Pharmacol Ther* 1997; **62**: 41–49.

334 Manez R, Martin M, Raman D, et al. Fluconazole therapy in transplant recipients receiving FK506. *Transplantation* 1994; **57**: 1521–1523.

335 Furlan V, Parquin F, Penaud JF, et al. Interaction between tacrolimus and itraconazole in a heart–lung transplant recipient. *Transplant Proc* 1998; **30**: 187–188.

336 Ptachcinski RJ, Carpenter BJ, Burckart GJ, Venkataramanan R, Rosenthal JT. Effect of erythromycin on cyclosporine levels. *N Engl J Med* 1985; **313**: 1416–1417.

337 Jensen C, Jordan M, Shapiro R, et al. Interaction between tacrolimus and erythromycin. *Lancet* 1994; **344**: 825.

338 Shaeffer MS, Collier D, Sorrell MF. Interaction between FK506 and erythromycin. *Ann Pharmacother* 1994; **28**: 280–281.

339 Wolter K, Wagner K, Philipp T, Fritschka E. Interaction between FK 506 and clarithromycin in a renal transplant patient. *Eur J Clin Pharmacol* 1994; **47**: 207–208.

340 Sadaba B, Lopez de Ocariz A, Azanza JR, Quiroga J, Cienfuegos JA. Concurrent clarithromycin and cyclosporin A treatment. *J Antimicrob Chemother* 1998; **42**: 393–395.

341 Boogaerts MA, Zachee P, Verwilghen RL. Cyclosporin, methylprednisolone, and convulsions. *Lancet* 1982; **2**: 1216–1217.

342 Keown PA, Laupacis A, Carruthers G, et al. Interaction between phenytoin and cyclosporine following organ transplantation. *Transplantation* 1984; **38**: 304–306.

343 Carstensen H, Jacobsen N, Dieperink H. Interaction between cyclosporin A and phenobarbitone. *Br J Clin Pharmacol* 1986; **21**: 550–551.

344 Freeman DJ, Laupacis A, Keown PA, Stiller CR, Carruthers SG. Evaluation of cyclosporin–phenytoin interaction with observations on cyclosporin metabolites. *Br J Clin Pharmacol* 1984; **18**: 887–893.

345 Maurer G. Metabolism of cyclosporine. *Transplant Proc* 1985; **17**(4 Suppl 1): 19–26.

346 Deray G, le Hoang P, Cacoub P, Assogba U, Grippon P, Baumelou A. Oral contraceptive interaction with cyclosporin. *Lancet* 1987; **1**: 158–159.

347 Ross WB, Roberts D, Griffin PJ, Salaman JR. Cyclosporin interaction with danazol and norethisterone. *Lancet* 1986; **1**: 330.

348 Passfall J, Schuller I, Keller F. Pharmacokinetics of cyclosporin during administration of danazol. *Nephrol Dial Transplant* 1994; **9**: 1807–1808.

349 Shapiro R, Venkataramanan R, Warty VS, et al. FK 506 interaction with danazol. *Lancet* 1993; **341**: 1344–1345.

350 Sacks FM, Pfeffer MA, Moye LA, et al. The effect of pravastatin on coronary events after myocardial infarction in patients with average cholesterol levels. Cholesterol and Recurrent Events Trial Investigators. *N Engl J Med* 1996; **335**: 1001–1009.

351 Long-Term Intervention with Pravastatin in Ischaemic Disease (LIPID) Study Group. Prevention of cardiovascular events and death with pravastatin in patients with coronary heart

disease and a broad range of initial cholesterol levels. *N Engl J Med* 1998; **339**: 1349–1357.

352 Shepherd J, Cobbe SM, Ford I, et al. Prevention of coronary heart disease with pravastatin in men with hypercholesterolemia. West of Scotland Coronary Prevention Study Group. *N Engl J Med* 1995; **333**: 1301–1307.

353 Norman DJ, Illingworth DR, Munson J, Hosenpud J. Myolysis and acute renal failure in a heart-transplant recipient receiving lovastatin. *N Engl J Med* 1988; **318**: 46–47.

354 Weise WJ, Possidente CJ. Fatal rhabdomyolysis associated with simvastatin in a renal transplant patient. *Am J Med* 2000; **108**: 351–352.

355 Ballantyne CM. Statins after cardiac transplantation: which statin, what dose, and how low should we go? *J Heart Lung Transplant* 2000; **19**: 515–517.

356 Keogh A, Macdonald P, Kaan A, Aboyoun C, Spratt P, Mundy J. Efficacy and safety of pravastatin vs simvastatin after cardiac transplantation. *J Heart Lung Transplant* 2000; **19**: 529–537.

357 Pochet JM, Pirson Y. Cyclosporin–diltiazem interaction. *Lancet* 1986; **1**: 979.

358 Robson RA, Fraenkel M, Barratt LJ, Birkett DJ. Cyclosporin–verapamil interaction. *Br J Clin Pharmacol* 1988; **25**: 402–403.

359 Boyd IW. Allopurinol–azathioprine interaction. *J Intern Med* 1991; **229**: 386.

360 Sheiner PA, Mor E, Chodoff L, et al. Acute renal failure associated with the use of ibuprofen in two liver transplant recipients on FK506. *Transplantation* 1994; **57**: 1132–1133.

361 Whiting PH, Simpson JG. The enhancement of cyclosporin A-induced nephrotoxicity by gentamicin. *Biochem Pharmacol* 1983; **32**: 2025–2028.

362 Termeer A, Hoitsma AJ, Koene RA. Severe nephrotoxicity caused by the combined use of gentamicin and cyclosporine in renal allograft recipients. *Transplantation* 1986; **42**: 220–221.

363 Kennedy MS, Deeg HJ, Siegel M, Crowley JJ, Storb R, Thomas ED. Acute renal toxicity with combined use of amphotericin B and cyclosporine after marrow transplantation. *Transplantation* 1983; **35**: 211–215.

364 Luber AD, Maa L, Lam M, Guglielmo BJ. Risk factors for amphotericin B-induced nephrotoxicity. *J Antimicrob Chemother* 1999; **43**: 267–271.

365 Thompson JF, Chalmers DH, Hunnisett AG, Wood RF, Morris PJ. Nephrotoxicity of trimethoprim and cotrimoxazole in renal allograft recipients treated with cyclosporine. *Transplantation* 1983; **36**: 204–206.

366 Morales JM, Muñoz MA, Fernandez Zatarain G, et al. Reversible acute renal failure caused by the combined use of foscarnet and cyclosporin in organ transplanted patients. *Nephrol Dial Transplant* 1995; **10**: 882–883.

367 Ahmad T, Simmonds M, McIver AG, McGraw ME. Reversible renal failure in renal transplant patients receiving oral acyclovir prophylaxis. *Pediatr Nephrol* 1994; **8**: 489–491.

368 Broeders N, Knoop C, Antoine M, Tielemans C, Abramowicz D. Fibrate-induced increase in blood urea and creatinine: is gemfibrozil the only innocuous agent? *Nephrol Dial Transplant* 2000; **15**: 1993–1999.

369 Barbir M, Hunt B, Kushwaha S, et al. Maxepa versus bezafibrate in hyperlipidemic cardiac transplant recipients. *Am J Cardiol* 1992; **70**: 1596–1601.

370 Brozena SC, Johnson MR, Ventura H, et al. Effectiveness and safety of diltiazem or lisinopril in treatment of hypertension after heart transplantation. Results of a prospective, randomized multicenter trail. *J Am Coll Cardiol* 1996; **27**: 1707–1712.

371 Marcus NJ, Breen JB, Yacoub MH, Banner NR. A randomised controlled trial of antihypertensive treatment with valsartan after heart transplantation [abstract]. *J Heart Lung Transplant* 2001; **20**: 246.

372 Halloran PF, Helms LM, Kung L, Noujaim J. The temporal profile of calcineurin inhibition by cyclosporine in vivo. *Transplantation* 1999; **68**: 1356–1361.

373 Sottong PR, Rosebrock JA, Britz JA, Kramer TR. Measurement of T-lymphocyte responses in whole-blood cultures using newly synthesized DNA and ATP. *Clin Diagn Lab Immunol* 2000; **7**: 307–311.

374 Barten MJ, Gummert JF, van Gelder T, Shorthouse R, Morris RE. Flow cytometric quantitation of calcium-dependent and -independent mitogen-stimulation of T cell functions in whole blood: inhibition by immunosuppressive drugs in vitro. *J Immunol Meth* 2001; **253**: 95–112.

375 Barten MJ, Gummert JF, van Gelder T, Shorthouse R, Morris RE. Assessment of mechanisms of action of immunosuppressive drugs using novel whole blood assays. *Transplant Proc* 2001; **33**: 2119–2120.

376 Holt DW, Johnston A, Roberts NB, Tredger JM, Trull AK. Methodological and clinical aspects of cyclosporin monitoring: report of the Association of Clinical Biochemists Task Force. *Ann Clin Biochem* 1994; **31**: 420–446.

377 Nankivell BJ, Hibbins M, Chapman JR. Diagnostic utility of whole blood cyclosporine measurements in renal transplantation using triple therapy. *Transplantation* 1994; **58**: 989–996.

378 Oellerich M, Armstrong VW, Kahan B, et al. Lake Louise Consensus Conference on cyclosporin monitoring in organ transplantation: report of the consensus panel. *Ther Drug Monit* 1995; **17**: 642–654.

379 Best NG, Trull AK, Tan KK, et al. Blood cyclosporin concentrations and the short-term risk of lung rejection following heart–lung transplantation. *Br J Clin Pharmacol* 1992; **34**: 513–520.

380 Inoue S, Beck Y, Nagao T, Uchida H. Early fluctuation in cyclosporine A trough levels affects long-term outcome of kidney transplants. *Transplant Proc* 1994; **26**: 2571–2573.

381 Keown P, Landsberg D, Halloran P, et al. A randomized, prospective multicenter pharmacoepidemiologic study of cyclosporine microemulsion in stable renal graft recipients. Report of the Canadian Neoral Renal Transplantation Study Group. *Transplantation* 1996; **62**: 1744–1752.

382 Johnston A, David OJ, Cooney GF. Pharmacokinetic validation of neoral absorption profiling. *Transplant Proc* 2000; **32**(3A Suppl): 53S–56S.

383 Belitsky P, Dunn S, Johnston A, Levy G. Impact of absorption profiling on efficacy and safety of cyclosporin therapy in transplant recipients. *Clin Pharmacokinet* 2000; **39**: 117–125.

384 Levy GA. C2 monitoring strategy for optimising cyclosporin immunosuppression from the Neoral formulation. *BioDrugs* 2001; **15**: 279–290.

385 Canadian Neoral Renal Transplantation Study Group. Absorption profiling of cyclosporine microemulsion (Neoral) during the first 2 weeks after renal transplantation. *Transplantation* 2001; **72**: 1024–1032.

386 Mahalati K, Belitsky P, West K, et al. Approaching the therapeutic window for cyclosporine in kidney transplantation: a prospective study. *J Am Soc Nephrol* 2001; **12**: 828–833.

387 Oellerich M, Armstrong VW, Schutz E, Shaw LM. Therapeutic drug monitoring of cyclosporine and tacrolimus. Update on Lake Louise Consensus Conference on cyclosporin and tacrolimus. *Clin Biochem* 1998; **31**: 309–316.

388 Taylor PJ, Jones A, Balderson GA, Lynch SV, Norris RL, Pond SM. Sensitive, specific quantitative analysis of tacrolimus (FK506) in blood by liquid chromatography–electrospray tandem mass spectrometry. *Clin Chem* 1996; **42**: 279–285.

389 Zhang Q, Simpson J, Aboleneen HI. A specific method for the measurement of tacrolimus in human whole blood by liquid chromatography/tandem mass spectrometry. *Ther Drug Monit* 1997; **19**: 470–476.

390 Tamura K, Fujimura T, Iwasaki K, et al. Interaction of tacrolimus (FK506) and its metabolites with FKBP and calcineurin. *Biochem Biophys Res Commun* 1994; **202**: 437–443.

391 Jusko WJ, Thomson AW, Fung J, et al. Consensus document: therapeutic monitoring of tacrolimus (FK-506). *Ther Drug Monit* 1995; **17**: 606–614.

392 Sher LS, Cosenza CA, Michel J, et al. Efficacy of tacrolimus as rescue therapy for chronic rejection in orthotopic liver transplantation: a report of the U.S. Multicenter Liver Study Group. *Transplantation* 1997; **64**: 258–263.

393 Jusko WJ, Piekoszewski W, Klintmalm GB, et al. Pharmacokinetics of tacrolimus in liver transplant patients. *Clin Pharmacol Ther* 1995; **57**: 281–290.

394 Wallemacq PE, Furlan V, Mollar A, et al. Pharmacokinetics of tacrolimus (FK506) in paediatric liver transplant recipients. *Eur J Drug Metab Pharmacokinet* 1998; **23**: 367–370.

395 Nowak I, Shaw LM. Mycophenolic acid binding to human serum albumin: characterization and relation to pharmacodynamics. *Clin Chem* 1995; **41**: 1011–1017.

396 Langman LJ, LeGatt DF, Yatscoff RW. Blood distribution of mycophenolic acid. *Ther Drug Monit* 1994; **16**: 602–607.

397 Beal JL, Jones CE, Taylor PJ, Tett SE. Evaluation of an immunoassay (EMIT) for mycophenolic acid in plasma from renal transplant recipients compared with a high-performance liquid chromatography assay. *Ther Drug Monit* 1998; **20**: 685–690.

398 Bullingham RE, Nicholls A, Hale M. Pharmacokinetics of mycophenolate mofetil (RS61443): a short review. *Transplant Proc* 1996; **28**: 925–929.

399 Shaw LM, Nicholls A, Hale M, et al. Therapeutic monitoring of mycophenolic acid. A consensus panel report. *Clin Biochem* 1998; **31**: 317–322.

400 Meiser BM, Pfeiffer M, Schmidt D, et al. The efficacy of the combination of tacrolimus and mycophenolate mofetil for prevention of acute myocardial rejection is dependent on routine monitoring of mycophenolic acid trough acid levels. *Transplant Proc* 1999; **31**: 84–87.

401 Holt DW, Lee T, Jones K, Johnston A. Validation of an assay for routine monitoring of sirolimus using HPLC with mass spectrometric detection. *Clin Chem* 2000; **46**: 1179–1183.

402 Kahan BD, Julian BA, Pescovitz MD, Vanrenterghem Y, Neylan J. Sirolimus reduces the incidence of acute rejection episodes despite lower cyclosporine doses in caucasian recipients of mismatched primary renal allografts: a phase II trial. Rapamune Study Group. *Transplantation* 1999; **68**: 1526–1532.

403 Norman DJ. Antilymphocyte antibodies in the treatment of allograft rejection: targets, mechanisms of action, monitoring, and efficacy. *Semin Nephrol* 1992; **12**: 315–324.

404 Henell KR, Norman DJ. Monitoring OKT3 treatment: pharmacodynamic and pharmacokinetic measures. *Transplant Proc* 1993; **25**(2 Suppl 1): 83–85.

405 Abouna GM, al-Abdullah IH, Kelly-Sullivan D, et al. Randomized clinical trial of antithymocyte globulin induction in renal transplantation comparing a fixed daily dose with dose adjustment according to T cell monitoring. *Transplantation* 1995; **59**: 1564–1568.

406 Cinti P, Cocciolo P, Evangelista B, et al. OKT3 prophylaxis in kidney transplant recipients: drug monitoring by flow cytometry. *Transplant Proc* 1996; **28**: 3214–3216.

407 Barlow CW, Moon MR, Green GR, et al. Rabbit antithymocyte globulin versus OKT3 induction therapy after heart–lung and lung transplantation: effect on survival, rejection, infection, and obliterative bronchiolitis. *Transpl Int* 2001; **14**: 234–239.

408 Palmer SM, Miralles AP, Lawrence CM, Gaynor JW, Davis RD, Tapson VF. Rabbit antithymocyte globulin decreases acute rejection after lung transplantation: results of a randomized, prospective study. *Chest* 1999; **116**: 127–133.

409 Kobashigawa JA, Stevenson LW, Brownfield E, et al. Does short-course induction with OKT3 improve outcome after heart transplantation? A randomized trial. *J Heart Lung Transplant* 1993; **12**: 205–208.

410 Guilinger RA, Paradis IL, Dauber JH, et al. The importance of bronchoscopy with transbronchial biopsy and bronchoalveolar lavage in the management of lung transplant recipients. *Am J Respir Crit Care Med* 1995; **152**: 2037–2043.

411 Yousem SA, Berry GJ, Cagle PT, et al. Revision of the 1990 Working Formulation for the classification of pulmonary allograft rejection: Lung Rejection Study Group. *J Heart Lung Transplant* 1996; **15**: 1–15.

412 Clelland CA, Higenbottam TW, Stewart S, Scott JP, Wallwork J. The histological changes in transbronchial biopsy after treatment of acute lung rejection in heart–lung transplants. *J Pathol* 1990; **161**: 105–112.

413 Shennib H, Mercado M, Nguyen D, et al. Successful treatment of steroid-resistant double-lung allograft rejection with orthoclone OKT3. *Am Rev Respir Dis* 1991; **144**: 224–226.

414 Kesten S, Maidenberg A, Winton T, Maurer J. Treatment of presumed and proven acute rejection following six months of lung transplant survival. *Am J Respir Crit Care Med* 1995; **152**: 1321–1324.

415 Meiser BM, Uberfuhr P, Fuchs A, et al. Tacrolimus: a superior agent to OKT3 for treating cases of persistent rejection after intrathoracic transplantation. *J Heart Lung Transplant* 1997; **16**: 795–800.

416 Rescue therapy with mycophenolate mofetil. The Mycophenolate Mofetil Renal Refractory Rejection Study Group. *Clin Transplant* 1996; **10**: 131–135.

417 Estenne M, Maurer JR, Boehler A, et al. Bronchiolitis obliterans syndrome 2001: an update of the diagnostic criteria. *J Heart Lung Transplant* 2002; **21**: 297–310.

418 Ross DJ, Lewis MI, Kramer M, Vo A, Kass RM. FK 506 'rescue' immunosuppression for obliterative bronchiolitis after lung transplantation. *Chest* 1997; **112**: 1175–1179.

419 Whyte RI, Rossi SJ, Mulligan MS, et al. Mycophenolate mofetil for obliterative bronchiolitis syndrome after lung transplantation. *Ann Thorac Surg* 1997; **64**: 945–948.

420 Kesten S, Rajagopalan N, Maurer J. Cytolytic therapy for the treatment of bronchiolitis obliterans syndrome following lung transplantation. *Transplantation* 1996; **61**: 427–430.

421 Date H, Lynch JP, Sundaresan S, Patterson GA, Trulock EP. The impact of cytolytic therapy on bronchiolitis obliterans syndrome. *J Heart Lung Transplant* 1998; **17**: 869–875.

422 Ross HJ, Gullestad L, Pak J, Slauson S, Valantine HA, Hunt SA. Methotrexate or total lymphoid radiation for treatment of persistent or recurrent allograft cellular rejection: a comparative study. *J Heart Lung Transplant* 1997; **16**: 179–189.

19

Chronic lung allograft dysfunction

Marshall I. Hertz

University of Minnesota, Minneapolis, Minnesota, USA

Introduction

Lung and heart–lung transplantation have now been performed in over 10 000 patients worldwide with two to three year survival rates of approximately 70%. Despite these remarkable successes, approximately one third of lung transplant recipients develop progressive airflow obstruction and deterioration of graft function, referred to as bronchiolitis obliterans syndrome (BOS). BOS is often associated with a specific histological lesion, obliterative bronchiolitis (OB), characterized by inflammation and fibrosis of small airways. Clinical and experimental evidence suggests that the alloimmune reaction plays a major role in disease pathogenesis, and OB/BOS is often considered to be synonymous with chronic lung rejection. OB/BOS is usually considered to be analogous to late graft loss after transplantation of other organs [1]. In general, this involves a fibroproliferative process leading to obliteration of tubular structures in the organ. In the heart this is manifested by the development of graft coronary artery stenosis, and in the kidney by chronic vascular and tubular fibrosis. All of these syndromes are believed to share a similar pathogenesis that includes an alloimmune response against donor targets, i.e. they represent forms of chronic graft rejection. However, multiple other factors, including ischaemia and infection, may also play important roles in some lung recipients. Much has been learned regarding chronic lung allograft dysfunction since it was first described in 1984 [2]. This brief review will summarize current understanding of the clinical features, pathogenesis, and treatment of OB/BOS.

Clinical features

The most consistent clinical manifestation of OB/BOS is progressive loss of lung function due to airflow obstruction

[3,4]. Several large multivariate analyses have identified prior episodes of severe or persistent acute rejection as being the most consistent clinical risk factor [5–7]. The clinical presentation and rate of progression are quite variable. The onset is frequently insidious, with the gradual development of exertional dyspnoea. In contrast, some patients develop an illness resembling viral or asthmatic bronchitis with acute or subacute onset of cough and wheezing, but the response to bronchodilators and oral corticosteroids is limited or absent. Although the term 'obliterative bronchiolitis' suggests that the disease is limited to small airways, involvement of large airways is common and is manifested clinically by bronchiectasis and superinfection with a variety of pathogens.

The chest radiograph is generally normal or shows mild hyperinflation. High resolution computed tomography (CT) scan findings commonly include bronchiectasis and may demonstrate a 'mosaic' pattern that is accentuated during exhalation, reflecting variable air trapping in different lung zones [8,9]. Pulmonary function tests demonstrate progressive airflow obstruction. In many cases, the forced expiratory flow (25–75%) (FEF_{25-75}) decreases weeks to months prior to the forced expiratory volume in 1 s (FEV_1), consistent with the widespread involvement of small airways. Daily home monitoring data demonstrate that decreases in FEF_{25-75} and FEV_1 can often be observed months before clinical disease is recognized. Cooper et al. [10] defined a staging system for BOS that is intended to provide uniform nomenclature and clinical staging for purposes of assessing and reporting results of transplantation and of treatment protocols. This system has recently been updated [11] (see also Chapter 16).

Obliterative bronchiolitis may be diagnosed by transbronchial biopsies of symptomatic or asymptomatic patients. However, there is considerable sampling error when transbronchial biopsies are performed, and many patients suffer progressive shortness of breath and decreased pulmonary function despite repeated negative biopsies. In addition, biopsies become more hazardous as the disease progresses. Therefore many patients are treated for OB/BOS without histological confirmation of OB.

Pathology and pathogenesis

Histopathologically, OB is characterized by inflammation and fibrosis of cartilaginous airways, with sparing of the alveoli and interstitium [12]. Although the most striking abnormalities are located in the bronchioles, large airway lesions are also present and include inflammation, peribronchial fibrosis and bronchiectasis. The bronchiolar component is characterized by inflammation and fibrosis of the lamina propria and lumen. The process is inhomogeneous and normal bronchioles often are present near areas of severe disease. In some airways, peribronchiolar lymphocytic inflammation and fibrosis lead to compromise of the airway lumen in a constrictive fashion. In other airways, disruption of the epithelium occurs and polyps of granulation tissue fill the lumen. As the process evolves, submucosal and intralumenal fibrous tissue proliferates with dense scar formation. The anatomical features of OB suggest that two interdependent but distinct pathogenetic processes are involved: inflammation and injury of airway structures and a fibroproliferative response that leads to progressive airflow obstruction and graft failure.

Alloimmune mechanisms

Several lines of evidence indicate that alloimmune mechanisms play an important role in OB/BOS pathogenesis. The single most important clinical risk factor for OB/BOS is acute vascular rejection, i.e. perivascular infiltration of activated lymphocytes into the graft tissue [5–7]. In one study, 90% of patients with one or more episodes of grade 3 or greater acute rejection, and 95% of patients with three or more episodes of grade 2 or greater acute rejection, developed OB/BOS; in contrast, among patients with fewer than three grade 2 acute rejection episodes, only 18% later developed OB/BOS [7]. Considerable clinical evidence suggests that acute vascular rejection is often, if not always, accompanied by airway inflammation and injury. In this regard, Kesten et al. [13] and Ross et al. [14] have reported that patients with acute rejection often suffer an irreversible reduction in airflow despite histological resolution of the vascular lesions. In addition, Yousem demonstrated that patients with untreated vascular rejection often had

associated small airway inflammation that also correlated with deteriorating pulmonary function [15]. More recently, Husain et al. have demonstrated that identification of lymphocytic bronchitis/bronchiolitis confers an even greater risk for subsequent OB/BOS than does acute vascular rejection [16].

Additional evidence for an alloimmune pathogenesis comes from results of the primed lymphocyte test, a variant of the mixed lymphocyte reaction, which measures alloreactivity stimulated by irradiated donor-derived antigen presenting cells. Donor-specific primed lymphocyte test reactivity of bronchoalveolar lavage-derived lymphocytes is increased in patients with OB/BOS as compared with recipients with normal graft function [17,18]. In addition, recipients with donor antigen-specific hyporeactivity of peripheral blood lymphocytes, evidenced by reduced or absent alloreactivity of peripheral blood lymphocytes when stimulated by cells bearing donor antigens in mixed lymphocyte culture assays, are less likely to develop OB/BOS than those with normal reactivity [19].

Nonalloimmune factors

Nonalloimmune factors may also play a role in OB/BOS pathogenesis. Cytomegalovirus (CMV)-related illness has been implicated in chronic rejection of nonpulmonary solid organ allografts; in some studies CMV pneumonitis, but not asymptomatic CMV bronchial shedding, has correlated with development of OB/BOS [20,21]. Other clinical reports, however, suggest no direct relationship between these diseases [22,23]. In a rat heterotopic tracheal transplant model, CMV infection also potentiates the development of obliterative airway disease [24,25].

The lung allograft is particularly susceptible to non-CMV viral infections, including respiratory syncytial virus, parainfluenza virus, and influenzas A and B [26], but so far these have not been associated causally with OB/BOS. However, patients with established OB/BOS are at high risk for developing these infections, with further compromise of lung function [27,28].

Patients who fail to reach a near-normal level of lung function in the early post-transplantation period are at high risk for OB/BOS [29]. Potential contributors to this phenomenon include ischaemic airway injury, ischaemia–reperfusion lung injury, infections, and early acute lung rejection. The role of airway ischaemia in the pathogenesis of OB/BOS is uncertain. In most transplant centres, the bronchial circulation is interrupted and not reanastamosed during the transplant procedure. Although this is compatible with adequate results in most patients, it is conceivable that chronic airway ischaemia predisposes the airways to subsequent injury and abnormal repair. Ya-coub et al. [30] and Pettersson et al. [31] have reported lung transplantation with reanastomosis of the bronchial arteries but long-term lung functional and histological outcomes are not yet known. In one study, acute is-chaemic airway injury at the time of transplantation has been implicated as a risk factor for OB/BOS [7]. This is to be distinguished from cold ischaemic time immedi-ately prior to transplantation, which has not been asso-ciated with OB/BOS, in most single-centre reports. How-ever, the United Network for Organ Sharing/International Society for Heart and Lung Transplantation Registry, the largest repository for lung transplant outcomes data, has recently identified cold ischaemic time as a significant risk factor for the OB/BOS at five years after transplantation [32].

Fibroproliferation

A fibroproliferative response follows airway injury, result-ing in accumulation of fibroblasts within the bronchiolar walls and lumens. Mesenchymal cell migration, replica-tion and connective tissue deposition are critical processes in fibroproliferation and are regulated by discrete sets of peptides, which include growth factors, cytokines, and ad-hesion molecules. Cytokines, including interferon gamma (IFN-γ), interleukin (IL) 1β, IL-2, IL-4, IL-6, IL-7, IL-8, and IL-10, have all been found to be involved in the com-plex cascade of events that comprise the acute rejection response [33] and probably contribute to the airway inflam-mation observed in acute lung rejection. Growth factor-mediated proliferation of fibrous tissue leads to airway constriction and lumenal obliteration as the OB/BOS pro-cess develops. In this regard, increased concentrations of platelet-derived growth factor (PDGF) [34], transforming growth factor (TGF) β [35], and insulin-like growth fac-tor 1 [36] are observed in bronchoalveolar lavage fluid of OB/BOS patients prior to irreversible bronchiolar obliter-ation. Although their involvement in OB/BOS has not yet been clarified, they probably contribute to alloactivation and lymphocyte recruitment, and, along with growth fac-tors, may mediate immune stimulation of fibroprolifera-tion. In addition, bronchoalveolar lavage fluid neutrophilia and increased IL-8 concentration and activity have been identified in patients with current or subsequent OB/BOS, suggesting a possible role in pathogenesis [37,38]. Integrins are also likely to be critical in the fibroproliferative pro-cess by virtue of their role in lymphocyte trafficking and in mediating mesenchymal cell adhesion to the extracellular matrix.

Preclinical models

Improved understanding of the pathogenesis of OB/BOS will probably depend, in part, on studies of animal mod-els of the disease. Several systems have been described, including orthotopic rat [39] and pig [40] lung transplant models. Our laboratory has reported fibroproliferative le-sions similar to OB in murine tracheal allografts harvested 21 days after heterotopic transplantation into the subcu-taneous tissue of allogeneically mismatched recipients. In addition to fibroproliferation, loss of the normal respiratory epithelium is a consistent finding. Similarly prepared syn-geneic isografts remain histologically normal [41]. Because the pathological changes occur in large airways rather than bronchioles, we refer to the observed lesion as obliterative airway disease (OAD). Similar results have been obtained after heterotopic tracheal transplants in rats [25,42] and pigs [43], and hamster to pig xenografts [44]. Studies to date in the heterotopic tracheal transplant models indi-cate that OAD results from a T-cell mediated response to class I MHC determinants [42,45]; the immune suppressive medications ciclosporin A and sirolimus (rapamycin) re-duce the fibroproliferation observed [46,47]; local applica-tion of the fibroblast growth factors (FGF) PDGF and FGF7 increase fibroproliferation [48]. Many laboratories are us-ing the OAD model to develop therapeutic approaches to OB/BOS by abrogating alloimmune injury and by limiting airway fibrosis.

Treatment

Treatment for established OB/BOS has been disappoint-ing. Although there have been reports of stabilization of early disease after administration of increased immune suppressive medications, recovery of lost lung function is unusual and progressive deterioration is common despite therapeutic efforts. These findings suggest that immune suppression interferes with airway inflammation and the development of new lesions, but is ineffective in amelio-rating airway fibroproliferation. This implies that improv-ing clinical outcomes of patients with OB/BOS will require treatment earlier in the course of the disease and the de-velopment of interventions designed to limit airway fibro-proliferation.

Current medical treatment

Current medical treatment of OB/BOS consists of efforts to attenuate the vigour of the alloimmune response. Many such treatments have been reported in small case series to be of some benefit in some patients. 'Benefit' in this setting is defined as stabilization of lung function; significant improvement in pulmonary function is unusual, presumably because the immune suppressive medications given are ineffective at inhibiting or reversing the fibroproliferative process occurring in the airways.

High dose intravenous methylprednisolone and antilymphocyte antibody preparations, including muromonab-CD3 (OKT-3) and antithymocyte globulin (ATG), have successfully stabilized the lung function of at least some patients with OB/BOS [49,50].

Tacrolimus is a macrolide immune suppressive compound that has been used in clinical kidney, liver, heart and lung transplantation. A recent nonrandomized series suggests that tacrolimus may stabilize pulmonary function of ciclosporin-treated patients with OB/BOS [51]. However, a larger compilation of cases did not show a similar benefit [52].

Methotrexate is effective for treatment of acute lung rejection that has been persistent after treatment with high-dose corticosteroids [53]. Methotrexate was also reported to help stabilize lung function in an open pilot study of 10 patients with OB/BOS [54]. In view of the potential toxicity of methotrexate, particularly pulmonary toxicity, the authors appropriately caution that methotrexate should not be used as first-line therapy for OB/BOS.

Mycophenolate mofetil is an inhibitor of the de novo purine synthesis pathway and thus inhibits lymphocyte proliferation, formation of cytotoxic lymphocytes, and both primary and secondary antibody formation. In experimental studies, mycophenolate mofetil was effective in preventing proliferative arteriopathy in aortic allografts [55], suggesting a role in the treatment of chronic rejection. At present, however, limited clinical data exist regarding the ability of mycophenolate mofetil to prevent or treat acute rejection or OB/BOS in lung transplant recipients. A multicentre controlled trial of mycophenolate mofetil in lung transplantation is currently in progress, but long-term results have not yet been published.

Retransplantation

Retransplantation for OB/BOS has been controversial in light of the very limited availability of donor lungs. Novick et al recently reported results of 230 retransplants, 63% of which were performed for patients with OB/BOS [56]. The report indicates that early survival after retransplantation is reduced as compared with first transplants, but good long-term results can be achieved in many patients. The results of retransplants performed for OB/BOS were not different from those done for other indications. Recurrent OB/BOS has been observed in a frequency similar to that seen after first transplants. Ventilator independence, ambulatory status, retransplant after 1991, and experience of the transplant centre in performing retransplants were predictors of good outcomes after retransplantation.

New approaches to therapy

In view of the disappointing results of currently employed medications, it is clear that new approaches are needed to reduce the incidence and impact of OB/BOS. Our current understanding of the pathogenesis of OB/BOS indicates that two general approaches may prove useful: (1) additional interference with the alloimmune response and (2) interference with the fibroproliferative response.

Locally administered immune suppressive medications
In an effort to reduce the unwanted effects of systemically administered medications while effectively inhibiting alloimmunity, interest has increased in delivering agents directly to the transplanted organ. The lung is a particularly attractive organ for local immune suppression in view of the potential for aerosolized drug delivery. Iacono et al. have reported that seven of nine patients with OB/BOS had histological improvement and stabilization of pulmonary function after treatment with inhaled ciclosporin A [57]. A larger clinical trial is currently in progress. In future studies, it will be important to demonstrate that these promising findings are the result of local effects of the inhaled ciclosporin, rather than reflecting increased circulating blood levels.

Inhaled corticosteroid medications are effective in the treatment of airway inflammation due to asthma. Consistent with the prominent component of airway inflammation in OB/BOS, some reports have suggested a role for inhaled steroids in preventing or treating that condition [58, 59]. However, recent studies have not confirmed a beneficial effect [60,61].

Other immune modulating strategies
Total lymphoid irradiation has been employed successfully to treat refractory or recurrent lung allograft rejection [62]. However, several of the treated lung transplant patients later developed OB/BOS, suggesting either that these patients were treated too late or that total lymphoid irradiation is not effective in preventing OB/BOS.

Photopheresis, or photochemotherapy, has also been employed in small numbers of patients. This immune modulating therapy involves apheresis with isolation of peripheral blood leukocytes, treatment of the leukocytes ex vivo with 8-methoxypsoralen and ultraviolet light, and subsequent reinfusion into the patient. Although its mechanism of immune modulation is poorly understood, photopheresis has been used in refractory acute cardiac and renal rejection and its use has been reported in several lung transplant recipients, with promising results [63]. Salerno et al. [64] recently reported results of photopheresis in seven patients with advanced OB/BOS; stabilization of pulmonary function was observed in all patients and survival was improved as compared with a group of patients with severe OB/BOS who were not treated with photopheresis. In addition, histological abnormalities, including peribronchial and perivascular inflammation, were reversed in two of the patients. It is possible, but unproven, that earlier treatment of patients with OB/BOS would be of greater clinical benefit than was observed in patients with far-advanced disease.

The development of bone marrow microchimerism, detected by identifying donor-derived cells in peripheral blood of allograft recipients, has been correlated with a reduced incidence of OB/BOS [19]. At this point it is unclear whether microchimerism induces graft tolerance, or is simply a marker of good graft acceptance. Pham et al. have reported that augmentation of donor cell chimerism can be achieved by infusing unmodified donor bone marrow in conjunction with heart or lung transplantation [65]; the long-term outcome of these patients will help to determine the efficacy of this approach.

Antifibroproliferative therapy

To date, treatment strategies for OB/BOS have focused on abrogation of alloimmune-induced airway injury. However, the chain of events linking airway injury to the fibroproliferative response that follows offers a number of additional potential targets for future therapy. For example, the migration of mesenchymal cells and endothelial cells from the airway wall into the lumen is probably regulated by interactions of integrins with fibronectin, fibrinogen and fibrin within the bronchiolar lumen. These interactions constitute potential loci for inhibition with antibodies, antisense ribonucleotides, or small peptide receptor antagonists. In that regard, blockade of $\alpha_4\beta_1$ integrin with a peptide analogue of the CS-1 region of fibronectin reduced coronary arteriopathy in rabbit cardiac allografts [66], possibly by interfering with smooth muscle cell migration into the graft.

Sirolimus (rapamycin, Rapamune®) and sirolimus-derivative (Certican®, currently in clinical trials) are structural analogues of tacrolimus and bind to the same intracellular target. However, unlike tacrolimus, they do not appear to inhibit IL-2 production, but rather inhibit the response of T cells to IL-2 and other cytokines [67]. Sirolimus has been shown to prolong graft survival in several animal transplant models and also is capable of reversing ongoing rejection. In addition to immune suppressive activity, sirolimus has also been shown to inhibit growth factor-induced endothelial cell and mesenchymal cell proliferation [68] and induce lymphoid cell apoptosis [69], implying that it may be useful in prevention and treatment of airway fibrosis in OB/BOS. A clinical trial comparing sirolimus-derivative with ATG in subjects with established OB/BOS is currently in progress.

REFERENCES

1 Tilney NL, Whitley WD, Diamond JR, Kupiec-Weglinski JW, Adams DH. Chronic rejection – an undefined conundrum. *Transplantation* 1991; **52**: 389–398.

2 Burke CM, Theodore J, Dawkins KD. Post-transplant obliterative bronchiolitis and other late lung sequelae in human heart–lung transplantation. *Chest* 1984; **86**: 824–829.

3 Kelly K, Hertz MI. Obliterative bronchiolitis. *Clin Chest Med* 1997; **18**: 319–338.

4 Trulock EP. Lung transplantation. *Am J Respir Crit Care Med* 1997; **155**: 789–818.

5 Scott JP, Higenbottam TW, Sharples L, et al. Risk factors for obliterative bronchiolitis in heart–lung transplant recipients. *Transplantation* 1991; **51**: 813–817.

6 Kroshus TJ, Kshettry VR, Savik K, John R, Hertz MI, Bolman RM III. Risk factors for the development of bronchiolitis obliterans syndrome after lung transplantation. *J Thorac Cardiovasc Surg* 1997; **114**: 195–202.

7 Bando K, Paradis IL, Similo S, et al. Obliterative bronchiolitis after lung and heart-lung transplantation. An analysis of risk factors and management. *J Thorac Cardiovasc Surg* 1995; **110**: 4–13.

8 Bankier AA, Van Muylem A, Knoop C, Estenne M, Gevenois PA. Bronchiolitis obliterans syndrome in heart–lung transplant recipients: diagnosis with expiratory CT. *Radiology* 2001; **218**: 533–539.

9 Ikonen T, Kivisaari L, Taskinen E, Piilonen A, Harjula AL. High-resolution CT in long-term follow-up after lung transplantation. *Chest* 1997; **111**: 370–376.

10 Cooper JD, Billingham M, Egan T. A working formulation for the standardization of nomenclature and for clinical staging of chronic dysfunction in lung allografts. *J Heart Lung Transplant* 1993; **12**: 713–716.

11 Estenne M, Maurer JR, Boehler A, et al. Bronchiolitis obliterans syndrome 2001: an update of the diagnostic criteria. *J Heart Lung Transplant* 2002; **21**: 297–310.

12 Tazelaar HD, Yousem SA. Pathologic findings in heart–lung transplantation. *Hum Pathol* 1988; **208**: 371–378.

13 Kesten S, Maidenberg A, Winton T, Maurer J. Treatment of presumed and proven acute rejection following six months of lung transplant survival. *Am J Respir Crit Care Med* 1995; **152**: 1321–1324.

14 Ross DJ, Marchevsky A, Kramer M, Kass RM. 'Refractoriness' of airflow obstruction associated with isolated lymphocytic bronchiolitis/bronchitis in pulmonary allografts. *J Heart Lung Transplant* 1997; **16**: 832–838.

15 Yousem SA. Lymphocytic bronchitis/bronchiolitis in lung allograft recipients. *Am J Surg Pathol* 1993; **17**: 491–496.

16 Husain AN, Siddiqui MT, Holmes EW, et al. Analysis of risk factors for the development of bronchiolitis obliterans syndrome. *Am J Resp Crit Care Med* 1999; **159**: 829–833.

17 Rabinowich H, Zeevi A, Yousem SA. Alloreactivity of lung biopsy and bronchoalveolar lavage-derived lymphocytes from pulmonary transplant patients: correlation with acute rejection and bronchiolitis obliterans. *Clin Transplant* (Copenhagen) 1990; **4**: 376–384.

18 Reinsmoen NL, Bolman RM, Savik K. Are multiple immunopathogenetic events occurring during the development of obliterative bronchiolitis and acute rejection? *Transplantation* 1993; **55**: 1040–1044.

19 McSherry C, Jackson A, Hertz MI, Bolman RM, Savik K, Reinsmoen NL. Sequential measurement of peripheral blood allogeneic microchimerism levels and association with pulmonary function. *Transplantation* 1996; **62**: 1811–1818.

20 Duncan SR, Paradis IL, Yousem SA. Sequelae of cytomegalovirus pulmonary infection in lung allograft recipients. *Am Rev Respir Dis* 1992; **146**: 1419–1425.

21 Rubin RH. The indirect effects of cytomegalovirus infection on the outcome of organ transplantation. *JAMA* 1989; **261**: 3607–3609.

22 Ettinger NA, Bailey TC, Trulock EP. Cytomegalovirus pneumonitis: impact following isolated lung transplantation. *Am Rev Respir Dis* 1993; **147**: 1017–1023.

23 Sharples LD, Scott JP, Dennis C. Risk factors for survival following combined heart–lung transplantation. *Transplantation* 1994; **57**: 218–223.

24 Koskinen PK, Kallio EA, Bruggeman CA, Lemstrom KB. Cytomegalovirus infection enhances experimental obliterative bronchiolitis in rat tracheal allografts. *Am J Respir Crit Care Med* 1997; **155**: 2078–2088.

25 Reichenspurner H, Soni V, Nitschke M, et al. Enhancement of obliterative airway disease in rat tracheal allografts infected with recombinant rat cytomegalovirus. *J Heart Lung Transplant* 1997; **17**: 439–451.

26 Wendt CH, Fox JM, Hertz MI. Paramyxovirus infection in lung transplant recipients. *J Heart Lung Transplant* 1995; **14**: 479–485.

27 Billings JL, Hertz MI, Wendt CH. Community respiratory virus infections following lung transplantation. *Transpl Infect Dis* 2001; **3**: 138–148.

28 Billings J, Hertz MI, Savik K, Wendt CH. Respiratory viruses do not predispose lung treansplant recipients to OB. *Am J Resp Crit Care Med* 1998; **157**: A759.

29 Sharples LD, Tamm M, McNeil K, Higenbottam TW, Stewart S, Wallwork J. Development of bronchiolitis obliterans syndrome in recipients of heart–lung transplantation – early risk factors. *Transplantation* 1996; **61**: 560–566.

30 Yacoub M, Al-Kattan KM, Tadjkarimi S, Eren T, Khaghani A. Medium term results of direct bronchial arterial revascularisation using IMA for single lung transplantation (SLT with direct revascularisation). *Eur J Cardiothorac Surg* 1997; **11**: 1030–1036.

31 Pettersson G, Norgaard MA, Arendrup H, et al. Direct bronchial artery revascularization and en bloc double lung transplantation – surgical techniques and early outcome. *J Heart Lung Transplant* 1997; **16**: 320–333.

32 Hosenpud JD, Bennett LE, Keck BM, Boucek MM, Novick RJ. The registry of the International Society for Heart and Lung Transplantation: 17th official report – 2000. *J Heart Lung Transplant* 2000; **19**: 909–931.

33 Tilney NL, Kupiec-Weglinski JW. The biology of acute transplant rejection. *Ann Surg* 1991; **214**: 98–106.

34 Hertz MI, Henke CA, Nakhleh RE. Obliterative bronchiolitis after lung transplantation: a fibroproliferative disorder associated with platelet-derived growth factor. *Proc Natl Acad Sci USA* 1992; **89**: 10385–10389.

35 Charpin JM, Valcke J, Kettaneh L, Epardean B, Stern M, Israel-Biet D. Peaks of transforming growth factor-beta mRNA in alveolar cells of lung transplant recipients as an early marker of chronic rejection. *Transplantation* 1998; **65**: 752–755.

36 Charpin JM, Stern M, Grenet D, Israel-Biet D. Insulinlike growth factor-1 in lung transplants with obliterative bronchiolitis. *Am J Respir Crit Care Med* 2000; **161**: 1991–1998.

37 Riise GC, Andersson BA, Kiellstrom C, et al. Persistent high BAL fluid granulocyte activation marker levels as early indicators of bronchiolitis obliterans after lung transplant. *Eur Respir J* 1999; **14**: 1123–1130.

38 DiGiovine B, Lynch JP, Martinez FJ, et al. Bronchoalveolar lavage neutrophilia is associated with obliterative bronchiolitis after lung transplantation: role of IL-8. *J Immunol* 1996; **157**: 4194–4202.

39 Uyama T, Winter JB, Groen G, Wildevuur CR, Monden Y, Prop J. Late airway changes caused by chronic rejection in rat lung allografts. *Transplantation* 1992; **54**: 809–812.

40 al-Dossari GA, Kshettry VR, Jessurun J, Bolman RM. Experimental large-animal model of obliterative bronchiolitis after lung transplantation. *Ann Thorac Surg* 1994; **58**: 34–39.

41 Hertz MI, Jessurun J, King MB. Reproduction of the obliterative bronchiolitis lesion after heterotopic transplantation of mouse airways. *Am J Pathol* 1993; **142**: 1945–1951.

42 Boehler A, Chamberlain D, Kesten S, Slutsky AS, Liu M, Keshavjee S. Lymphocytic airway infiltration as a precursor to fibrous obliteration in a rat model of bronchiolitis obliterans. *Transplantation* 1997; **64**: 311–317.

43 Ikonen T, Taskinen E, Uusitalo M, Aarnio P, Hayry P, Harjula AL. Chronic vascular changes and obliterative bronchiolitis in an experimental porcine lung transplantation model. *Transplant Proc* 1995; **27**: 2117.

44 Reichenspurner H, Soni V, Nitschke M, et al. Obliterative airway disease after heterotopic tracheal xenotransplantation. *Transplantation* 1997; **64**: 373–383.

45 Kelly KE, Hertz MI, Mueller DL. T-cell and major histocompatibility complex requirements for obliterative airway disease in heterotopically transplanted murine tracheas. *Transplantation* 1998; **66**: 764–771.

46 King MB, Jessurun J, Savik SK, Murray JJ, Hertz MI. Cyclosporine reduces development of obliterative bronchiolitis in a murine heterotopic airway model. *Transplantation* 1997; **63**: 528–532.

47 Fahrini JA, Berry GJ, Morris RE, Rosen GD. Rapamycin inhibits development of obliterative airway disease in a murine heterotopic airway transplant model. *Transplantation* 1997; **63**: 533–537.

48 al-Dossari G, Jessurun J, Bolman RM. Pathogenesis of obliterative bronchiolitis. *Transplantation* 1995; **59**: 143–145.

49 Snell GI, Esmore DS, Williams TJ. Cytolytic therapy for the bronchiolitis obliterans syndrome complicating lung transplantation. *Chest* 1996; **109**: 874–878.

50 Kesten S, Rajagopalan N, Maurer J. Cytolytic therapy for the treatment of bronchiolitis obliterans syndrome following lung transplantation. *Transplantation* 1996; **61**: 427–430.

51 Ross DJ, Lewis MI, Kramer M, Vo A, Kass RM. FK 506 'rescue' immunosuppression for obliterative bronchiolitis after lung transplantation. *Chest* 1997; **112**: 1175–1179.

52 Klepetko W, Estenne M, Glanville A, et al. A multicenter study to assess outcome following a switch in the primary immunosuppressant from cyclosporin (CYA) to tacrolimus (TAC) in lung recipients. *J Heart Lung Transplant* 2001; **20**: 208.

53 Cahill BC, O'Rourke MK, Strasburg KA, et al. Methotrexate for lung transplant recipients with steroid-resistant acute rejection. *J Heart Lung Transplant* 1996; **15**: 1130–1137.

54 Dusmet M, Maurer J, Winton T, Kesten S. Methotrexate can halt the progression of bronchiolitis obliterans syndrome in lung transplant recipients. *J Heart Lung Transplant* 1996; **15**: 948–954.

55 Steele DM, Hullett DA, Bechstein WO. The effects of immunosuppressive therapy on the rat aortic allograft model. *Transplant Proc* 1993; **25**: 754.

56 Novick RJ, Stitt LW, Al-Kattan K, et al. Pulmonary retransplantation: predictors of graft function and survival in 230 patients. Pulmonary Retransplant Registry. *Ann Thorac Surg* 1998; **65**: 227–234.

57 Iacono AT, Keenan RJ, Duncan SR, et al. Aerosolized cyclosporine in lung recipients with refractory chronic rejection. *Am J Respir Crit Care Med* 1996; **153**: 1451–1455.

58 Speich R, Boehler A, Russi EW, Weder W. A case report of a double-blind, randomized trial of inhaled steroids in a patient with lung transplant bronchiolitis obliterans. *Respiration* 1997; **64**: 375–380.

59 Takao M, Higenbottam TW, Audley T. Effects of inhaled nebulized steroids (Budesonide) on acute and chronic lung function in heart–lung transplant patients. *Transplant Proc* 1995; **27**: 1284–1285.

60 Whitford HM, Orsida B, Ward C, et al. Inhaled fluticasone propionate (FP) does not alter inflammation in the airway of lung allografts: a double blind placebo controlled trial. *J Heart Lung Transplant* 2000; **19**: A54.

61 Klauss V, Pethig K, Kalies H, et al. The effect of inhaled steroids on inflammatory markers associated with obliterative bronchiolitis. *J Heart Lung Transplant* 2000; **19**: A53.

62 Valentine VG, Robbins RC, Wehner JH, Patel HR, Berry GJ, Theodore J. Total lymphoid irradiation for refractory acute rejection in heart–lung and lung allografts. *Chest* 1996; **109**: 1184–1189.

63 Slovis B, Loyd J, King JL. Photopheresis for chronic rejection of lung allografts. *N Engl J Med* 1995; **6**: 962.

64 Salerno CT, Park SJ, Kreykes NS, et al. Adjuvant treatment of refractory lung transplant rejection with extracorporeal photopheresis. *J Thorac Cardiovasc Surg* 1999; **117**: 1063–1069.

65 Pham SM, Keenan RJ, Rao AS. Perioperative donor bone marrow infusion augments chimerism in heart and lung transplant recipients. *Ann Thorac Surg* 1995; **60**: 1015–1020.

66 Molossi S, Elices M, Arrhenius T. Blockade of very late antigen-4 integrin binding of fibronectin with connecting segment-1 peptide reduces accelerated coronary arteriopathy. *J Clin Invest* 1995; **95**: 2601–2610.

67 Morris RE. Rapamycins: antifungal, antitumor, antiproliferative, and immunosuppressive macrolides. *Transplant Rev* 1992; **6**: 39–87.

68 Gregory CR, Hule P, Billingham ME. Rapamycin inhibits arterial intimal thickening caused by both alloimmune and mechanical injury. Its effect on cellular, growth factor and cytokine response in injured vessels. *Transplantation* 1993; **55**: 1409–1418.

69 Muthukkumar S, Ramesh TM, Bondada S. Rapamycin, a potent immunosuppressive drug, causes programmed cell death in B lymphoma cells. *Transplantation* 1995; **60**: 264–270.

20

Infectious complications

Keith McNeil[1], Juliet Foweraker[1] and Tim Wreghitt[2]

[1]Papworth Hospital, Cambridgeshire, UK
[2]Addenbrookes Hospital, Cambridge, UK

Introduction

Infection is the major cause of both morbidity and mortality post lung transplantation [1,2]. It is usually the final common pathway complicating any significant insult to the allograft, be that in the early postoperative period, when ischaemia–reperfusion injury and high levels of immunosuppression increase the risk, through to the end-stages of the transplant marked by the presence of obliterative bronchiolitis.

Throughout the life of the transplant, even when patients are well with normal allograft function, the risk of infection is ever present. This is in part because of the ongoing need for immunosuppression, but also because of unique features associated with the lung. The lung allograft is unique among solid organ transplants in that it remains in direct contact with the external environment. This exposes the allograft to the numerous potential infectious agents and allergens that cause many of the problems encountered both immediately post-transplantation and in the longer term. In addition, the normal physiological and anatomical mechanisms that help to prevent infection in the healthy lung (such as coughing and mucociliary clearance) are disrupted by the transplantation operation, adding to the risk of developing infection. This is a particular problem in the immediate postoperative period.

Here, the infectious complications of lung transplantation will be considered in two ways. First, we will look at the issues relevant to the different phases of transplantation, by considering the assessment and management of infection associated with the recipient, donor, perioperative phase and long-term survival. Second, we will consider individual organisms and the features associated with their presentation, diagnosis and treatment in lung transplant recipients.

Recipient issues

Recipient suitability for lung transplantation [3] is determined by two factors, the underlying disease indication and the severity of that disease. Broadly speaking, there are four disease groups that cover the majority of lung transplant indications. These are obstructive lung diseases (e.g. emphysema, chronic obstructive pulmonary disease), pulmonary fibrosis, pulmonary vascular diseases (primary pulmonary hypertension, Eisenmenger's syndrome) and septic lung disease (cystic fibrosis (CF), non-CF bronchiectasis).

The pulmonary vascular diseases are not generally associated with infectious problems as the airways and lung parenchyma are structurally normal. The obstructive and fibrotic groups of diseases are associated with community acquired respiratory pathogens such as the pneumococcus, *Haemophilus influenzae*, *Moraxella catarrhalis*, etc. In the septic lung diseases where bronchiectasis is present, *Pseudomonas aeruginosa* is the predominant organism, but with the increasing use of antibiotics, especially in CF, a wide variety of Gram-negative organisms can be encountered.

In considering patients for transplantation, certain infections such as pan-resistant *Pseudomonas aeruginosa*, *Burkholderia cepacia*, and *Aspergillus* involving the pleural surface confer an increased risk in the peri-transplant period. These are discussed in greater detail in a later section. Most centres have individual policies regarding the suitability for transplantation of patients infected with these organisms. In general, none of these is an absolute contraindication to transplantation [4], but each case must be considered carefully with due regard to the unit's overall level of experience and expertise.

Table 20.1. Laboratory markers for chronic/latent infections for which all potential transplant candidates should be tested

- HBsAg (hepatitis B surface antigen)
- HIV (human immunodeficiency virus) antibody
- HCV (hepatitis C virus) antibody
- CMV (cytomegalovirus) antibody
- HSV (herpes simplex virus) antibody
- VZV (varicella-zoster virus) antibody
- *Toxoplasma gondii* antibody

Recipient assessment

All potential transplant patients should be tested for the pathogens listed in Table 20.1. Hepatitis B and C are likely to progress to severe disease in immunosuppressed transplant recipients [5,6]. Patients who are positive for markers of these diseases should be carefully assessed before transplantation, and only those with a low risk of disease progression should be considered for lung transplantation. This is a specialized area and referral to a hepatologist with transplant experience is advisable.

Cytomegalovirus (CMV) antibody status should be tested by two assays [7]. Accurate determination of CMV status is important in order that the risk of donor-acquired CMV infection and CMV reactivation can be assessed and appropriate antiviral prophylaxis (e.g. oral ganciclovir), or pre-emptive treatment can be provided.

Primary herpes simplex virus (HSV) infection is rare in transplant patients but reactivation can be fatal if it presents as post-transplantation pneumonitis [8]. Thus HSV antibody-positive recipients, not receiving ganciclovir for CMV prophylaxis, should be given either aciclovir or famciclovir prophylaxis.

Varicella zoster virus (VZV) antibody status is determined so that those (5%) who are VZV antibody negative can be advised to seek urgent medical review if they come into contact with chickenpox or shingles after transplantation. Treatment with zoster immune globulin (ZIG) and aciclovir is required to prevent life-threatening haemorrhagic chickenpox [9]. Pretransplant vaccination against VZV is an option for seronegative patients, but as this is a live attenuated vaccine, listing for transplantation would need to be deferred because of the risk of reactivation should a transplant be given. There are, however, no data as to the length of time that should be allowed between live vaccination and transplantation.

Toxoplasma gondii antibody status is determined so that if *T. gondii* antibody-positive donor organs are given to

a *T. gondii* antibody-negative recipient appropriate prophylaxis can be given [10,11]. Co-trimoxazole prophylaxis is given routinely for *Pneumocystis* infection beginning within the first week after transplantation and this is also effective in preventing toxoplasma reactivation. In the occasional patient who is allergic or intolerant of co-trimoxazole, consideration needs to be given to the toxoplasma status (see below).

Screening of potential organ donors

Guidelines from the UK Department of Health UK [12] indicate which infections should be tested for in the donor, and how to assess donor suitability. The range of infections that can be transmitted by a donor organ is considerable [1,13,14,]. Our experience, and that of others [1] is that donor-related infections are uncommon following lung transplantation. This reflects the care and attention given in selecting organs for transplantation, and the use of effective prophylactic antimicrobial strategies. However, with the increasing use of more compromised (so-called 'marginal') donor organs, other centres report a higher incidence of donor-acquired infections [13].

A serum sample from all organ donors should be tested for the pathogens listed in Table 20.2. Whenever possible, clotted blood samples should accompany organs so that the host laboratory can conduct confirmatory tests. Organ donors who are positive for hepatitis B surface antigen (HBsAg), human immunodeficiency virus (HIV) or hepatitis C virus (HCV) antibody should not be considered for transplantation except in acutely life-saving situations after all implications have been discussed with the potential recipient and/or his or her family [5,12].

Postoperative care

The first 24–48 hours are critical to the long-term outcome of the transplantation. The principal aim of immediate

Table 20.2. Laboratory markers for which a serum sample from all organ donors should be tested

- HBsAg
- HIV antibody
- HCV antibody
- CMV antibody
- *Toxoplasma gondii* antibody

Note: For abbreviations, see Table 20.1.

postoperative care is to reduce allograft injury during this critical period. The allograft sustains an endothelial injury because of ischaemia and preservation. This causes a breakdown of the capillary endothelial barrier, resulting in leakage of fluid into alveoli. Increasing damage leads to a progressive impairment in gas exchange. This may necessitate prolonged mechanical ventilatory support, with an increased risk of infection and barotrauma often resulting in irreversible damage to the allograft.

Bacterial infection remains the most significant problem encountered in the early phase and is responsible for most deaths during the perioperative period. In the majority of cases the organism is recipient derived [1,13]. Antibiotic prophylaxis may be administered until the patient is mobile, all drains have been removed and respiratory secretions are clear. Subsequent antibiotic therapy is determined by the culture results of the perioperative microbiology specimens.

The underlying disease and/or pretransplant microbiology findings dictate the choice of antibiotic prophylaxis. In cystic fibrosis and other septic lung diseases, the antibiotics used cover *Pseudomonas aeruginosa* and *Staphylococcus aureus*. In other patients, community-acquired respiratory pathogens (*Streptococcus pneumoniae, Haemophilus influenzae*, etc.) and *Staph. aureus* are targeted. In cystic fibrosis patients, extensive pretransplant microbiology results are usually available to guide perioperative antibiotic selection. Intraoperative specimens should be taken (recipient and donor airway swabs) and the antibiotic regimen re-evaluated when the results of these are known, usually 48 hours later. In patients colonized with *Pseudomonas*, in addition to intravenous antibiotics, it is our usual practice to administer inhaled (nebulized) colistin 1–2 MU twice daily, for the first two to four weeks. There is, however, no evidence that this decreases the incidence of postoperative infective complications or improves outcome.

Methicillin-resistant *Staph. aureus* (MRSA) colonization has become a major problem for many transplant units around the world and vancomycin is often administered in the perioperative period until the MRSA status of both the donor and recipient is known.

Fungal infection in the form of oropharyngeal candidiasis is common post-transplantation and prophylaxis with topical nystatin or amphotericin is effective. Systemic prophylaxis against *Candida* is not generally necessary but this will be determined by local experience. *Aspergillus* is the commonest cause of invasive fungal disease (see below). In single and bilateral lung transplantation, nebulized amphotericin (5 mg three times per day), given for the first month post-transplantation is effective in reducing

Aspergillus-related problems. Routine use of itraconazole prophylaxis is dependent on local policy and experience. In contrast to single and bilateral lung transplants (which employ a bronchial anastamosis), it is very uncommon for combined heart–lung transplant recipients to have problems with *Aspergillus* in this period. Unlike the bronchial anastamosis, the tracheal anastomosis is not ischaemic and routine prophylactic strategies are therefore not required.

Viral infections (specifically herpes viruses) tend to occur later in the recovery period [5] but prophylaxis must be administered from the early stages to be effective. Ganciclovir is very effective in reducing both the incidence and severity of CMV and other herpes virus-related illness [15]. There is no consensus, however, on the optimal prophylaxis regimen. Most units opt for a combination of intravenous and oral therapy for one to three months, given to any recipient who is serologically CMV positive, or receives an allograft from a CMV-positive donor. Alternatively, so-called 'pre-emptive' therapeutic strategies can be employed for those at risk, utilizing either antigenaemia or polymerase chain reaction (PCR) monitoring of CMV activity. HSV commonly causes mucocutaneous infection. In the case of CMV-negative donor/recipient pairs (where ganciclovir is unnecessary), aciclovir or famciclovir should be used as prophylaxis in HSV seropositive individuals [8].

Co-trimoxazole prophylaxis is used to prevent both *Pneumocystis* and toxoplasma infection [16] reactivation. Standard therapy is 480 mg daily or 960 mg three times per week. Therapy is given for a minimum of 12 months or until corticosteroid therapy has been reduced to physiological replacement doses. If co-trimoxazole is not tolerated, nebulized pentamidine (300 mg per month) is an effective alternative [17]. Pentamidine is not, however, effective at preventing toxoplasma reactivation, which must be covered separately with pyrimethamine in this situation [11].

Long-term management

Early recognition and treatment of infection is vitally important if allograft dysfuction is to be minimized over the long term. Monitoring of symptoms, chest X-ray and spirometry are the basis of allograft surveillance. When allograft dysfunction occurs, transbronchial biopsies are performed and bronchoalveolar fluid taken for culture of bacteria, fungi and viruses. Particularly in the early stages of the transplant, it is not possible to distinguish acute rejection and infection on clinical grounds. Indeed they often occur simultaneously. Histopathological diagnosis of the cause of dysfunction is therefore highly desirable, especially in the first three to six months when the incidences of acute rejection and infection are highest.

Once out of hospital, patients are at risk of contracting community-acquired viral and 'atypical' infections. Of these, influenza, respiratory syncytial virus (RSV), adenovirus, and mycoplasma can have devastating consequences leading to significant losses in lung function and reduced survival prospects. It should be noted that these organisms are also acquired as nosocomial infections at any time post-transplantation, and therefore should be considered in the differential diagnosis of any hospital-acquired infection. These organisms are discussed in more detail below. Public Health Laboratories are able to provide data regarding concurrent community infection problems (such as influenza epidemics and outbreaks of RSV and mycoplasma, etc.), allowing early diagnosis and intervention. The role of organisms such as human herpes virus 6 and *Chlamydia* in causing acute and chronic allograft dysfunction is not yet clear but these and other 'atypical' organisms are attracting more attention as more reliable diagnostic techniques become available for routine clinical application.

Yearly influenza, and five-yearly pneumococcal vaccines should be administered to all patients on the waiting list and all lung transplant recipients as per the recommendations for any immunosuppressed patient or patient with severe lung disease. There are no data to attest to the efficacy of these vaccines in this population; however, if infection can be avoided or attenuated, then the potential to minimize allograft damage is very significant.

Obliterative bronchiolitis

Obliterative bronchiolitis (OB) is a fibroproliferative scarring process that results in either total or subtotal obliteration of the affected airway lumen. It affects 50% of lung transplant recipients between three and five years post-transplantation [18]. Its pathogenesis is discussed elsewhere in this volume (see Chapter 19).

OB confers an increased risk of death. In patients with OB, the main cause of death is infection, and one of the main risks for progression of the disease is the number of infective episodes complicating the OB [18]. Inevitably, bronchiectasis develops in association with the airway scarring, and consequently organisms such as *Pseudomonas aeruginosa*, *Aspergillus* and atypical mycobacteria become problematic. Therapy should be aimed at reducing the risk of infection with the use of infection prophylaxis strategies as well as reducing the level of immunosuppression to the lowest safe level. Appropriate vaccination has already been discussed. Inhaled colistin or tobramycin is effective in reducing *Pseudomonas* exacerbations. *Aspergillus* is effectively controlled with long-term itraconazole, and there is increasing experience with the use of long-term terbinafine therapy in this situation. None of these therapies has been subjected to clinical trials and recommendations are therefore based on anecdotal evidence and the experience of large centres.

Specific infections

Infection with *Pseudomonas aeruginosa* and related organisms prior to transplantation

Pseudomonas aeruginosa is the predominant organism causing infection late in the course of CF-associated lung disease and other types of bronchiectasis [19]. The strains are usually mucoid, an adaptation to chronic colonization, and may have acquired many resistance genes after years of antibiotics. Strains may be multiresistant, which is defined as resistant to all antibiotics in two of the three groups: cell wall agents (penicillins, cephalosporins and penems), aminoglycosides (e.g. gentamicin and tobramycin) and quinolones. Pan-resistant organisms are resistant to all three groups. Pan- and multi-resistant *Pseudomonas* as defined by conventional laboratory sensitivity may, however, still respond in vivo to the antibiotics to which the *Pseudomonas* is resistant. This may be because antibiotics at subinhibitory concentration may reduce bacterial pathogenicity, or because of the synergistic effect of certain antibiotic combinations. The exclusion of patients with pan-resistant organisms is controversial [20]. Some units such as ours have shown that such patients may do just as well post-transplantation [21]. In addition, the antibiotic sensitivity patterns of bacteria cultured from operative respiratory tract samples are often different from those grown during the pretransplantation period [21].

Studies with molecular typing methods have shown that patients often have late infections, with strains of *Ps. aeruginosa* found in their lungs at explant, despite appropriate prophylaxis [19]. This suggests carriage post-transplantation in the upper respiratory and/or gastrointestinal tracts.

Two antipseudomonal antibiotics should be used to treat infections with *Ps. aeruginosa*. The combination of a cell wall active agent (penicillin or cephalosporin) and an aminoglycoside is thought to be synergistic. A more compelling reason for combination therapy, however, is the frequent occurrence in CF patients of strains of *Ps. aeruginosa* with a high spontaneous mutation rate (antibiotic resistance mutations at a frequency of 10^{-3}) [19].

Other 'pseudomonads'

CF patients in particular may be infected with other *Pseudomonas*-like organisms such as *Stenotrophomonas maltophilia* and *Alkaligenes* species. The pathogenicity of these organisms in CF is still poorly understood and there is insufficient information to assess their importance in the post-transplantation period. Like *Ps. aeruginosa*, however, they may be pan- or multiresistant. *Stenotrophomonas* is intrinsically resistant to the penems (imipenem and meropenem) and both organisms can become resistant to colistin. Where *Stenotrophomonas* has been problematic post-transplantation (and not responsive to conventional antipseudomonal antibiotics), we have found that high dose intravenous co-trimoxazole (1440 mg twice daily) can be effective.

Burkholderia cepacia

Burkholderia cepacia is an important cause of infection late in CF. Some strains can cause a rapid deterioration, the so-called 'cepacia syndrome'. Certain types of *B. cepacia* (genomovar III) have been associated with a poor prognosis following lung transplantation [22]. *Burkholderia cepacia* may be resistant to many antibiotics, and all are intrinsically resistant to colistin. It is still debated whether patients who carry *B. cepacia* should be accepted for transplantation [4] or whether there are sufficient data to exclude only those carrying genomovar III.

Clostridium difficile

All patients receive antibiotics post-transplantation and *Clostridium difficile* should be considered in the differential diagnosis of any case of diarrhoea or large bowel problems. CMV is the only other common infective gastrointestinal complication in lung transplant recipients. Standard *C. difficile* toxin assays are used for diagnosis but on occasions the diagnosis will be evident only after colonoscopy and biopsy. It is our practice to commence oral metronidazole or vancomycin therapy in any patient currently or recently treated with antibiotics, who develops diarrhoea. Treatment is started before the *C. difficile* toxin result is available. If a response to therapy is seen in this situation, a full treatment course is given regardless of the toxin assay result. We have seen a number of cases of pseudomembranous colitis diagnosed on colonoscopic biopsy where the *C. difficile* toxin assay was repeatedly negative.

Cytomegalovirus

CMV is the commonest opportunistic pathogen to affect lung transplant patients; it is discussed elsewhere in this volume (see Banner, Chapter 21). There are several points,

however, that relate specifically to lung transplant recipients and should be mentioned here.

Before the introduction of ganciclovir, CMV pneumonitis had a high mortality rate, particularly in CMV naive lung transplant recipients [23,24,25]. This led to a policy of matching CMV-negative recipients with CMV-negative donors to prevent primary (donor acquired) infection. Ganciclovir therapy (both treatment and prophylaxis) has proved very effective in reducing both the morbidity and mortality associated with this infection and thus CMV matching is not deemed necessary in the current transplant era [15]. Prophylaxis appears effective in both delaying the onset of clinical infection and reducing the severity of subsequent infective episodes. CMV has also been identified as a risk factor for the development of OB [18]. The exact link between the virus and OB is unclear. Consequently it is not known whether or not treatment and/or prophylaxis of CMV will prove effective in reducing this risk.

Nocardia asteroides

Although given prominence in reviews of infection in lung transplants, this organism is an uncommon opportunistic pathogen in lung transplantation. This may in part be because of the use of co-trimoxazole for the prevention of *Pneumocystis carinii* infection. *Nocardia* may disseminate [26], the most serious consequence being cerebral disease. If suspected, it is important to warn the microbiology laboratory as cultures need to be kept longer than usual and special growth medium employed to isolate the organism. If *Nocardia* infection is suspected or diagnosed, standard treatment regimens apply.

Legionella pneumophila

Early in solid organ transplantation there were several outbreaks of nosocomial (hospital-acquired) legionellosis. Animal studies have shown that lung transplantation predisposes to early and severe pneumonia with *Legionella pneumophila* [27]. This is an infection that can and should be prevented by introducing optimal engineering controls to reduce the presence of the organism in hospital water systems and commercial premises. It is usual to perform serological and immunofluorescence testing for *Legionella* in any case of severe infection complicating a lung transplant. If infection does occur, standard treatment regimens should be applied.

Aspergillus infections

Aspergillus infection occurs in pulmonary and extrapulmonary forms. There are several forms of pulmonary infection ranging from invasive parenchymal (*Aspergillus* pneumonia and chronic necrotizing pulmonary aspergillosis) and invasive airways disease (necrotizing ulcerative tracheobronchitis), to allergic manifestations (mucous plugging, eosinophilic bronchitis and allergic bronchopulmonary aspergillosis) and simple saprophytic colonization [28,29]. Extrapulmonary disease is always invasive. There are significant differences in the timing and pattern of *Aspergillus* infection related to the type of transplant. In single and bilateral lung transplants where the bronchial anastomosis is ischaemic, *Aspergillus*-related problems tend to occur early (most within the first three months) [30,31]. In addition, there is a very high risk of developing an airway problem if *Aspergillus* is present in this setting [31]. In contrast, in heart–lung transplantation the tracheal anastomosis is not ischaemic (due to a collateral blood supply from the coronary arteries). Early *Aspergillus*-related problems are uncommon. Most occur later with the onset of the airflow obstruction and bronchiectasis associated with OB.

Aspergillus infection of any sort must be diagnosed and treated early. Airway manifestations and early invasive parenchymal disease generally have a good prognosis. Late stage or disseminated disease is almost invariably fatal. Treatment with systemic amphotericin in high doses is used. Liposomal amphotericin B (LAB) is our preferred therapy because of its much improved side effect profile as compared to the conventional preparation (CAB). This is very evident in the setting of calcineurin-induced renal dysfunction, which severely limits therapy with CAB. Treatment with LAB can be started at a single dose of 5 mg/kg per day. It is generally well tolerated and can be given via a peripheral line. Other forms of amphotericin such as the colloidal dispersion also have a reduced side effect profile but experience with their use in lung transplantation is limited. There have been no comparative trials of CAB and the newer preparations in lung transplant patients and, as is often the case in this population, recommendations are based on retrospective reviews, anecdotal series, and the experience of larger centres.

The role of azoles (predominantly itraconazole) as primary treatment of *Aspergillus* infection in this population is not established. Itraconazole is generally reserved for prolonged treatment following a course of amphotericin, or where long-term prophylaxis is required. The latter situation usually arises where *Aspergillus* is repeatedly isolated in the setting of an airway complication, or in the presence of OB. It is important to ensure that adequate levels of itraconazole are achieved. Itraconazole must be taken on an empty stomach to ensure the acid environment necessary for its absorption. Experience with terbinafine and voriconazole is limited.

Other fungi

Candida species are a common contaminant in sputum and bronchoalveolar lavage, usually originating in the oropharynx. Treatment of such an isolate is not necessary in the absence of disease and may actually be counterproductive because of the concerns over the development of fluconazole resistance. *Candida* has been associated with airway dehisence (both as a cause and a complication) and may be acquired from the donor [1,13]. It is, however, an exceedingly rare cause of pneumonia except as part of the spectrum of disseminated disease from a blood-borne source.

Patients in the endemic areas are at risk of the systemic mycoses – coccidioidomycosis, histoplasmosis and paracoccidioidomycosis. *Cryptococcus neoformans* is an uncommon cause of infection in solid organ transplantation, as are the mucorales (*Mucor, Absidia, Rhizopus*). These all have a characteristic appearance on biopsy and treatment requires higher doses of amphotericin than do *Aspergillus* species. Excision of infected tissue needs also to be considered [31]. *Scedosporium* species resemble *Aspergillus* on biopsy but are intrinsically resistant to amphotericin. Voriconazole is (anecdotally) proving effective in the treatment of this infection.

It is essential that careful culture and identification of fungi be performed in the investigation of any infection in a lung transplant recipient [33].

Pneumocystis pneumonia

Pneumocystis infection is now an uncommon occurrence following the introduction of specific (co-trimoxazole) prophylaxis [16,29]. Infection usually occurs when prophylaxis is not taken [34] or when large doses of steroids are prescribed late after transplantation when prophylaxis may have been stopped. *Pneumocystis carinii* pneumonia (PCP) in lung transplant recipients presents in a very different manner to PCP in acquired immune deficiency syndrome (AIDS) patients, and if not recognized can be fatal. The onset is often insidious. The usual presentation is with a low grade febrile illness and mild to moderate dyspnoea, often only on exertion. Chest X-ray film may be normal or show subtle alveolar shadowing, usually in the upper lobes. High resolution computed tomography (CT) scanning often shows a groundglass pattern [35]. Severe hypoxaemia and gross radiographic changes are uncommon. Transbronchial biopsies typically show a granulomatous pneumonitis. On occasions, the histology mimics acute rejection and if special staining is not performed and the slides assiduously searched, the organisms will be missed [Dr S. Stewart, personal communication]. In distinct contrast to PCP in AIDS, the organism load in lung transplant recipients can be very low. Pneumocysts are not usually recovered from bronchoalveolar lavage fluid [29] and indeed can be very difficult to find in biopsy tissue. Repeated transbronchial biopsies may be necessary to diagnose this illness. Treatment regimens are the same as those employed in human immunodeficiency virus (HIV)-infected patients, although very high dose therapy is usually not required with the low organism loads. Co-trimoxazole 960 mg twice daily, either intravenously or orally, has been effective in the treatment of some of our patients with milder forms of this disease. In patients with more severe disease, however, full dose regimens are recommended (e.g. intravenous co-trimoxazole 960 mg six-hourly).

Toxoplasma gondii

Toxoplasma gondii can be transmitted from the organ donor to the recipient, causing fever, encephalitis, pneumonia and/or myocarditis [10]. In heart recipients, 60% of T. gondii antibody negative recipients who receive organs from T. gondii antibody positive donors acquire infection. Infection can be treated with sulfadiazine and pyrimethamine but providing co-trimoxazole or pyrimethamine prophylaxis to patients at risk of primary infection will prevent severe infection [11]. Whilst this should be considered in the differential diagnosis of patients with fever, malaise, encephalitis, pneumonia or myocarditis, T. gondii reactivation in lung recipients is rare probably because of the widespread use of co-trimoxazole prophylaxis.

Listeria monocytogenes

Although rare, this organism can cause meningitis in the lung transplant recipient. Dietary advice similar to that given to pregnant women (avoidance of unpasteurized cheeses and pâté, etc.), may help to prevent infection, especially in the early post-transplantation period when the patients are most heavily immunosuppressed.

It is common for a third generation cephalosporin such as cefotaxime to be used as first-line (empirical) treatment of meningitis in an adult. This antibiotic does not, however, act against Listeria and a penicillin should, therefore, always be part of the empirical treatment of meningitis in a transplant recipient.

Mycobacterial infection

Tuberculous (MTB) and nontuberculous (NTM) mycobacterial disease occur at an increased frequency in lung transplant recipients as compared with the general population [36,37]. Occult mycobacterial disease is sometimes found unexpectedly in explanted organs. In single lung transplantation, unsuspected disease may remain in the native lung. Rarely, MTB is transmitted from the donor [38]. With previous inadequately or untreated MTB infection, prophylaxis with isoniazid (INAH) should be considered. Unless there is documented exposure to INAH-resistant MTB, the use of rifampicin as a chemoprophylactic agent is not advisable because of the profound interaction with ciclosporin. If full treatment is required, standard robust antituberculous regimens are indicated. Rifampicin has a profound effect of inducing hepatic metabolism, and ciclosporin and corticosteroid doses must be adjusted (increased) accordingly. Ciclosporin levels in this setting are markedly reduced and dose increases of four to five times are usually required to maintain adequate immunosuppression levels. Regimens that do not contain rifampicin can be used [36], but these are by necessity much longer (a year or more) and less robust in achieving control than the modern short course treatments used for the treatment of tuberculosis.

NTM infections tend to occur later in the post-transplantation course than MTB. The indications to treat these organisms are the same as in the non-transplant population. Patients with intermittent isolation of NTM not associated with evidence of allograft dysfunction or progressive disease may be safely observed. Treatment should be reserved for those with evidence of disease directly attributable to the mycobacteria, or those in which the cause of allograft dysfunction is unclear.

Treatment of most NTM's is difficult and based largely on experiential data. Chemotherapy regimens depend on the species of Mycobacterium, but in general, are usually based on ethambutol and rifampicin with the addition of a macrolide (clarithromycin or azithromycin) and/or ciprofloxacin [39]. There are no data to guide the choice or length of treatment, but a minimum of 12 months' therapy is usually required depending on the organism and response to therapy. Intolerance of medication is a significant problem, which often limits treatment options in the longer term.

Nontuberculous mycobacteria can cause infection at other sites in the immunocompromised patient, most commonly the skin. This is, however, rarely reported in lung transplant patients [37].

There have been radical improvements in the laboratory diagnosis of mycobacterial disease. Direct differentiation of TB from NTM on respiratory samples can be achieved by PCR, and identification and sensitivity testing can be performed in days rather than weeks using rapid culture systems. Early diagnosis in the transplant patient can allow appropriate drugs to be given and reduce the risk of cross-infection [40].

Epstein–Barr virus

Approximately 95% of adult transplant recipients have had previous infection with Epstein–Barr virus (EBV), thus primary infection in adults is rare. EBV-negative patients who receive organs from EBV-positive donors will, however, experience primary EBV infection. Transplant patients do not experience glandular fever-like symptoms. They present with nonspecific symptoms such as fever, malaise, coryza and cough [41]. The most serious disease manifestation is post-transplantation lymphoproliferative syndrome, which results from EBV-driven B-cell replication.

Infection can be diagnosed by the detection of EBV DNA by PCR, or by serological methods. Since most infections are reactivations, if serological diagnosis is attempted, a rise in EBV virus capsid antibody (VCA) is sought. EBV nuclear antigen (EBNA) antibody is not reliably produced in transplant recipients and is not useful. EBV-specific immunoglobulin (Ig)M is also not useful for diagnosis, since this antibody is often not produced in reactivation states.

Other herpes virus infections

Herpes simplex virus (HSV) can produce skin and genital lesions, encephalitis and pneumonitis in lung transplant recipients [8]. Primary VZV infection (chickenpox) can be fatal in transplant recipients, especially if the haemorrhagic form, encephalitis or pneumonia develop [9]. VZV reactivation, often occurring in the first few weeks after transplantation, manifests as skin lesions (shingles). This usually affects one dermatome; however, generalized shingles can occur. The appropriate samples and tests used for diagnosis of HSV and VZV are shown in Table 20.3. Treatment is with standard courses of either aciclovir or famciclovir.

Other 'atypical' organisms

The most commonly identified of the other so-called 'atypical' organisms causing infectious problems in lung transplant recipients are *Mycoplasma*, adenovirus and respiratory syncytial virus (RSV). All have the potential to cause a spectrum of illness from relatively mild upper and lower respiratory tract infections, through to severe pneumonitis. The more severe manifestations can be associated with irreversible allograft dysfunction. *Mycoplasma* is treated with macrolide antibiotics or doxycycline. Treatment options for the viral infections are limited and unproven in the lung transplant population. Ribavirin, has been used to treat RSV in bone marrow [42,43] and lung transplant [44] recipients. If this is to be of benefit, therapy should be instituted early. The role of steroids in the treatment of viral pneumonitis is again unproven, but

Table 20.3. Laboratory diagnosis of virus and atypical organism infection in lung transplant recipients

Organism	Samples	Laboratory tests
HSV	Vesicle fluid	Electron microscopy[a], PCR, virus culture
	BAL	PCR, virus culture, IF
	Throat swab in VTM	PCR, virus culture
	Lung biopsy	PCR, virus culture
	CSF	PCR
VZV	Vesicle fluid	Electron microscopy[a], PCR, virus culture
	CSF	PCR
EBV	Serum	Paul Bunell test, specific EBV antibody, PCR
Influenza viruses	BAL/NPA	Virus culture, IF
Adenoviruses	Throat swab in VTM	Virus culture, IF
	BAL	Virus culture, IF
Respiratory syncytialvirus	Serum	Virus-specific antibody[b]
	Throatswab in VTM BAL	Virus culture
Parainfluenza viruses		Virus culture, IF
Mycoplasma pneumoniae *Chlamydia psittaci* *Chlamydia pneumoniae* *Coxiella burnetii*	Serum	Specific antibody[b]
Legionella pneumophila	Serum	Specific antibody[c]
	Urine	Antigen detection[d]
	BAL/lung biopsy	*Legionella* culture
Papillomaviruses	Biopsy	PCR
Toxoplasma gondii	Serum	*T. gondii*, IgG, IgM

Note: HSV, herpes simplex virus; PCR, polymerase chain reaction; BAL, bronchoalveolar lavage; IF, immunofluorescence; CSF, cerebrospinal fluid; VZV, varicella-zoster virus; EBV, Epstein–Barr virus; NPA, nasopharyngeal aspirate; VTM, virus transport medium; Ig, immunoglobulin.

[a] All herpes viruses have identical morphology. Presence of herpes virus particles could indicate presence of HSV or VZV.

[b] Allow 10 days for specific antibody to be produced.

[c] May take one month for antibody to be produced.

[d] Take in the first five days after onset of symptoms.

many clinicians will use pulsed methylprednisolone in this situation, in an attempt to reduce inflammation and the subsequent scarring.

Laboratory diagnosis of virus and atypical organism infection in lung transplant recipients

Viruses can cause respiratory infections at any time of year but most (in particular influenza and RSV) are more prevalent in the winter months. Lung transplant recipients may have mixed infections with viruses and bacteria, and knowledge of the infecting organisms is important for guiding the choice of the most appropriate (antibiotic) treatment. It is important to take samples for virus culture or immunofluorescence (IF) from patients with respiratory symptoms. Specimens must be taken in virus transport medium. IF should be performed on a nasopharyngeal aspirate (NPA), and/or a bronchoalveolar lavage fluid if available. Cells from the specimens are fixed onto a microscope slide and fluorescein-labelled monoclonal antibodies are used to detect specific viruses (influenza A virus, influenza B virus, RSV, adenoviruses, parainfluenzaviruses 1–3).

Specific antibodies to several viruses and atypical organisms can be detected in the complement fixation test (see Table 20.3). It is important to remember that it takes at least 10 days for these antibodies to be produced. Paired serum samples tested in parallel, one taken in the first week of illness and a second taken at least 10 days after onset of symptoms are necessary to best achieve a serological diagnosis. Interpretation of single sample virus titres is often difficult.

Clinical approach to the lung transplant patient with infection

Given the frequency of infectious complications and the potential for loss of allograft function, it is important that infection is considered, investigated and treated as soon as possible after the onset of symptoms. Initial symptoms may be nonspecific and thus patients must be educated to communicate with the transplant service in the event of any significant problems developing at any stage post-transplantation.

It is highly desirable for suitable specimens to be obtained for microbiological and virological testing before treatment is commenced. However, empirical treatment (see below) should not be withheld until results are available. The results of a transbronchial lung biopsy can be available in hours, with the pattern of histology often diagnostic, or at the very least giving valuable clues as to the likely aetiology. CMV and other herpes virus infections

are associated with distinctive viral inclusions. Bacterial infection is suspected when neutrophilic infiltration of the bronchial mucosa or pulmonary interstitium is present. Characteristic fungal hyphae allow the identification of *Aspergillus* and other fungal species. The presence of granulomatous inflammation prompts a hunt for mycobacteria or pneumocysts. Appropriate anti-infective treatment can therefore be commenced on the basis of the histology, pending the results of cultures and immunofluorescence testing of lavage samples.

On occasions, it will not be possible nor practical to biopsy these patients. Appropriate material should still be collected for culture, etc., and empirical therapy started to cover likely pathogens.

In the majority of cases, lung transplant patients presenting with an acute infective illness will have either a bacterial or viral infection. In these circumstances it is useful to consider the following. First, was the (potential) infection acquired in the community or in hospital? Community-acquired infections are well covered by the combination of a third generation cephalosporin such as cefotaxime or ceftriaxone, and a macrolide antibiotic. Dosing of cephalosporins may need modification according to renal function. Immunosuppressive drug levels (ciclosporin, tacrolimus and sirolimus) need to be monitored if macrolides are used (levels increase on macrolide therapy because of competitive enzyme inhibition).

Empirical treatment of hospital-acquired infection requires Gram-negative organisms (particularly *Pseudomonas*) to be covered. This also applies to patients with cystic fibrosis, or those with bronchiectasis complicating OB where recurrent *Pseudomonas* infection is very common. The combination of an antipseudomonal beta-lactam antibiotic with an aminoglycoside is usually effective. If patients have previously isolated MRSA from their respiratory tract it is our practice to use vancomycin in addition to the above antibiotics until culture results are available. Renal function must be considered in the choice and dosing of antibiotics, but the choice of optimal anti-infective therapy should not be compromised because of concerns regarding renal function. Short-term renal dysfunction is usually recoverable in this situation.

The combination of upper or lower gastrointestinal symptoms with a low white blood cell count is suggestive of CMV infection, and in this situation consideration should be given to commencing ganciclovir therapy pending CMV antigen (pp65) or PCR results.

Obviously not every potential pathogen can be covered in the acute setting. For this reason, and because of the not infrequent co-existence of multiple processes in these patients, the value of early diagnosis via bronchoscopy, bronchoalveolar lavage (with culture, immunofluorescence, PCR, etc.) together with transbronchial lung biopsy cannot be overemphasized.

REFERENCES

1 Zenati M, Dowling RD, Dummer JS, et al. Influence of the donor lung on development of early infections in lung transplant recipients. *J Heart Transplant* 1990; **9**: 502–509.

2 Chapparo C, Maurer JR, Chamberlain D. Causes of death in lung transplant recipients. *J Heart Lung Transplant* 1994; **13**: 758–766.

3 Anonymous. International guidelines for the selection of lung transplant candidates. The American Society for Transplant Physicians (ASTP)/American Thoracic Society (ATS)/European Respiratory Society (ERS)/International Society for Heart and Lung Transplantation (ISHLT). *Am J Respir Crit Care Med* 1998; **158**: 335–339.

4 Egan JJ, McNeil K, Bookless B, et al. Post-transplantation survival of cystic fibrosis patients infected with *Pseudomonas cepacia. Lancet* 1994; **344**: 552–553.

5 Fishman JA, Rubin RH. Infection in organ-transplant recipients. *New Engl J Med* 1998; **338**: 1741–1751.

6 Hosenpud JD, Pamidi SR, Fiol BS, Cinquegrani MP, Keck BM. Outcomes in patients who are hepatitis B surface antigen positive before transplantation: an analysis using the joint ISHLT/UNOS thoracic registry. *J Heart Lung Transplant* 2000; **19**: 781–785.

7 Farrington M, Tedder R, Kibbler C, Wreghitt T, Gould K, Tremlett CH. Pre-transplantation testing: who when and why? *J Hosp Inf* 1999; **43**: 5243–5252.

8 Smyth RL, Higenbottam TW, Scott JP, et al. Herpes simplex virus infection in heart–lung transplant recipients. *Transplantation* 1990; **49**: 735–739.

9 Bradley JR, Wreghitt TG, Evans DB. Chickenpox in adult renal transplant recipients. *Nephrol Dial Transplant 1987*; **1**: 242–245.

10 Wreghitt TG, Hakim M, Gray JJ, et al. Toxoplasmosis in heart and lung transplant recipients. *J Clin Pathol* 1989; **42**: 194–199.

11 Wreghitt TG, Gray JJ, Pavel P, et al. Efficacy of pyrimethamine for the prevention of donor-acquired *Toxoplasma gondii* infection in heart and lung transplant patients. *Transpl Int* 1992; **5**: 197–200.

12 *Guidance on the Microbiological Safety of Human Organs, Tissues and Cells used in Transplantation.* UK Department of Health, August 2000.

13 Low DE, Kaiser LR, Haydock DA, Trulock E, Cooper JD. The donor lung: infectious and pathologic factors affecting outcome in lung transplantation. *J Thorac Cardiovasc Surg* 1993; **106**: 614–621.

14 Eastlund T. Infectious disease transmission through cell, tissue, and organ transplantation: reducing the risk through donor selection. *Cell Transplant* 1995; **4**: 455–477.

15 Wreghitt TG, Abel SJ, McNeil K, et al. Intravenous ganciclovir prophylaxis for cytomegalovirus in heart, heart–lung, and lung transplant recipients. *Transpl Int* 1999; **12**: 254–260.

16 Kramer MR, Stoehr C, Lewiston NJ, Starnes VA, Theodore J. Trimethoprim-sulfamethoxazole prophylaxis for *Pneumocystis carinii* infections in heart–lung and lung transplantation – how effective and for how long? *Transplanation* 1992; **53**: 586–589.

17 Nathan SD, Ross DJ, Zakowski P, Kass RM, Koerner SK. Utility of inhaled pentamidine prophylaxis in lung transplant recipients. *Chest* 1994; **105**: 417–420.

18 Heng D, Sharples LD, McNeil K, Stewart S, Wreghitt T, Wallwork J. Bronchiolitis obliterans syndrome: incidence, natural history, prognosis, and risk factors. *J Heart Lung Transplant* 1998; **17**: 1255–1263.

19 Walter S, Gudowius P, Bosshammer J, et al. Epidemiology of chronic *Pseudomonas aeruginosa* infections in the airways of lung transplant recipients with cystic fibrosis. *Thorax* 1997; **52**: 318–321.

20 Egan TM, Detterbeck FC, Mill MR, et al. Improved results of lung transplantation for patients with cystic fibrosis. *J Thorac Cardiovasc Surg* 1995; **109**: 224–235.

21 Smith SR, Foweraker J, et al. Impact of antibiotic-resistant *Pseudomonas* on the survival of cystic fibrosis (CF) patients following heart–lung transplantation. *J Heart Lung Transplant* 2001; **209**: 224 (Abstract 219).

22 Aris RM, Routh JC, LiPuma JJ, Heath DG, Gilligan PH. Lung transplantation for cystic fibrosis patients with *Burkholderia cepacia* complex. Survival linked to genomovar type. *Am J Respir Crit Care Med* 2001; **164**: 2102–2106.

23 Hutter JA, Scott J, Wreghitt T, Higenbottam T, Wallwork J. The importance of cytomegalovirus in heart–lung transplant recipients. *Chest* 1989; **95**: 627–631.

24 Smyth RL, Scott JP, Borysiewicz LK, et al. Cytomegalovirus infection in heart–lung transplant recipients: risk factors, clinical associations, and response to treatment. *J Infect Dis* 1991; **164**: 1045–1050.

25 Smyth RL, Sinclair J, Scott JP, et al. Infection and reactivation with cytomegalovirus strains in lung transplant recipients. *Transplantation* 1991; **52**: 480–482.

26 McNeil KD, Johnson DW, Oliver WA. Endobronchial nocardial infection. *Thorax* 1993; **48**: 1281–1282.

27 Aeba R, Stout JE, Francalancia NA, et al. Aspects of lung transplantation that contribute to increased severity of pneumonia. An experimental study. *J Thorac Cardiovasc Surg* 1993; **106**: 449–457.

28 Kramer MR, Denning DW, Marshall SE, et al. Ulcerative tracheobronchitis after lung transplantation. A new form of invasive aspergillosis. *Am Rev Respir Dis* 1991; **144**: 552–556.

29 Shreeniwas R, Schulman LL, Berkman YM, McGregor CC, Austin JH. Opportunistic bronchopulmonary infections after lung transplantation: clinical and radiographic findings. *Radiology* 1996; **200**: 349–356.

30 Higgins R, McNeil K, Dennis C, et al. Airway stenoses after lung transplantation management with expanding metal stents. *J Heart Lung Transplant* 1994; **13**: 774–778.

31 Herrera JM, McNeil KD, Higgins RS, et al. Airway complications after lung transplantation: treatment and long-term outcome. *Ann Thorac Surg* 2001; **71**: 989–994.

32 Zander DS, Cicale MJ, Mergo P. Durable cure of mucormycosis involving allograft and native lungs. *J Heart Lung Transplant* 2000; **19**: 615–618.

33 Paradowski LJ. Saprophytic fungal infections and lung transplantation – revisited. *J Heart Lung Transplant* 1997; **16**: 524–531.

34 Gryzan S, Paradis IL, Zeevi A, et al. Unexpectedly high incidence of *Pneumocystis carinii* infection after lung–heart transplantation. Implications for lung defense and allograft survival. *Am Rev Respir Dis* 1988; **137**: 1268–1274.

35 Bergin CJ, Wirth RL, Berry GJ, Castellino RA. *Pneumocystis carinii* pneumonia: CT and HRCT observations. *J Comput Assist Tomogr* 1990; **14**: 756–759.

36 Dromer C, Nashef SA, Velly JF, Martigne C, Couraud L. Tuberculosis in transplanted lungs. *J Heart Lung Transplant* 1993; **12**: 924–927.

37 Malouf MA, Glanville AR. The spectrum of mycobacterial infection after lung transplantation. *Am J Respir Crit Care Med* 1999; **160**: 1611–1616.

38 Ridgeway AL, Warner GS, Phillips P, et al. Transmission of *Mycobacterium tuberculosis* to recipients of single lung transplants from the same donor. *Am J Respir Crit Care Med* **153**: 1166–1168.

39 Campbell IA. The management of lung disease caused by opportunistic mycobacteria. *Proc R Coll Physic Edinb* 1999; **29**: 315–318.

40 American Thoracic Society. Diagnostic standards and classification of tuberculosis in adults and children. *Am J Respir Care Med* 2000; **161**: 1376–1395.

41 Wreghitt TG, Sargaison M, Sutehall G, et al. A study of Epstein–Barr virus infections in heart and lung transplant recipients. *Transplant Proc* 1989; **21**: 2502–2503.

42 McColl MD, Corser RB, Bremner J, Chopra R. Respiratory syncytial virus infection in adult BMT recipients: effective therapy with short duration nebulised ribavirin. *Bone Marrow Transplant* 1998; **21**: 423–425.

43 Whimbey E, Champlin RE, Englund JA, et al. Combination therapy with aerosolized ribavirin and intravenous immunoglobulin for respiratory syncytial virus disease in adult bone marrow transplant recipients. *Bone Marrow Transplant* 1995; **16**: 393–399.

44 Doud JR, Hinkamp T, Garrity ER Jr. Respiratory syncytial virus pneumonia in a lung transplant recipient: case report. *J Heart Lung Transplant* 1992; **11**: 77–79.

21

Cytomegalovirus infection

Nicholas R. Banner

Harefield Hospital, Harefield, Middlesex, UK

Introduction

Nonspecific pharmacological immunosuppression has to be used after transplantation to prevent rejection of the allograft (see Chapter 18); this puts the recipient of a transplant at risk from a number of medical complications including infection. Cytomegalovirus (CMV) is currently the most common opportunistic pathogen to affect this patient group. CMV infection typically becomes apparent one to four months after transplantation [1]. Prior to the development of strategies to control CMV, this infection had a high mortality rate, especially in those lung transplant recipients who developed respiratory failure due to CMV pneumonitis [2,3]. Currently, CMV still causes considerable morbidity, and occasional mortality, in thoracic organ transplant recipients and adds to the cost of transplantation [4]. In addition, CMV infection appears to predispose to some of the long-term complications of transplantation including transplant-associated coronary vascular disease and bronchiolitis obliterans syndrome [5–7].

Cytomegalovirus

CMV is a human herpes virus of the beta subfamily, systematically designated as human herpesvirus 5 (HHV-5) [8]. Like other members of the family, it is a double-stranded DNA virus and has a large genome. Initial CMV infection in an immunocompetent individual is often asymptomatic or only mildly symptomatic. Infection results, however, in a life-long latent infection that can be reactivated or transmitted in circumstances such as organ transplantation.

CMV is a ubiquitous virus and about 60% of the adult population are seropositive indicating prior (and latent) infection. A number of clinical syndromes are associated with CMV, including congenital infection, an infectious

mononucleosis-like illness and more severe disease in those immunocompromised after solid organ or bone marrow transplantation or by cancer or human immunodeficiency virus (HIV) infection.

The structure of CMV and its growth cycle are now understood in some detail [9]. Productive viral infection results from the sequential expression of groups of viral genes that can be divided according to the order of their activation: α immediate-early, β early (delayed-early) and γ late. The pattern of gene expression during latent infection is restricted to early gene products (Figure 21.1).

CMV infection in transplant recipients

Before effective drug therapy became available, CMV disease caused significant morbidity and mortality in transplant patients (Figure 21.2) [3]. Improvements in diagnosis and the availability of effective antiviral drug therapy have greatly reduced the risk of mortality but CMV infection still causes substantial morbidity. Surveillance for CMV infection, diagnostic investigations, drug therapy and hospital care all contribute to the health care costs caused by this infection. In addition, the late sequelae of CMV infection may reduce the long-term benefits of transplantation.

It has become apparent that early treatment greatly reduces the risk from CMV infection. The trend towards earlier 'pre-emptive' therapy and prophylactic therapy has led to a larger proportion of patients receiving treatment and increased potential for drug toxicity. It is to be hoped that, in the future, a better understanding of the complex relationship between the transplant patient, the virus, the graft and the immunosuppression used will enable us to reduce the burden of CMV infection.

The infection can vary greatly in its severity and clinical manifestations. Even in immunosuppressed patients some

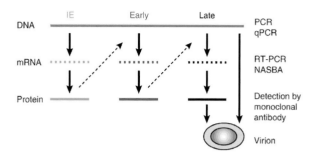

Figure 21.1 Sequence of gene expression during CMV infection and methods available to detect genomic DNA or gene expression at mRNA and protein levels. IE, intermediate early; PCR, polymerase chain reaction; qPCR, quantitative PCR; RT-PCR, reverse transcriptase PCR; NASBA, nucleic acid sequence-based amplification.

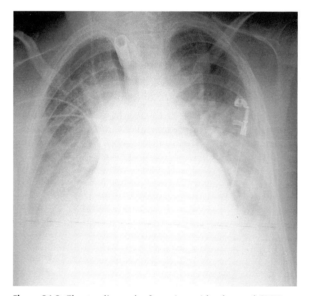

Figure 21.2 Chest radiograph of a patient with advanced CMV pneumonitis and respiratory failure. CMV pneumonitis was a common and severe complication of lung transplantation until rapid diagnostic tests and effective drug therapy became available; such cases are now uncommon.

episodes may be mild and self limited. The likelihood of serious disease depends on the host's ability to mount an effective immune response. This, in turn, is influenced by previous exposure to the virus (immunological memory), the level of immunosuppression, and type of transplant received [10].

Attempts have been made to clarify the literature by standardizing the definitions of various manifestations of CMV infection [11,12]. 'Active CMV infection' implies laboratory evidence of productive viral replication or the presence of a host response to viral infection (e.g. seroconversion). Such an infection may be primary or secondary (reactivation or superinfection). 'CMV disease' refers to the presence of symptoms or signs related to infection or organ dysfunction coupled with evidence of active CMV infection in that organ. 'Tissue invasive disease' appears to have a predilection for the transplanted organ that may cause problems in separating the effects of infection from the possibility of coexisting rejection. Histological examination of a biopsy coupled, when necessary, with immunohistochemistry or in situ hybridization will usually confirm the presence of invasive CMV disease.

The sample that most commonly reveals the presence of CMV infection is blood. Detection of virus by culture, with or without accelerated detection techniques, is defined as viraemia whereas the presence of viral protein antigens, demonstrated by monoclonal antibody techniques, is referred to as antigenaemia. The detection of viral genomic material, by molecular biological methods, requires further clarification, since this could merely reflect latent infection.

The term 'CMV syndrome' refers to the presence of a persistent (otherwise unexplained) fever, bone marrow suppression and constitutional symptoms coupled with CMV antigenaemia or viraemia. Chronic uncontrolled infection can lead to a debilitating wasting syndrome. In most cases infection progresses from an asymptomatic stage with local viral replication to viraemia followed by the CMV syndrome and finally severe tissue invasive disease. Early or 'pre-emptive' therapy may interrupt the process at the stage of asymptomatic viraemia (Figure 21.3) [13].

Pathogenesis

Recognized sources of CMV infection after transplantation are: reactivation of latent virus in the recipient; infection from the donor organ (which can cause a primary infection in a naive recipient or may cause a superinfection in a patient who has had previous infection) [14–16]; there is also a small risk of infection from white cells present in blood products [17].

The mechanisms by which T cells recognize the allograft are similar to those by which virally infected cells are recognized [18]. The alloimmune response is believed to be an example of molecular mimicry in which mechanisms that have developed to protect against viral infection are inappropriately triggered by the allograft. Therefore, the immunosuppressive agents used to prevent rejection also reduce the host immune response to CMV infection. Primary immune responses are affected most severely,

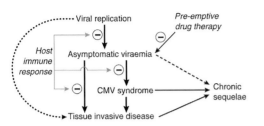

Figure 21.3 Hypothetical model of development of CMV infection after transplantation. Local viral replication spills over into the blood causing asymptomatic viraemia. An increasing viral load results in systemic symptoms (CMV syndrome) and may progress to tissue invasive disease. Instances where local viral replication results in serious disease without viraemia are uncommon (curved dotted arrow). Even in the absence of treatment some episodes of infection will be controlled by the host immune response and will not progress to cause serious disease. Early diagnosis at the time of viraemia (CMV antigenaemia) will allow pre-emptive treatment that usually prevents serious disease but will also result in the treatment of some patients who would not have developed symptoms. CMV disease has been linked to chronic rejection but it has not been determined whether asymptomatic, low level, viraemia is an important risk factor for chronic rejection.

thereby rendering patients who are immunologically naive to CMV at greatest risk. Immunological memory (antibody and cytotoxic T cells) can play a protective role in those experiencing reactivation of CMV or superinfection [19].

The incidence of CMV infection peaks one to four months after surgery, owing to several factors. The intensity of pharmacological immunosuppression is greatest at this time. In addition a primary infection, or superinfection with a new CMV strain, will become apparent at this time. Activation of the immune system after transplantation, the proinflammatory response in the allograft and the effect of some immunosuppressive agents can also lead to reactivation of latent CMV infection [20]. The type and intensity of immunosuppression used can affect the risk of CMV disease. Cyclophosphamide and azathioprine can reactivate CMV [21]. Antithymocyte globulin (ATG) and the monoclonal antibody muromonab-CD3 (OKT3) increase the risk of CMV infection after transplantation [22,23]. Both cause transient T-cell activation and the release of cytokines including tumour necrosis factor alpha (TNF-α) [24]. TNF-α can act as a promoter for the expression of CMV immediate-early genes probably via the nuclear factor kappa B (NF-κB) pathway of the host cell. Increased gene expression may then trigger transition from the latent to the active state. Potentially this mechanism could be blocked by antibody to TNF-α or by pharmacologically inhibiting

the NF-κB pathway [24]. The newer immunosuppressive monoclonal antibodies directed against the α-chain of the interleukin (IL) 2 receptor do not activate T cells and would not be expected to activate CMV by this mechanism [25].

Clinical aspects of CMV infection

CMV infection can result in an acute inflammatory process within most body organs. The severity and type of disease depends on the clinical setting. After transplantation there appears to be an increased risk that disease will localize in the transplanted organ. This may be because of the injury caused during organ preservation or because of immune dysregulation within the graft. Lung transplant recipients who have a complete human leukocyte antigen (HLA) class II (DR) mismatch with their graft appear to be at greater risk of developing CMV pneumonitis, perhaps because of impaired immune surveillance by the host immune system [7].

In general, renal transplant recipients experience the least severe disease, while liver and heart patients are at intermediate risk, and lung and bone marrow recipients experience the most severe disease. In thoracic organ transplant recipients CMV pneumonitis and myocarditis are the most commonly encountered serious manifestations. Currently, the use of early or pre-emptive therapy limits most infections to episodes of CMV syndrome rather than tissue invasive disease.

The importance of CMV infection is not limited to its direct manifestations. CMV appears to increase the patient's net state of immunosuppression and the risk of other opportunistic coinfections occurring [26]. There has been controversy about whether CMV infection can cause acute rejection. Certainly episodes of acute graft dysfunction may occur where it is difficult to separate out the effects of CMV infection and rejection. A recent study of CMV prophylaxis in renal transplantation produced the intriguing observation that treatment with valaciclovir not only reduced the incidence of CMV infection but also reduced the frequency of acute rejection in seronegative patients who received a graft from a seropositive donor [27]. CMV infection has been associated with the subsequent development of chronic rejection [5–7].

Diagnostic methods

One of the first methods for diagnosis was the detection of anti-CMV antibody in the blood. Such serological tests are performed on both the organ donor and the potential transplant recipient to avoid, when possible, the risk of primary CMV and to stratify the patient's risk of CMV disease after transplantation. Since an antibody response is a host reaction to infection, serological diagnosis is usually delayed until well after the patient has developed symptoms and early treatment is therefore impossible [28], although serological changes after transplantation can be useful to retrospectively classify patients for research purposes. Similarly, conventional cell culture techniques do not provide timely clinical information because viral cytopathic effects can take up to three weeks to develop and cell cultures only become positive after a mean of 9.2 days [29].

Rapid diagnosis and early treatment first became possible with the development of monoclonal antibody techniques to accelerate detection of virus replication in cell culture using the detection of early antigen fluorescent foci (DEAFF) [30] or the shell vial centrifugation tests [31]. False negative results can occur, however, when the patient has received prior antiviral therapy [29]. The next advance came with direct detection of the viral matrix protein pp65 in circulating white cells using monoclonal antibodies [32,33]. This approach avoids the need for technically demanding cell culture techniques and allows the result to be read on the same day. Since there is no amplification in a cell culture, the test provides a quantitative estimate of the level of circulating virus [29]. This allows a threshold to be chosen for initiating therapy and also for the effect of therapy to be monitored. The level of antigenaemia or viraemia correlates with the probability of a patient developing symptomatic infection [34,35]. This method is restricted to studying circulating virus within peripheral blood leukocytes and cannot be applied to other clinical specimens (samples such as bronchoalveolar lavage fluid can be examined by the DEAFF test). In addition, neutropenia, which may occur as a result of immunosuppressive drug therapy or as a complication of CMV infection or its treatment, may interfere with this test.

More recently, molecular biological approaches have been applied to diagnosis (Figure 21.1). The polymerase chain reaction (PCR) allows rapid, selective, amplification of target DNA. It can be used to detect DNA from a variety of infectious agents including CMV. The specificity of the process is determined by the oligonucleotide primers used in the reaction [36]. The PCR method has been used to detect CMV genomic DNA in clinical samples [37]. The amplification achieved with PCR provides a high level of sensitivity but the detection of CMV DNA does not distinguish between latent and productive infection. This reduces the specificity of PCR for active infection. Nevertheless, PCR can be applied to a variety of clinical samples and, since

DNA is relatively stable in peripheral blood, the method can provide a robust clinical test [38].

Two approaches have been used to overcome the limited specificity of the PCR technique. The first is quantification of the level of DNA present (or 'viral load'), while the second is to detect transcription of viral genes indicating active infection. The PCR technique can be modified to provide a quantitative estimate of the amount of DNA present in the sample. High levels of DNA usually reflect active infection [39,40].

Reverse transcription PCR (RT-PCR) can be used to detect the presence of mRNA transcribed from specific viral genes. This approach requires either the elimination of genomic DNA from the sample, with DNase digestion, or selective reverse transcription of the mRNA, with poly(dT) priming. Alternatively amplifying the transcript of a gene where the mRNA is spliced will allow differentiation of amplified mRNA from amplified genomic DNA [41]. These approaches have shown that CMV immediate-early gene transcription may occur in the absence of productive infection whereas late gene expression correlates with antigenaemia and active infection [42]. Detection of mRNA expression usually occurs before that of protein expression (antigenaemia), potentially allowing earlier initiation of treatment. Although RT-PCR enables the detection of viral gene transcription, the method is labour intensive, requires specialized laboratory equipment and necessitates stringent laboratory conditions. Therefore, although it is useful in the research setting, it is not ideal for routine diagnostic work. Newer, alternative methods for mRNA amplification such as nucleic acid sequence-based amplification (NASBA) may overcome these problems and could make detection of mRNA the method of choice to diagnose active CMV infection [43,44].

The presence of tissue invasive disease is often inferred from organ dysfunction developing in the context of a CMV infection. Other causes must be considered, however, such as drug toxicity. Particular care must be exercised when considering the transplant organ to differentiate CMV infection from rejection. The 'gold standard' in evaluating invasive disease is a tissue biopsy with histological examination for cells containing typical CMV intranuclear inclusion bodies (Figure 21.4) combined, when necessary, with immunohistochemistry to confirm the presence of viral antigen. Nevertheless rejection can sometimes coexist with CMV infection and there is an overlap in the histological features of the two conditions. In the lung or heart, rejection cannot be diagnosed with confidence in the presence of active CMV disease and in these circumstances histology cannot be used to confidently exclude an element of rejection [45,46] (see Chapter 23).

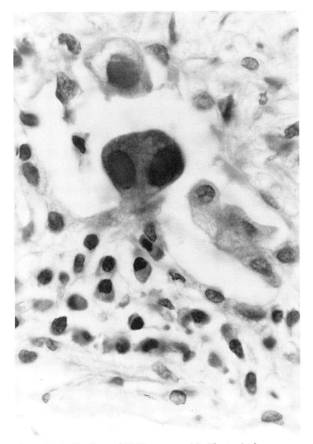

Figure 21.4 Histology of CMV pneumonitis. The typical intranuclear inclusions of CMV are seen in the cell at the centre of the field. The alveolar interstitium beneath this cell has been infiltrated by plasma cells. At the top left of the picture there is a small pneumocyte containing a few small cytoplasmic viral inclusions. (Haematoxylin and eosin; original magnification 620×.)

Management of CMV infection and tissue invasive disease

Several pharmacological agents with activity against CMV are available for clinical use. Aciclovir was the first antiviral agent to be effective against herpes virus infections. It is highly effective against α-herpes viruses but is less active against β-herpes viruses such as CMV [8]. Aciclovir is no longer used in the treatment of CMV disease but may still have a role in prophylaxis against infection. Its main toxicity is renal dysfunction, particularly when administered intravenously.

Ganciclovir is a homologue of aciclovir which has greater activity against CMV and became the first drug to be effective in the treatment of CMV disease [47]. Intravenously

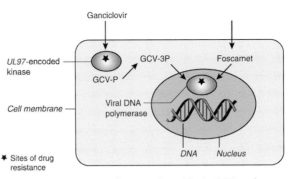

Figure 21.5 Mechanisms of action of ganciclovir (GCV) and foscarnet. After uptake into the cell, ganciclovir is phosphorylated (GCV-P) by the CMV *UL97*-encoded kinase. After further phosphorylation, GCV-3P inhibits the action of the virally encoded DNA polymerase. Foscarnet is a direct inhibitor of the DNA polymerase. Mutations in the *UL97*-encoded kinase can result in ganciclovir resistance, while mutations in the DNA polymerase could cause resistance to either drug.

administered ganciclovir is the first-line agent for the treatment of CMV infection after organ transplantation. Ganciclovir is converted to ganciclovir phosphate within the CMV-infected cell by a viral protein kinase (coded for by CMV gene *UL97*) and then to the triphosphate by cellular kinases. The triphosphate inhibits viral DNA polymerase, competitively inhibiting the incorporation of deoxyguanosine triphosphate into viral DNA (Figure 21.5). Ganciclovir has been a successful therapy for CMV pneumonitis in renal transplant patients [48]. In more highly immunosuppressed bone marrow transplant recipients, ganciclovir monotherapy was less successful but uncontrolled studies using the combination of ganciclovir and high titre anti-CMV immunoglobulin have produced more favourable results [49]. The main dose-limiting toxicity of ganciclovir is bone marrow suppression, although renal impairment may also occur during therapy. The oral formulation of ganciclovir has a low bioavailability and the blood level achieved after oral administration is inadequate for the treatment of CMV infection, although the preparation can be used for prophylaxis against infection [50].

Foscarnet acts as a direct inhibitor of CMV DNA polymerase that is coded for by the *UL54* gene of the virus. Its use in the solid organ transplant recipients is limited by renal toxicity; it may also cause hypocalcaemia, seizures and other metabolic disturbances [51,52]. It remains a second-line agent that is used when ganciclovir has failed or resistance to ganciclovir has developed.

A number of newer agents with activity against CMV have been developed including the valine esters of aciclovir (valaciclovir) [27] and ganciclovir (valganciclovir) [53,54].

These have better absorption than their parent compounds and act as prodrugs that are rapidly hydrolysed to yield the parent after absorption. Both appear suitable for prophylaxis against CMV and, since orally administered valganciclovir can produce ganciclovir levels similar to those achieved after the intravenous administration of ganciclovir, it may also be effective for the treatment of CMV infection.

Cidofovir is a nucleotide analogue with broad antiviral activity including activity against CMV; its main toxicity is renal. Patients receiving cidofovir must receive prophylactic prehydration and be treated with probenecid. It has been effective in some cases of CMV infection that have been refractory to ganciclovir or foscarnet [55].

Failure to respond to antiviral therapy (clinical resistance) can reflect the patient's degree of immunosuppression but may also reflect viral resistance to the drug therapy. Ganciclovir resistance often arises from mutation in the *UL97* gene that can also lead to resistance to cidofovir [56,57]. Resistance due to mutation in *UL97* can be overcome by foscarnet (Figure 21.5), although resistance to this agent can be caused by mutation in *UL54* [58].

Antiviral drugs control CMV replication without eliminating the virus. The final outcome of an infection depends on the host response. In transplant recipients, there is the option of modifying the intensity of the immunosuppressive drug therapy to allow an increase in this response. A reduction in the level of immunosuppression always carries the risk of allograft rejection. There are no routine laboratory tests that inform the clinician of the patient's current level of alloreactivity or potential reactivity when immunosuppression is reduced. Therefore the decision to reduce immunosuppression remains one of clinical judgement. In cases of refractory or relapsing CMV syndrome, where there is good allograft function and no previous history of rejection, cautiously reducing immunosuppression while monitoring graft function may aid recovery. In other cases, where there has been previous rejection or where the graft is involved by CMV disease (and it is difficult to separate infection from possible rejection), the situation can be problematic; the management of immunosuppression in a lung transplant recipient with CMV pneumonitis is especially difficult.

Although pharmacological immunosuppression impairs the host response to CMV infection, it has recently been found that the immunosuppressive agent mycophenolate mofetil can potentiate the antiviral activity of drugs such as ganciclovir or aciclovir [59] and so it may be of help in managing such infection.

An alternative approach is to selectively enhance the host defence mechanisms against CMV. The use of passive immunization using high titre anti-CMV immunoglobulin (CMV-Ig) has had some success when combined with antiviral drug therapy [49,60–62]. Another potential approach involves the administration of CMV-specific cytotoxic (CD8+) T cells to selectively reconstitute cellular immunity against CMV [63,64]. In principle, this approach is straightforward in bone marrow transplantation, where T-cell clones can be derived from the marrow donor, but is more problematic in solid organ transplantation. The logistics, risks and benefits of using T-cell clones from HLA-matched third party donors have not yet been explored. Nevertheless, this approach offers a potential method of selectively enhancing anti-CMV immunity without compromising the level of overall immunosuppression and increasing the risk of allograft rejection.

Adjunctive therapy in the management of CMV disease

Bone marrow suppression, particularly neutropenia, is common in CMV syndrome and can be aggravated by ganciclovir. It usually responds to granulocyte–macrophage colony stimulating factor (GM-CSF), so allowing the continuation of ganciclovir therapy [65]. Patients with respiratory failure due to CMV pneumonitis require supplemental oxygen therapy and often mechanical ventilatory support. Such patients require intensive anti-CMV therapy such as the combination of ganciclovir and CMV-Ig.

Respiratory dysfunction in CMV pneumonitis is partly due to the host immunological response [66] and a brief period of more intense immunosuppression (with intravenous corticosteroids) in combination with antiviral therapy may be beneficial. Liver dysfunction due to CMV may necessitate the temporary withdrawal of hepatotoxic drugs such as azathioprine. Gastrointestinal CMV may produce complications such as gastrointestinal haemorrhage or perforation that require specific intervention. Superinfection with bacteria or fungi is a common complication of CMV disease that requires both diagnostic vigilance and active treatment.

Refractory and relapsing infection

Early diagnosis and treatment has reduced the risk of patients developing severe tissue invasive disease. However, infection that fails to respond adequately to standard treatment or relapses following the cessation of therapy remains an important problem.

In refractory infection, laboratory tests for phenotypic or genotypic viral resistance may define the mechanism of treatment failure. Therapy usually consists of either the use of an alternative agent such as foscarnet or of combination therapy such as ganciclovir combined with either CMV-Ig or foscarnet. Foscarnet acts synergistically with ganciclovir and can be used at a lower dose with ganciclovir to reduce the risk of toxicity [67,68].

Relapse after treatment is especially common in those with primary infection. A standard course of intravenous ganciclovir may be inadequate to suppress viral replication in such patients. Monitoring using molecular biological techniques may help to tailor the duration of therapy to the needs of the individual patient. Antigenaemia (pp65) can persist after viral gene transcription has ceased and the presence of pp65 in peripheral leukocytes after infection may reflect uptake by phagocytosis rather than de novo synthesis [69]. Monitoring viral load by quantitative PCR [70] or late gene mRNA expression by NASBA [44] may provide a means of determining when therapy should cease.

Clinical strategies for preventing or controlling CMV disease

The high levels of morbidity and mortality associated with CMV tissue invasive disease have led to a variety of approaches to either prevent active CMV infection or to treat it at an early, asymptomatic, stage. The data available have been obtained in a variety of clinical settings with a number of different approaches to prophylaxis and monitoring. Unfortunately, few satisfactory studies have been conducted in thoracic organ transplantation and we have to rely quite heavily on data derived from other organ transplants.

Primary infection results in the most severe form of disease, which is also the most difficult to treat [71]. Primary infection can be avoided by using organs from seronegative donors for seronegative transplant recipients and using blood products from CMV-negative blood donors [72]. This was essential in the era before rapid diagnostic methods and effective antiviral therapy were available. Although the avoidance of primary CMV infection is still highly desirable, the limited supply of organs available for transplantation and the need to allocate many organs on the basis of clinical urgency and other important criteria have eroded our ability to avoid CMV-mismatched transplants. Not only are patients with primary infection at risk of the most severe disease, they are also more likely to relapse after therapy and to develop drug-resistant disease [73,74].

For transplant recipients who have latent CMV infection, or who are at risk of infection from the donor, two approaches have been used: either prophylactic drug therapy aimed at preventing symptomatic infection or laboratory surveillance with the aim of beginning treatment early during infection to attenuate the clinical severity of infection (pre-emptive therapy) [13,75].

Prophylaxis

Primary prophylaxis has been attempted with several agents. A number of factors will influence the outcome after prophylaxis, including the type of transplant and the degree of immunosuppression present. Therefore caution must be used when attempts are made to extrapolate from results obtained in one setting to those obtained in another. Many of the studies that have been performed in the field of thoracic organ transplantation have limitations in their study design, either relying on small numbers of patients or lacking appropriate control groups and randomization of treatment allocation.

Passive immunization with an immunoglobulin preparation containing high titre anti-CMV antibodies had been shown to reduce the incidence of CMV disease in renal transplant recipients at risk of primary infection [76]. There was a trend toward a reduction in the frequency of CMV infection in the CMV-Ig group that was not statistically significant. Therefore, CMV-Ig was beneficial in attenuating the clinical impact of CMV infection rather than in preventing infection. CMV-Ig was well tolerated, with a low incidence of serious side effects. It lacked the haematological and renal toxicity that limits the use of antiviral drugs. Nevertheless, the use of CMV-Ig as a prophylactic agent has important limitations. Supplies of immunoglobulin preparations are often limited and are very expensive. As a biological preparation, standardization between different suppliers' products and batch-to-batch variability are a concern. Over recent years there have been concerns about the safety of products derived from blood with respect to HIV and HCV infection and, most recently, prion disease, which have episodically disrupted product availability.

Aciclovir has only moderate activity against CMV but has a lower bone marrow toxicity than ganciclovir. It is now available as a generic preparation and so high dose oral aciclovir can be administered at relatively low cost. Several studies have found that aciclovir can reduce the burden of CMV disease. Balfour and colleagues found that high dose (3.2 g/day) oral aciclovir for three months after renal transplantation reduced the incidence of symptomatic CMV disease from 29% to 7.5%. Side effects were minimal and graft/patient survival was similar in treatment and control groups [77]. Some other studies have found similar results, while others have not, and the use of aciclovir as prophylaxis after organ transplantation has remained controversial.

Ganciclovir is a more potent inhibitor of CMV in vitro than is aciclovir and is the drug of choice for treating symptomatic infections in transplant patients. A number of studies have investigated its use as a prophylactic agent. Early reports of brief courses of ganciclovir treatment (one to three weeks) were not encouraging [78]. Merigan and colleagues found that a 28 day course of prophylactic intravenous ganciclovir reduced the incidence of CMV disease from 46% to 9% in recipients of heart transplants [79]. There appeared to be no benefit, however, in those at risk of primary infection (donor seropositive for anti-CMV antibodies and recipient seronegative). Virus shedding appeared to occur later in the primary infections than in secondary infection. This led to the hypothesis that ganciclovir prophylaxis should be continued for a longer period at least in those at risk of primary infection. Ganciclovir toxicity was minimal, with mild renal impairment occurring transiently. There was no significant increase in the number of episodes of significant neutropenia. This protocol appeared to be a step forward in CMV prophylaxis but involved a significant cost for both the drug and prolonged intravenous access while not effectively addressing the most serious problem of primary CMV infection [79].

In a nonrandomized study, Seu and colleagues found that prolonged intravenous ganciclovir (up to 100 days) after liver transplantation could prevent CMV disease in high risk seronegative liver transplant recipients who had received organs from seropositive donors [80]. Ganciclovir also appeared to be effective in a high risk group who required muromonab-CD3 treatment for refractory rejection [81]. Although prolonged intravenous ganciclovir appears to provide effective prophylaxis, the need for administration via a central venous access makes this treatment difficult and expensive to apply to all patients at risk of CMV disease.

More recently, an oral formulation of ganciclovir has become available which allows simple out-patient treatment [82,83]. A small study in renal transplant recipients found that oral ganciclovir reduced CMV infection [84]. A randomized clinical trial, comparing oral ganciclovir with placebo to prevent CMV infection after liver transplantation, demonstrated that ganciclovir (administered from the early postoperative period up to day 98 after transplantation) was highly effective in reducing CMV disease [85]. CMV infection was reduced from an incidence of 52% to 25%. CMV disease fell from 19% to 5%. In the placebo group 8.5% developed invasive disease as compared with 0.7% in the ganciclovir group [85]. Oral ganciclovir was very effective in this population but a number of issues remain to be considered.

Although oral ganciclovir is convenient, the cost of universal prophylaxis is high. By analogy with other antimicrobial therapy, there must be concern about using the best therapeutic agent available against an organism as prophylaxis because of the danger of drug resistance developing. Initially ganciclovir-resistant strains of CMV were seen mainly in HIV-infected patients receiving long-term therapy [86], but resistance has also been reported in transplant patients [57,73]. The limited bioavailability of oral ganciclovir results in peak levels of drug that are near the typical inhibitory concentrations for viral replication. This may create conditions where selective pressure can lead to the emergence of drug-resistant strains especially in patients with high viral loads due to primary infection or intense immunosuppression [74]. The efficacy of valaciclovir and valganciclovir has not been studied yet in lung or heart transplantation.

Short courses of intravenous ganciclovir appear to be ineffective in preventing CMV infection after lung transplantation [78]. A small clinical trial compared intravenous ganciclovir prophylaxis for three months with ganciclovir for two weeks followed by oral aciclovir for the same time period; the three month treatment with ganciclovir resulted in a lower incidence of symptomatic infection and seroconversion but this did not seem to translate into any long-term clinical benefit [87]. A more recent study that used either intravenous ganciclovir for 90 days or two weeks of intravenous ganciclovir followed by oral ganciclovir up to 90 days found a low incidence of CMV disease in both groups compared to historical controls [88]. Another observational study found that even longer prophylaxis with intravenous ganciclovir (up to 20 weeks after lung transplantation) further reduced the incidence of CMV infection [89] but the protocol did not appear to be cost effective. The optimum approach to CMV prophylaxis after lung transplantation will be identified only through adequately powered randomized controlled trials [90].

A meta-analysis of prophylaxis with antiviral agents in solid organ transplant recipients concluded that both aciclovir and ganciclovir could reduce CMV disease [91]. The relative risk of infection was 0.74 whereas the relative risk for CMV disease was 0.5, indicating that prophylaxis is more effective at reducing symptomatic disease than infection per se. In this analysis the benefits of aciclovir and ganciclovir appeared to be similar [91]. However, a trial in liver transplants, directly comparing aciclovir and ganciclovir prophylaxis, found ganciclovir to be a more effective prophylactic agent [92], as did a study in lung transplant patients [87].

Direct evidence for efficacy of prophylactic aciclovir in thoracic organ transplantation is lacking. Nevertheless, it has relatively little toxicity and an oral preparation is now available at low cost; so aciclovir prophylaxis may merit further investigation particularly in patients treated with mycophenolate. Overall, ganciclovir appears to be more effective than aciclovir in preventing CMV infection, reflecting its greater activity in vitro against CMV [93]. Prophylaxis with ganciclovir appears to be an effective approach to preventing CMV disease but the cost of this approach is considerable.

Targeted drug treatment may reduce the cost of prophylaxis. This approach can be of value in high risk situations such as patients at risk of primary infection or those who require treatment with T-cell activating antilymphocyte antibody preparations (ATG or muromonab-CD3) because of severe rejection [81].

Pre-emptive therapy

An alternative approach is to prevent serious CMV infection by early diagnosis and treatment of infection before symptoms have developed. This requires a surveillance strategy to detect infection at an asymptomatic stage. This pre-emptive approach was first used in bone marrow transplant recipients where a routine surveillance bronchoscopy, bronchoalveolar lavage and shell-vial culture at day 35 after transplantation was used to detect subclinical CMV infection in the lung before clinical pneumonitis had developed [94]. Patients who had subclinical CMV infection were randomized to pre-emptive treatment with intravenous ganciclovir or observation. Ganciclovir treatment reduced the incidence of CMV pneumonitis (or death) from 70% to 25%.

The pre-emptive strategy has subsequently been developed using less invasive methods for early diagnosis, usually based on the detection of viraemia by monoclonal antibody or molecular biological techniques [13,33]. The appeal of this approach is that it avoids exposing patients who will not develop CMV infection to unnecessary prophylactic therapy. In addition, since therapy is only started at the time that subclinical infection is detected, and the response to therapy can be monitored, the duration of treatment needed is usually shorter than that for primary prophylaxis. This approach has limitations. Its effectiveness depends on the monitoring protocol and the performance characteristics of the test procedure. Since viraemia currently triggers treatment with intravenous ganciclovir (as for symptomatic infection), asymptomatic patients have to be hospitalized to establish central venous access and then to undergo intravenous drug therapy and monitoring for several weeks.

The basis of the pre-emptive approach is that patients with a sufficient load of replicating CMV to produce clinical disease will have viraemia (Figure 21.3); however, not all viraemic patients will become symptomatic. The number of leukocytes that are pp65 antigen positive correlates with risk of disease [95]. Attempts have been made to determine an appropriate level of antigenaemia to trigger therapy, with the aim of preventing clinical disease while minimizing unnecessary treatment. This will depend on the patients serological status (primary or secondary infection), the immunosuppression used and type of transplant received. The diagnostic methodology used in a particular laboratory will also influence the threshold and there will be a trade off between sensitivity (to avoid serious CMV disease) and specificity (and positive predictive value for CMV disease in the absence of pre-emptive therapy) [29].

A wide range of thresholds have been suggested in the literature varying between 1 and 100 positive cells within a sample of 2×10^5 cells [29,34,35,96,97]. This reflects variation in methodology as well as in the clinical context of the studies. Antigen levels may rise rapidly within a few days of the onset of an infection so that, if an initial positive result does not initiate pre-emptive treatment, close follow-up is indicated. Increasing the threshold used to trigger pre-emptive therapy will delay the start of therapy and may increase the chance of symptoms developing before treatment can become effective.

Iberer and colleagues studied the effect of pre-emptive therapy in 22 heart transplant patients who had received induction therapy with ATG. Treatment was started as soon as antigenaemia was detected. Ten of 19 patients who became CMV positive developed symptomatic, albeit mild, disease [96]. Thus, although pre-emptive therapy can attenuate the severity of disease and prevent tissue invasive disease, it does not always prevent symptomatic infection. The relationship of these modified episodes to the risk of long-term complications of CMV infection has not been determined.

PCR detection of CMV genome is highly sensitive and can detect low levels of virus unlikely to be correlated with CMV disease, including cases of latent infection. Pre-emptive treatment based solely on PCR can lead to the unnecessary treatment of some patients and increased cost [38]. In addition PCR does not correlate well with the clinical course of the disease and the effect of therapy [28]. PCR does, however, detect viraemia at an earlier stage than the antigenaemia test, giving the potential for earlier therapy [28]. Quantification of the level of viraemia by PCR has been used to assess the need for treatment [39,98,99].

Another approach has been to focus on viral gene transcription [42,97]. Immediate-early genes are transcribed in both productive and nonproductive (latent) infection [100]. Late gene transcripts provide an index of viral replication that may allow early treatment without unnecessary therapy [41,44].

Thus pre-emptive therapy is effective in preventing severe disease and allows a shorter period of treatment and reduced drug cost. The cost and logistic issues of regular laboratory monitoring must be weighed against this. In addition, since pre-emptive treatment requires intravenous therapy and many patients still develop symptoms requiring medical evaluation, hospital costs will be higher than for effective oral prophylaxis administered as an outpatient. However, in the future, treatment with a therapeutic dose of oral valganciclovir may allow effective pre-emptive therapy of an evolving CMV infection [54].

At present we do not have adequate data on the use of oral ganciclovir for prophylaxis in thoracic organ transplant patients. No direct comparison of pre-emptive and prophylactic therapy has been made. The role of virological monitoring and the interpretation of results in asymptomatic patients who are already receiving anti-CMV prophylaxis has not been established. Therefore, the most cost-effective strategy for the prevention of CMV disease and its sequelae remains uncertain.

Summary and future directions

Substantial progress has been made in the management of CMV infection after transplantation. The introduction of effective antiviral agents combined with rapid diagnostic techniques have greatly reduced the mortality related to this infection and have also diminished morbidity. Preemptive therapy can prevent severe disease but many patients continue to experience symptoms or require extended antiviral therapy. The resource implications of CMV infection after transplantation remain a serious problem. Primary prophylaxis with oral ganciclovir has been successful in liver transplantation but has not been adequately studied in the thoracic transplant population. Such prophylaxis still allows a substantial number of patients to experience asymptomatic infection. It is uncertain whether this predisposes them to long-term complications such as chronic rejection. Indeed, whether any of the approaches currently available will reduce long-term complications after thoracic organ transplantation is unknown.

The limited number of drugs effective against CMV, and the similarity in their mode of action, is a cause for concern. The high level of drug exposure in the transplant population could result in drug resistance emerging as a major problem in the future. Our increasing understanding of the factors that trigger CMV replication and the interrelationship between the virus and the host immune system are leading to new approaches. Immunosuppressive monoclonal antibodies that do not activate T cells may replace muromonab-CD3 and ATG in immunosuppression protocols and reduce the risk of CMV disease. It may become possible to selectively block pathways that trigger CMV replication. The hope of establishing a method that can produce graft-specific tolerance, without generalized immunosuppression and the consequent risk of infection, remains a long-term goal for the transplant community. Selective enhancement of the host immune response to CMV may become possible in the foreseeable future.

REFERENCES

1 Fishman JA, Rubin RH. Infection in organ transplant recipients. *N Engl J Med* 1998; **338**: 1741–1751.

2 Soghikian MV, Valentine VG, Berry GJ, Patel HR, Robbins RC, Theodore J. Impact of ganciclovir prophylaxis on heart–lung and lung transplant recipients. *J Heart Lung Transplant* 1996; **15**: 881–887.

3 Dummer JS, White LT, Ho M, Griffith BP, Hardesty RL, Bahnson HT. Morbidity of cytomegalovirus infection in heart or heart–lung transplants who received cyclosporin. *J Infect Dis* 1985; **152**: 1182–1191.

4 McCarthy JM, Karim MA, Keown PA, Krueger H. The cost impact of cytomegalovirus disease in renal transplant recipients. *Transplantation* 1993; **55**: 1277–1282.

5 Smith MA, Sundaresan S, Mohanakumar T, et al. Effect of development of antibodies to HLA and cytomegalovirus mismatch on lung transplantation survival and development of bronchiolitis obliterans syndrome. *J Thorac Cardiovasc Surg* 1998; **116**: 812–820.

6 Grattan MT, Moreno-Cabral CE, Starnes VA, Oyer PE, Stinson EB, Shumway NE. Cytomegalovirus infection is associated with cardiac allograft rejection and atherosclerosis. *JAMA* 1989; **261**: 3561–3566.

7 Schulman LL, Weinberg AD, McGregor CC, Suciu-Foca NM, Itescu S. Influence of donor and recipient HLA locus mismatching on development of obliterative bronchiolitis after lung transplantation. *Am J Respir Crit Care Med* 2001; **163**: 437–442.

8 Griffiths P. Update on herpesvirus infections. *J Roy Coll Physic Lond* 1998; **32**: 199–202.

9 Mocarski ES. Cytomegalovirus biology and replication. In: Roizman B, Whitely RJ, Lopez C, eds. *The human herpes viruses*. Raven Press Ltd; New York, 1993: 173–226.

10 Peterson PK, Balfour HH Jr, Fryd DS, Ferguson R, Kronenberg R, Simmons RL. Risk factors in the development of cytomegalovirus-related pneumonia in renal transplant recipients. *J Infect Dis* 1983; **148**: 1121.

11 Ljungman P, Griffiths P. Definitions of cytomegalovirus infection and disease. In: Michelson S, Plotkin SA, eds. *A multidisiplinary approach to understanding cytomegalovirus disease.* Elsevier Science Publishers BV, Amsterdam, 1993: 233–237.

12 Lungman P, Plotkin SA. Workshop on CMV disease: definitions, clinical severity scores, and new syndromes. *Scand J Infect Dis* 1995; **99**(Suppl): 87–89.

13 Rubin RH. Preemptive therapy in immunocompromised hosts. *N Engl J Med* 1991; **324**: 1057–1059.

14 Ho M, Suwansirikul S, Dowling JN, et al. The transplanted kidney as a source of cytomegalovirus infection. *N Engl J Med* 1975; **293**: 1109–1112.

15 Chou SW. Acquisition of donor strains of cytomegalovirus by renal-transplant recipients. *N Engl J Med* 1986; **314**: 1418–1423.

16 Grundy JE, Lui SF, Suoer M, et al. Symptomatic cytomegalovirus infection in seropositive patients: reinfection with donor virus rather than reactivation of recipient virus. *Lancet* 1988; **ii**: 132–135.

17 Prince AM, Szmuness W, Millian SJ, et al. A serologic study of cytomegalovirus infections associated with blood transfusions. *N Engl J Med* 1971; **284**: 1125–1131.

18 Krensky AM. Immune response to allografts. In: Norman DJ, Suki WN, eds. *Primer on transplantation*. American Society of Transplant Physicians, Thorofare, NJ, 1998: 21–31.

19 Reusser P, Cathomas G, Attenhofer R, Tamm M, Thiel G. Cytomegalovirus (CMV)-specific T cell immunity after renal transplantation mediates protection from CMV disease by limiting the systemic virus load. *J Infect Dis* 1999; **180**: 247–253.

20 Rubin RH. Impact of cytomegalovirus infection on organ transplant recipients. *Rev Infect Dis* 1990; **12**(Suppl 7): S754–S766.

21 Dowling JN, Saslow AR, Ho M, et al. Cytomegalovirus infection in patients receiving immunosuppressive therapy for rheumatologic disorders. *J Infect Dis* 1976; **133**: 399–408.

22 Singh N, Dummer JS, Kusne S, et al. Infections with cytomegalovirus and other herpesviruses in 121 liver transplant recipients: transmission by donated organ and the effect of OKT3 antibodies. *J Infect Dis* 1988; **158**: 124–131.

23 Portela D, Patel R, Larso-Keller JJ, et al. OKT3 treatment for allograft rejection is a risk factor for cytomegalovirus disease in liver transplantation. *J Infect Dis* 1995; **171**: 1014–1018.

24 Fietze E, Prosch S, Reinke P, et al. Cytomegalovirus infection in transplant recipients. The role of tumor necrosis factor. *Transplantation* 1994; **58**: 675–680.

25 Nashan B, Moore R, Amlot P, et al. Randomised trial of basiliximab versus placebo for control of acute cellular rejection in renal allograft recipients. *Lancet* 1997; **250**: 1193–1198.

26 Rand KH, Pollard RB, Merigan TC. Increased pulmonary superinfections in cardiac transplants patients undergoing primary cytomegalovirus infection. *N Engl J Med* 1978; **298**: 951–953.

27 Lowance D, Neumayer HH, Legendre CM, et al. Valacyclovir for the prevention of cytomegalovirus disease after renal transplantation. International Valacyclovir Cytomegalovirus Prophylaxis Transplantation Study Group. *N Engl J Med* 1999; **340**: 1462–1470.

28 Tanabe K, Tokumoto T, Ishikawa N, et al. Comparative study of cytomegalovirus (CMV) antigenemia assay, polymerase chain reaction, serology, and shell vial assay in the early diagnosis and monitoring of CMV infection after renal transplantation. *Transplantation* 1997; **64**: 1721–1725.

29 Niubo J, Perez JL, Martinez Lacasa JT, et al. Association of quantitative cytomegalovirus antigenemia with symptomatic infection in solid organ transplant patients. *Diagn Microbiol Infect Dis* 1996; **24**: 19–24.

30 Griffiths PD, Panjwani DD, Stirk PR, et al. Rapid diagnosis of cytomegalovirus infection in immunocompromised patients by detection of early antigen fluorescent foci. *Lancet* 1984; **ii**: 1242–1245.

31 Gleaves CA, Smith TF, Schuster EA, Pearson GR. Rapid detection of cytomegalovirus in MRC-5 cells inoculated with urine specimens by using slow speed centrifugation and monoclonal antibody to early antigen. *J Clin Microbiol* 1984; **19**: 917–919.

32 van der Bij W, Torensma R, van Son WJ, et al. Rapid immunodiagnosis of active cytomegalovirus infection by monoclonal antibody staining of blood leucocytes. *J Med Virol* 1988; **25**: 179–188.

33 van der Bij W, Torensma R, van Son WJ, et al. Antigen test for early diagnosis of active cytomegalovirus infection in heart transplant recipients. *J Heart Transplant* 1988; **7**: 106–109.

34 Egan JJ, Barber L, Lomax H, et al. Detection of human cytomegalovirus antigenaemia: a rapid diagnostic technique for predicting CMV infection/pneumonitis in lung and heart transplant recipients. *Thorax* 1995; **50**: 9–13.

35 Grossi P, Minoli L, Percivalle E, Irish W, Vigano M, Gerna G. Clinical and virological monitoring of human cytomegalovirus infection in 294 heart transplant recipients. *Transplantation* 1995; **59**: 847–851.

36 Day IN. Polymerase chain reaction. *Br J Hosp Med* 1997; **57**: 170–171.

37 Evans MJ, Edwards Spring Y, Myers J, et al. Polymerase chain reaction assays for the detection of cytomegalovirus in organ and bone marrow transplant recipients. *Immunol Invest* 1997; **26**: 209–229.

38 Brennan DC, Garlock KA, Lippmann BJ, et al. Polymerase chain reaction-triggered preemptive or deferred therapy to control cytomegalovirus-associated morbidity and costs in renal transplant patients. *Transplant Proc* 1997; **29**: 809–811.

39 Imbert-Marcille B-M, Cantarovich D, Ferre-Aubineau V, Richet B, Soulillou J-P, Billaudel S. Usefulness of DNA viral load quantification for cytomegalovirus disease monitoring in renal and pancreas/renal transplant recipients. *Transplantation* 1997; **63**: 1476–1481.

40 Humar A, Gregson D, Caliendo AM, et al. Clinical utility of quantitative cytomegalovirus viral load determination for predicting cytomegalovirus disease in liver transplant recipients. *Transplantation* 1999; **68**: 1305–1311.

41 Nelson PN, Rawal BK, Boriskin YS, Mathers KE, Powles RL. A polymerase chain reaction to detect a spliced late transcript of human cytomegalovirus in the blood of bone marrow transplant recipients. *J Virol Meth* 1996; **56**: 139–148.

42 Lam KMC, Oldenburg N, Khan MA, et al. Significance of reverse transcription polymerase chain reaction in the detection of human cytomegalovirus gene transcripts in thoracic organ transplant recipients. *J Heart Lung Transplant* 1998; **17**: 555–565.

43 Compton J. Nucleic acid sequence-based amplification. *Nature* 1991; **350**: 91–92.

44 Oldenburg N, Lam KM, Khan MA, et al. Evaluation of human cytomegalovirus gene expression in thoracic organ transplant recipients using nucleic acid sequence-based amplification. *Transplantation* 2000; **70**: 1209–1215.

45 Yousem SA, Berry GJ, Brunt EM, et al. A working formulation of the standardization of nomenclature in diagnosis of heart and lung rejection: Lung Rejection Study Group. *J Heart Lung Transplant* 1990; **9**: 593–601.

46 Nakhleh RE, Bolman RM, Henke CA, Herz MI. Lung transplant pathology: a comparative study of pulmonary acute rejection and cytomegaloviral infection. *Am J Surg Pathol* 1991; **15**: 1197–1201.

47 Crumpacker CS. Ganciclovir. *N Engl J Med* 1996; **335**: 721–729.

48 Hecht DW, Snydman DR, Crumpacker CS, Werner BG, Heinze-Lacey B. Ganciclovir for treatment of renal transplant associated primary cytomegalovirus pneumonia. *J Infect Dis* 1988; **157**: 187–190.

49 Emanuel D, Cunningham I, Jules-Elysee K, et al. Cytomegalovirus pneumonia after bone marrow transplantation successfully treated with the combination of ganciclovir and high dose intravenous immune globulin. *Ann Intern Med* 1988; **109**: 777–782.

50 Noble S, Faulds D. Ganciclovir. An update of its use in the prevention of cytomegalovirus infection and disease in transplant recipients. *Drugs* 1998; **56**: 115–146.

51 Jayaweera DT. Minimising the dosage-limiting toxicities of foscarnet induction therapy. *Drug Saf* 1997; **16**: 258–266.

52 Deray G, Martınez F, Katlama C, et al. Foscarnet nephrotoxicity: mechanism, incidence and prevention. *Am J Nephrol* 1989; **9**: 316–321.

53 Brown F, Banken L, Saywell K, Arum I. Pharmacokinetics of valganciclovir and ganciclovir following multiple oral dosages of valganciclovir in HIV- and CMV-seropositive volunteers. *Clin Pharmacokinet* 1999; **37**: 167–176.

54 Pescovitz MD, Rabkin J, Merion RM, et al. Valganciclovir results in improved oral absorption of ganciclovir in liver transplant recipients. *Antimicrob Agents Chemother* 2000; **44**: 2811–2815.

55 Ljungman P, Deliliers GL, Platzbecker U, et al. Cidofovir for cytomegalovirus infection and disease in allogeneic stem cell transplant recipients. The Infectious Diseases Working Party of the European Group for Blood and Marrow Transplantation. *Blood* 2001; **97**: 388–392.

56 Harada K, Eizuru Y, Isashiki Y, Ihara S, Minamishima Y. Genetic analysis of a clinical isolate of human cytomegalovirus exhibiting resistance against both ganciclovir and cidofovir. *Arch Virol* 1997; **142**: 215–225.

57 Rosen HR, Benner KG, Flora KD, et al. Development of ganciclovir resistance during treatment of primary cytomegalovirus infection after liver transplantation. *Transplantation* 1997; **63**: 476–478.

58 Sarasini A, Baldanti F, Furione M, et al. Double resistance to ganciclovir and foscarnet of four human cytomegalovirus strains recovered from AIDS patients. *J Med Virol* 1995; **47**: 237–244.

59 Neyts J, Andrei G, De Clercq E. The novel immunosuppressive agent mycophenolate mofetil markedly potentiates the anti-herpesvirus activities of acyclovir, ganciclovir, and penciclovir in vitro and in vivo. *Antimicrob Agents Chemother* 1998; **42**: 216–222.

60 Reed EC, Bowden RA, Dandliker PS, Lilleby KE, Myers JD. Treatment of cytomegalovirus pneumonia with ganciclovir and intravenous cytomegalovirus immunoglobulin in patients with bone marrow transplants. *Ann Intern Med* 1988; **109**: 783–788.

61 George MJ, Snydman DR, Werner BG, et al. Use of ganciclovir plus cytomegalovirus immune globulin to treat CMV pneumonia in orthotopic liver transplant recipients. The Boston Center for Liver Transplantation CMVIG-Study Group. *Transplant Proc* 1993; **25**(5 Suppl 4): 22–24.

62 Enright H, Haake R, Weisdorf D, et al. Cytomegalovirus pneumonia after bone marrow transplantation. Risk factors and response to therapy. *Transplantation* 1993; **55**: 1339–1346.

63 Riddell SR, Watanabe KS, Goodrich JM, Li CR, Agha ME, Greenber PD. Restoration of viral immunity in immunodeficient humans by the adoptive transfer of T-cell clones. *Science* 1992; **257**: 238–241.

64 Riddell SR, Greenberg PD. Therapeutic reconstitution of human viral immunity by adoptive transfer of cytotoxic T lymphocyte clones. *Curr Top Microbiol Immunol* 1994; **189**: 9–34.

65 Hardy WD. Combined ganciclovir and recombinant human granulocyte-macrophage colony stimulating factor in the treatment of cytomegalovirus retinitis in AIDS patients. *J Acquir Immune Defic Syndr* 1991; **4**(Suppl 1): S22–S28.

66 Grundy JE, Shanley JD, Griffiths PD. Is cytomegalovirus interstitial pneumonitis in transplant recipients an immunopathological condition? *Lancet* 1987; **ii**: 996–999.

67 Manischewitz JF, Quinnan GV Jr, Lane HC, Wittek AE. Synergistic effect of ganciclovir and foscarnet on cytomegalovirus replication in vitro. *Antimicrob Agents Chemother* 1990; **34**: 373–375.

68 Combination foscarnet and ganciclovir therapy vs monotherapy for the treatment of relapsed cytomegalovirus retinitis in patients with AIDS. The Cytomegalovirus Retreatment Trial. The Studies of Ocular Complications of AIDS Research Group in Collaboration with the AIDS Clinical Trials Group. *Arch Ophthalmol* 1996; **114**: 23–33.

69 Grefte A, Harmsen MC, van der Giessen M, Knollema S, van Son WJ, The Th. The presence of human cytomegalovirus (HCMV) immediate early mRNA but not ppUL83 (lower matrix protein pp65) mRNA in polymorphonuclear and mononuclear leucocytes during active HCMV infection. *J Gen Virol* 1994; **75**: 1989–1998.

70 Sia IG, Wilson JA, Groettum CM, Espy MJ, Smith TF, Paya CV. Cytomegalovirus (CMV) DNA load predicts relapsing CMV infection after solid organ transplantation. *J Infect Dis* 2000; **181**: 717–720.

71 Smiley ML, Wlodaver CG, Grossman RA, et al. The role of pretransplant immunity in protection from cytomegalovirus disease following renal transplantation. *Transplantation* 1985; **40**: 157–161.

72 Wreghitt T. Cytomegalovirus infection in heart and heart–lung transplant recipients. *J Antimicrob Chemother* 1989; **23**(Suppl E): 49–60.

73 Limaye AP, Corey L, Koelle DM, Davis CL, Boeckh M. Emergence of ganciclovir-resistant cytomegalovirus disease among recipients of solid-organ transplants. *Lancet* 2000; **356**: 645–649.

74 Drew WL. Ganciclovir resistance: a matter of time and titre. *Lancet* 2000; **356**: 609–610.

75 Griffiths PD. Prophylaxis against CMV infection in transplant patients. *J Antimicrob Chemother* 1997; **39**: 299–301.

76 Snydman DR, Werner BG, Heinze-Lacey B, et al. Use of cytomegalovirus immune globulin to prevent cytomegalovirus disease in renal transplant recipients. *N Engl J Med* 1987; **317**: 1049–1054.

77 Balfour HH, Chace BA, Stapleton JT, Simmons RL, Fryd DS. A randomized placebo controlled trial of oral acyclovir for the prevention of cytomegalovirus disease in recipients of renal allografts. *N Engl J Med* 1989; **320**: 1381–1387.

78 Bailey TC, Trulock EP, Ettinger NA, Storach GA, Cooper JD, Powderly WG. Failure of prophylactic ganciclovir to prevent cytomegalovirus disease in the recipients of lung transplants. *J Infect Dis* 1992; **165**: 548–552.

79 Merigan TC, Renlund DG, Keay S, et al. A controlled trial of ganciclovir to prevent cytomegalovirus disease after heart transplantation. *N Engl J Med* 1992; **326**: 1182–1186.

80 Seu P, Winston DJ, Holt CD, Kaldas F, Busuttil RW. Long-term ganciclovir prophylaxis for successful prevention of primary cytomegalovirus (CMV) disease in CMV-seronegative liver transplant recipients with CMV-seropositive donors. *Transplantation* 1997; **64**: 1614–1617.

81 Winston D, Imagawa D, Holt C, Kaldas F, Shaked A, Busuttil R. Long term ganciclovir prophylaxis eliminates serious cytomegalovirus disease in liver transplant recipients receiving OKT3 therapy for rejection. *Transplantation* 1995; **60**: 1357–1360.

82 Spector SA, Busch DF, Follansbee S, et al. Pharmacokinetic, safety and antiviral profiles of oral ganciclovir in persons infected with human immunodeficiency virus: a phase I/II study. AIDS clinical trials group and cytomegalovirus cooperative study group. *J Infect Dis* 1995; **171**: 1431–1471.

83 Spector S, McKlinley G, Lalezari JP, et al. Oral ganciclovir for the prevention of cytomegalovirus disease in patients with AIDS. *N Engl J Med* 1996; **334**: 1491–1497.

84 Ahsan N, Holman MJ, Yang HC. Efficacy of oral ganciclovir in prevention of cytomegalovirus infection in post-kidney transplant patients. *Clin Transplant* 1997; **11**: 633–639.

85 Gane E, Saliba F, Valdecasa GJC, et al. Randomised trial of efficacy and safety of oral ganciclovir in the prevention of cytomegalovirus disease in liver transplant recipients. *Lancet* 1997; **350**: 1729–1733.

86 Erice A, Chou S, Biron KK, Stanat SC, Balfour HH Jr, Jordan MC. Progressive disease due to ganciclovir resistant cytomegalovirus in immunocompromised patients. *N Engl J Med* 1989; **320**: 289–293.

87 Duncan SR, Grgurich WF, Iacono AT, et al. A comparison of ganciclovir and acyclovir to prevent cytomegalovirus after lung transplantation. *Am J Respir Crit Care Med* 1994; **150**: 146–152.

88 Speich R, Thurnheer R, Gaspert A, Weder W, Boehler A. Efficacy and cost effectiveness of oral ganciclovir in the prevention of cytomegalovirus disease after lung transplantation. *Transplantation* 1999; **67**: 315–320.

89 Gerbase MW, Dubois D, Rothmeier C, Spiliopoulos A, Wunderli W, Nicod LP. Costs and outcomes of prolonged cytomegalovirus prophylaxis to cover the enhanced immunosuppression phase following lung transplantation. *Chest* 1999; **116**: 1265–1272.

90 Orens JB. Cytomegalovirus prophylaxis with IV ganciclovir in lung transplant recipients: the long and the short of it! *Chest* 1999; **116**: 1152–1153.

91 Couchoud C, Cucherat M, Haugh M, Pouteil Noble C. Cytomegalovirus prophylaxis with antiviral agents in solid organ transplantation: a meta-analysis. *Transplantation* 1998; **65**: 641–647.

92 Winston DJ, Wirin D, Shaked A, Busuttil R. Randomised comparison of ganciclovir and high dose acyclovir for long term cytomegalovirus prophylaxis in liver-transplant recipients. *Lancet* 1995; **346**: 69–74.

93 Faulds D, Heel RC. Ganciclovir: a review of its antiviral activity, pharmacokinetic properties and therapeutic efficacy in cytomegalovirus infections. *Drugs* 1990; **39**: 597–638.

94 Schmidt GM, Horak DA, Niland JC, et al. A randomized controlled trial of prophylactic ganciclovir for cytomegalovirus pulmonary infection in recipients of allogeneic bone marrow transplants. The City of Hope–Stanford–Syntex CMV Study Group. *N Engl J Med* 1991; **324**: 1005–1011.

95 Gerna G, Ziepeto D, Parea M, et al. Monitoring of human cytomegalovirus infections and ganciclovir in heart transplant recipients by determination of viraemia, antigenaemia and DNAemia. *J Infect Dis* 1991; **164**: 488–498.

96 Iberer F, Tscheliessnigg K, Halwachs G, et al. Definitions of cytomegalovirus disease after heart transplantation: antigenemia as a marker for antiviral therapy. *Transpl Int* 1996; **9**: 236–242.

97 Gaeta A, Nazzari C, Angeletti S, Lazzarini M, Mazzei E, Mancini C. Monitoring for cytomegalovirus infection in organ transplant recipients: analysis of pp65 antigen, DNA and late mRNA in peripheral blood leukocytes. *J Med Virol* 1997; **53**: 189–195.

98 Fox JC, Kidd IM, Griffiths PD, Sweny P, Emery VC. Longitudinal analysis of cytomegalovirus load in renal transplant recipients using a quantitative polymerase chain reaction: correlation with disease. *J Gen Virol* 1995; **76**: 309–319.

99 Rawal BK, Booth JC, Fernando S, Butcher PD, Powles RL. Quantification of cytomegalovirus DNA in blood specimens from bone marrow transplant recipients by the polymerase chain reaction. *J Virol Meth* 1994; **47**: 189–202.

100 Taylor-Wiedeman J, Sissons P, Sinclair J. Induction of human cytomegalovirus gene expression after differentiation of monocytes from healthy carriers. *J Virol* 1994; **68**: 1597–1604.

22

Imaging

R. Jane Chambers

Harefield Hospital, Harefield, Middlesex, UK

Introduction

The expected radiological appearances and potential surgical complications of lung transplantation vary depending on the type of transplantation that has been performed (see Chapters 13 and 14). Whereas the appearances of medical complications such as rejection, infection and malignancy are common to all types of lung transplant. Some findings are unique to lung transplantation whereas others are related to the effects of cardiothoracic surgery in general. Radiological investigation may provide a specific diagnosis but many pulmonary complications have a nonspecific appearance and their differential diagnosis must be established from the clinical context and from laboratory investigation (see Chapters 20, 21 and 23). Therefore close correlation with time-related clinical and pathological findings is essential.

Postoperative complications

Early complications of lung transplant surgery include haemothorax, pneumothorax, effusion, infection and wound complications.

Haemothorax

This is usually related to surgical bleeding, which is more likely to occur in patients who have undergone previous surgery and those who underwent cardiopulmonary bypass as part of the surgical procedure. Computed tomography (CT) of the chest can localize the extent of a haemothorax and define any underlying parenchymal abnormality.

Pneumothorax

This may occur in all types of lung transplantation and was found in 10% of one series of 138 patients [1]. In heart–lung transplantation it may be bilateral due to the communication between the two pleural spaces; in bilateral sequential lung transplantation performed through an anterior clam shell incision, a similar communication between the pleural spaces occurs anteriorly. Postoperative pneumothoraces may be therefore be unilateral, bilateral and may shift between sides with changes in the patient's posture. Importantly, early postoperative chest films obtained with the patient in the supine position may not demonstrate the true size of the pneumothorax, which will be revealed by CT (Figure 22.1). Iatrogenic causes of pneumothorax that may occur later after surgery include complication of transbronchial biopsy, central venous line insertion, transthoracic aspiration or thoracentesis.

In unilateral lung transplants, performed for emphysema, pneumothorax may be due to a ruptured bulla in the native lung; a persistent air leak may complicate concurrent lung volume reduction surgery on the native lung. A tension pneumothorax is a potentially life-threatening complication, which may cause compression of the transplanted lung or cause cardiovascular collapse due to 'respiratory tamponade'.

Pleural effusion

Effusions are common in the first seven days postoperatively and are related to disruption of the lymphatic drainage via the visceral pleura, a positive fluid balance, or reperfusion lung injury. Appearances are entirely nonspecific so that the aetiology in a single instance is not apparent on the chest film. Experience has shown that the effusion usually decreases in size during the first week

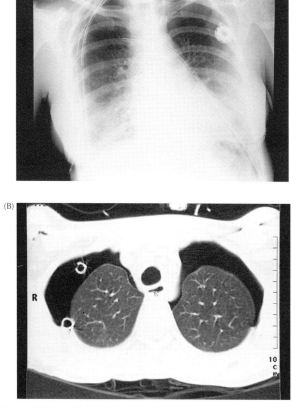

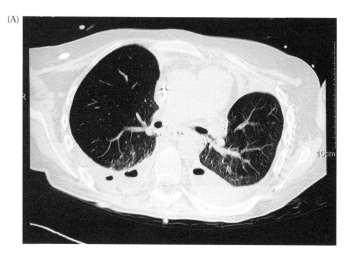

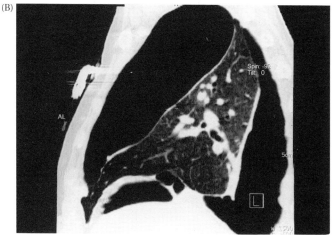

Figure 22.1 (A) Chest radiograph of a supine patient obtained seven days following heart–lung transplantation, showing small bilateral apical pneumothoraces. (B) High resolution computed tomography (HRCT) scan performed the same day because of an unexplained decline in respiratory function, demonstrated unsuspected large bilateral pneumothoraces that extended bilaterally to the lung bases anteriorly.

Figure 22.2 (A) HRCT scan from a patient following a bilateral lobe transplant, with bilateral empyema due to *Enterococcus*. (B) Multiplanar reconstruction following surgical drainage, demonstrating large left pneumothorax with thickened visceral pleura.

postoperatively; increase in size beyond day 7 usually indicates an alternative aetiology, usually infection or acute rejection. Rarely frankly chylous effusions occur. Ultrasound or CT examination may be necessary to define the nature and the extent of the fluid; a diagnostic or therapeutic aspiration, usually under ultrasound control, may be required; fluid samples should be submitted for microscopy and culture together with biochemical and immunocytological examination.

Infection

Infections within the chest in the early postoperative period include pneumonia, empyema and mediastinitis; the incidence of the latter two is low but they are associated with a high mortality rate.

Infection is one of the main differential diagnoses of pulmonary infiltrates and consolidation. Plain film examination should usually be followed by bronchoscopy to obtain sputum for culture together with a bronchoalveolar lavage with a transbronchial biopsy to look for evidence of infection or rejection.

A CT scan can define the extent and location of an empyema collection, so allowing for optimal placement of drainage tubes. Delayed removal of empyema fluid may result in significant pleural fibrosis, with subsequent failure of the underlying lung to re-expand (Figure 22.2).

(A)

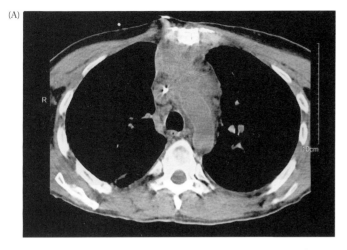

(B)

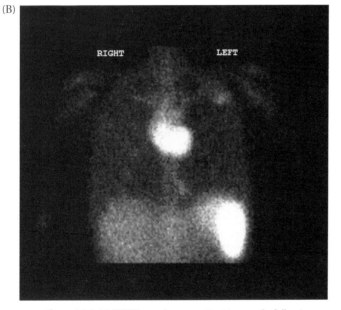

Figure 22.3 (A) HRCT scan from a patient two weeks following transplant surgery, with nonspecific chest radiograph; blood cultures were positive for *Acinetobacter*; the scan shows nonspecific heterogeneous retrosternal soft-tissue density. (B) A radionuclide ^{99m}Tc white blood cell scan demonstrates a large retrosternal abscess.

Mediastinitis is rare, less common than following cardiac transplantation, and is usually not specifically identifiable on the plain chest film. In a patient with a persistent pyrexia of unknown aetiology, or a positive blood culture, a CT scan of the chest is indicated for evaluation of the lung, pleura and mediastinum, although the mediastinal appearances may be inconclusive as they usually do not resolve the differential diagnosis between mediastinal haematoma or infection. A technetium-99m (^{99m}Tc) white blood cell scan

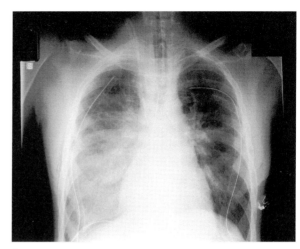

Figure 22.4 Ischaemia–reperfusion injury (the 'reimplantation response'). Chest radiograph taken 12 hours following bilateral lung transplantation, showing asymmetric diffuse right mid and lower zone parenchymal opacity, which subsequently resolved in 16 days.

can be performed, to localize the focus of infection (Figure 22.3). Needle aspiration of a retrosternal soft tissue density under CT guidance may therefore be necessary for diagnosis.

Pulmonary ischaemia–reperfusion injury

Ischaemia–reperfusion injury to the transplanted lung (also known as the pulmonary reimplantation response or reperfusion pulmonary oedema) is a form of noncardiogenic pulmonary oedema that has a nonspecific radiological appearance. It is a diagnosis of exclusion, and alternative diagnoses to be considered include fluid overload, hyperacute and early acute lung rejection, infection, postoperative atelectasis and left ventricular failure. The appearances in a postoperative radiograph taken in a recumbent ventilated patient can be exaggerated by the presence of concomitant pleural effusions that may lie behind the lungs. A clue to this possibility is unexpected good pulmonary gas exchange; the situation can be easily clarified by ultrasound examination or a CT scan.

In ischaemia–reperfusion injury, the spectrum of radiological appearances of interstitial and air space oedema varies from a mild perihilar haze to interstitial oedema, or dense alveolar consolidation, usually in the mid and lower lung zones, which may be asymmetric in bilateral lung transplants (Figure 22.4). The time interval following surgery is of diagnostic importance; some changes are usually seen in the first postoperative chest film, the abnormalities usually become most intense at three to four days and typically resolve within 5–14 days. New radiological abnormalities that occur more than five days after surgery are likely to be due to another cause. In one study of 105 lung transplant patients, radiographic abnormalities occurred on the first postoperative chest radiograph in 141 of 148 (95%) transplanted lungs, with changes by day 3 in 97% [2]. However, in a few instances of severe pulmonary injury, residual reticulonodular changes persisted for up to six months [3]. The radiological appearances were a poor predictor of the degree of functional impairment.

The pathogenesis of ischaemia–reperfusion injury involves increased pulmonary vascular permeability and pulmonary inflammation related to the duration of organ preservation as well as other factors including surgical trauma, denervation, interruption of the pulmonary lymphatics, and the use of cardiopulmonary bypass in the recipient.

Hyperacute and acute rejection

Hyperacute rejection is an uncommon complication of lung transplantation (see Chapter 23), which usually presents with severe pulmonary oedema and grossly impaired pulmonary compliance and gas exchange either in the operating room or soon after the patient has been transferred to the intensive care unit. The principal differential diagnosis is severe ischaemia–reperfusion injury.

Acute rejection occurs in the majority of lung transplant recipients, being observed as early as one to two weeks after surgery, with the great majority of first rejection episodes occur within the first three months after transplantation, the incidence subsequently decreasing with time. Pathologically, acute rejection is a cell-mediated response, with a mononuclear inflammatory infiltrate surrounding venules and arterioles; the bronchial and alveolar walls may also be involved. The radiographic appearances reflect this pathology, with interlobular septal thickening, a fine reticular pattern, ill-defined perihilar nodular densities extending to the lower lung zones, frank lower zone consolidation and pleural effusions (Figure 22.5). Pleural effusions commonly occur during early rejection episodes either

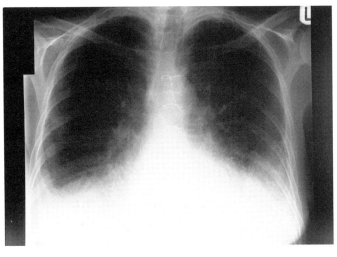

(A)

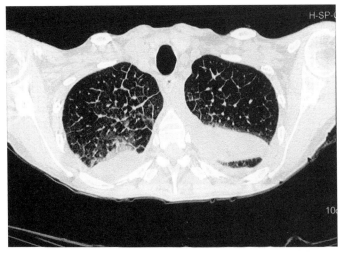

(B)

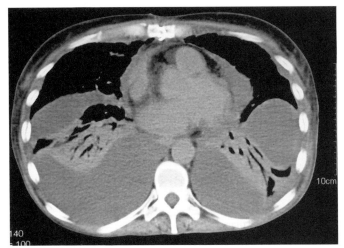

(C)

Figure 22.5 (A) Acute lung rejection. Chest radiograph four weeks following a bilateral single lung transplantation with new bilateral pleural effusions. (B and C) HRCT scan obtained two days later, showing large basal effusions with a small pericardial effusion and prominent interlobular septa. A transbronchial biopsy confirmed acute rejection.

alone or associated with septal lines; CT appearances may include peribronchial cuffing, interlobular septal thickening and groundglass attenuation. Thus the radiographic appearances mimic hydrostatic pulmonary oedema and are nonspecific, with no particular finding enabling differentiation from reimplantation response, fluid overload or certain infections. The timing of changes is useful in that if they occur more than one week after surgery, particularly with a new or enlarging pleural effusion, they most likely represent acute rejection rather than the ischaemia–reperfusion injury. However, the diagnosis of rejection can be confirmed only by bronchoscopy and transbronchial biopsy; a bronchoalveolar lavage must also be performed to exclude concomitant infection; abnormalities present in the chest radiograph may be useful in choosing the target site for the lavage and biopsy

Studies have correlated transbronchial biopsy findings with plain chest radiographs. In patients with a biopsy diagnosis of rejection, associated radiographic changes are more likely to be present during episodes that occurred in the early postoperative period. For example, in one study abnormal radiographs were present during 17 of 23 (74%) of rejection episodes that occurred in the first month after surgery, but only in 5 of 22 (22%) episodes that occurred later than this [4]. Acute rejection may therefore be present with a normal chest radiograph, as was found in 48% of biopsy-proven acute rejection episodes in another series [5]. Therefore, chest radiographs are not a sensitive method for diagnosing rejection beyond the early postoperative period and other investigations such as serial spirometric measurements are used to detect rejection at an early stage. Conversely, the occurrence of new pulmonary infiltrates more than a month after lung transplantation strongly favours an infective aetiology.

Anastomotic complications

Bronchus

In single lung and bilateral sequential lung transplantations the bronchial anastomoses are made as near to the hilum of the transplanted lung as possible to minimize the length of extrapulmonary bronchus that is transplanted (see Chapter 13). In the combined heart–lung transplantation procedure the three organs are transplanted en bloc and an anastomosis is made between the donor trachea, which has been transected just above the carina, and the lower most portion of the recipient's trachea; in this case the viability of the extrapulmonary bronchi is preserved through

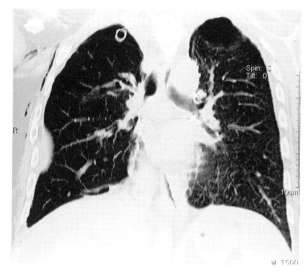

Figure 22.6 Bronchial stenosis due to infection; a coronal multiplanar reconstruction image demonstrating severe right main bronchial stenosis six weeks following bilateral lung transplantation.

collaterals between the coronary arteries of the donor heart and the bronchial circulation of the donor lung (see Chapter 14).

Major bronchial airway complications can occur in lung transplantation; dehiscence and stenosis occurred in 10–20% and 12–17% of anastomoses in early series [6,7], but have become less frequent with increasing surgical experience and the refinement of surgical methods; for example, in a review of 229 patients complications developed in only 5 of 126 (4%) anastomoses performed in the most recent group of transplant recipients, compared with 13% in the initial group [8].

Dehiscence of the bronchial anastomosis is an early complication, with bronchial ischaemia and infection contributing to its aetiology (Figure 22.6). Other possible contributing factors may include low collateral flow from the pulmonary arterial circulation to the bronchus during any perioperative periods of low cardiac output, the effects of ischaemia–reperfusion injury or acute rejection, and mucosal injury if positive pressure ventilation is required. The radiographic appearances that may be present in the plain chest film are nonspecific, namely pneumothorax or pneumomediastinum; in contrast, CT imaging is highly specific, with a sensitivity of 100% in a series of 21 patients, and specificity of 94% [9]. The usual appearance of bronchial dehiscence in thin section (1–3 mm) axial CT images consists of varying sized collections of extraluminal air in the soft tissues adjacent to a bronchial wall defect at the site of

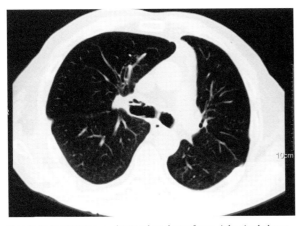

Figure 22.7 HRCT scan obtained 26 days after a right single lung transplantation (this patient had had a previous left single lung transplant). An anterior right bronchial wall defect is present, with extraluminal air within a soft tissue mass that was due to *Aspergillus fumigatus* infection at the anastomotic site. The patient had presented with haemoptysis.

the anastomosis (Figure 22.7). The bronchial defect may be confined or obscured by an abnormal adjacent soft tissue density consisting of granulation or necrotic tissue. Mediastinal air may be present with pneumothorax, but these additional findings are nonspecific; the presence of some extraluminal air alone does not definitely indicate a dehiscence, since this may remain from the time of the surgery.

CT interpretation has pitfalls, and awareness of the surgical technique is important. Early attempts to prevent dehiscence consisted of placing an omental flap around the anastomosis, producing a soft tissue mass adjacent to the anterior bronchial wall; this technique is no longer used. Telescoping at the anastomotic site has been performed in some transplant units, consisting of overlapping the anterior wall but with an end-to-end anastomosis posteriorly. This may result in a linear soft tissue intraluminal flap with a subjacent crescent of air along the anterior bronchial margin, giving the appearance of dehiscence, but this a normal finding with this operative technique. However, since this operative procedure does not involve overlap of the posterior bronchial wall, a linear flap with subjacent air indicates true dehiscence when present posteriorly. A small spherical anastomotic diverticulum adjacent to the medial and inferior aspect of the anastomosis is also a normal finding; the three appearances of flaps, air menisci and diverticula are more numerous in relation to the right rather than the left bronchus, possibly related to the increased angulation of the right main bronchus relative to the axial imaging plane [10]. Newer techniques of CT imaging, with oblique

multiplanar reconstructions, improve the definition of these early bronchial anastomotic appearances. Surgical intervention is required for a major dehiscence, but small defects 4 mm in size or less have been shown to heal without sequelae; topical application of methyl methacrylate glue has been used successfully to obliterate a small defect [11].

Historically, a high incidence of ischaemic breakdown of the tracheal anastomosis occurred in en bloc double lung transplantation. Subsequently, direct bronchial artery revascularization was performed by anastomosis between a donor bronchial artery and the left internal mammary artery (LIMA) of the recipient. Selective angiography could be used to demonstrate vascularity extending throughout the entire tracheobronchial tree that was associated with early airway healing and absence of anastomotic complications [12] (Figure 22.8). Bronchial artery perfusion scintigraphy with selective injection of ^{99m}Tc macroaggregated albumen into the LIMA in a similar group of patients confirmed preservation of bronchial arterial supply to the mediastinal structures, with vascularity extending to the peripheral lung fields in many. Norgaard et al. suggest that preservation of the bronchial arterial supply significantly contributed to the lower incidence of anastomotic and infective complications in 70 lung transplant patients, not only in en bloc double lung transplant but also in recipients of heart–lung and single lung transplants [13]. However such bronchial revascularization procedures are surgically demanding and prone to technical failure, which may lead to bronchial dehiscence; hence such methods are no longer routinely used in most transplant centres.

Bronchial wall stenoses may be due to strictures (Figure 22.9), bronchomalacia, or to the presence of excessive granulation tissue, which usually occurs during the first few months after surgery. Symptoms of cough and dyspnoea are present often associated with malaise or fever; there will be a decline in the results of spirometric tests with biphasic flow volume loop reflecting unilateral obstruction, or limitation of both in inspiratory and expiratory phases reflecting central airway obstruction. CT imaging is essential both to confirm the diagnosis and to define the site and extent of the stenosis; paired inspiratory and expiratory images may be required to demonstrate bronchomalacia. Thin-section axial images together with multiplanar reconstructions are recommended (Figure 22.10); a reduction of more than 50% in the luminal diameter of a main bronchus is usually considered to be functionally significant. Minor stenotic lesions may be missed, both on CT axial images and with multiplanar reconstruction.

Radionuclide ventilation scintigraphy using ^{99m}Tc DTPA (diethylene triamine penta-acetic acid) can demonstrate

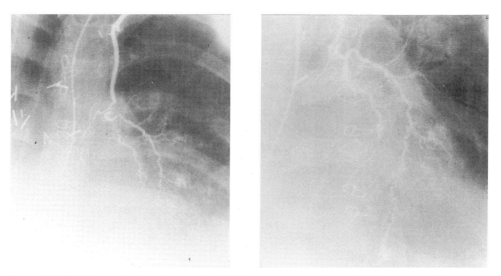

Figure 22.8 Selective contrast injection into the left internal mammary artery, which had been used to revascularize the bronchial circulation at the time of transplantation.

the relative distribution of inspired air between the two lungs and quantitative values indicate the severity of bronchial stenosis by the extent of diversion of ventilation to the opposite lung (Figure 22.9c).

Balloon dilatation alone for annular fibrotic lesions results in a high recurrence rate, and so the insertion of a bronchial stent is usually necessary; stents are always required for bronchomalacia (Figure 22.11). CT imaging contributes to the assessment of the length, severity and nature of the stricture prior to stent implantation and, following an implant, can define the site of any recurrent stenosis, reveal stent migration (Figure 22.12), or the presence of segmental bronchial obstruction caused by such migration. Other treatment methods for bronchial stenosis include laser therapy, cryotherapy or alternatively, brachytherapy with an iridium source (^{192}Ir), which has been used for treatment of recurrent excessive granulation tissue [14].

Axial thin section (1–3 mm) CT images have traditionally been used to assess airway stenosis; newer techniques of volumetric CT provide the possibility of multiplanar and three-dimensional images that are particularly useful for assessing the severity and longitudinal extent of the intraluminal component. Virtual bronchoscopy (VB) is a three-dimensional reconstruction technique that renders the axial CT data into simulated endobronchial views. Recent studies comparing the VB with fibreoptic bronchoscopy in lung transplant patients indicated that 97% of right main bronchial lesions and 92% of left main bronchial

lesions were detected with VB. This imaging method has the potential advantages of being noninvasive and providing a method for the evaluation of severe lesions that cannot be traversed by bronchoscopy. Disadvantages include the inability to detect mucosal lesions such as a flat ulcer, and the absence of samples for diagnosis of associated infection; VB can therefore provide information that is complementary to conventional bronchoscopy but is unlikely to replace it [15].

Pulmonary vessels

Complications related to major vascular anastomoses are uncommon. Transoesophageal echocardiography allows assessment of the pulmonary veins and right pulmonary artery anastomosis, but the left pulmonary artery is not visualized. Decreased perfusion to the lung can also be identified with pulmonary scintigraphy using ^{99m}Tc-labelled albumen. Contrast-enhanced CT or pulmonary angiography are required for an anatomical assessment, with direct measurement of the pressure gradient across the stenosis at cardiac catheterization. Balloon dilatation of the pulmonary arterial anastomosis may be performed if appropriate (Figures 22.13 and 22.14).

Rarely pulmonary vein stenosis has been associated with graft dysfunction, and lobar torsion has been described. Postoperative deep vein thrombosis and pulmonary embolism may occur as in any other postoperative patient.

(A)

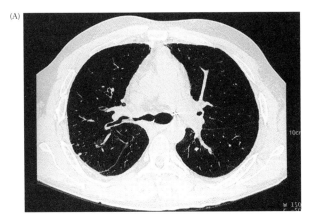

(B)

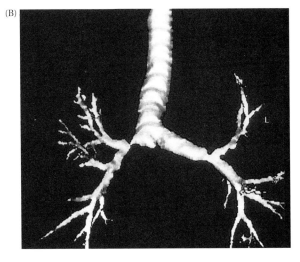

(C)

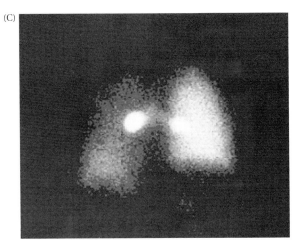

(A)

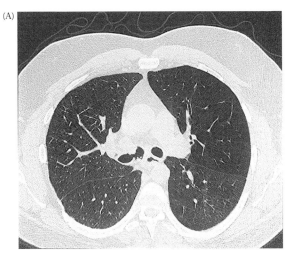

(B)

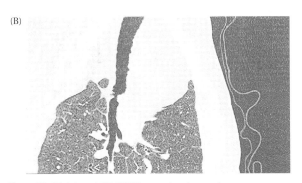

Figure 22.10 (above) (A) HRCT scan showing exuberant granulation tissue at a bronchial anastomotic site after right single lung transplantation. (B) Coronal multiplanar reconstruction image indicating the extent and severity of the stenosis.

Figure 22.9 (left) (A) Bronchial stenosis. HRCT scan performed seven weeks after a bilateral lung transplantation because of chest tightness and wheezing. Severe right focal and moderate left bronchial stenoses are present; bronchoscopy and biopsy showed granulation tissue only. (B) Three-dimensional reconstruction image showing the stenotic bronchial lesions. (C) Diethylene triamine penta-acetic acid (DTPA) ventilation scan demonstrating aerosol deposition at stenotic sites, aerosol deposition within the lung parenchyma was 24% in the right lung and 76% in the left lung, reflecting the functional severity of the two stenoses.

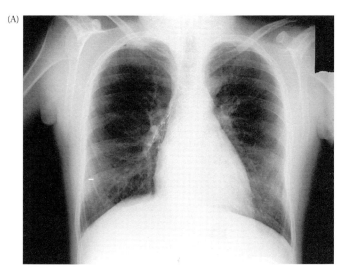

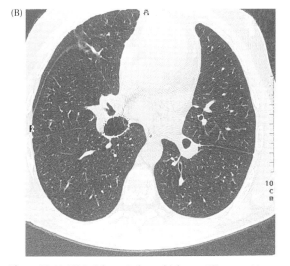

Figure 22.11 (A) A right main bronchial stent (Gianturco) inserted for focal stenosis. (B) HRCT scan with stent in situ; images lower in the chest showed patent segmental bronchi in the mid and lower lobes.

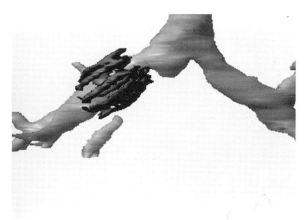

Figure 22.12 Maximal intensity projection image showing stent migration beyond a focal right bronchial stenosis in a patient following bilateral lobe transplants. Image artefacts in axial images may obscure lesions within or adjacent to stents; such reconstruction techniques are therefore useful for evaluation.

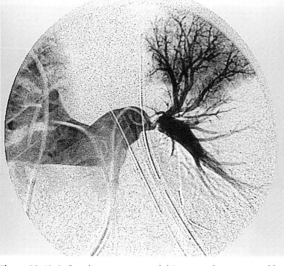

Figure 22.13 Left pulmonary artery dehiscence, demonstrated by selective left pulmonary angiogram two days after a left single lung transplantation.

Infections

Infection is an important cause of both morbidity and mortality after lung transplantation. Multiple factors account for the high incidence of infection in this patient group; these include loss of the cough reflex in the denervated transplanted lung, interruption of pulmonary lymphatic drainage, altered function of the mucociliary escalator and immune dysregulation within the lung, including impaired function of alveolar macrophages. In addition the host response to infection will be impaired by the pharmacological immunosuppression that is required to prevent rejection of the lung allograft.

An unrecognized infective process may be present in the donor lung at the time of surgery, and organisms related to subclinical aspiration in the donor before lung harvesting have been implicated. In contrast to other organ transplants, the transplanted lung is in direct communication

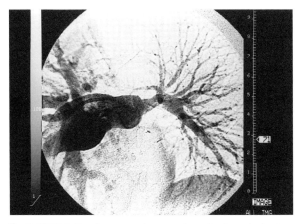

Figure 22.14 Left pulmonary artery anastomotic stenosis due to mismatch between donor and recipient vessels demonstrated by selective pulmonary angiography six weeks after surgery; the pressure gradient was 6 mmHg (800 Pa).

with the atmosphere and is particularly exposed to the risk of infection during the postoperative period of mechanical ventilation. In single allografts the transplanted lung shows a significantly higher infection rate as compared with the native lung.

Infection accounts for 48% of early postoperative mortality [16]. In the first month following surgery, bacterial and fungal infections are most common, possibly acquired during or immediately following the operative procedure, or from the donor organ. In one study, bacterial pneumonias accounted for 16 (36%) of 45 pneumonias after lung transplantation, usually involving a single organism, although mixed infections can occur. In the following three months, viral and fungal infections have the highest frequency.

Plain chest radiographs usually show nonspecific patchy infiltrates, often with a pleural effusion of varying size and most commonly in the transplanted lung in those with single lung transplants. CT appearances consist of any combination of consolidation, groundglass opacification, tree-in-bud pattern, and varying sized nodules, also with septal thickening and pleural effusions. Consolidation is commonest in the middle and lower lobes. CT appearances are usually nonspecific because of the overlap with other pulmonary processes such as rejection and fluid overload; however, some features such as the cavitating nodules that are seen occasionally with *Pseudomonas* infection may favour an infective process. Purulent bronchitis has no specific imaging findings, but may be associated with loss of volume or atelectasis on the plain chest radiograph. The diagnosis is usually made using bronchoscopy coupled with bronchoalveolar lavage and transbronchial biopsy (see Chapters 20 and 23).

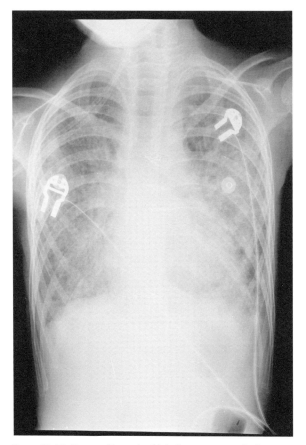

Figure 22.15 Chest radiograph of fulminant cytomegalovirus (CMV) pneumonitis in a seven year old boy following heart–lung transplantation.

Viral infections typically occur one to four months post-transplantation, and are related to impaired immunity due to pharmacological immunosuppression. In lung transplant patients, infection with the herpes group of viruses is the most common, particularly infection with cytomegalovirus (CMV). Without either antiviral prophylaxis or monitoring to allow early (pre-emptive) therapy, CMV can result in severe pneumonitis in lung transplant recipients (see Chapter 21); this is one of the most serious forms of CMV infection (Figure 22.15). Untreated, CMV pneumonitis is reported to have a 75% mortality, and it predisposes to bacterial and fungal superinfection of the lung as well as being associated with obliterative bronchiolitis. Early recognition and treatment is therefore essential.

In early CMV pneumonitis, the plain chest film may be normal, or show only mild interstitial infiltrates. The CT appearances consist of multiple, often coalescing, nodules with areas of groundglass attenuation, consolidation, bronchial wall thickening with dilatation, and small

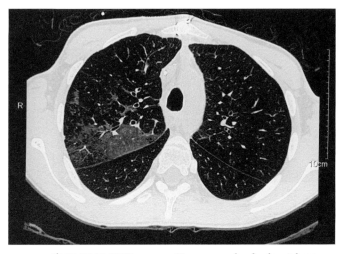

Figure 22.16 CMV pneumonitis seven weeks after heart–lung transplant. HRCT scan shows areas of groundglass attenuation in both lungs.

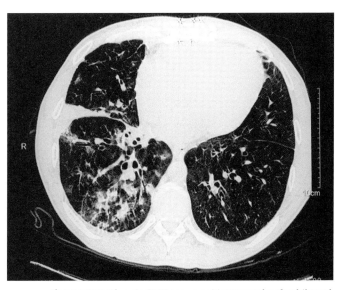

Figure 22.17 Chronic CMV pneumonitis 20 months after bilateral lung transplant. HRCT scan shows irregular peribronchial nodules, a small area of subpleural consolidation and interlobular septal thickening.

pleural effusions. These abnormalities may be present in either the transplanted or nontransplanted lungs, although CMV preferentially affects the transplanted lung. Septal thickening and tree-in-bud appearances may also be present, so that overall findings are not specific for this infective agent (Figures 22.16 and 22.17).

Other viral infections include the community-acquired respiratory syncytial virus (RSV) and adenovirus, both of which are acquired by aerosol inhalation. The CT appear-

ances of these infections are similar to CMV pneumonitis but with no pleural effusions or lymph node enlargement. RSV infection usually presents in adult patients who have a normal chest radiograph [17]. Herpes simplex pneumonia produces diffuse alveolar infiltrates that may resemble the acute respiratory distress syndrome.

Fungal spores are ubiquitous in the environment and are inhaled into the tracheobronchial tree; these organisms do not usually cause disease in immunocompetent individuals but may colonize immunosuppressed transplant recipients and may cause serious tissue invasive disease. *Aspergillus fumigatus* is the most usual organism and this opportunistic infection usually presents two to six months following transplantation. Airways colonization occurs in 40–90% of lung transplant patients, with invasive aspergillosis subsequently occurring in 3% [18]. A recent survey, however, found infections much later after surgery, the mean time for *Aspergillus* infection to occur being 15 months after transplantation surgery [19]. Tissue invasion may occur via the bronchial anastomotic site, usually within the first four months after surgery; CT imaging may reveal a polypoid intraluminal nodule or ulcerative lesion penetrating the bronchial wall (Figure 22.7). *Aspergillus* pneumonia with spread through the bronchial tree, angioinvasive aspergillosis, empyema, or an aspergilloma within a cavity (the latter particularly in a nontransplanted contralateral lung) may all occur (Figure 22.18). CT appearances of *Aspergillus* pneumonia may be highly suggestive, with multiple nodules surrounded by a halo of groundglass attenuation; other features include wedge-shaped subpleural areas of consolidation, or groundglass attenuation in association with septal thickening with pleural effusions. Rarely an air-crescent sign may be present.

The diagnosis of colonization with *Aspergillus* is normally made from a bronchoalveolar lavage. Evidence of colonization in association with strongly suggestive radiological appearances may sometimes be taken as sufficient evidence to diagnose tissue invasive disease. In view of the toxicity associated with intensive antifungal therapy, however, a firm diagnosis is highly desirable and this requires a lung biopsy (either transbronchial or CT guided); however, there is a risk of haemorrhage complicating a biopsy taken from areas of angioinvasive disease. Despite therapy, invasive aspergillosis has a high mortality rate in lung transplant patients.

Other fungal parenchymal infections include *Candida*, *Cryptococcus*, and rarely mucormycosis, the latter occurring almost only in diabetic patients. All produce varying sized pulmonary nodules, which may be solitary or multiple. Any fungal infection may become disseminated

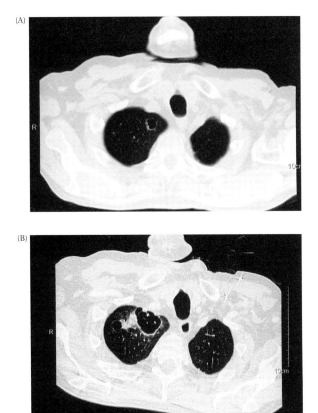

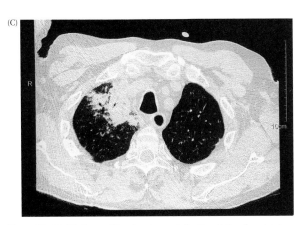

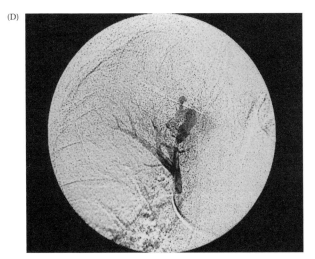

Figure 22.18 (cont.)

Figure 22.18 (A) *Aspergillus fumigatus* infection following right single lung transplantation. Small right apical cyst 26 days after surgery, present at the same time as the right bronchial wall defect (see Figure 22.7). (B) HRCT scan showing enlarging cyst with peribronchial density, two weeks after (A). (C) Increased parenchymal infiltrate, presumed to represent haemorrhage, with the patient developing worsening haemoptysis. (D) One week after (C), selective right upper pulmonary angiogram showing a mycotic aneurysm due to angioinvasive aspergillosis. Subsequent massive haemoptysis necessitated right upper lobectomy.

to other organs. *Cryptococcus* infection can present with subacute meningitis.

Pneumocystis carinii was a common infection causing pneumonitis in the lung transplant population and the disease had a high mortality rate. However, prophylactic antimicrobial therapy has very significantly reduced the incidence of this infection. The chest film usually demonstrates faint hazy infiltrates that are characterized in a CT scan as diffuse alveolar consolidation resembling pulmonary oedema.

Mycobacterium tuberculosis occurs in 2–4% of lung transplant patients [20]. Radiographic appearances are nonspecific, with multiple nodules that may cavitate, consolidation, septal thickening, pleural effusions and mediastinal node enlargement. Nontuberculous mycobacterium infection also occurs, appearing on CT scan as multiple small nodules.

Patients who are long-term survivors after lung transplantation and who have good lung function remain at increased risk of infection, but the organisms encountered are more similar to those in community-acquired pneumonia occurring within the general population. In contrast, patients who have developed obliterative bronchiolitis (see below) are prone to recurrent bacterial infections, particularly with Gram-negative organisms, related to the development of bronchiectasis together with a wide range of opportunistic infections due to the increased intensity of immunosuppression used to treat this condition.

Infection is therefore an ongoing and important cause of morbidity and mortality in lung transplant patients (Figures 22.19 and 22.20). The plain chest radiograph is frequently abnormal but may even appear normal in some instances (particularly early viral infection); however, the appearance of a new pulmonary infiltrate in a

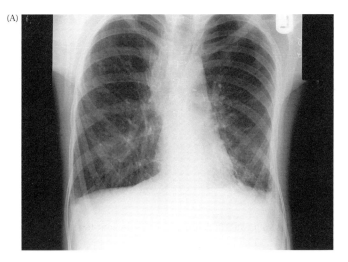

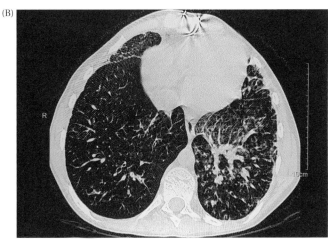

Figure 22.19 (A) *Haemophilus influenzae.* Chest radiograph showing nonspecific left basal patchy infiltrate. (B) HRCT scan with peribronchial infiltrates and interlobular septal thickening representing nonspecific finding two years following bilateral lung transplantation.

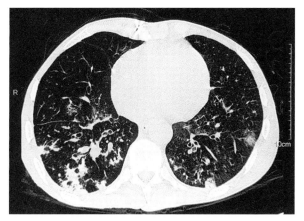

Figure 22.20 *Pseudomonas aeruginosa* infection in heart–lung transplant patient 12 years after transplantation and two years after a renal transplant. Peribronchial consolidation is present with slightly dilated and thick-walled bronchi.

lung transplant recipient more than a month after surgery favours an infective process rather than rejection. The radiological findings are usually nonspecific and the differential diagnosis is therefore wide; however, the most likely type of infection can often be assessed by the clinical picture coupled with consideration of the time after the transplant, level of pulmonary function and the intensity of the patient's current immunosuppression. CT findings are also usually nonspecific but can help to define the nature, extent and severity of the disease as well as providing a useful guide for targeting a transbronchial biopsy.

Obliterative bronchiolitis

Obliterative bronchiolitis is a major cause of morbidity and mortality after lung transplantation; it is a progressive process that leads to obstruction of the small airways owing to concentric bronchiolar fibrosis. Obliterative bronchiolitis is generally considered to be a form of chronic allograft rejection; it has been reported to occur eventually in 70% of lung transplant patients and it is associated with a high mortality rate [21]. Obliterative bronchiolitis is a pathological diagnosis but the involvement of bronchioles is patchy and may be missed with a transbronchial biopsy. Consequently, a functional syndrome 'bronchiolitis obliterans syndrome' has been defined, which refers to a progressive deterioration in the function of the transplanted lung due to airways obstruction; this diagnosis can be made only after the exclusion of other causes of pulmonary dysfunction including large airways obstruction, acute rejection and infection.

The functional changes in bronchiolitis obliterans syndrome are those of progressive airflow obstruction, with a progressive fall in expiratory flow rates, the forced expiratory volume in 1 s (FEV_1), forced vital capacity (FVC) and FEV_1:FVC ratio. The findings in the plain chest radiograph are nonspecific and usually do not contribute to the diagnosis, although there may be decreased peripheral vascular markings, increased (or less commonly decreased) lung volumes, or evidence of bronchiectasis. In advanced bronchiolitis obliterans the chest radiograph may show marked hyperinflation resembling severe chronic obstructive pulmonary disease.

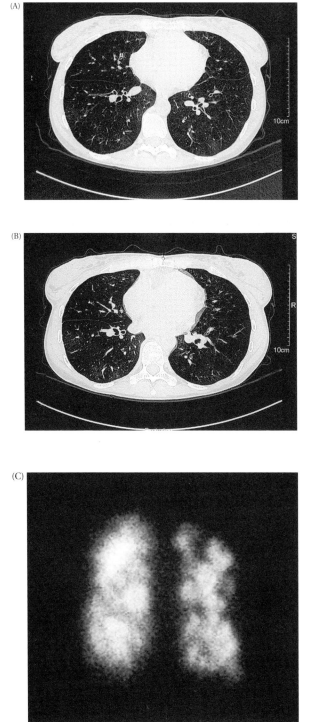

Several studies have been performed to define the value of high resolution CT (HRCT) scans obtained in both inspiration and expiration to demonstrate the presence of obliterative bronchiolitis. Since the site of fundamental abnormality occurs within the respiratory bronchioles, which are beyond the resolution of HRCT, the diagnostic findings depend on effects secondary to the bronchiolar obstruction and associated changes within the larger airways. In biopsy-proven obliterative bronchiolitis, inspiratory images demonstrate bronchial dilatation, mainly involving the segmental and subsegmental bronchi; dilatation is present when the internal diameter of the bronchus is greater than the diameter of the adjacent artery. Bronchial wall thickening may be present together with a mosaic pattern of both attenuation and perfusion; this latter phenomenon is due to hypoxic vasoconstriction of the poorly ventilated lung regions of lung subtended by obstructed bronchioles, which results in diversion of blood flow to adjacent normally ventilated regions, thus producing patchy areas of low and normal attenuation, respectively. Bronchiolar obstruction also causes air trapping that can be demonstrated in expiratory views, with regions of decreased volume loss in expiration again producing patchy areas of decreased attenuation (Figure 22.21). This air trapping was found to be the most sensitive and accurate radiological finding for the diagnosis of obliterative bronchiolitis in two studies [22,23] and may be present when no definite abnormality can be identified in images obtained during inspiration. Extensive bronchiectasis throughout both lung fields is a feature of advanced obliterative bronchiolitis (Figure 22.22), and extensive and progressive apical fibrosis may occur that is unrelated to infection or other known cause (Figure 22.23).

Since both the onset and the clinical course of obliterative bronchiolitis are variable, and since HRCT findings may not be definitive and transbronchial biopsy will not always establish the diagnosis, serial spirometric evaluations of lung function are used to screen patients for this condition [24]. When symptoms or spirometric abnormalities appear, HRCT and transbronchial biopsy are useful both

Figure 22.21 (A) Obliterative bronchiolitis. HRCT scan obtained 16 years after heart–lung transplantation showing bronchial wall thickening but no major dilatation. (B) Expiratory HRCT scan at same anatomical level as (A) demonstrates only minimal volume reduction and no significant change in parenchymal density, indicating widespread air trapping. (C) DTPA ventilation scan shows patchy parenchymal aerosol deposition consistent with diffuse severe obliterative bronchiolitis.

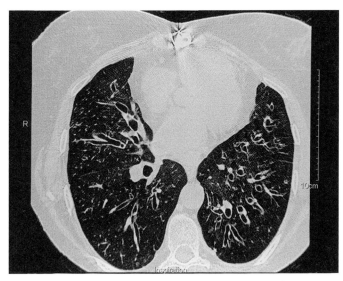

Figure 22.22 Obliterative bronchiolitis. HRCT scan showing severe bronchiectasis nine years after a bilateral lung transplant.

to demonstrate the presence of obliterative bronchiolitis and, importantly, to exclude other treatable lung pathology. The contribution of long-term follow-up with HRCT was demonstrated in a study of a group of 13 lung transplant patients [25] in whom obliterative bronchiolitis developed in eight cases; in these cases, HRCT findings of decreased lung volume, decreased peripheral markings and interlobular septal thickening appeared within 7–11 months of surgery. The mean interval to the finding of bronchial dilatation was 12 months, and decreased attenuation with mosaic perfusion appeared between 16 and 21 months. In that particular study no expiratory views were available.

Post-transplantation lymphoproliferative disorder

Post-transplantation lymphoproliferative disorder (PTLD) is a serious complication of transplantation that occurs in 2–8% of adult lung transplant recipients [26]; a higher incidence of 15% has been reported in paediatric patients due to their susceptibility to primary infection with Epstein–Barr virus (EBV) [27]. PTLD can occur at any stage after transplantation but those cases related to a primary infection with EBV usually occur several months after surgery and generally within the first year. The pathogenesis of most cases is related to EBV-induced B-cell proliferation, combined with reduced immunosurveillance of the B-cell population by T cells due to post-transplantation immunosuppression. A spectrum of disease can occur, ranging from virally driven hyperplasia to high grade malignant

(A)

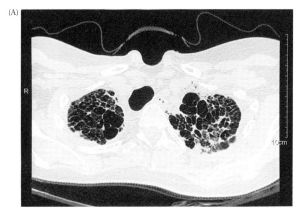

(B)

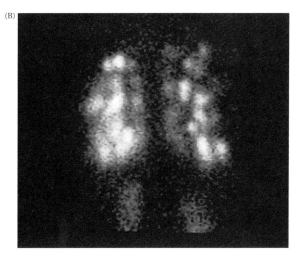

Figure 22.23 (A) HRCT scan nine years after a bilateral lung transplant showing severe bilateral apical fibrosis in a patient with obliterative bronchiolitis. (B) DTPA lung scan demonstrating aerosol deposition throughout both lung fields consistent with obliterative bronchiolitis, with rapid alveolar clearance resulting in early renal opacification.

lymphoma and cases that present more than a year after transplantation are more likely to follow a malignant clinical course. In lung transplant patients PTLD is usually manifest within the thorax, thus showing a predilection for involvement of the allograft but disseminated disease may occur.

The patient may be asymptomatic, with the abnormality being a chance finding on the chest radiograph or CT, there may be symptoms resembling a virus infection or those typical of a non-Hodgkin's lymphoma such as lymphadenopathy or weight loss. The chest radiograph may show solitary or multiple pulmonary nodules (Figure 22.24). CT findings most commonly show randomly distributed nodules 1–4 cm in diameter, well defined or surrounded by

(A)

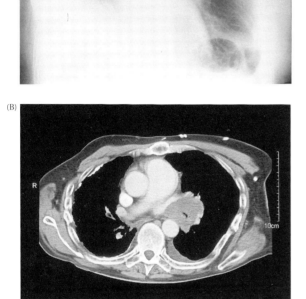

(B)

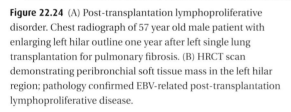

Figure 22.24 (A) Post-transplantation lymphoproliferative disorder. Chest radiograph of 57 year old male patient with enlarging left hilar outline one year after left single lung transplantation for pulmonary fibrosis. (B) HRCT scan demonstrating peribronchial soft tissue mass in the left hilar region; pathology confirmed EBV-related post-transplantation lymphoproliferative disease.

groundglass attenuation as a 'halo sign', but rarely having an air bronchogram within them. The nodules may be subpleural and are usually more widespread in the lower lung zones, with peribronchial distribution. Cavitation is usually absent, although central low attenuation necrosis has been reported. Mediastinal involvement occurs in 25% of patients and may be discreet node enlargement or a diffuse mass (Figure 22.25); an area of consolidation, groundglass attenuation and solitary endobronchial lesions has also been reported, together with mild pericardial or pleural thickening or a small effusion. These CT appearances are nonspecific and may mimic infection so that tissue biopsy is required for diagnosis. Extrathorax sites may be involved including the brain, head and neck, and particularly abdominal nodes (Figure 22.26) [28].

(A)

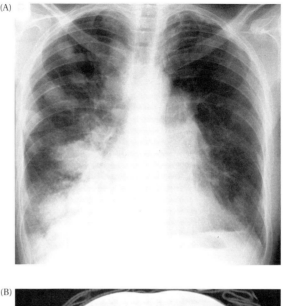

(B)

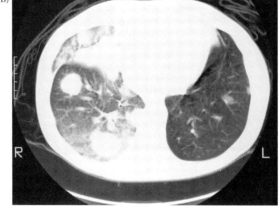

Figure 22.25 (A) Post-transplantation lymphoproliferative disease. Multiple pulmonary nodules on a chest radiograph four months following a right single lung transplant for emphysema. The patient presented with increasing dyspnoea. This case was related to a primary infection with Epstein–Barr virus (EBV), the transplant recipient having been EBV negative and the organ donor being EBV positive. (B) HRCT scan showing numerous parenchymal nodules, also present in the nontransplanted left lung. Complete resolution followed a reduction in the intensity of pharmacological immunosuppression and treatment with intravenous ganciclovir.

Complications related to the native lung

Native lung complications in patients who have undergone single lung transplants vary in incidence from 15% to 25%, and are associated with both morbidity and mortality. In one series abnormalities occurred in 17 of 111 single lung transplants (15%) with infection confined to the native lung being the commonest problem, which usually presented

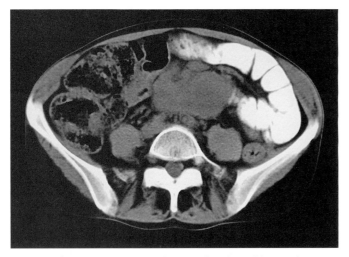

Figure 22.26 Post-transplantation lymphoproliferative disease. HRCT scan of abdomen demonstrating a large lymph node mass representing a B-cell lymphoma in a 26 year old female patient 11 years following heart–lung transplant for cystic fibrosis.

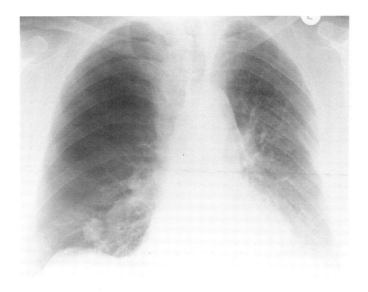

Figure 22.27 Squamous cell carcinoma presenting as a right basal nodule in the emphysematous right lung of a patient eight years following left single lung transplantation.

with symptoms and segmental or lobar opacities in the plain chest radiographs or CT images [29]. Organisms included *Pseudomonas aeruginosa*, *Haemophilus influenzae*, *Aspergillus fumigatus* and other fungi, *M. tuberculosis* and *M. avium intracellulare* but, in contrast to infections commonly seen in lung allografts, no viral infections were seen.

Nonsmall cell cancer in the native emphysematous lung occurred in 2 of 86 patients with chronic obstructive airway disease who had undergone single lung transplantation (2.3%) and in 1 of 15 patients with pulmonary fibrosis (6.5%); both of these conditions known to be associated with increased prevalence of cancer [30] (Figure 22.27). Pretransplant surveillance with CT imaging showed no evidence of these tumours, or of TB prior to surgery, but has been recommended post-transplantation to exclude unsuspected lung malignancies [31]. Rarer complications in the native lung include pulmonary embolism and infarction, which occurred in two patients in this series. PTLD rarely involves the native lung, unless widely disseminated.

Single lung transplantation, particularly for emphysema, may result in herniation of the native lung across the midline, resulting in compression of the allograft. In the acute early postoperative setting, selective intubation and ventilation of each lung may be required (see Chapter 15). More frequently a gradual progressive compression of the graft occurs, associated with impaired function, particularly an increase in pulmonary vascular resistance and subsequent diversion of pulmonary blood flow away from the graft [32] (Figure 22.28). Lung volume reduction surgery (LVRS) on the native lung is now sometimes performed at the time of single lung transplantation in an attempt to avoid this complication. Occasionally, this has also been performed after the initial transplant; in this situation, however, case selection is difficult because over expansion of the native lung may be secondary to intrinsic changes in lung allograft such as fibrosis, or the development of obliterative bronchiolitis.

Recurrent disease

Recurrence of the original pulmonary disease within the transplanted lung is most commonly seen in sarcoidosis, but has also been observed with lymphangioleiomyomatosis, Langerhans cell histiocytosis, diffuse panbronchiolitis, alveolar proteinosis and giant cell pneumonitis. Recurrent disease must therefore be considered in differential diagnosis of abnormal finding in the allograft on CT imaging [33].

Complications of ciclosporin therapy

Immunosuppression with ciclosporin or tacrolimus may be associated with impairment of renal function and with neurological complications. Data from the International Society for Heart and Lung Transplantation Registry indicates that 34% of lung transplant patients develop renal

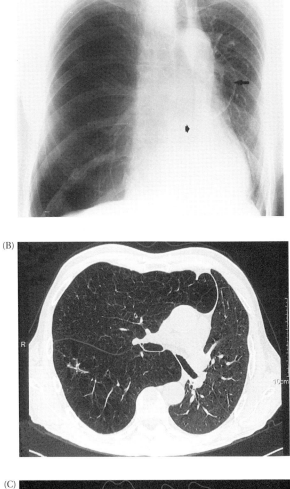

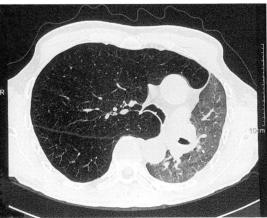

insufficiency within five years of transplantation, with end-stage disease requiring dialysis occurring in fewer than 5% of cases [34]. Injury to preglomerular and glomerular microvasculature causes glomerular, vascular and tubular defects, and other associated risk factors for toxicity include concomitant use of other nephrotoxic drugs. Ultrasound images usually show slightly small kidneys with significant increase in cortical echogenicity and loss of the corticomedullary margin, but with no evidence of pelvicaliceal obstruction. Further imaging may be required to exclude other causes of renal dysfunction such as renovascular disease or obstructive uropathy. In cases where the diagnosis is uncertain renal biopsy may be indicated (see Chapter 23)

Ciclosporin neurotoxicity has many features in common with hypertensive encephalopathy, and may produce headaches, seizures and visual disturbances, transient aphasia and weakness [35]. CT and magnetic resonance (MR) images show oedema in the subcortical white matter, most commonly of the occipital lobes, with occasional involvement of parietal, temporal and frontal regions (Figure 22.29). The clinical, CT and MR findings are reversible with a reduction in the dose of ciclosporin and treatment of hypertension. Imaging is important, since similar clinical symptoms may occur with intracerebral infection in the immunosuppressed patient (meningitis, abscess or viral encephalitis) and rarely with intracerebral haemorrhage.

Miscellaneous findings

Transbronchial lung biopsy is frequently performed in lung transplant patients, both as a surveillance procedure for rejection and for tissue diagnosis for new bronchial or parenchymal densities. The biopsy procedure itself may produce small parenchymal nodules [36], which usually resolve completely, but occasionally these cavitate and leave a thin-walled cyst in the lung parenchyma (Figure 22.30). Diaphragmatic paralysis due to injury of the phrenic nerve

Figure 22.28 (A) Compression of a left single lung transplant owing to herniation of the native right lung; chest radiograph shows the anterior junction line to be significantly displaced leftward (small arrow) and right lung extending leftward across the azygos-oesophageal recess to extend beyond the lateral margin of the descending aorta (large arrow). (B) HRCT scan in inspiration showing small volume of left lung, with leftward position of the anterior junction line. (C) HRCT scan in expiration with extremely small left lung volume.

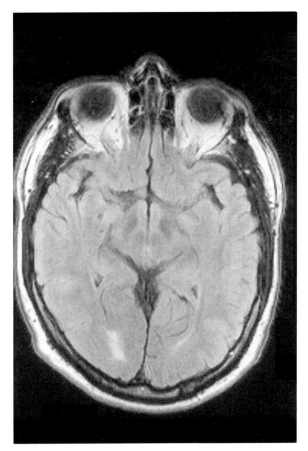

Figure 22.29 Ciclosporin neurotoxicity. A 36 year old patient who had presented with blurred vision and headache three months post-transplantation. An axial magnetic resonance FLAIR (fluid attenuated inversion recovery) image at the level of the occipital lobes, showing high signal in the white matter, with no grey matter involvement; this is a nonspecific vascular effect that was related to ciclosporin therapy in this instance.

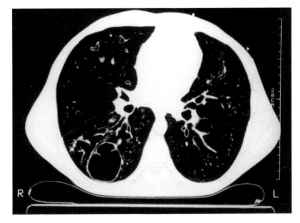

Figure 22.30 Lung cyst remaining following a previous transbronchial biopsy.

may occur following either single or double lung transplantation; it was present in 6 of 185 patients in one series and resulted in prolonged stay in intensive care and hospitalization [37].

REFERENCES

1 Herridge MS, de Hoyos AL, Chaparro C, et al. Pleural complications in lung transplant recipients. *J Thorac Cardiovasc Surgery* 1995; **110**: 22–26.
2 Anderson DC, Glazer HS, Semenkovitch JW, et al. Lung transplant oedema: chest radiography after lung transplantation. The first 10 days. *Radiology* 1995; **195**: 275–281.
3 Herman SJ. Radiologic assessment after lung transplantation. *Clin Chest Med* 1990; **11**: 333–346.
4 Millett B, Higenbottam TW, Flower CDR, et al; The radiographic appearances of infection and acute rejection of the lung after heart–lung transplantation. *Am Rev Respir Dis* 1989; **140**: 62–67.
5 Kindu S, Herman SJ, Larhs A, et al. Correlation of chest radiographic findings with biopsy-proven acute lung rejection. *J Thorac Imag* 1999; **14**: 178.
6 Truelock EP: Lung transplantation. *Am J Respir Crit Care Med* 1997; **155**: 789–818.
7 Ramirez J, Patterson GA. Airway complications after lung transplantation. *Semin Thorac Cardiovasc Surg* 1992; **4**: 122–125.
8 Date H, Trulock EP, Arcidi JM, et al. Improved airway healing after lung transplantation. An analysis of 348 bronchial anastomoses. *J Thorac Cardiovasc Surg* 1995; **110**: 1424–1433.
9 Semenkovich JW, Glazer HS, Anderson DC, et al. Bronchial dehiscence in lung transplantation: CT evaluation. *Radiology* 1995; **194**: 205–208.
10 McAdams HP, Murray JG, Erasmus JJ, et al. Telescoping bronchial anastomoses for unilateral or bilateral sequential lung transplantation: CT appearances. *Radiology* 1997; **203**: 202–206.
11 Collins J, Kuhlman JE, Love RB. Acute life threatening complications of lung transplantation. *Radiographics* 1998; **18**: 21–43.
12 Daly RC, Tadjkarimi S, Khaghani A, et al. Successful double lung transplantation with direct bronchial artery revascularization. *Ann Thorac Surg* 1993; **56**: 885–892.
13 Norgaard MA, Gadsboll N, Efson F, et al. Bronchial artery perfusion scintigraphy to assess bronchial artery blood flow after lung transplantation. *J Nucl Med* 1999; **40**: 290–295.
14 Kennedy AS, Sonett JR, Orens JB, et al. High dose rate brachytherapy to prevent recurrent benign hyperplasia in lung transplant bronchi: theoretical and clinical considerations. *J Heart Lung Transplant* 2000; **19**: 155–159.
15 McAdams HP, Palmer SM, Evasmus JJ, et al. Bronchial anastomotic complications in lung transplant recipients: virtual bronchoscopy for non-invasive assessment. *Radiology* 1998; **209**: 689–695.
16 Collins J, Kuhlman JE, Lowe RB. Acute life threatening complications of lung transplantation. *Radiographics* 1998; **18**: 21–43.
17 Ko JP, Shepard JO, Sproule MW, et al. CT manifestations of

respiratory syncytial virus infection in lung transplant recipients. *J Comput Assist Tomogr* 2000; **24**: 235–241.

18 Cahill BC, Hibbs JR, Savik K, et al. *Aspergillus* airway colonisation and invasive disease after lung transplantation. *Chest* 1997; **112**: 1160–1164.

19 Diederich S, Scadeng M, Dennis C, et al. *Aspergillus* infections of the respiratory tract after lung transplantation: chest radiographic and CT findings. *Eur Radiol* 1998; **8**: 306–312.

20 Kesten S, Chaparro C. Mycobacterial infections in lung transplant patients. *Chest* 1999; **115**: 741–745.

21 Boehler A, Keston S, Weder W, et al. Bronchiolitis obliterans after lung transplantation. *Chest* 1998; **114**: 1411–1426.

22 Leung AN, Fisher K, Valentine V, et al. Bronchiolitis obliterans after lung transplantation detection using expiratory HRCT. *Chest* 1998; **113**: 365–370.

23 Worthy SA, Park CS, Kim JS, Müller NL. Bronchiolitis obliterans after lung transplantation: high resolution CT findings in 15 patients. *Am J Roentgenol* 1997; **169**: 673–677.

24 Cooper J D, Billingham M, Egan T, et al. A working formula for the standardisation of nomenclature and for clinical staging of chronic dysfunction in lung allografts. *J Heart Lung Transplant* 1993; **12**: 713–716.

25 Ikonen T, Kivisaari L, Taskinen E, et al. High resolution CT in long term follow up after lung transplantation. *Chest* 1997; **111**: 370–376.

26 Collins J, Müller NL, Leung AN, et al. Epstein–Barr-virus associated lymphoproliferative disease of the lung: CT and histological findings. *Radiology* 1998; **208**: 749–759.

27 Pickhardt PJ, Siegel MJ, Hayashi RJ, et al. Post transplant lymphoproliferative disorder in children. Clinical, histopathologic and imaging features. *Radiology* 2000; **217**: 16–25.

28 Rappaport DC, Chamberlain DW, Shepherd FA, et al. Lymphoproliferative disorders after lung transplantation. Imaging features. *Radiology* 1998; **206**: 519–524.

29 Speziali G, McDougall JC, Midthun DE, et al. Native lung complications after single lung transplantations for emphysema. *Transpl Int* 1997; **10**: 113–115.

30 McAdams HP, Erasmus JJ, Palmer SM. Complications (excluding hyperinflation) involving native lung after single lung transplantation. Incidence, radiological features and clinical importance. *Radiology* 2001; **218**: 233–341.

31 Kazerooni EA, Chow LC, Whyte RI, et al. Pre-operative examination of lung transplant candidates. Value of chest CT compared with chest radiography. *Am J Roentgenol* 1995; **165**: 1343–1348.

32 Murray JG, McAdams HP, Erasmum JJ, et al. Complications of lung transplantation. Radiologic findings. *Am J Roentgenol* 1996; **166**: 1405–1411.

33 Collins J, Hartman MJ, Warner TF, et al. Frequency and CT findings of recurrent disease after lung transplantation. *Radiology* 2001; **219**: 503–509.

34 Hosenpud JD, Bennet LE, Keck BM. The Registry of International Society for Heart and Lung Transplantation: 17th official report – 2000. *J Heart Lung Transplant* 2000; **19**: 909–932.

35 Schwartz RB, Bravo SM, Klufas RA. Cyclosporine neurotoxicity in relationship to hypertensive encephalopathy. CT & MR findings in 16 cases. *Am J Roentgenol* 1995; **165**: 627–631.

36 Kazerooni EA, Cascade PN, Gross BH. Transplanted lungs: nodules following transbronchial biopsy. *Radiology* 1995; **194**: 209–211.

37 Maqiak DE, Maurer JR, Kesten S. Diaphragmatic paralysis. A complication of lung transplantation. *Ann Thorac Surg* 1996; **61**: 170–173.

23

Transplant pathology

Margaret M. Burke

Harefield Hospital, Harefield, Middlesex, UK

Introduction

The Registry of the International Society for Heart and Lung Transplantation (ISHLT) has reported survival rates of 64% and 18% at 1 and 14 years, respectively, for heart–lung transplantation and of 70%, 45% and 20% at 1, 5 and 10 years, respectively, for lung transplantation [1]. Despite the increasing range and sophistication of immunosuppressive and antimicrobial drugs, the main causes of morbidity and mortality occurring after the immediate postoperative period remain acute rejection, infection and, in late survivors, obliterative bronchiolitis. In order to improve the results of lung transplantation, early diagnosis and treatment of postoperative complications are essential. The histopathologist has a role to play in this process in terms of biopsy diagnosis of, and research into, the pulmonary and systemic complications (Table 23.1) and in contributing to clinical audit through postmortem examination [2]. In addition, review of lung biopsies taken prior to transplantation may confirm the referral diagnosis, which, in turn, is audited by histological examination of the explanted lung. In a small number of cases this may reveal a different, or an additional diagnosis, sometimes in the context of systemic disease, with implications for post-transplantation management [3] (see Chapter 10).

Technical aspects of lung allograft pathology

The histopathologist must ensure that the clinical requirement for a rapid biopsy reporting service, including an on-call service, can be met. In addition to standard technology, he/she should have access to a variety of specialist techniques including immunohistochemistry (IHC) and molecular techniques such as in situ hybridization

(ISH) and the polymerase chain reaction (PCR). Review of biopsies at regular joint clinical pathology meetings is important in patient management.

Lung biopsies

Bronchoscopy and transbronchial biopsies (TBBx) are used for diagnostic and routine surveillance of the lung allograft. The procedure may be done under local or general anaesthesia. Morbidity is low, but complications such as haemorrhage and pneumothorax may occur. Routinely processed tissue is sectioned at multiple levels and selected sections are stained with haematoxylin–eosin (H&E). Additional stains for connective tissue (e.g. elastic Van Gieson) and for fungi and *Pneumocystis carinii* (e.g. Grocott's silver methenamine) should be done. Interpretation should take account of the adequacy of the specimen, artefacts of biopsy and 'incidental' pathological abnormalities. Open lung biopsies may be submitted for evaluation in ill patients in whom other investigations have failed to yield a diagnosis [4].

Cytology

Cytological specimens such as bronchoalveolar lavage (BAL) and pleural fluid are routinely submitted for an infection screen. Cytological examination of BAL may supplement TBBx in the diagnosis of rejection and some infections but on its own is not sufficiently reliable [5]. It may, however, have a role to play in monitoring graft function [6]. Cytospin preparations should be stained with the H&E or Papanicolaou stains and with a May–Gruenwald–Giemsa stain. Sufficient unstained preparations should be made in case further tests for infections or cell phenotyping are required.

Table 23.1. Common complications of lung transplantation relevant to the pathologist

Immediate (<2 days)
Immediate graft failure
Reimplantation injury
Hyperacute rejection
Haemorrhage and other surgical complications

Postoperative (<30 days)
Infection
Multiorgan failure
Acute rejection

Early (1–6 months)
Infection
Acute rejection
Drug toxicity (NB nephrotoxicity)
Lymphoproliferative disorder
Graft-versus-host disease

Late (>6 months)
Infection
Obliterative bronchiolitis
Drug toxicity (NB nephrotoxicity)
Acute rejection
Neoplasia (including lymphoproliferative disorder)
Disease recurrence in the graft

Other specimens

Other specimens may include bronchial biopsies for the diagnosis of mass lesions in the larger airways, located either distal to the airway anastomosis or at the anastomosis itself; endomyocardial biopsies to exclude the rare complication in heart–lung recipients of acute cardiac allograft rejection [7]; lymph node or other biopsies for tumours such as post-transplantation lymphoproliferative disease and for infections; skin biopsies for graft-versus-host disease, drug-related rash, infections or neoplasia; biopsy of viscus such as stomach or colon for viral infections or neoplasia, and of other sites such as kidney and liver as clinically indicated. All may require further investigation and specialist reporting depending on the nature of the pathological findings.

Autopsies

Clinical governance in the UK now recommends that all deaths in hospital should be audited. Experience at our institute has shown that autopsy examination in lung transplantation may yield much information of value for the family of the deceased and for clinicians about graft failure and other complications. Consent from the next of kin is required for comprehensive sampling of all organs and tissues and for retention of organs as appropriate. Appropriate sampling of tissue for microbiological investigations should also be done. It is helpful to know the donor details, including the cause of death and serological status for evidence of cytomegalovirus (CMV) and *Toxoplasma gondii* infection. The type of transplant, graft ischaemic time, complications, circumstances surrounding death and specific clinical points to be clarified should also be noted.

Perioperative lung allograft pathology

The International Society of Heart–Lung Transplantation (ISHLT) reports a 30 day mortality for lung transplantation overall of 17% [8]. The main causes of death include haemorrhage, early graft failure and infection, with previous cardiac or thoracic surgery, pretransplantation intubation and pulmonary infections being major risk factors.

Transbronchial biopsy (TBBx) of the recently implanted lung may show a number of minor morphological changes, referred to as reimplantation injury [9,10]. They include perivascular and peribronchial oedema, lymphatic dilatation and the intra-alveolar accumulation of proteinaceous fluid, macrophages and scanty clusters of neutrophils. Contributory factors include preimplantation injury of the donor lung, surgical trauma, ischaemia, denervation and interruption of lymphatic drainage. Light microscopic and ultrastructural features consistent with alveolar proteinosis have recently been described [11], and are thought to result from impaired function of alveolar macrophages due to repeated alveolar injury and drug-induced immunosuppression. An unusual neutrophil-rich histological pattern of mixed interstitial pneumonitis was reported by McDonald et al. [12], who considered it to be a novel response to acute allograft injury. It should be differentiated from hyperacute lung allograft rejection (see below). Diffuse alveolar damage may occur as part of the reimplantation response, rejection, and infection and for no obvious cause [9] (Figure 23.1), and may progress to parenchymal fibrosis [13]. Its occurrence in biopsies has been associated with a significantly reduced survival at one year [14]. Acute bronchitis and bronchiolitis may indicate secondary airway infection in severe reimplantation injury [15].

Lung allograft rejection

Lung allograft rejection is classified as hyperacute, acute and chronic, and affects the vasculature and the airways. The recipient's immune system recognizes class I and class II major histocompatibility (MHC) and other, as yet incompletely characterized, antigens in the tissue of the

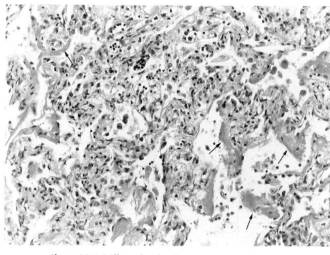

Figure 23.1 Diffuse alveolar damage in a lung biopsy due to severe reimplantation injury one week following transplantation. Note hyaline membranes (arrows) and thickened septae due to oedema and inflammation. (Haematoxylin–eosin (H&E), original magnification 110×.)

donor organs [16]. The resulting rejection process may involve humoral/antibody-mediated and cell-mediated immune mechanisms but the extent to which each contributes to the development of rejection varies in that hyperacute rejection is antibody-mediated whereas acute rejection is regarded as predominantly a cell-mediated process (see Chapter 17).

Hyperacute lung allograft rejection

Hyperacute rejection is a clinicopathological entity requiring the appropriate clinical, serological, histological and immunofluorescence findings to confirm the diagnosis. It has only recently been described in the lung [17–19]. It occurs within 24 to 48 hours of graft implantation and should be suspected if the lungs become markedly congested and oedematous, with the production of copious frothy bloodstained sputum from the bronchial orifice of the allograft. Microscopy shows marked pulmonary oedema, intra-alveolar haemorrhage, vascular platelet/fibrin thrombi, capillary engorgement and interstitial infiltration by neutrophils, and endothelial and epithelial damage (Figure 23.2). The diagnosis is confirmed histologically by the detection, using immunofluorescence, of immunoglobulin (Ig) G deposition on endothelium, along vessel walls and in alveolar spaces, and immunologically by a strongly positive IgG-mediated lymphocytotoxic cross-match to donor T and/or B lymphocytes. If the patient survives, diffuse alveolar damage may develop.

Hyperacute rejection may occur against a clinical background of previous multiple transfusions, pregnancy,

surgery or a previous transplant. Pretransplant screening of potential recipients for panel-reactive lymphocytotoxic antibody (PRA) status against a wide range of class I and class II human leukocyte antigens (HLA) should identify those in a whom a donor-specific T- and B-lymphocytotoxic antibody cross-match is required prior to transplantation [20,21], as there is a significant risk not only of hyperacute rejection but also of later, accelerated graft loss [20]. A positive cross-match is a contraindication to transplantation with organs from that donor.

Pulmonary capillaritis and alveolar haemorrhage similar to that seen in hyperacute rejection has recently been described in five patients between three weeks and several months after transplantation [22]. Although two patients died, treatment with plasmapheresis, augmentation of immunosuppression and, in one instance of clinical recurrence, total lymphoid irradiation was effective in the remaining three patients, two of whom later developed acute rejection, which was successfully treated. Although a humoral component was not documented, the possibility that this represented a form of humoral/vascular rejection akin to that described in cardiac allograft recipients requires further investigation.

Diagnosis and grading of acute and chronic lung allograft rejection – the ISHLT Working Formulation

In 1990 Yousem et al. [23] published a Working Formulation for the biopsy diagnosis and grading of lung allograft rejection under the aegis of the ISHLT (Table 23.2). It was subsequently revised in 1996 [24] and has proved to be easy to use, reliable and reproducible as a means of monitoring the graft. It is now in use in lung transplant centres worldwide.

The utility of the ISHLT Working Formulation hinges on the adequacy of lung tissue taken at transbronchial biopsy. In the early days of lung transplantation, the number of specimens ranged from three pieces from one lobe of lung in some centres [25] to as many as 17 pieces from both lungs in others [26]. With experience, it is now recommended that five pieces of alveolated lung parenchyma is considered as adequate, and that to achieve this more than five pieces of lung may need to be taken in order to minimize the risk of sampling error. If fewer than five pieces are taken or are adequate, the report should state that the biopsy findings might not be fully representative of significant allograft pathology. The laboratory handling of the biopsies has already been described [24]. It is important to note that the differential diagnosis includes rejection and infection, and that both may be present in the lung contemporaneously and show overlapping histological features. Therefore final interpretation of the biopsy findings should always be in

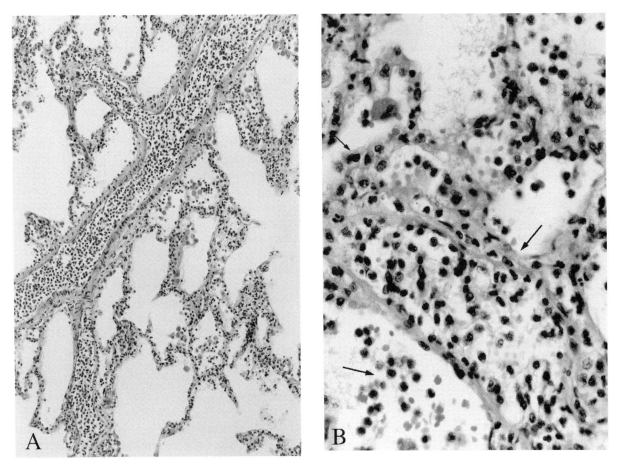

Figure 23.2 Hyperacute lung allograft rejection in the autopsied lung allograft of a patient who died intraoperatively: (A) there is marked engorgement of arterial, capillary and venous blood vessels by neutrophils; (B) neutrophils are seen in capillaries, interstitium and alveoli (arrows), with focal desquamation of hyperplastic alveolar epithelial cells (short arrow). The panel reactive lymphocytotoxic antibody was positive (80%) and the donor-specific lymphocytotoxic cross-match was strongly positive for T and B lymphocytes. ((A) H&E 150×; (B) H&E 300×.)

the light of the clinical and radiological findings, previous biopsy findings and the results of current microbiological and serological investigations, including microscopy and culture of the BAL fluid. It is recommended that acute rejection should be diagnosed and graded *only* in the absence of infection [24].

While acute rejection tends to occur early in the recipient's postoperative course, and chronic rejection is rarely seen before six months, the pathological features probably form a continuum, often with temporal overlap. The features have been allocated to four grades [24]. The cellular infiltrate of acute rejection involving lung parenchyma (grade A) is graded separately from that involving airways (grade B), as similar airway infiltrates may also occur in the presence of chronic infection, ischaemia, aspiration and obliterative bronchiolitis (13,15,27–29). None the less, the presence of an airway infiltrate is worth noting as, in the absence of infection, it may be a harbinger of

chronic rejection. Chronic allograft rejection is defined as dense hyaline fibrous scarring of submucosa of the smaller airways (grade C). It may also involve intima of vessels (grade D). While the fibroproliferative process of chronic airway rejection is often missed on biopsy because of its random distribution, its identification in biopsies is the key discriminator between acute and chronic rejection [24].

Acute allograft rejection

Acute allograft rejection involving lung parenchyma (grade A)

The biopsy diagnosis and grading of acute allograft rejection is based exclusively on the presence of perivascular and interstitial mononuclear cell infiltrates in lung parenchyma *in the absence of infection*. The infiltrates tend to be sparse, patchy and confined to the perivascular

Table 23.2. Revised ISHLT Working Formulation for classification and grading of lung allograft rejection

Grade A: Acute rejection

Grade 0   No rejection
Grade 1   Minimal acute rejection
Grade 2   Mild acute rejection   } with/without grade B
Grade 3   Moderate acute rejection
Grade 4   Severe acute rejection

Grade B[a]: Airway inflammation – lymphocytic bronchitis/bronchiolitis

Grade 0   No airway inflammation
Grade 1   Minimal airway inflammation
Grade 2   Mild airway inflammation
Grade 3   Moderate airway inflammation
Grade 4   Severe airway inflammation
Grade BX   Ungradable (sampling problems, infection, tangential sectioning)

Grade C: Chronic airway rejection – bronchiolitis obliterans
(a) Active
(b) Inactive

Grade D: Chronic vascular rejection – accelerated graft vascular sclerosis

[a] Pathologist may choose to grade airway inflammation.
Source: From ref. 24.

adventitia in early acute rejection, becoming more intense and diffuse as rejection progresses. In the early stages it comprises small lymphoid cells with sparse plasma cells. In higher grades of rejection the infiltrates include medium and large lymphoid cells, plasma cells, eosinophils, mast cells, macrophages and, occasionally, neutrophils, the proportion of large lymphoid cells and eosinophils increasing as rejection progresses in severity. The endothelium is infiltrated by lymphoid cells ('endothelialitis') and shows hyperplasia.

Immunohistochemical studies show that the majority of the lymphoid cells express CD3 and hence are of T-cell origin. There is inversion of the normal CD4/CD8 ratio, with predominance of CD8 positive cells regardless of the grade of rejection [30]. The activated lymphoid cells are often pyroninophilic and may express the lymphocyte activation antigen CD30 and the proliferation antigen Ki-67. B lymphocytes are usually sparse; their presence in significant numbers in acute rejection early after transplantation may predict nonresponsiveness to increased immunosuppression, possibly the result of humoral/antibody-mediated rejection [31]. Eosinophils may predominate in moderate to severe acute rejection, in association with peripheral blood and BAL

eosinophilia [32]. However, their presence in significant numbers, especially late after rejection, should prompt investigations to exclude other entities such as chronic eosinophilic pneumonia and fungal infections. Both vascular and alveolar epithelium show upregulation of HLA class II (HLA-DR) antigens in acute rejection [16]. Some of these findings are illustrated in Figure 23.3.

Figure 23.4 illustrates the different grades of acute rejection. In minimal acute rejection (grade A1), the infiltrates are not obvious at low magnification, comprising one or two perivascular layers of small lymphocytes with occasional plasma cells and macrophages. In mild acute rejection (grade A2), the infiltrate increases in intensity but is still confined to the perivascular space and is obvious at low magnification. It now includes activated medium and large lymphoid cells, and endothelialitis is easily seen (Figure 23.3A). In moderate acute rejection (grade A3) the infiltrate spills over into the alveolar septae and spaces. Large lymphoid cells now predominate and there are eosinophils, macrophages and, occasionally, neutrophils. In severe acute rejection (grade A4), the alveolar epithelium undergoes necrosis, with the development of diffuse alveolar damage, including hyaline membrane formation and intrapulmonary haemorrhage. At this stage residual perivascular lymphoid infiltrates may be the only clue to acute rejection as the underlying cause. Follow-up biopsies after successful treatment of acute rejection tend to show reduction or resolution of the infiltrate. They should be graded as 'resolving rejection/lower grade' or 'resolved rejection/grade A0', respectively.

Acute allograft rejection involving airways (grade B)
Involvement of small airways – lymphocytic bronchitis/bronchiolitis – in the acute rejection process is held to be a harbinger of chronic rejection. The changes range from sparse airway cuffing by small lymphoid cells, to diffuse infiltration of lamina propria and epithelium by medium and large lymphoid cells (Figure 23.5) with epithelial apoptosis, to dense lymphoid cell infiltration, epithelial ulceration and fibrinopurulent exudation. The pathologist should note the presence or absence of airways in the biopsy specimen and, when present, if there is airway inflammation (grade B). The infiltrate may be graded at the pathologist's discretion. Airways changes cannot be graded if there are sampling problems, infection or tangential sectioning. The significance of isolated bronchitis in the absence of infection and acute rejection remains uncertain but could be the result of subclinical infections, smoking-related chronic bronchitis, aspiration [27,29] and chronic rejection.

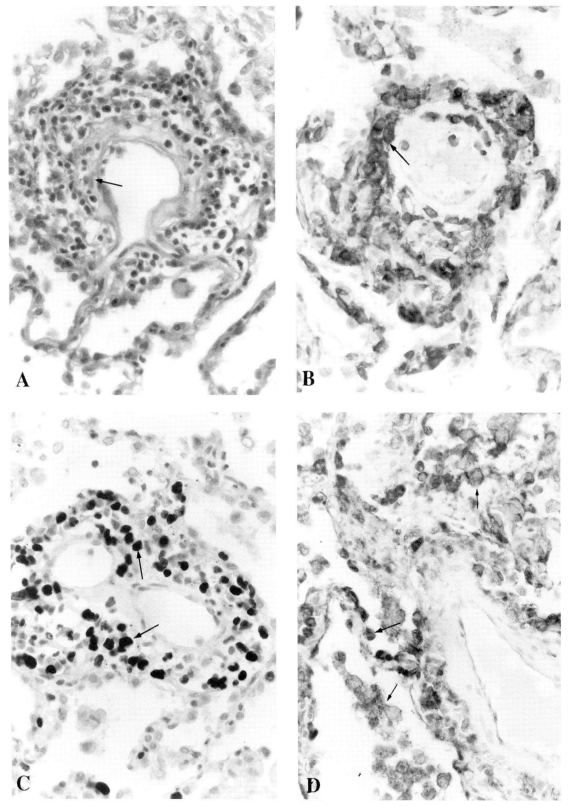

Figure 23.3 Immunohistology of acute lung allograft rejection: (A) perivascular cuffing by lymphoid cells, with focal endothelialitis (arrow); using IHC the lymphoid cells express (B) the pan T-lymphocyte marker CD3 (arrow) and (C) the proliferation marker Kiel-67 (arrow); (D) HLA class II antigens are strongly expressed by alveolar epithelium (arrow) and macrophages (short arrows). ((A) H&E 280×; (B), (C), (D) streptavidin-biotin (SAB)/diaminobenzidine (DAB), monoclonal antibodies (MAbs) to CD3, Kiel-67 and HLA-DR, respectively (Dako Ltd), all 280×.)

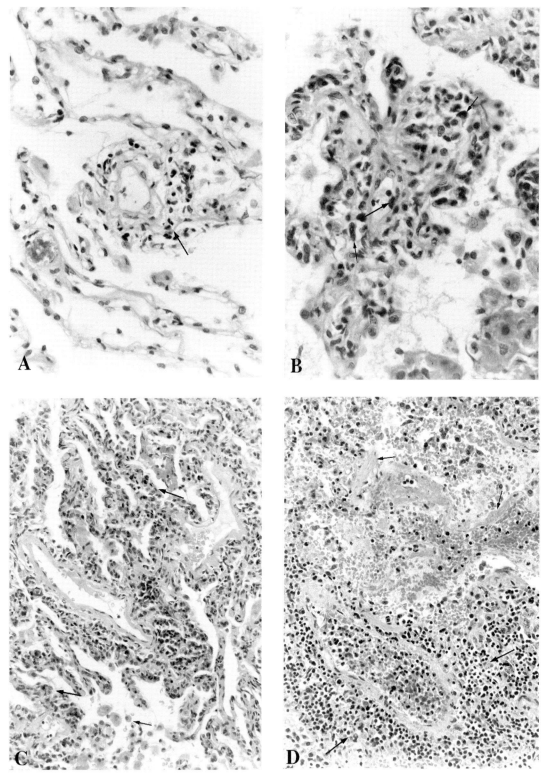

Figure 23.4 The ISHLT biopsy grading of acute lung allograft rejection: (A) minimal acute rejection (grade A1) showing a sparse perivascular infiltrate of lymphoid cells (arrow); surrounding lung is normal; (B) mild acute rejection (grade A2) with several layers of lymphoid cells cuffing a vessel. There is focal endothelialitis (arrow) and large lymphoid cells are seen in the infiltrate (short arrows). (C) and (D): low power (LP) views showing (C) the pattern of moderate acute rejection (grade A3), with spread of the infiltrate into interstitium of surrounding alveolar septae (arrows), and small clusters of macrophages in alveoli (short arrow); (D) severe acute rejection (grade A4) in an autopsied lung, resulting in diffuse alveolar damage with perivascular and interstitial lymphoid cell infiltration (confirmed on IHC as T cells) (arrows), parenchymal haemorrhage and hyaline membranes (short arrows). ((A), (B) H&E 280×; (C), (D) H&E 140×.)

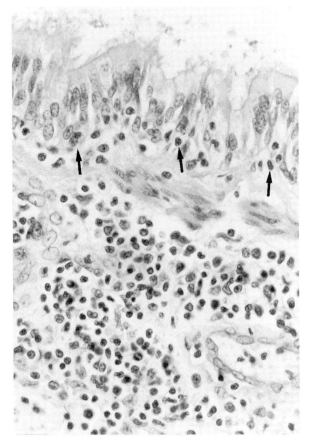

Figure 23.5 Early lymphocytic bronchiolitis (ISHLT grade B1): occasional small lymphocytes infiltrate into bronchiolar epithelium (arrows) and there is a dense lymphoplasmacytic infiltrate in underlying lamina propria. (H&E 150×.)

Chronic lung allograft rejection

Chronic lung allograft dysfunction is associated with the development of obliterative bronchiolitis (OB), which affects the membranous and respiratory bronchioles and is associated with obstructive lung disease. Acute rejection early after transplantation is a major risk factor for the development of OB [33,34], which, in this context, has an immunological basis and is analogous to that occurring in other clinical situations, for example connective tissue diseases, drug toxicity and following bone marrow transplantation [35]. Other causes such as CMV pneumonitis [33,36], ischaemia and denervation may contribute. Recently, Norgaard et al. [37] have shown that bronchial artery revascularization at the time of transplantation – originally devised at our institute by Daly et al. [38] to improve airway healing – may delay the onset of OB.

Chronic airway rejection (grade C)

The pathological diagnosis of chronic airway rejection – OB – refers to dense eosinophilic hyaline fibrous plaques in the bronchiolar submucosa that encroach on the airway lumen to produce partial, and eventually total, occlusion (Figure 23.6). It is associated with an obstructive pattern of respiratory function tests, specifically, reduction in forced expiratory volume in 1 s (FEV_1). Residual bronchiolar epithelium may show squamous metaplasia. The fibrous plaques may be concentric or eccentric, and cause fragmentation and destruction of the smooth muscle wall, with extension into nearby interstitium. The process may be active (i.e. associated with ongoing lymphocytic bronchiolitis) or inactive (i.e. dense fibrous scarring with minimal or no inflammation). The infiltrating cells are of T-lymphocytic origin [39]. Adjacent lung may be normal, show focal obstructive pneumonitis distal to the occluded bronchiole or show concomitant acute rejection (Figure 23.7). The presence of chronic inflammation in the absence of infection implies that there may have been previous airway rejection (grade B) that has progressed to OB [28]. Concomitant acute airway inflammation suggests postobstructive infection [15]. The significance of fibrosis in the larger airways is unknown and is currently regarded as nonspecific.

Bronchiolitis obliterans syndrome

OB is randomly distributed throughout the lungs and hence may be missed in transbronchial and even in open lung biopsies. Conversely, its presence in biopsies may not always correlate with clinical graft function. Hence in 1993 a Working Formulation was agreed (and subsequently updated in 2001), under the aegis of the ISHLT, for the definition and clinical staging of chronic lung allograft dysfunction [40a,b]. The outcome was the bronchiolitis obliterans syndrome (BOS), which is defined as graft deterioration due to progressive airways disease for which there is no other cause. Its diagnosis and staging is based on serial evaluation of lung function using the FEV_1 as the most reliable and consistent indicator of lung function. It is recognized that causes other than chronic rejection can affect the FEV_1 and that the role of the transbronchial lung biopsy is to exclude treatable causes of deterioration in lung function rather than to confirm the diagnosis of OB (see Chapter 19).

Chronic allograft vasculopathy (grade D)

Chronic allograft vasculopathy – accelerated graft vascular disease – refers to fibrointimal thickening of arteries and veins analogous to that occurring in the coronary arteries

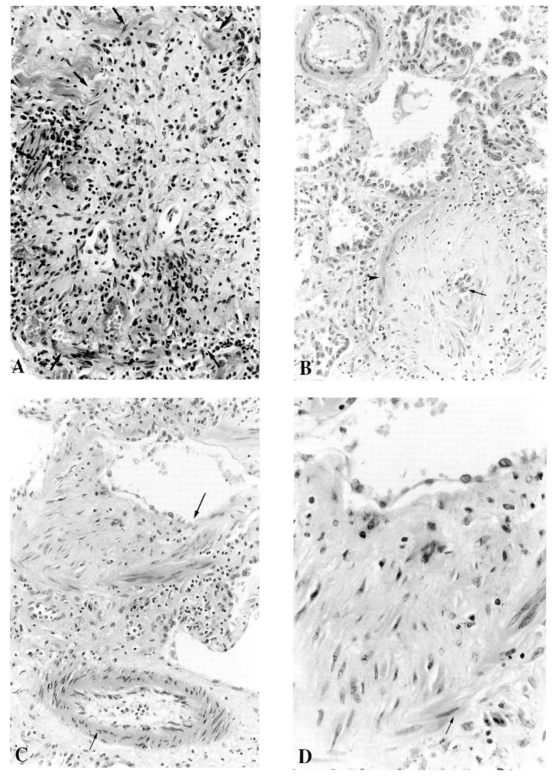

Figure 23.6 Chronic airway rejection (obliterative bronchiolitis, ISHLT grade C) in an explanted allografted lung: (A) active obliterative bronchiolitis, with lymphoplasmacytic infiltration of a totally occluded bronchiole (outlined by arrows); (B) a bronchiole almost totally obliterated by constricting intramural fibrosis, with a tiny central lumen (arrow); note residual muscle fibres at the outer rim of the bronchiole (arrowhead), the normal vessel and intervening lung with alveolar cell hyperplasia; (C) subtotal occlusion of a bronchiole by plaque-like fibrosis of lamina propria (arrow), contrasting with the normal artery nearby (short arrow); note the adjacent normal lung. (D) the fibrous plaque expands the lamina propria, splitting and infiltrating residual bronchiolar smooth muscle (arrow) and leading to flattening of the overlying epithelium. ((A) H&E 140×; (B) H&E 70×; (C) H&E 70×; (D) H&E 280×.)

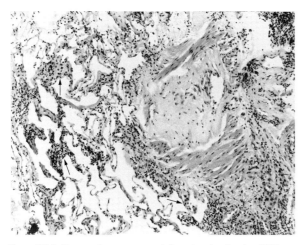

Figure 23.7 Concomitant acute and chronic rejection in a TBBx: obliterative bronchiolitis (centre) with evidence of acute rejection in surrounding lung and in adventitia of bronchiole (arrows). (H&E 65×.)

of heart and heart–lung allografts. It may be active or inactive (Figure 23.8). While it may be seen in association with OB – which dominates the clinical picture – its appearance in biopsies is regarded as nonspecific as it may also follow ischaemic damage during preservation, healed acute rejection, nonrejection-related pulmonary inflammation or donor-related factors. It may also be associated with accelerated graft coronary artery disease in heart–lung allografts [41,42].

Cryptogenic organizing pneumonia

Parenchymal fibrosis often accompanies end-stage obliterative bronchiolitis and is regarded by many as a host response to infection, aspiration, severe reimplantation injury and ischaemia [13,43] (Figure 23.9). However, histological findings akin to the steroid-responsive condition cryptogenic organizing pneumonia (COP)/bronchiolitis obliterans-organizing pneumonia (BOOP) may be seen in TBBx in the absence of infection or aspiration and in association with graft dysfunction [44,45]. The pattern of intraluminal buds of fibrous tissue in bronchioles and alveoli ('Masson buds') in this condition (Figure 23.10) is in contrast to the plaque-like intramural fibrosis illustrated above (Figure 23.6), which gradually obliterates the lumen of the bronchiole in transplant-associated OB, sparing the lung. COP/BOOP developing in the first year is said to be a risk factor for the subsequent development of OB, especially when it coexists with acute rejection [44,46]. It has been suggested that COP/BOOP should be acknowledged within

the Working Formulation [44]. However, this view has been challenged by other workers who regard COP/BOOP-like changes as a nonspecific tissue response in association with coexistent pathology such as infection, aspiration and diffuse alveolar damage [43,47], and which may coexist with OB typical for BOS [43]. A significant increase in the incidence of subsequent BOS has not been detected in those patients in whom COP/BOOP-like changes have been detected as compared with those patients in whom they were absent [47].

Pitfalls in the histological diagnosis of lung allograft rejection

Differential diagnosis of parenchymal and airway lymphoid infiltrates

Although perivascular lymphoid cell infiltration is the hallmark of acute rejection, similar infiltrates may be seen in patients with infections and other conditions for which augmented immunosuppression is inappropriate. The infections include CMV pneumonitis [48], *P. carinii* pneumonia [49] and chronic fungal and bacterial pneumonias [10,25]. Recent biopsy site scars, reimplantation injury, post-transplantation lymphoproliferative disorders and recurrence in the allograft of diseases such as sarcoidosis and Langerhans cell histiocytosis [2] may also be misinterpreted as acute rejection. The differential diagnosis of lymphocytic bronchiolitis includes transplanted bronchus-associated lymphoid tissue of donor origin, low grade infections of viral, mycoplasmal, fungal, bacterial or chlamydial origin and the consequences of aspiration [28,50]. Further tests on the biopsy and careful correlation with the clinical history, radiology, microbiology and serology should minimize the risk of misdiagnosis.

Concomitant rejection and infection

Airway and parenchymal infection, notably CMV (Figure 23.11), may be present in the biopsy simultaneously with acute rejection [10,25]. In such cases, rejection should not be graded [24]. The pathologist may be able to favour one diagnosis over the other but further tests on the biopsy, such as IHC for CMV or *P. carinii*, and the results of microbiology and serological investigations, such as measurement of peripheral blood CMV pp65 antigen, may be required to resolve the differential diagnosis [51]. A repeat biopsy should be done to evaluate the grade of acute rejection once the infection has been treated [24].

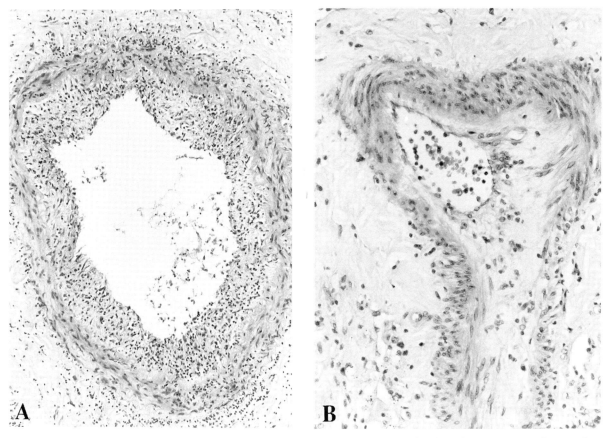

Figure 23.8 Chronic lung allograft vasculopathy (ISHLT grade D) in an explanted allograft: (A) florid lymphocytic intimitis of a muscular pulmonary artery; (B) intimal sclerosis involving a venule, with associated mild lymphocytic intimitis. ((A) H&E 70×; (B) H&E 140×.)

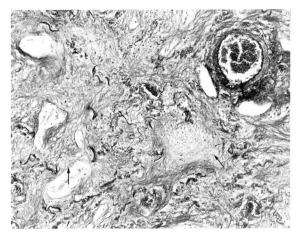

Figure 23.9 Organizing pneumonia in an autopsied lung: extensive intra-alveolar fibrosis, often seen following infections, aspiration and previous diffuse alveolar damage. The intact artery (thick arrow) contrasts with extensive intra-alveolar fibrosis ('Masson buds') (thin arrows). (H&E 65×.)

Histological and cytological monitoring of lung allografts

Over the last decade many studies have demonstrated that monitoring of the lung allograft for rejection and infection by TBBx is safe and reliable, provided recommendations about adequacy and appropriate tissue handling are met [24]. Surveillance TBBx may also yield information predictive for the development of OB, notably subclinical acute rejection, the aggressive treatment of which may delay the onset and progression of BOS [52–54] (see Figure 23.7). Clinically indicated biopsies may be triggered by clinical symptoms, abnormal radiology or an acute reduction in lung function studies, notably the FEV$_1$, and should form part of a range of investigations such as screening of BAL fluid for infections and of peripheral blood for CMV pp65 antigen. The main limitations of TBBx are the lack of specificity of the mononuclear infiltrate and the presence of concomitant pathologies such as infection, thus widening the differential diagnosis beyond that of rejection alone.

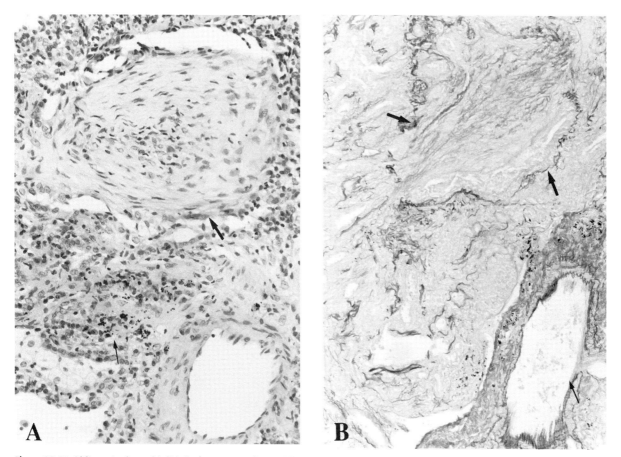

Figure 23.10 Obliterative bronchiolitis in the context of organizing pneumonia (BOOP-like reaction) in an explanted allograft: (A) intraluminal fibrosis of a bronchiole (thick arrow) with extensive interstitial inflammation in adjacent alveolar septae (thin arrow); (B) an elastic Van Gieson stain for fibrous tissue shows the outline of the bronchiole (thick arrows), which is plugged with fibrous tissue, in contrast to the normal artery nearby (thin arrow). ((A) H&E 160×; (B) elastic Van Gieson (EVG) 80×.)

A high diagnostic yield is often obtained from clinically indicated biopsies [29,55]. However, the sensitivity and specificity of TBBx is often diagnosis dependent. Pomerance et al. [25] found a specificity (clinical agreement with TBBx diagnosis) of 93% and a sensitivity (clinical rejection confirmed by TBBx) of 61% for the procedure for the diagnosis of acute rejection when three pieces from one lobe were subjected for analysis. Sensitivity increased to 77% if unsatisfactory specimens were excluded. When the number of biopsies increased to 17, taken from three lobes, Scott et al. [26] found that specificity and sensitivity increased to 90% and 94%. Sensitivity and specificity for infections (excluding fungal infection) were also high at 83.5% and 91% for CMV and 88% and 100% for *P. carinii* infection [25]. However, sensitivity for OB was poor (25%) [25], although specificity was 75%, confirming other authors' findings of 18% and 85%, respectively [56]. Increasing the number of biopsies increased the sensitivity of the

procedure to 71% [53]. This is not surprising as OB is a patchy focal process, resulting in sampling error, which should decrease the greater the number of biopsies taken [57]. Many studies also confirmed the lack of specificity of the lymphoid infiltrates, which were seen frequently in patients with proven infection and which often resolved with treatment for infection alone [10]. When TBBx suggested both rejection and infection without favouring either, specificity (clinical agreement with TBBx diagnosis) for concomitant infection and rejection was 66%, but where one was favoured over the other the clinical impression was almost always rejection [25].

Many studies have confirmed that serial TBBx and BAL, as dictated by lung function studies and clinical status, facilitate early diagnosis and treatment of rejection and infection [10,55,58,59]. Surveillance biopsies may reveal subclinical minimal (grade A1) or mild (grade A2) acute rejection [10,55,59], which may resolve spontaneously or

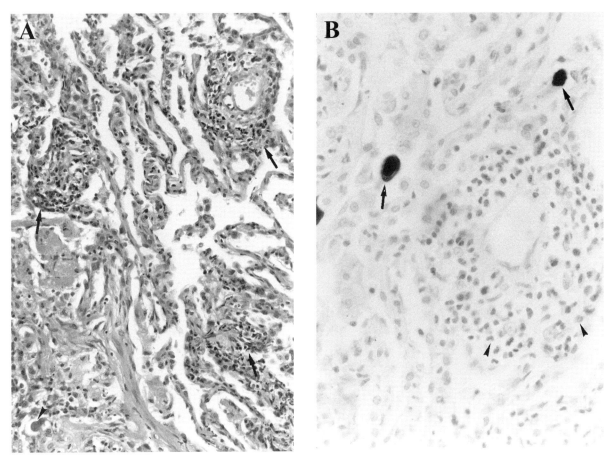

Figure 23.11 Acute rejection and coexisting CMV infection in a follow-up TBBx from a patient recently treated for CMV pneumonitis; chest radiograph shadowing and FEV₁ had worsened despite treatment with ganciclovir and return of peripheral blood CMV pp65 antigen level to zero; note (A) perivascular and interstitial lymphocytic infiltration suggestive of acute rejection (arrows), with a CMV inclusion noted on the H&E stain (arrowhead); (B) IHC for CMV early antigen confirmed several inclusions (arrows) adjacent to a vessel with a pronounced perivascular infiltrate (arrowheads). The patient improved after treatment with high dose corticosteroids, the peripheral blood CMV antigen levels remaining at zero. ((A) H&E 70×; (B) SAB/DAB, MAb to CMV CCH2 (delayed early antigen p52), 70×.)

progress to a higher grade of rejection, necessitating treatment. Histological abnormalities in follow-up biopsies after treatment may include reduction in the infiltrate of rejection [60], persistence of acute rejection despite treatment or the development of opportunistic infections such as CMV pneumonitis. Prompt treatment of both is important, as they are risk factors for the development of later OB [33,34,36]. Lymphocytic bronchiolitis may also be predictive for OB [53], as may the presence of mast cells [61].

BAL is pivotal to the diagnosis and management of most infections occurring in lung transplant recipients. However, its role in the diagnosis of acute rejection and in differentiating between rejection and infection is less clear. In studies correlating differential cell counts in BAL fluid with TBBx as the 'gold standard', eosinophils, basophils, lymphocytes and neutrophils were all increased in rejection [5] as well as infection [62–64]. Eosinophils, basophils and

lymphocytes were all increased in acute rejection in the first postoperative month with a specificity of 77% and sensitivity of 64% [64]. Lymphocytes, mainly of CD8+ (T-cell suppressor) phenotype predominated in acute rejection, and neutrophils in infection, although no clear distinction could be made between the two groups owing to the considerable overlap in differential cell counts and lymphocyte phenotype [62]. High BAL lymphocyte counts are supportive, only, of acute rejection and supplement TBBx in reaching a definitive diagnosis.

However, BAL cell counts may have a role to play in predicting the development of OB. Follow-up biopsies after treatment of acute rejection showed that total inflammatory cell and lymphocyte counts remained raised albeit at a level lower than in acute rejection [62], suggestive of continuing subclinical immunological injury and perhaps the cytological correlate of the biopsy finding of lymphocytic bronchiolitis. Prospective studies in patients who subsequently developed OB may show: elevated eosinophil counts and interleukin 6 (IL-6) levels as compared with those who remained free from OB [65]; airway neutrophilia, which may predict for the later development of OB [6,66]; and increased BAL fluid levels of cytotoxic eosinophil cationic protein, IL-6, IL-8 and myeloperoxidase [6,66]. Airway neutrophilia has also been shown to correlate with exhaled nitric oxide (NO) and expression of inducible nitric oxide synthase (iNOS) in bronchial epithelium of stable lung transplant recipients [67]. iNOS has also been demonstrated in the damaged epithelium of OB and in inflammatory cells [68]. This suggests a role for NO in the development of OB by formation, from NO and superoxide, of the oxidant peroxynitrite, detected in tissues as nitrotyrosine and a potential indicator of cellular damage [67,68]. The above findings imply on-going production, even in clinically stable patients, of inflammatory mediators with chemoattractant, cytotoxic and profibrotic properties central to the development of the fibroproliferative response that characterizes OB (see Chapter 19).

BAL examination is a valuable adjunct to diagnosis of lung tumours in transplanted and nonimmunosuppressed individuals. However, it should be noted that the presence of epithelial cell atypia in BAL specimens from lung transplant recipients does not necessarily signify neoplasia, as similar cytological features may be seen in a range of reactive conditions such as diffuse alveolar damage, acute rejection and infections such as CMV pneumonitis [69], which are much more commonly encountered in this group of patients.

Therefore overall sensitivity of TBBx in the diagnosis of acute rejection early after transplantation is good provided specimens are adequate and infection has been excluded [10,25]. BAL supplements, but does not replace, TBBx in reaching a definitive diagnosis of acute rejection [5,62]. Diagnosis of acute rejection in surveillance and clinically indicated biopsies should prompt aggressive treatment because of the risk of progression to later OB [52–54]. Because of its low sensitivity in OB, TBBx in this condition is better directed to excluding other treatable pathology such as subclinical acute rejection and infection such as CMV rather than attempting to confirm the diagnosis of OB. Monitoring of BAL differential cell counts and inflammatory markers may predict the development of subsequent OB.

The heart in combined heart–lung transplantation

The number of combined heart and lung transplantation (HLT) procedures peaked in the late 1980s and started to decrease from 1995 onwards as more single lung and double lung transplantations were done [1], reflecting improved

management of complications related to the airway anastomosis. Monitoring of the heart in HLT using surveillance endomyocardial biopsy (EMBx) has shown a low incidence of acute cardiac allograft rejection such that EMBx is recommended only if clinically indicated [7]. Significant cardiac graft vascular disease may occur in association with pulmonary vascular disease and OB, but the degree of concordance between all three is not absolute [40,41]. A later study of chronic rejection in paediatric HLT recipients found that, although cardiac graft vascular disease in HLT occurred, it is infrequent, the clinical picture in long-term survivors being dominated by BOS [70].

Airway complications in lung and heart–lung allografts

Surgical intervention may be required for airway complications in the lung allograft recipient [71]. Ischaemia due to interruption of the bronchial artery supply may be a contributing factor. Bronchial artery revascularization at the time of transplantation has been shown to reduce the incidence of early complications such as infection and dehiscence of the airway anastomosis [37] (Figure 23.12). Late airway complications include stenosis (Figure 23.13) and bronchomalacia (Figure 23.14), in which weakening of the bronchial wall due to fibrovascular ingrowth into, and destruction of, the normally avascular cartilaginous plate may lead to its collapse [72]. In both conditions, insertion of intraluminal stents may be required to maintain airway patency and reduce the risk of infection.

Acute and chronic airway inflammation may result from nonimmunological causes such as severe reimplantation injury, infection and aspiration [15,27,28]. Scarring and, in some instances, complete airway obliteration may result. Granulation tissue reactions manifest as intrabronchiolar and intra-alveolar plugs of fibromyxoid connective tissue (see Figure 23.10), and may develop following previous infection, rejection and diffuse alveolar damage [13,27] as well as in cryptogenic organizing pneumonia (COP) [44,46].

Bronchiectasis is a feature of advanced BOS, the associated infections often leading to the demise of the patient [8]. Factors contributing to its development and progression include ischaemia due to interruption of the bronchial blood supply at the time of transplantation and denervation of airways leading to loss of the cough reflex, increasing the risk of subclinical aspiration [27]. Subsequent pooling of secretions in a progressively dilating, distally obstructed bronchial tree may lead to recurrent airway infections, with destruction of intramural mucus glands and loss of the mucociliary defence mechanism due to squamous cell metaplasia of airway epithelium.

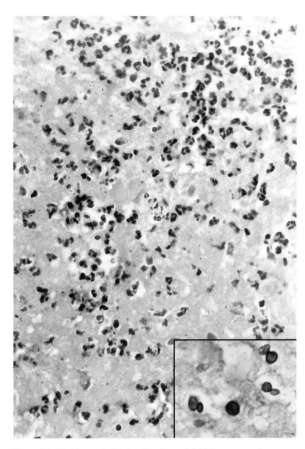

Figure 23.12 Airway infection in a bronchial biopsy: purulent exudate at a bronchiolar anastomosis containing fungal yeasts (inset) typical for infection with *Candida* species, confirmed on culture as *Candida albicans*. (H&E 300×, inset: Grocott's silver methenamine 750×.)

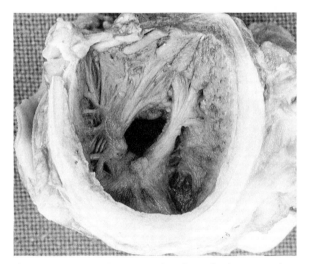

Figure 23.13 Severe airway stenosis at the tracheal anastomosis following heart–lung transplantation (3×.)

Infections in lung and heart–lung allograft recipients

The lung allograft shows increased susceptibility to bacterial and opportunistic infections [73]. Multiple infections are common. Microbiological screening of BAL specimens remains the mainstay of diagnosis as, in many instances, the histopathological features are nonspecific and management depends on precise identification of the causative organism. However, in some infections TBBx in addition to BAL may increase the likelihood of their detection [74].

It is important to remember that, in the context of infection, problems in biopsy interpretation may arise in three areas, namely: differentiation of acute rejection from infections such as CMV and *P. carinii*; differentiation between colonization, subclinical infection and clinically significant disease; and identification of infections with histological patterns that may differ from those observed in the nontransplanted, immune-competent patient [2].

Cytomegalovirus infection

CMV infection may cause significant morbidity and mortality in lung transplant recipients. Primary infection, through blood transfusion or transmitted in the graft, may result in aggressive disease in the graft with systemic spread. Reactivation in a seropositive recipient may cause clinical disease, which is less severe than in the seronegative recipient. Prophylactic regimens reduce the severity of clinical illness regardless of serological status but they also modify the histological pattern of the disease, giving rise to diagnostic problems for the histopathologist [50].

The diagnosis of clinically significant disease is made on biopsy evidence of an appropriate tissue inflammatory reaction and the detection of CMV in the biopsy, using IHC, and of CMV pp65 antigen in peripheral blood by monoclonal antibody staining of peripheral blood leukocytes [75]. Several studies have confirmed the value of this test in the diagnosis and monitoring of CMV infection and disease in heart and lung transplant recipients [52,76,77], with a high sensitivity (100%) and specificity (93.7%), and a positive predictive value for CMV infection of 94.1% [76] (see Chapter 21).

The histological appearances of CMV pneumonitis are those of interstitial pneumonitis and bronchiolitis [78]. In the early stages of infection there is acute interstitial pneumonitis, with alveolar cell hyperplasia (Figure 23.15) and microabscess formation. CMV inclusions are sparse but may be detected using IHC for CMV early antigen. In the later stage of infection, the infiltrate becomes mixed,

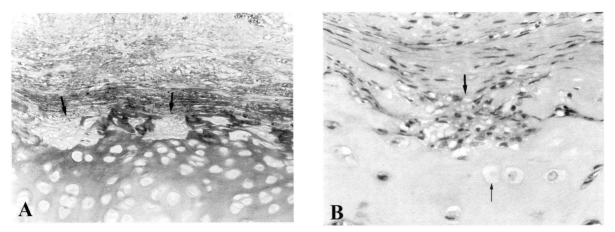

Figure 23.14 Bronchomalacia in a lung allograft explanted because of bronchiectasis: (A) note the irregular outline of the perichondrium around the cartilaginous ring (arrows); (B) there is a fibrovascular reaction at the area of erosion (thick arrow) with focal necrosis of cartilage, demonstrated by lysis of nuclei in lacunae (thin arrow). ((A) EVG 140×; (B) H&E 280×.)

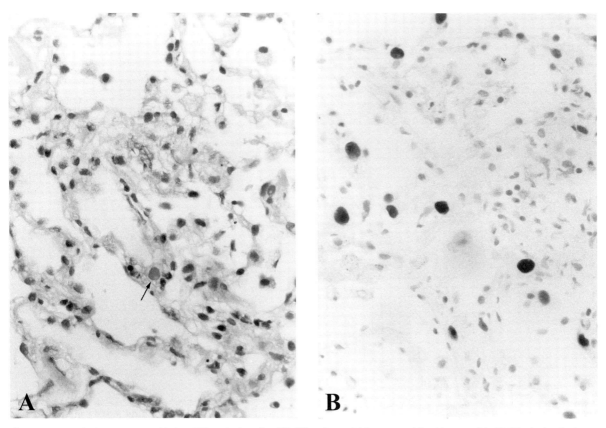

Figure 23.15 Early CMV pneumonitis in a TBBx: (A) there is mild diffuse interstitial pneumonitis with a possible CMV inclusion in the centre of the field (arrow); (B) IHC shows many more CMV inclusions than expected in endothelial and alveolar epithelial cells. ((A) H&E 280×; (B) SAB/DAB, MAb to CMV 280×.)

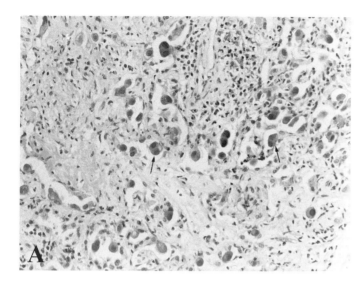

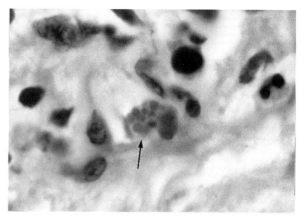

Figure 23.17 Fragmented CMV inclusions (arrow) in a follow-up TBBx of a patient treated for recurrent CMV pneumonitis. (H&E 640×.)

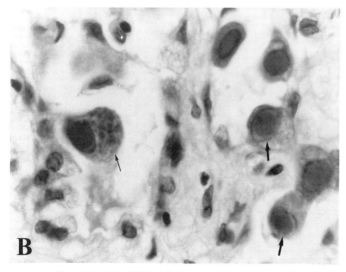

Figure 23.16 Established CMV pneumonitis in a TBBx from a seronegative recipient of a seropositive graft: (A) florid interstitial inflammation and alveolar cell hyperplasia with numerous CMV inclusions (arrows); (B) both intranuclear (thick arrows) and cytoplasmic (thin arrow) viral inclusions were seen. ((A) H&E 120×; (B) H&E 600×.)

showing an increase in macrophages and lymphocytes with numerous intranuclear and cytoplasmic inclusions (Figure 23.16A). Although the characteristic 'owl's-eye' CMV inclusions may be seen in epithelial and endothelial cells along with eosinophilic granular cytoplasmic inclusions (Figure 23.16B), classical inclusions may be sparse early in the disease. The histological picture may be difficult to differentiate from acute rejection, especially if both diseases coexist and inclusions are sparse [49] (see Figure 23.10). Poorly formed granulomas may be seen, raising the

differential diagnosis of infection due to mycobacteria, fungi or *P. carinii*. In severe infection, diffuse alveolar damage may dominate the histological picture. CMV prophylaxis alters the histological picture in the lung in that there is focal acute neutrophilic pneumonitis, which may be detected only on screening of multiple sections. Inclusions in alveolar cells at this stage are often cytoplasmic, fragmented and degenerate without evidence of alveolar cell hyperplasia [50] (Figure 23.17). Again, IHC for CMV early antigen will aid in their detection.

CMV infection is known to be associated with an increased incidence of allograft rejection, possibly through upregulation of MHC class I and class II antigens in alveolar lining cells in the lung allograft [16,79]. Evidence in support of this is the encoding of a protein with homology to MHC class I and class II antigens in experimental CMV infection [80,81]. CMV bronchiolitis may also be a harbinger of OB [33,36,43,78].

Pneumocystis carinii infection

Pneumocystis carinii pneumonia is now rare in lung transplantation owing to chemoprophylaxis. In one survey from our institute [82] it was diagnosed in 14 (0.9%) of 1433 thoracic transplant recipients, most within six months of transplantation and following augmentation of immunosuppression for the treatment of acute rejection. The classical intra-alveolar foamy exudate containing numerous cysts and a mild lymphohistiocytic pneumonitis is rarely encountered, perhaps because immunosuppression in the solid organ transplant recipient is not as profound as in the human immunodeficiency virus (HIV)-positive patient with acquired immune deficiency syndrome (AIDS). The histological patterns observed include a predominantly

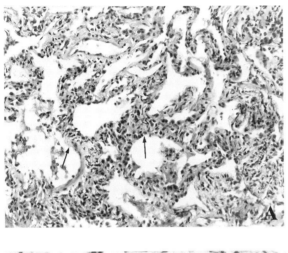

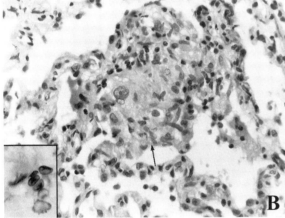

Figure 23.18 Patterns of *Pneumocystis carinii* infection observed in TBBx from lung allografts: (A) a diffuse interstitial pneumonitis-like reaction resembling moderate acute rejection (arrows) (cf. Figure 23.4 C) with virtually no exudate; (B) small interstitial noncaseating granulomas (arrow); only sparse clusters of *P. carinii* cysts (inset) were found. ((A) H&E 200×; (B) H&E 240×; inset: Grocott's silver methenamine 600×.)

lymphoplasmacytic interstitial pneumonitis with scanty exudate, and a granulomatous pneumonitis with virtually no exudates; the cysts of *P. carinii* are sparse (Figure 23.18). When the lymphoplasmacytic pattern is present, the perivascular component resembles acute rejection and differentiation depends on the demonstration of *P. carinii*, hence the mandatory use of silver staining techniques in all transbronchial lung allograft biopsies [49,24] and the routine screening of all BAL specimens using IHC or PCR [83].

Fungal infections

Fungal infections may cause serious morbidity in lung allograft recipients, including colonization of bronchiectatic

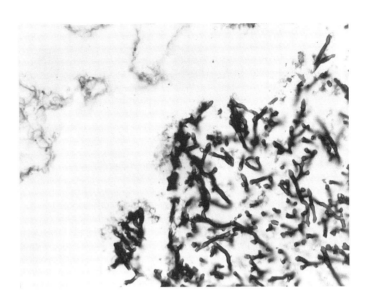

Figure 23.19 Fungal airway infection picked up in a TBBx: clumps of branching septate fungal hyphae (bottom right), confirmed on BAL culture as *Aspergillus fumigatus*. Note that the fungal colony is separate from adjacent normal lung (top left), which shows no evidence of invasive aspergillosis. (Grocott's silver methenamine 280×.)

airways (Figure 23.19), cavitating pneumonia, bronchocentric granulomatosis, invasive infection with mediastinitis, infection of the airway anastomosis with dehiscence (see Figure 23.12) and bloodborne dissemination with multiple organ involvement, including brain abscesses [73]. Fungal infections due to *Candida* and *Aspergillus* species are the main culprits. The histopathological features range from aspergillomas, to suppuration with abscess formation, to granulomatous inflammation, which may be suppurative. The pathologist should always have a high index of suspicion for fungal infection if these patterns of inflammation are seen. Except in aspergillomas, fungal hyphae may be sparse and silver staining techniques may be required for their demonstration.

Toxoplasmosis

Infection of the lung allograft with *T. gondii* is rare, usually occurring in the context of systemic disease in a graft mismatch [84]. From experience in AIDS [85], the pathological changes fall into two groups – interstitial pneumonitis/diffuse alveolar damage and necrotizing bronchopneumonia. Identification of the organism in biopsy material may be difficult as cysts of *T. gondii* are sparse and extracellular tachyzoites may be mistaken for haematoxyphil debris [86]. The diagnosis may be confirmed by IHC on tissue samples or by PCR on tissue, body fluids or peripheral

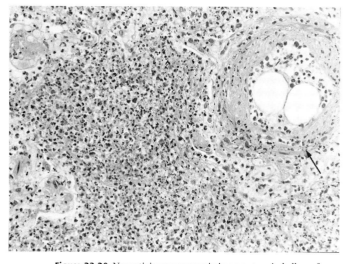

Figure 23.20 Necrotizing pneumonia in an autopsied allograft due to *Legionella pneumoniae*: note the extensive suppurative necrosis of lung parenchyma associated with septic vasculitis (arrow). (H&E 125×.)

blood [87]. Infection with *T. gondii* has largely been eliminated in seronegative solid organ transplant recipients due to prophylaxis with pyrimethamine.

Other infections

Infection due to herpes simplex virus is infrequently encountered but may cause necrotizing tracheobronchitis with pneumonitis, which must be differentiated from CMV and *T. gondii* pneumonitis by its distribution, the nature of the infiltrate, the extent of necrosis and, if necessary, by the use of IHC and molecular techniques [88]. *Mycobacterium tuberculosis* and nontuberculous mycobacterial infections such as *M. kansaii* are rare [89–91] and may originate in the donor or recipient. Atypical mycobacteria may colonize the graft without disease, posing a difficult therapeutic problem. Other infections that may be encountered by the pathologist include nocardiosis, acute necrotizing pneumonia due to Legionnaire's disease (Figure 23.20) and systemic infection due to varicella-zoster and to mucormycosis (Figure 23.21). Hepatitis C virus infection has been diagnosed in a small number of patients, all of whom received transplants in the 1980s prior to the introduction of screening of organ and blood donors for this infection (see Chapter 24).

Graft-versus-host disease

Graft-versus-host disease is rare following solid organ transplantation [92] but has been reported in the lung [93].

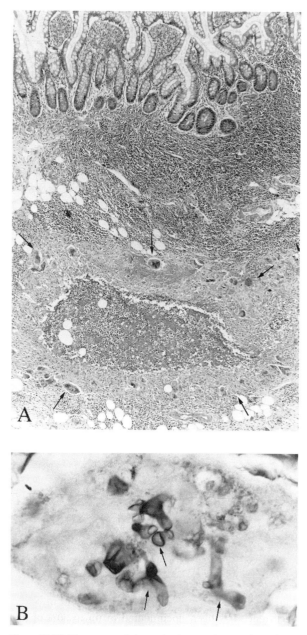

Figure 23.21 Mucormycosis in a colonic resection specimen from a heart–lung transplant recipient: (A) marked expansion of colonic submucosa by an abscess surrounded by many multinucleated giant cells (arrows); (B) the giant cells contain many folded, irregularly branching, broad thick-walled hyphae (arrows) consistent with *Mucorales* (and contrasting with *Aspergillus fumigatus*, illustrated in Figure 23.19). ((A) H&E 35×; (B) Grocott's silver methenamine 660×.)

It is thought to occur because immunocompetent donor mucosa-associated lymphoid tissue reacts to recipient tissue that expresses HLA class I antigens. The clinical features

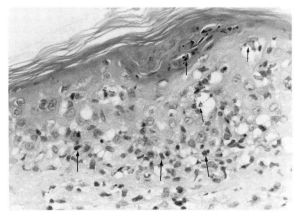

Figure 23.22 Suspected graft-versus-host disease (GVHD) in a biopsy of a skin rash six weeks after heart–lung transplantation: there is vacuolation of the basal epithelium of epidermis, exocytosis of lymphocytes into epidermis (arrows) and scattered shrunken necrotic keratinocytes (short arrows), all features of a lichenoid skin reaction with a differential diagnosis of GVHD or lichenoid drug eruption. The demonstration of chimerism in peripheral blood is proof of GVHD. (H&E 220×.)

and pathological findings resemble that occurring in bone marrow allograft transplantation [94] but are not as severe, perhaps because immunosuppression is not so profound [95]. Biopsy diagnosis is difficult because the histological appearances in skin – the most frequently biopsied site – resemble those of a lichenoid drug reaction (Figure 23.22). The diagnosis is confirmed by demonstrating donor and recipient chimerism on HLA typing of peripheral blood lymphocytes (see Chapter 24).

Disease recurrence in the graft

Lung transplantation may be done for a wide range of primary lung disorders, some of which may be associated with extrapulmonary disease and may recur in the graft. Recurrence has been documented in up to 60% of patients receiving transplants to relieve sarcoidosis [50,96] (Figure 23.23) but does not seem to be associated with clinical deterioration, progression of the disease or an increase in the incidence of acute rejection or BOS. There are anecdotal instances of recurrent Langerhans cell histiocytosis [97,98] (Figure 23.24), one patient showing a good and sustained response to chemotherapy [98]. Instances of recurrent lymphangioleiomyomatosis [99–101] have been reported – one recurrence, in a female recipient of a lung from a male donor, associated with a renal lymphangiomyoma and confirmed to be of donor origin using in situ hybridization for the Y chromosome [99]. Instances of recurrent giant

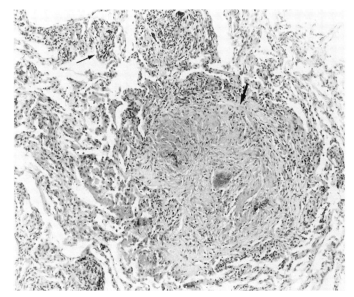

Figure 23.23 Recurrence of sarcoidosis in a TBBx from a double lung transplant recipient: noncaseating granulomas (thick arrow) with a surrounding interstitial lymphoid inflammatory infiltrate (thin arrow), which may be confused with acute rejection. Infection was excluded in this patient prior to augmentation of immunosuppression with corticosteroids. (H&E 65×.)

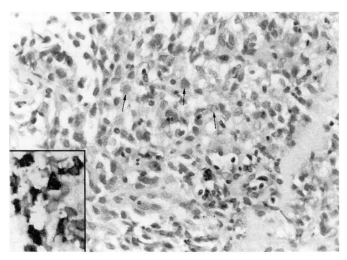

Figure 23.24 Recurrence of Langerhans cell histiocytosis, seen in a TBBx from a double lung transplant recipient: aggregates of Langerhans cells with large folded nuclei, small nucleoli and abundant cytoplasm (arrows), amongst which were scattered eosinophils (not clearly seen in this frame). IHC for S100 (inset) confirmed the diagnosis, with strong cytoplasmic positivity of the Langerhans cells. (H&E 230×; inset: SAB/DAB, Polyclonal Ab to S100, 230×.)

cell interstitial pneumonitis [102] and alveolar proteinosis [103] have also been described.

Problems encountered in biopsy diagnosis of disease recurrence include: the exclusion of infective causes of granulomas in sarcoidosis; the recognition of Langerhans cells in small biopsies and their differentiation from granulomas; the differentiation of both entities from acute rejection when lymphocytes are conspicuous; differentiation of the proliferating smooth muscle that characterizes lymphangioleiomyomatosis from post-transplantation smooth muscle nodules (104) and from tangentially sectioned bronchiolar and bronchial walls; and the evaluation of the potential significance of exudates in recurrent alveolar proteinosis. Immunohistochemical investigation of the biopsy and careful clinical and radiological correlation should minimize the risk of diagnostic error.

Histopathological aspects of immunosuppressive drug toxicity

All immunosuppressive drugs are associated with an increased risk of post-transplantation lymphoproliferative disorder, to be discussed in the next section. The histopathological features of other drug side effects are described here, with special reference to nephrotoxicity and hepatotoxicity.

Nephrotoxicity

Ciclosporin and tacrolimus (previously known as FK506) are associated with significant nephrotoxicity, which is usually dose related and may lead to chronic renal failure, necessitating haemodialysis. Mild renal dysfunction in the absence of morphological abnormalities is common soon after the onset of therapy, whether ciclosporin or tacrolimus is used. There is a slight increase in serum creatinine, which responds to dose reduction. In more severe forms of short-term nephrotoxicity a number of tubular epithelial lesions may occur such as inclusion bodies in epithelial cells of the convoluted portion of the proximal tubules, shown ultrastructurally to be giant mitochondria [105,106]; isometric vacuolation, which mainly involves the straight segments of the proximal tubule [106,107]; and microcalcification. Tubular and myocyte vacuolation may also occur with tacrolimus therapy [106,108].

The morphological lesions of long-term ciclosporin nephrotoxicity are thought to be vascular in origin, resulting from injury to medium-sized arteries, preglomerular arterioles and glomerular capillaries [109]. Ascribing these lesions to ciclosporin may be difficult in the presence of

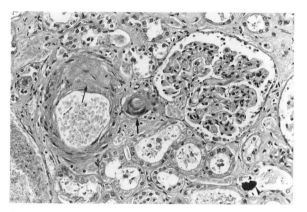

Figure 23.25 Acute tacrolimus-associated vascular nephropathy in an autopsied kidney from a heart transplant recipient who developed the haemolytic-uraemic syndrome: arcuate artery in cortex of kidney shows intimal swelling (thin arrow), with fibrinoid necrosis of an afferent arteriole (thick arrow). The glomerulus in this frame is normal. Calcium deposits are noted in a tubule (arrowhead). (Mallory's trichrome, 110×.)

hypertension (which occurs in up to 50% of patients receiving ciclosporin) and diabetes mellitus, in both of which the vascular changes are indistinguishable from those of chronic ciclosporin vasculopathy. Similar changes have been reported in tacrolimus-related nephrotoxicity [108].

Acute and chronic forms of vascular nephrotoxicity are described. In the acute form, the clinical picture is that of thrombotic microangiopathy/haemolytic-uraemic syndrome [108–110]. Pathological changes include arteriolar occlusive concentric oedematous intimal thickening and, occasionally, fibrinoid necrosis (Figure 23.25). Glomeruli show thrombosis, fibrinoid necrosis and mesangiolysis, often focal and associated with cellular crescents and segmental endocapillary and extracapillary proliferation. It is potentially reversible with cessation of therapy [111].

The chronic form of vascular toxicity is most frequently observed [107,109]. In its most severe form there is arteriolar hyalinosis, reflecting myocyte necrosis, and/or arterial intimal fibrous proliferation. There is also focal segmental glomerulosclerosis and glomerular hyalinosis (Figure 23.26), and occasional glomeruli show ischaemic collapse. Uninvolved glomeruli may be hypertrophied, with enlargement of juxtaglomerular apparatus. An increase in number of renin-containing cells may be observed that diminishes after cessation of ciclosporin [112]. Tubules may show atrophy alternating with hypertrophy. There is often interstitial chronic inflammation. In the study of Griffiths et al. [109] of 22 patients from the Harefield programme, less severe forms of glomerular and tubular injury were often seen, but overall the severity of tubular

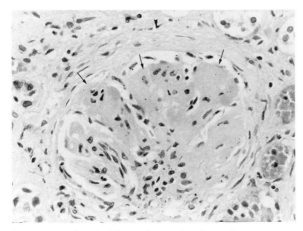

Figure 23.26 Chronic ciclosporin-associated vascular nephropathy in an autopsied kidney from a heart transplant recipient with end-stage renal failure on haemodialysis: the glomerulus shows nodular segmental hyaline sclerosis (arrows) and there is fibrosis of Bowman's capsule (arrowhead). (H&E, 240×.)

atrophy tended to parallel that of glomerular sclerosis. Ultrastructural changes include thickening of the glomerular basement membrane and basal lamina reduplication in arterioles, both of which may be specific for ciclosporin toxicity [109]. Areas of tubular atrophy, interstitial inflammation and fibrosis were band-like, alternating with areas of tubular hypertrophy – the 'striped fibrosis' lesion noted by some authors [106], presumably reflecting the anatomy of the vascular changes.

Hepatotoxicity

Ciclosporin may be associated with cholestasis and, possibly, with the formation of biliary calculi. A range of hepatotoxic reactions attributed to azathioprine is known to occur [113,114] and is thought to result from injury to the endothelial cells lining the sinusoids and venules [114]. Biochemical abnormalities include asymptomatic rise in serum transaminase activity and cholestasis.

Chronic azathioprine hepatotoxicity is associated with veno-occlusive disease, portal hypertension, peliosis hepatis and nodular regenerative hyperplasia [115,116]. The most frequently encountered changes on liver biopsy are sinusoidal congestion with perivenular hepatocellular necrosis, suggesting vascular outflow obstruction, which regresses with cessation of the drug and recurs with drug challenge [114]. Portal hypertension may develop, with a histological picture of veno-occlusive disease including nonthrombotic partial or total obliteration of the lobular

and sublobular venules by subintimal fibrosis, often with sparse chronic inflammation. In some cases, peliosis hepatitis may be seen adjacent to occluded veins [113]. In all autopsied cases, nodular regenerative hyperplasia was noted. Early diagnosis of azathioprine hepatotoxicity is important, as established veno-occlusive disease may not respond to cessation of the drug. Nodular regenerative hyperplasia may also occur with steroid therapy [115].

Other drug reactions of note

Myelosuppression is the most frequently encountered side effect of azathioprine; it is dose related and can be reversed by dose adjustment. Hypertension, hypertrichosis, tremor, headache and tinnitus are known side-effects of ciclosporin, as is gum hypertrophy, which may need removal on clinical grounds. The squamous mucosa of the gum typically shows papillary hyperplasia, with a dense polyclonal plasma cell infiltrate in underlying stroma (Figure 23.27). The infiltrate should be differentiated from soft tissue involvement by post-transplant lymphoproliferative disorder (see below). Cushing's syndrome, diabetes mellitus, osteoporosis, avascular necrosis of the hip and, in children, growth retardation are all well-known side effects of steroid therapy given as part of maintenance triple immunosuppression. Rhabdomyolysis (Figure 23.28) has been described in three patients, two of whom were lung transplant recipients receiving ciclosporin, one of whom suffered a possible ciclosporin-mediated reaction while on statins [117]. The third occurred in a child receiving tacrolimus following bone marrow transplantation [118].

A hypertrophic cardiomyopathy (HCM)-like syndrome has been described in children receiving tacrolimus following liver and/or small bowel transplants [119] who were routinely followed up with two-dimensional echocardiography. Autopsy studies in one patient [119] showed myofibre hypertrophy with some myocyte disarray, said to be distinct from that observed in hypertrophic cardiomyopathy occurring in the general population. However, the existence of tacrolimus-associated HCM as a distinct entity has been questioned by a follow-up study in paediatric heart transplant recipients maintained on either tacrolimus or ciclosporin [120]. Factors such as the hypertrophic effect of steroids in children, a tendency to use oversized donors in younger children, undetected ambulatory hypertension (difficult to diagnose in younger children) and ventricular volume overload (known to be associated with end-stage liver failure) may all contribute to the echocardiographic abnormalities observed. Scott et al. [120] concluded from their study that, while the implanted heart is thicker than normal, with decreased end-diastolic

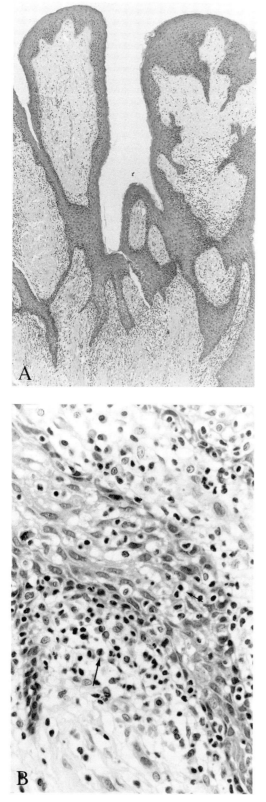

Figure 23.27 Ciclosporin-associated gingival hyperplasia in a resection specimen: (A) marked papillary hyperplasia of squamous mucosa of the gum; (B) there is a florid plasma cell infiltrate involving the submucosa (arrow), infiltrating into the basal layer of mucosa (short arrow). ((A) H&E 35×; (B) H&E 300×.)

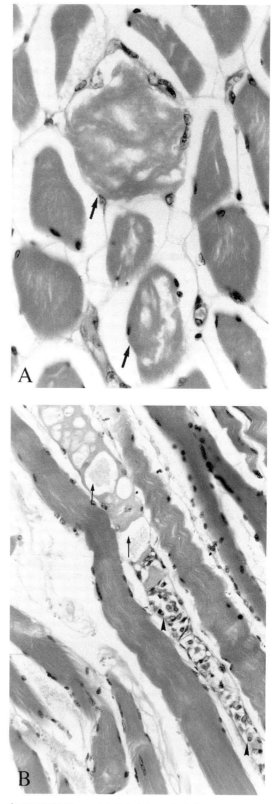

Figure 23.28 Drug-related rhabdomyolysis in a postmortem biopsy of skeletal muscle: (A) there is extensive vacuolation of myocytes (arrows); (B) in a longitudinal section of skeletal fibres, some appear 'empty' (thin arrows), with an associated inflammatory reaction (arrowheads). ((A) H&E 75×; (B) H&E 160×.)

volume, this is most apparent early after transplantation and gradually diminishes over the first year. No difference was observed between patients on ciclosporin and those on tacrolimus.

Neoplasia in solid organ transplantation

Penn [121] reviewed the clinical features of all tumours in transplant recipients reported to the Cincinnati Transplant Tumor Registry (CTTR) since its establishment in 1968. After chronic rejection, malignant tumours are the most significant limiting factor for long-term survival in solid organ transplantation [121], including lung allograft recipients. The overall incidence in the transplant population ranges from 6% to 11% [122,123], some tumours such as post-transplantation lymphoproliferative disorders (PTLDs) showing a three- to four-fold increase in incidence as compared with age-matched controls in the general population [124]. They include tumours arising de novo in transplant recipients, a small number of tumours inadvertently 'transplanted' with the allograft, and recipient tumours treated prior to transplantation [121]. The most frequently observed are squamous carcinomas of the skin and lips, PTLDs, lymphomas, Kaposi's sarcoma (KS) and genitourinary carcinomas. The majority of tumours, with the exception of most cases of PTLD, occur late after transplantation and behave more aggressively than similar tumours in the general population. Predisposing factors include immunosuppression, ultraviolet irradiation in skin tumours and activation of oncogenic viruses such as Epstein–Barr virus (EBV) in PTLD and smooth muscle tumours, human papilloma virus (HPV) in skin and lower genital tract tumours and human herpes virus (HHV) in KS.

Post-transplantation lymphoproliferative disorders

An important and clinically challenging group of tumours in the transplant population are the PTLDs, many associated with EBV infection and, since the landmark publication by Starzl et al. [125], recognized as potentially reversible once immunosuppression is reduced. PTLDs constitute a spectrum of lymphoproliferation that follows immunosuppression for solid organ and bone marrow transplantation [126]. Specific risk factors include the type of transplant, young age, number of rejection episodes, multiagent immunosuppression, use of T-cytolytic therapy and pretransplant EBV seronegativity [124].

The overall incidence of PTLDs in solid organ transplantation is 1–2%, ranging from < 1 % in renal recipients to 9% for lung and heart–lung recipients to 17% for intestinal recipients [127]. The majority of cases occur in the first four years following transplantation and are associated with active or latent EBV infection [128]. The source of EBV in early PTLD is usually primary infection in the recipient, especially in children [129], although PTLD of donor origin may rarely occur [127]. PTLD is thought to result from uncontrolled proliferation of EBV-immortalized B cells owing to loss of cytotoxic T-cell control because of immunosuppression for the prevention and treatment of acute allograft rejection [128]. Disease regression may occur once underlying immunosuppression is reduced or reversed [125,126], although the graft may be compromised due to acute rejection. PTLD may also develop several years after transplantation, often lacks EBV and tends to behave more aggressively [124,130,131]. Disease may be nodal or extranodal, and may involve the graft, notably the lung [132]. The nontransplanted lung may be involved by PTLD in recipients of other solid organ transplants. One instance of primary effusion PTLD of pleura in a liver transplant recipient has recently been reported [133].

Classification of PTLD

The morphology of PTLD ranges from plasma cell hyperplasia and infectious mononucleosis-like changes to appearances identical with large B-cell lymphomas. Classification systems developed over the past 20 years have identified three major morphological groups – 'early', polymorphic and monomorphic. The majority are of B-cell origin [126]. Initial correlation with biological behaviour was poor but more reproducible and clinically applicable classification schemes evolved when the results of molecular studies of immunoglobulin and EBV clonality were taken into account [134]. Monomorphous monoclonal lesions with clonal EBV expression tend to have a worse prognosis than polymorphous polyclonal lesions with nonclonal EBV expression, although this correlation is not absolute [135]. Hodgkin's disease-like PTLD [136] and EBV-negative non-Hodgkin's lymphomas, often with rearranged oncogenes such as c-*myc* [130,131] have also been described. It is noteworthy that endemic-type Burkitt's lymphoma-like PTLD is rare, with only anecdotal cases of this condition [137] and of Burkitt-type B-acute lymphoblastic leukaemia [138] reported. Jaffe et al. [139] acknowledge the overlap between PTLD and true lymphoma, identifying PTLD in the World Health Organization (WHO) classification of lymphomas as a specific category on the basis of their distinctive biological and clinical features (Table 23.3).

Tissue diagnosis of PTLD

The pathological diagnosis of PTLD is made on evaluation of cell morphology and immunophenotype, immunoglobulin clonality and detection of tissue EBV DNA or RNA.

Table 23.3. WHO classification of post-transplant lymphoproliferative disorders

---

1. Early lesions
Reactive plasmacytic hyperplasia
Infectious mononucleosis

2. PTLD – polymorphic
Polyclonal (rare)
Monoclonal

3. PTLD monomorphic (classify according to lymphoma classification)
- B-cell lymphomas
  Diffuse large B-cell lymphoma (immunoblastic, centroblastic, anaplastic)
  Burkitt/Burkitt-like
  Plasma cell myeloma
- T-cell lymphomas
  Peripheral T-cell lymphoma, not otherwise categorized
  Other types (hepatosplenic, gamma-delta, T/NK)

4. Other types (rare)
Hodgkin's disease-like lesions
Plasmacytoma-like lesions

Note: PTLD, post-transplantation lymphoproliferative disease; NK, natural killer cell.
Source: From ref. 139.

Immunoglobulin clonality should be determined using IHC or ISH, although in cases of doubtful clonality PCR for heavy chain gene rearrangement is the gold standard [126,134]. Detection of EBV should be done using ISH for EBV-encoded RNA (EBERs) on paraffin sections [140], or IHC for EBV nuclear antigens 1–6 (EBNA) on cryostat sections [141]. The histopathological report should include a full description of the findings and a diagnosis using the WHO classification [139]. Final interpretation should be 'in the clinical setting of immunosuppression'. Synchronous and metachronous lesions should be fully investigated as variations in clonality and morphology may occur both within an individual lesion and between simultaneous or subsequent lesions in individual patients [126].

Histopathological appearances of PTLD in the lung
PTLD may involve the transplanted or native lung in isolation or as part of disseminated disease [132]. When confined to the lung, it may be asymptomatic or associated with cough, fever and malaise. Chest radiography and CT scan may show diffuse infiltrates or single or multiple nodules. Tissue may be obtained by transthoracic needle biopsy or, rarely, by thoracoscopic wedge biopsy.

The histopathological appearance of pulmonary PTLD is variable and, clinical setting apart, may resemble lym-

phomatoid granulomatosis in that it is usually angio-invasive and shows extensive necrosis. Infiltration of septal and pleural lymphatics, terminal bronchioles and visceral pleura may also be seen. Early lesions may be rich in mature plasma cells or show changes suggestive of infectious mononucleosis. Polymorphous infiltrates may include plasma cells and lymphoplasmacytoid cells, resembling the spectrum of appearances in lymphoplasmacytoid lymphomas. Monomorphous infiltrates may include transformed blasts, centroblast-like and centrocyte-like cells and immunoblasts, show a high proliferation index and resemble large B-cell lymphomas (Figure 23.29A). Single cell necrosis is common. There is a background population of interstitial histiocytes and T lymphocytes, often cuffing the tumour. Uninvolved lung may show lymphocytic bronchiolitis and patchy organizing pneumonia. Immunoglobulin clonality is variable; however, while 'early' lesions tend to be polyclonal and most monomorphous lesions are monoclonal, polymorphous lesions may be either [134,135]. Virtually all B-cell lesions contain EBV demonstrated by ISH for EBERs (Figure 23.29B) or by IHC for EBNAs. EBV-negative lesions resembling B-cell, T-cell or anaplastic large cell lymphomas may be seen [130,131] in long-term lung allograft survivors.

Difficulties encountered in diagnosis, especially on core biopsies, stem from the small size of the sample, the risk of crush artefact and the tendency for pulmonary PTLD to show extensive necrosis because of angioinvasion. The differential diagnosis of PTLD includes infections such as cytomegalovirus or *P. carinii*, inflammation related to previous biopsy sites, other pulmonary lymphoid disorders such as lymphoid interstitial pneumonia, bronchus-associated lymphoid tissue and, in the transplanted lung, acute allograft rejection and, rarely, graft-versus-host disease.

Disease management
Regression of pulmonary PTLD occurring early after transplantation is rapid and usually complete after reduction of immunosuppression and treatment with antiviral agents [132]. Disease relapse or progression may require treatment with radio- or chemotherapy. Recent research into the molecular biology of EBV infection has led to the development of newer, less toxic, more physiological treatments such as cytotoxic T-lymphocyte infusions [142,143], interferon alpha [144] or antibodies to B cells (anti-CD20) [145,146].

There are currently no reliable clinical, radiological or serological methods available to monitor PTLD. However, recent studies using the polymerase chain reaction to measure EBV DNA load in peripheral blood are of potential value in predicting and monitoring EBV-related PTLD.

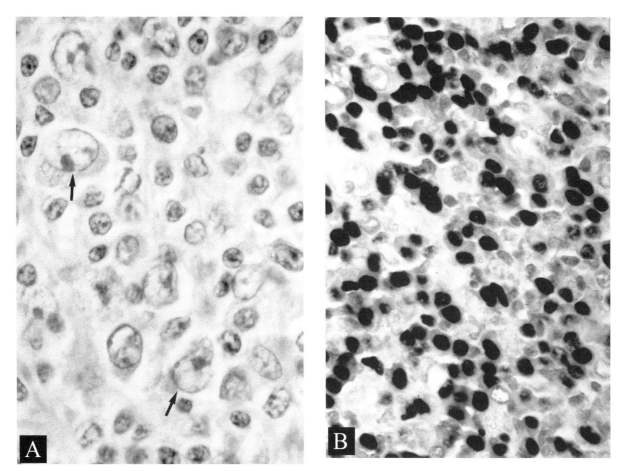

Figure 23.29 EBV-driven PTLD in a lung allograft mass biopsy: (A) a monomorphous infiltrate of large lymphoid cells, many with immunoblastic features (arrows) and classified as large B-cell lymphoma-like PTLD (139) ((A) H&E 310×); (B) ISH for EBERs shows uniform nuclear positivity (150×) (courtesy of Dr J.A. Thomas, London School of Hygiene and Tropical Medicine, London, UK; first published in *CPD Cellular Pathology* 2000; **21**(3): 142–147, by Rila Publications Ltd, London.)

Results vary according to how frequently patients are tested and whether serum, plasma or whole blood is used [147–149]. Standardization of the methodology is needed and larger prospective studies on high risk patients are required to establish baseline levels for infection and clinically significant disease. Rowe et al. [150] have recently reviewed current work in this field.

Other tumours

In the CTTR's experience [121], the most frequently encountered de novo tumours (excluding PTLD) are cutaneous in origin, notably squamous cell carcinomas and premalignant skin lesions that are often multiple, frequently develop metastases and often contain human papilloma virus (HPV) [151]. This contrasts with the general population, in whom skin cancer (with the exception of melanoma) is a disease of the seventh decade and over, and in whom basal cell carcinoma predominates. Intraepithelial neoplasia and squamous cell carcinomas of the uterine cervix, vulva and perineum, also known to be associated with HPV infection, may occur. Other carcinomas said to occur with greater frequency than in the general population include renal tumours [152] and lung carcinomas [153], which often present at an advanced clinical stage.

Until the AIDS epidemic in the 1980s, KS was rarely seen outside tropical Africa. In the immunosuppressed solid organ transplant population KS comprised 6% of tumours reported to the CTTR [121], most occurring in renal transplant recipients of Afro-Caribbean or Mediterranean origin. In Penn's series, in 61% of patients, the tumours were nonvisceral, affecting skin or oropharynx, and regressed completely in 54%; in 36% reduction in immunosuppression, only, was required. In 41% of patients, tumours were visceral, affecting mainly the gastrointestinal tract and lungs, but were often disseminated. Tumour regression was seen in only 30%, in half of whom reduction of immunosuppression was the only therapy required. Fifty-four per cent of patients with visceral tumours died, three-quarters from malignancy per se. Only one case of KS has been reported in a lung transplant recipient, of African origin, in whom a KS lesion was found in the native lung contemporaneously with CMV pneumonitis in the transplanted lung six months after single lung transplantation for end-stage chronic obstructive airways disease [154]. The association of KS with HHV-8 infection has been well documented [155].

While smooth muscle tumours associated with intralesional clonal EBV have been reported in liver allograft recipients [156], only one case of asymptomatic bronchial smooth muscle nodules in a lung allograft has been reported [104]. The lesions were negative for EBV and were undetectable bronchoscopically and radiologically.

Conclusion

Lung transplantation is a successful method of treatment for end-stage lung disease. Complications may involve the lung, as in rejection, infection and disease recurrence, or be systemic, as in PTLD and immunosuppressive drug toxicity. Most of the complications discussed and illustrated in this chapter are diagnosed by the histopathologist who, as a member of the multidisciplinary team, has an important role to play in the clinical management of this challenging group of patients.

Acknowledgements

I thank Alan Crabtree and colleagues, Photography Unit, Mount Vernon Hospital, for assistance with the illustrations.

REFERENCES

1 Hosenpud JD, Bennett LE, Keck BM, Boucek MM, Novick RJ. The Registry of the International Society for Heart and Lung Transplantation – 18th official report – 2001. *J Heart Lung Transplant* 2001; **20**: 805-815.
2 Burke MM. Complications of heart and lung transplantation and of cardiac surgery. In: Anthony P, MacSween RNM, eds. *Recent advances in histopathology*, vol 16 Churchill Livingstone, London, 1994: 95–122.
3 Stewart S, McNeil K, Nashef SA, Wells FC, Higenbottam TW, Wallwork J. Audit of referral and explant diagnoses in lung transplantation: a pathologic study of lungs removed for parenchymal disease. *J Heart Lung Transplant* 1995; **14**: 1173–1186.
4 Weill D, McGiffin DC, Zorn GL Jr, et al. The utility of open lung biopsy following lung transplantation. *J Heart Lung Transplant* 2000; **19**: 852–857.
5 Selvaggi S. Bronchoalveolar lavage in lung transplant patients. *Acta Cytolog* 1992; **36**: 674–679.
6 Riise GC, Andersson BA, Kjellstrom C, et al. Persistent high BAL fluid granulocyte activation marker levels as early indicators of bronchiolitis obliterans after lung transplant. *Eur Respir J* 1999; **14**: 1123–1130.
7 Glanville AR, Imoto E, Baldwin JC, Billingham ME, Theodore J, Robin ED. The role of right ventricular endomyocardial biopsy in the long-term management of heart-lung transplant recipients. *J Heart Transplant* 1987; **6**: 357–361.
8 Kriett JM, Kaye M. The Registry of the International Society for Heart and Lung Transplantation: 8th official report – 1991. *J Heart Lung Transplant* 1991; **10**: 491–498.
9 Tazelaar HD, Yousem SA. The pathology of combined heart–lung transplantation: an autopsy study. *Hum Pathol* 1988; **19**: 1403–1416.
10 Sibley RK, Berry GJ, Tazelaar HD, et al. The role of transbronchial biopsies in the management of lung transplant recipients. *J Heart Lung Transplant* 1993; **12**: 308–324.
11 Yousem SA. Alveolar lipoproteinosis in lung allograft recipients. *Hum Pathol* 1997; **28**: 1383–1386.
12 McDonald JW, Keller CA, Ramos RR, Brunt EM. Mixed (neutrophil-rich) interstitial pneumonitis in biopsy specimens of lung allografts: a clinicopathologic evaluation. *Chest* 1998; **113**: 117–123.
13 Yousem SA, Duncan SR, Griffith BP. Interstitial and airspace granulation tissue reactions in lung transplant recipients. *Am J Surg Pathol* 1992; **16**: 877–884.
14 Gammie JS, Stukus DR, Pham SM, et al. Effect of ischemic time on survival in clinical lung transplantation. *Ann Thorac Surg* 1999; **68**: 2015–2019.
15 Ohori NP, Iacono AT, Grgurich WF, Yousem SA. Significance of acute bronchitis/bronchiolitis in the lung transplant recipient. *Am J Surg Pathol* 1994; **18**: 1192–1204.
16 Taylor PM, Rose ML, Yacoub MH, et al. Expression of MHC antigens in normal human lungs and transplanted lungs with obliterative bronchiolitis. *Transplantation* 1989; **48**: 506–510.
17 Frost AE, Jammal CT, Cagle PT. Hyperacute rejection following lung transplantation. *Chest* 1996; **110**: 559–562.
18 Choi JK, Kearns J, Palevsky HI, et al. Hyperacute rejection of a pulmonary allograft. Immediate clinical and pathologic findings. *Am J Resp Crit Care Med* 1999; **160**: 1015-1018.
19 Bittner HB, Dunitz J, Hertz M, Bolman MR, Park SJ. Hyperacute rejection in single lung transplantation – case report of successful management by means of plasmapheresis and antithymocyte globulin treatment. *Transplantation* 2001; **71**: 649–651.
20 Smith JD, Danskine AJ, Laylor RM, Rose ML, Yacoub MH. The effect of panel-reactive antibodies and the donor-specific

crossmatch on graft survival after heart and heart–lung transplantation. *Transplant Immunol* 1993; **1**: 60–65.

21 Scornik JC, Zander DS, Baz MA, Donnelly WH, Staples ED. Susceptibility of lung transplants to preformed donor-specific HLA antibodies as detected by flow cytometry. *Transplantation* 1999; **68**: 1542–1546.

22 Badesch DB, Zamora M, Fullerton D, et al. Pulmonary capillaritis: a possible histologic form of acute pulmonary allograft rejection. *J Heart Lung Transplant* 1998; **17**: 415–422.

23 Yousem SA, Berry GJ, Brunt EM, et al. A Working Formulation for the standardization of nomenclature in the diagnosis of heart and lung rejection: Lung Rejection Study Group. *J Heart Transplant* 1990; **9**: 593–601.

24 Yousem SA, Berry GJ, Cagle PT, et al. Revision of the 1990 Working Formulation for the classification of pulmonary allograft rejection: Lung Rejection Study Group. *J Heart Lung Transplant* 1996; **15**: 1–15.

25 Pomerance A, Madden B, Burke MM, Yacoub MH. Transbronchial biopsy in heart and lung transplantation: clinicopathologic correlations. *J Heart Lung Transplant* 1995; **14**: 761–773.

26 Scott JP, Fradet G, Smyth RL, et al. Prospective study of transbronchial biopsies in the management of heart–lung and single lung transplant patients. *J Heart Lung Transplant* 1991; **10**: 626–637.

27 Yousem SA, Paradis IL, Dauber JA, et al. Large airway inflammation in heart–lung transplant recipients – its significance and prognostic implications. *Transplantation* 1990; **49**: 654–656.

28 Yousem SA. Lymphocytic bronchitis/bronchiolitis in lung allograft recipients. *Am J Surg Pathol* 1993; **17**: 491–496.

29 Foerster A, Bjortuft O, Geiran O, Rollag H, Leivestad T, Froysaker T. Single lung transplantation. Morphological surveillance by transbronchial biopsy. *APMIS* 1993; **101**: 455–466.

30 de Blic J, Peuchmaur M, Carnot F, et al. Rejection in lung transplantation – an immunohistochemical study of transbronchial biopsies. *Transplantation* 1992; **54**: 639–644.

31 Yousem SA, Martin T, Paradis IL, Keenan R, Griffith BP. Can immunohistological analysis of transbronchial biopsy specimens predict responder status in early acute rejection of lung allografts? *Hum Pathol* 1994; **25**: 525–529.

32 Yousem SA. Graft eosinophilia in lung transplantation. *Hum Pathol* 1992; **23**: 1172–1177.

33 Heng D, Sharples LD, McNeil K, Stewart S, Wreghitt T, Wallwork J. Bronchiolitis obliterans syndrome: incidence, natural history, prognosis, and risk factors. *J Heart Lung Transplant* 1998; **17**: 1255–1263.

34 Clelland C, Higenbottam T, Otulana B, et al. Histologic prognostic indicators for the lung allografts of heart–lung transplants. *J Heart Lung Transplant* 1990; **9**: 177–186.

35 Yousem SA. The histological spectrum of pulmonary graft-versus-host disease in bone marrow transplant recipients. *Hum Pathol* 1995; **26**: 668–675.

36 Kroshus TJ, Kshettry VR, Savik K, John R, Hertz MI, Bolman RM. Risk factors for the development of bronchiolitis obliterans syndrome after lung transplantation. *J Thorac Cardiovasc Surg* 1997; **114**: 195–202.

37 Norgaard MA, Andersen CB, Pettersson C. Does bronchial artery revascularization influence results concerning bronchiolitis obliterans syndrome and/or obliterative bronchiolitis after lung transplantation? *Eur J Cardiothorac Surg* 1998; **14**: 311–318.

38 Daly R, Tadjkarimi S, Khagani A, Banner NR, Yacoub MH (1992). Successful double lung transplantation with direct bronchial artery revascularization. *Ann Thorac Surg* 1992; **56**: 885–892.

39 Milne DS, Gascoigne A, Wilkes J, et al. The immunohistopathology of obliterative bronchiolitis following lung transplantation. *Transplantation* 1992; **54**: 748–750.

40a Cooper JD. Billingham M, Egan T, et al. A Working Formulation for the standardization of nomenclature and for clinical staging of chronic dysfunction in lung allografts. *J Heart Lung Transplant* 1993; **12**: 713–716.

40b Estenne M, Maurer JR, Boehler A, et al. Branchiolitis obliterans syndrome 2001: an update of the diagnostic criteria. *J Heart Lung Transplant* 2002; **21**: 297–310.

41 Dawkins KD, Jamieson SW, Hunt SA, et al. Long-term results, haemodynamics and complications after combined heart and lung transplantation. *Circulation* 1985; **71**: 919–926.

42 Pucci A, Forbes RDC, Berry GJ, Rowan RA, Billingham ME. Accelerated posttransplant coronary atherosclerosis in combined heart–lung transplantation. *Transplant Proc* 1991; **23**: 1228–1229.

43 Abernathy EC, Hruban RH, Baumgartner WA, Reitz BA, Hutchins GM. The two forms of bronchiolitis obliterans in heart–lung transplant recipients. *Hum Pathol* 1991; **22**: 1102–1110.

44 Egan JJ, Sarker S, Hasleton PS, Woodcock AA, Younan N, Deiraniya AK. Should cryptogenic organising pneumonia be included in the classification of pulmonary allograft rejection? *J Heart Lung Transplant* 1996; **15**: 1268–1269.

45 Chaparro C, Chamberlain D, Maurer J, Winton T, Dehoyos A, Kesten S. Bronchiolitis obliterans organizing pneumonia (BOOP) in lung transplant recipients. *Chest* 1996; **110**: 1150–1154.

46 Milne DS, Gascoigne AD, Ashcroft T, Sviland L, Malcolm AJ, Corris PA. Organizing pneumonia following pulmonary transplantation and the development of obliterative bronchiolitis. *Transplantation* 1994; **57**: 1757–1762.

47 Siddiqui MT, Garrity ER, Husain AN. Bronchiolitis obliterans organising pneumonia-like reactions. A non-specific response or an atypical form of rejection or infection in lung allograft recipients? *Hum Pathol* 1996; **27**: 714–719.

48 Nakhleh RE, Bolman RM, Henke CA, Hertz MI. Lung transplant pathology: a comparative study of pulmonary acute rejection and cytomegalovirus infection. *Am J Surg Pathol* 1991; **15**: 1197–1201.

49 Tazelaar HD. Perivascular inflammation in pulmonary infections: implications for the diagnosis of lung rejection. *J Heart Lung Transplant* 1991; **10**: 437–441.

50 Stewart S, Cary NRB. The pathology of heart and lung transplantation. *Curr Diag Pathol* 1996; **3**: 69–79.

51 van der Bij W, van Son WJ, van Dijk RB, et al. Antigen test for early diagnosis of active cytomegalovirus infection in heart transplant recipients. *J Heart Transplant* 1988; **7**: 106–109.

52 Keenan RJ, Konishi H, Kawai A, et al. Clinical trial of tacrolimus versus cyclosporine in lung transplantation. *Ann Thorac Surg* 1995; **60**: 580–585.

53 Reichenspurner H, Girgis RE, Robbins RC, et al. Stanford experience with obliterative bronchiolitis after lung and heart–lung transplantation. *Ann Thorac Surg* 1996; **62**: 1467–1472.

54 Kesten S, Chaparro C, Scavuzzo M, Gutiérrez C. Tacrolimus as rescue therapy for bronchiolitis obliterans syndrome. *J Heart Lung Transplant* 1997; **16**: 905–912.

55 Boehler A, Vogt P, Zollinger A, Weder W, Speich R. Prospective study of the value of transbronchial lung biopsy after lung transplantation. *Eur Respir J* 1996; **9**: 658–662.

56 Chamberlain D, Maurer J, Chaparro C, Idolor L. Evaluation of transbronchial lung biopsy specimens in the diagnosis of obliterative bronchiolitis after lung transplantation. *J Heart Lung Transplant* 1994; **13**: 963–971.

57 Kramer MR, Stoehr C, Whang JL, et al. The diagnosis of obliterative bronchiolitis after heart–lung and lung transplantation: low yield of transbronchial lung biopsy. *J Heart Lung Transplant* 1993; **12**: 675–681.

58 Starnes VA, Theodore J, Oyer PE, et al. Evaluation of heart–lung transplant recipients with prospective serial transbronchial biopsies and pulmonary function studies. *J Thorac Cardiovasc Surg* 1989; **98**: 683–690.

59 Scott JP, Higenbottam T, Clelland CA, et al. Natural history of chronic rejection in heart–lung transplant recipients. *J Heart Transplant* 1990; **9**: 510–515.

60 Clelland CA, Higenbottam TW, Stewart S, Scott JA, Wallwork J. The histological changes in transbronchial biopsy after treatment of acute lung rejection in heart–lung transplants. *J Pathol* 1990; **161**: 105–112.

61 Yousem SA. The potential role of mast cells in lung allograft rejection. *Hum Pathol* 1997; **28**: 179–182.

62 Clelland C, Higgenbottam T, Stewart S, et al. Bronchoalveolar lavage and transbronchial lung biopsy during acute rejection and infection in heart–lung transplant patients. *Am Rev Respir Dis* 1993; **147**: 1386–1392.

63 Paradis IL, Duncan SR, Dauber JH, Yousem S, Hardesty R, Griffiths B. Distinguishing between infection, rejection and the adult respiratory distress syndrome after human lung transplantation. *J Heart Lung Transplant* 1992; **11**: S232–S236.

64 Tikkanen J, Lemstrom K, Halme M, Pakkala S, Taskinen E, Koskinen P. Cytological monitoring of peripheral blood, bronchoalveolar lavage fluid, and transbronchial biopsy specimens during acute rejection and cytomegalovirus infection in lung and heart–lung allograft recipients. *Clin Transplant* 2001; **15**: 77–88.

65 Scholma J, Slebos D-J, Boezen HM, et al. Eosinophilic granulocytes and interleukin-6 level in bronchoalveolar lavage fluid are associated with the development of obliterative bronchiolitis after lung transplantation. *Am J Respir Crit Care Med* 2000; **162**: 2221–2225.

66 Zheng L, Walters EH, Ward C, et al. Airway neutrophils in stable and bronchiolitis obliterans syndrome patients following lung transplantation. *Thorax* 2000; **55**: 53–59.

67 Gabbay E, Walters EH, Orsida B, et al. In stable lung transplant recipients, exhaled nitric oxide levels positively correlate with airway neutrophilia and bronchial epithelial iNOS. *Am J Respir Crit Care Med* 1999; **160**: 2093–2099.

68 Mason NA, Springall DR, Pomerance A, Evans TJ, Yacoub MH, Polak JM. Expression of inducible nitric oxide synthase and formation of peroxynitrite in posttransplant obliterative bronchiolitis. *J Heart Lung Transplant* 1998; **17**: 710–714.

69 Ohori NP. Epithelial cell atypia in bronchoalveolar lavage specimens from lung transplant recipients. *Am J Clin Pathol* 1999; **112**: 204–210.

70 Radley-Smith RC, Burke M, Pomerance A, Yacoub MH. Graft vessel disease and obliterative bronchiolitis after heart/lung transplantation in children. *Transplant Proc* 1995; **27**: 2017–2018.

71 Kshettry VR, Kroshus TJ, Hertz MI, et al. Early and late airway complications after lung transplantation: incidence and management. *Ann Thorac Surg* 1997; **63**: 1576–1583.

72 Yousem SA, Dauber JH, Griffith B. Bronchial cartilage alterations in lung transplantation. *Chest* 1990; **98**: 1121–1124.

73 Fishman JA, Rubin RH. Infection in organ-transplant recipients. *New Engl J Med* 1998; **338**: 1741–1751.

74 Patterson A, Stewart S, Cary NRB. Bronchoalveolar lavage and transbronchial biopsies are complementary in the assessment of opportunistic infections in heart–lung transplant (HLT) recipients. *J Pathol* 1991; **163**: 164A.

75 van der Bij W, Torensma R, van Son WJ, et al. Rapid immunodiagnosis of active cytomegalovirus infection by monoclonal antibody staining of blood leucocytes. *J Med Virol* 1988; **25**: 179–188.

76 Egan JJ, Barber L, Lomax J, et al. Detection of human cytomegalovirus antigenaemia: a rapid diagnostic technique for predicting CMV infection/pneumonitis in lung and heart transplant recipients. *Thorax* 1995; **50**: 9–13.

77 Niubo J, Perez JL, Martínez-Lacasa JT, et al. Association of quantitative cytomegalovirus antigenaemia with symptomatic infection in solid organ transplant patients. *Diagn Microbiol Infect Dis* 1996; **24**: 19–24.

78 Fend F, Prior C, Margreiter R, Mikuz G. Cytomegalovirus pneumonitis in heart–lung transplant recipients: histopathology and clinicopathologic considerations. *Hum Pathol* 1990; **21**: 918–926.

79 Arbustini E, Morbini P, Grasso M, et al. Human cytomegalovirus early infection, acute rejection and major histocompatibility class II expression in transplanted lung: molecular, immunocytochemical and histopathologic investigations. *Transplantation* 1996; **61**: 418–427.

80 Sissons JG, Borysiewicz LK. Human cytomegalovirus infection. *Thorax* 1989; **44**: 241–246.

81 You X-M, Stainmuller C, Wagner TOF, Bruggeman CA, Haverich A, Steinhoff G. Enhancement of cytomegalovirus infection and acute rejection after allogeneic lung transplantation in the rat: virus-induced expression of major histocompatibility complex class II antigens. *J Heart Lung Transplant* 1996; **15**: 1108–1119.

82 Scoones DJ, Burke MM. The spectrum of histological appearances of *Pneumocystis carinii* pneumonia in transbronchial lung biopsies from heart and lung transplant recipients. *J Pathol* 1993; **169**(Suppl): 165A.

83 Wakefield AE, Miller RF, Guiver LA, Hopkin JM. Granulomatous *Pneumocystis carinii* pneumonia: DNA amplification studies on bronchoscopic alveolar lavage samples. *J Clin Pathol* 1994; **47**: 664–666.

84 Wreghitt TG, Hakim M, Gray JJ, et al. Toxoplasmosis in heart and heart and lung transplant recipients . *J Clin Pathol* 1989; **42**: 194–199.

85 Nash G, Kerschmann RL, Herndier B, Dubey JP. The pathological manifestations of pulmonary toxoplasmosis in the acquired immunodeficiency syndrome. *Hum Pathol* 1994; **25**: 652–658.

86 Holliman R, Johnson J, Burke M. Toxoplasmosis. In: Geraint JD, Zumla A, eds. The *granulomatous disorders*. Cambridge University Press, Cambridge, 1998: 257–275.

87 Holliman RE, Johnson J, Savva D, Cary N, Wreghitt T. Diagnosis of *Toxoplasma* infection in cardiac transplant recipients using the polymerase chain reaction. *J Clin Pathol* 1992; **45**: 931–932.

88 Smyth RL, Higenbottam TW, Scott JP, et al. Herpes simplex virus infection in heart–lung transplant recipients. *Transplantation* 1990; **49**: 735–739.

89 Dromer C, Nashef SAM, Velly J-F, Martigne C, Couraud L. Tuberculosis in transplanted lungs. *J Heart Lung Transplant* 1993; **12**: 924–927.

90 Schulman LL, Scully B, McGregor CC, Austin JHM. Pulmonary tuberculosis after lung transplantation. *Chest* 1997; **111**: 1459–1462.

91 Kesten S, Chaparro C. Mycobacterial infections in lung transplant recipients. *Chest* 1999; **115**: 741–745.

92 Heaton ND, Reece AS, Tan KC. Graft-versus-host disease following liver transplantation. *J Roy Soc Med* 1992; **85**: 313–314.

93 Chau EM, Lee J, Yew WW, Chiu CS, Wang EP. Mediastinal irradiation for graft-versus-host-disease in a heart–lung transplant recipient. *J Heart Lung Transplant* 1997; **16**: 974–979.

94 Sloane JP, Norton J. The pathology of bone marrow transplantation. *Histopathology* 1993; **22**: 201–209.

95 Herman JG, Beschorner WE, Baughman KL, Boitnott JK, Vogelsang GB, Baumgartner WA. Pseudo-graft-versus-host disease in heart and heart–lung transplant recipients. *Transplantation* 1988; **46**: 93–98.

96 Walker S, Mikhail G, Banner N, et al. Medium term results of lung transplantation for end stage pulmonary sarcoidosis. *Thorax* 1998; **53**: 281–284.

97 Habib SB, Congleton J, Carr D, et al. Recurrence of recipient Langerhans cell histiocytosis following bilateral lung transplantation. *Thorax* 1998; **53**: 323–325.

98 Gabbay E, Dark JH, Ashcroft T, et al. Recurrence of Langerhans cell granulomatosis following lung transplantation. *Thorax* 1998; **53**: 326–327.

99 Nine JS, Yousem SA, Paradis IL, Keenan R, Griffiths B. Lymphangioleiomyomatosis: recurrence after lung transplantation. *J Heart Lung Transplant* 1994; **13**: 714–719.

100 O'Brien JD, Lium JH, Parosa JF, Deyoung BR, Wick MR, Trulock EP. Lymphangioleiomyomatosis recurrence in the allograft after single-lung transplantation. *Am J Respir Crit Care Med* 1995; 151: 2033–2036.

101 Bittmann I, Dose TB, Muller C, Dienemann H, Vogelmeier C, Lohrs U. Lymphangioleiomyomatosis: recurrence after single lung transplantation. *Hum Pathol* 1997; **26**: 1420–1423.

102 Frost AE, Keller CA, Brown RW, et al. Giant cell interstitial pneumonitis. Disease recurrence in the transplanted lung. *Am Rev Respir Dis* 1993; **148**: 1401–1404.

103 Parker LA, Novotny DB. Recurrent alveolar proteinosis following double lung transplantation. *Chest* 1997; **111**: 1457–1458.

104 Flint A, Lynch JP, Martínez FJ, Whyte RI. Pulmonary smooth muscle proliferation occurring after lung transplantation. *Chest* 1997; **112**: 283–284.

105 Myers BD, Ross J, Newton L, Luetscher J, Perlroth M. Cyclosporine-associated chronic nephropathy. *N Engl J Med* 1984; **311**: 699–705.

106 Palestine AG, Austin HA, Balow JE, et al. Renal histopathologic alterations in patients treated with cyclosporin for uveitis. *N Engl J Med* 1986; **314**: 1293–1298.

107 Mihatsch MJ, Thiel G, Ryffel B. Morphologic diagnosis of cyclosporine nephrotoxicity. *Semin Diag Pathol* 1988; **5**: 104–121.

108 Randhawa PS, Shapiro R, Jordan ML, Starzl TE, Demetris AJ. The histopathological changes associated with allograft rejection and drug toxicity in renal transplant recipients maintained on FK506. Clinical significance and comparison with cyclosporine. *Am J Sug Pathol* 1993; **17**: 60–68.

109 Griffiths MH, Crowe AV, Papadaki L, et al. Cyclosporine nephrotoxicity in heart and lung transplant patients. *Q J Med* 1996; **89**: 751–763.

110 Cummins D, Jenkins G, Hall A, Banner N, Burke M. Thrombotic thrombocytopenic purpura in association with acute toxoplasmosis after cardiac transplantation. *Br J Haematol* 1999; **105**(Suppl 1): 40.

111 Wolfe JA, McCann RL, Sanfilippo F. Cyclosporine-associated microangiopathy in renal transplantation. A severe but potentially reversible form of early graft injury. *Transplantation* 1986; **41**: 541–544.

112 Gardiner DS, Watson MA, Junor BJR, Briggs JD, More IAR, Lindop GBM. The effect of conversion from cyclosporin to azathioprine on renin-containing cells in renal allograft biopsies. *Nephrol Dial Transplant* 1991; **6**: 363–367.

113 Weitz H, Golek JM, Loeschke K, Possinger K, Eder M. Veno-occlusive disease of the liver in patients receiving

immunosuppressive therapy. *Virchows Arch (Pathol Anat)* 1982; **395**: 245–256.

114 Sterneck M, Wiesner R, Ascher N, et al. Azathiaprine hepatotoxicity after liver transplantation. *Hepatology* 1991; **14**: 806–810.

115 Stromeyer FW, Ishak KG. Nodular transformation (nodular 'regenerative' hyperplasia) of the liver. *Hum Pathol* 1981; **12**: 60–71.

116 Ihara H, Ichikawa Y, Nagano S, Fukunishi T, Shinji Y. Peliosis hepatitis and nodular regenerative hyperplasia of the liver in renal transplant recipients. *Med J Osaka Univ* 1982; **33**: 13–18.

117 Cohen E, Kramer MR, Maoz C, Ben-Dayan D, Garty M. Cyclosporin drug-interaction-induced rhabdomyolysis. A report of two cases in lung transplant recipients. *Transplantation* 2000; **70**: 119–122.

118 Hibi S, Misawa A, Tamai M, et al. Severe rhabdomyolysis associated with tacrolimus. [letter] *Lancet* 1995; **346**: 702.

119 Atkison P, Joubert G, Barron A, et al. Hypertrophic cardiomyopathy associated with tacrolimus in paediatric transplant patients. *Lancet* 1995; **345**: 894–895.

120 Scott JS, Boyle GJ, Daubenay PE, et al. Tacrolimus: a cause of hypertrophic cardiomyopathy in paediatric heart transplant recipients? *Transplant Proc* 1999; **31**: 82–83.

121 Penn I. Occurrence of cancers in immunocompromised organ transplant recipients. *Clin Transplant* 1998; 147–158.

122 Mihalov ML, Gattuso P, Abraham K, Holmes EW, Reddy V. Incidence of post-transplant malignancy among 674 solid-organ-transplant recipients at a single center. *Clin Transplant* 1996; **10**: 248–255.

123 Rinaldi M, Pellegrini C, D'Armini AM, et al. Neoplastic disease after heart transplantation. Single center experience. *Eur J Cardiothorac Surg* 2001; **19**: 696–701.

124 Swerdlow AJ, Higgins CD, Hunt BJ, et al. Risk of lymphoid neoplasia after cardiothoracic transplantation. A cohort study of the relation to Epstein–Barr virus. *Transplantation* 2000; **69**: 897–904.

125 Starzl TE, Nalesnik MA, Porter KA, et al. Reversibility of lymphomas and lymphoproliferative lesions developing under cyclosporin-steroid therapy. *Lancet* 1984; **1**: 583–587.

126 Swerdlow SH. Post-transplant lymphoproliferative disorders: a working classification. *Curr Diag Pathol* 1997; **4**: 28–35.

127 Nalesnik MA. Clinical and pathological features of post-transplant lymphoproliferative disorders. *Springer Sem Immunopathol* 1998; **20**: 325–342.

128 Thomas JA, Crawford DH, Burke M. Clinicopathologic implications of Epstein–Barr virus related B-cell lymphoma in immunocompromised patients. *J Clin Pathol* 1995; **48**: 287–290.

129 Weissmann DJ, Ferry JA, Harris NL, Louis DN, Delmonico F, Spiro L. Posttransplant lymphoproliferative disorders in solid organ recipients are predominantly aggressive tumours of host origin. *Am J Clin Pathol* 1995; **103**: 748–755.

130 Dotti G, Fiocchi R, Motta T, et al. Epstein–Barr virus-negative lymphoproliferative disorders in long-term survivors after

heart, liver and kidney transplant. *Transplantation* 2000; **69**: 827–833.

131 Nelson BP, Nalesnik MA, Bahler DW, Locker J, Fung JJ, Swerdlow S. Epstein–Barr virus-negative post-transplant lymphoproliferative disorders: a distinct entity? *Am J Surg Pathol* 2000; **24**: 375–385.

132 Yousem SA, Randhawa P, Locker J, et al. Posttransplant lymphoproliferative disorders in heart–lung transplant recipients: primary presentation in the allograft. *Hum Pathol* 1989; **20**: 361–369.

133 Ohori NP, Whisnant RE, Nalesnik MA, Swerdlow SH. Primary pleural effusion posttransplant lymphoproliferative disorder: distinction from secondary involvement and effusion lymphoma. *Diagn Cytopathol* 2001; **25**: 50–53.

134 Locker J, Nalesnik MA. Molecular genetic analysis of lymphoid tumours arising after organ transplantation. *Am J Pathol* 1989; **135**: 977–987.

135 Knowles DM, Cesarman E, Chadburn A, et al. Correlative morphologic and molecular genetic analysis demonstrates three distinct categories of posttransplantation lymphoproliferative disorders. *Blood* 1995; **85**: 552–565.

136 Tinguely M, Vonlanthen R, Muller E, et al. Hodgkin's disease-like lymphoproliferative disorders in patients with different underlying immunodeficiency states. *Modern Pathol* 1998; **11**: 307–312.

137 Hunt BJ, Thomas JA, Burke M, Walker H, Yacoub M, Crawford DH. Epstein–Barr virus associated Burkitt lymphoma in a heart transplant recipient. *Transplantation* 1996; **62**: 869–872.

138 Tweddle DA, Gennery AR, Reid MM, et al. Posttransplantation B lymphoblastic leukaemia with Burkitt-like features. *Transplantation* 1999; **67**: 1379–1380.

139 Jaffe ES, Harris NL, Stein H, Vardiman JW, eds. Immunodeficiency associated lymphoproliferative disorders. In: *Tumours of haemopoietic and lymphoid tissues. Pathology and genetics.* WHO Classification of Tumours series. International Agency for Research on Cancer (IARC), Lyons, 2001: 264–269.

140 Thomas JA, Allday MJ, Crawford DH. Epstein–Barr virus-associated lymphoproliferative disorders in immunocompromised individuals. *Adv Cancer Res* 1991; **57**: 329–380.

141 Thomas JA, Hotchin NA, Allday MJ, et al. Immunohistology of Epstein–Barr virus-associated antigens in B cell disorders from immunocompromised individuals. *Transplantation* 1990; **49**: 944–953.

142 Gustafsson A, Levitsky V, Zou JZ, et al. Epstein–Barr virus (EBV) load in bone marrow transplant recipients at risk to develop posttransplant lymphoproliferative disease: prophylactic infusion of EBV-specific cytotoxic T cells. *Blood* 2000; **95**: 807–814.

143 Khanna R, Bell S, Sherritt M, et al. Activation and adoptive transfer of Epstein–Barr virus-specific cytotoxic T cells in solid organ transplant patients with posttransplant lymphoproliferative disease. *Proc Natl Acad Sci USA* 1999; **96**: 10391–10396.

144 Davis CL, Wood BL, Sabath DE, Joseph JS, Stehman-Breen C, Broudy VC. (1998) Interferon-alpha treatment of

posttransplant lympho-proliferative disorder in recipients of solid organ transplants. *Transplantation* 1998; **66**: 1770–1779.

145 Milpied N, Vasseur B, Parquet N, et al. Humanized anti-CD20 monoclonal antibody (Rituximab) in post transplant B-lymphoproliferative disorder: a retrospective analysis on 32 patients. *Ann Oncol* 2000; **11**(Suppl 1): S113–S116.

146 Reynaud-Gaubert M, Stoppa AM, Gaubert J-Y, Thomas P, Fuentes P. Anti–CD20 monoclonal antibody therapy in Epstein–Barr virus-associated B cell lymphoma following lung transplantation. *J Heart Lung Transplant* 2000; **19**: 492–495.

147 Limaye AP, Huang ML, Atienza EE, Ferrenberg JM, Corey L. Detection of Epstein–Barr virus DNA in sera from transplant recipients with lymphoproliferative disorders. *J Clin Microbiol* 1999; **37**: 1113–1116.

148 Stevens SJ, Verschuuren EA, Pronk I, et al. Frequent monitoring of Epstein–Barr virus DNA load in unfractionated whole blood is essential for early detection of posttransplant lymphoproliferative disease in high-risk patients. *Blood* 2001; **97**: 1165–1171.

149 Wagner HJ, Wessel M, Jabs W, et al. Patients at risk for development of posttransplant lymphoproliferative disorder: plasma versus peripheral blood mononuclear cells as material for quantification of Epstein–Barr viral load by using real-time quantitative polymerase chain reaction. *Transplant* 2001; **72**: 1012–1019.

150 Rowe DT, Webber S, Schauer EM, Reyes J, Green M. Epstein–Barr virus load monitoring: its role in the prevention and management of posttransplant lymphoproliferative disease. *Transpl Infect Dis* 2001; **3**: 79–87.

151 Harwood CA, Surentheran T, McGregor JM, et al. Human papillomavirus infection and non-melanoma skin cancer in immunosuppressed and immunocompetent individuals. *J Med Virol* 2000; **61**: 289–297.

152 Torbenson M, Wang J, Nichols L, Randhawa P, Nalesnik MA. Renal cortical neoplasms in long-term survivors of solid organ transplantation. *Transplantation* 2000; **15**: 864–868.

153 Curtil A, Robin J, Tronc F, Ninet J, Boissonnat P, Champsaur G. Malignant neoplasms following cardiac transplantation. *Eur J Cardiothorac Surg* 1997; **12**: 101–106.

154 Sleiman C, Mal H, Roue C, et al. Bronchial Kaposi's sarcoma after single lung transplantation. *Eur Respir J* 1997; **10**: 1181–1183.

155 Knowles DM, Cesarman E. The Kaposi's sarcoma-associated herpesvirus (human herpesvirus-8) in Kaposi's sarcoma, malignant lymphoma and other diseases. *Ann Oncol* 1997; **8**(Suppl 2): 123–129.

156 Lee ES, Locker J, Nalesnik M, et al. The association of Epstein–Barr virus with smooth muscle tumours occurring after organ transplantation. *N Engl J Med* 1995; **332**: 19–25.

24

Haematology

David Cummins

Harefield Hospital, Harefield, Middlesex, UK

Introduction

Haematological abnormalities are common in patients referred for lung transplantation and are among the most frequently observed complications of transplant surgery and immunosuppressive treatment. This chapter provides an overview of the most important haematological aspects of lung transplantation.

Haematological abnormalities in patients referred for lung transplantation

Cystic fibrosis

Cystic fibrosis (CF) may be associated with liver disease [1], secondary hypersplenism and vitamin K deficiency [2,3]. The former tends to be relatively uncommon in CF patients referred for lung transplantation, because of selection effects. (CF-related liver cirrhosis tends to develop before puberty [1], before major lung damage has had a chance to develop.) When present, liver disease may not be an absolute contraindication to isolated lung transplantation if the prothrombin time and other measures of hepatic synthetic function are normal [4]. Where liver and pulmonary function are both severely compromised, heart–lung–liver transplantation is an option [5].

Vitamin K is a fat-soluble vitamin required for synthesis of the procoagulant factors II, VII, IX and X. Deficiency of vitamin K may develop in CF because of pancreatic insufficiency, liver disease, inadequate dietary intake of the vitamin, or the effects of antibiotics on vitamin K synthesis by gut flora. The frequency of vitamin K deficiency in CF patients is unclear: some believe it to be common [2], while others believe it to be very uncommon [3]. In most vitamin K deficient patients, the prothrombin time and

other haemostatic variables remain normal [2]; thus, any CF patient who develops unexplained bleeding should receive vitamin K therapy regardless of the results of routine coagulation tests.

Finally, CF is of considerable importance to the transfusionist, because repeated pulmonary infections in CF patients lead to pleural and pericardial adhesions, increasing the risk of haemorrhage during transplant surgery [6].

Alpha-1-antitrypsin deficiency

Alpha-1-antitrypsin (AAT) deficiency, like CF, is an important cause of acquired liver disease. Cirrhosis and hepatic carcinoma are reported to affect at least 25% of AAT-deficient adults over the age of 50 years and may be unaccompanied by overt clinical manifestations [7]. Though severe lung and liver disease rarely coexist in patients with AAT, the author has seen one AAT-deficient patient who developed profound coagulopathy after lung transplantation and was found at autopsy to have unsuspected cirrhosis.

Pulmonary hypertension

Longstanding pulmonary arterial hypertension (whether primary or due to Eisenmenger's syndrome) is important haematologically because of its association with chronic hepatic venous congestion and cardiac cirrhosis. Studies have shown that the presence of severe liver abnormalities prior to surgery is a strong predictor of haemorrhage and death in patients undergoing heart–lung transplantation [8,9].

Many patients with chronic respiratory failure develop secondary polycythaemia; those affected should be regarded as potentially suitable candidates for isovolaemic haemodilution immediately prior to the transplant procedure.

Heparin-induced thrombocytopenia

Type II heparin-induced thrombocytopenia (HIT) is a serious complication of heparin treatment [10–12]. Its pathogenesis involves the development of a heparin-dependent antibody that causes widespread platelet agglutination in vivo. Patients who develop HIT antibody are at risk of developing arterial and venous thrombosis if they are re-exposed to heparin. Safe anticoagulation of such patients during cardiopulmonary bypass can be achieved with danaparoid (an inhibitor of factor Xa) or lepirudin (recombinant hirudin, a direct thrombin inhibitor) [10,12].

Antiphospholipid antibodies and other prothrombotic abnormalities

Lung transplantation has been carried out in patients with pulmonary hypertension associated with systemic lupus erythematosus and/or antiphospholipid antibodies, but these patients may be at increased risk for thrombotic complications postoperatively [13]. A lupus anticoagulant was the commonest haemostatic abnormality identified in a series of 72 patients who underwent lung transplantation or other surgical treatment for unresolved pulmonary embolism [14]. The requirement for long-term oral anticoagulation in lung transplant patients with prothrombotic states has implications for the management of transbronchial lung biopsies and other invasive procedures. Such interventions can generally be performed after temporary discontinuation of warfarin and substitution of low molecular weight heparin.

Haematological malignancies

Lung transplantation has been used as a treatment for radiation-induced lung damage in a patient cured of Hodgkin's disease [15], for bleomycin-induced lung fibrosis in a patient cured of acute lymphoblastic leukaemia [16], and for chronic graft-versus-host disease following allogeneic bone marrow transplantation [17]. Potentially, chemotherapy administered prior to lung transplantation may diminish bone marrow reserve, increasing patients' sensitivity to myelosuppressive agents.

Haematological aspects of donor-recipient matching

Donor-recipient ABO matching

Except where infants [18] are concerned, hearts and lungs must be transplanted only from donors who are ABO-compatible with the prospective recipient. Otherwise, the graft may undergo hyperacute rejection, a process in which host anti-A and/or anti-B antibodies bind to ABO antigens on donor endothelial cells and provoke an acute vascular injury. In a survey of 4895 heart transplants performed at 66 centres worldwide, eight patients (0.16%) received ABO-incompatible hearts, five (63%) of which underwent hyperacute rejection [19]. Transplant units must therefore establish effective procedures to guard against the possibility of inadvertently transplanting across a major ABO barrier. (Why some ABO-incompatible organs do not get rejected is unclear, but in some cases may reflect weak expression of ABO antigens [20] on donor vascular endothelium.)

Passenger lymphocyte syndrome

Because of the shortage of suitable donors, hearts and lungs are sometimes transplanted into patients that are ABO-incompatible with the donor (i.e. group O organs are given to an A, B or AB recipient). Such 'minor' ABO-mismatched transplants are of no clinical consequence in heart transplant patients, but about two thirds of heart–lung recipients develop immune-mediated red cell destruction 4–12 days after surgery [21]. This phenomenon, which has also been reported after single lung transplantation [22,23], is caused by antigenic stimulation of lymphoid tissue transferred with the graft. Generally the haemolysis is short lived, though donor ABO antibodies may persist in the recipient for over one year post-transplantation [21]. Thus all ABO-mismatched lung and heart–lung transplant patients should be carefully monitored for evidence of immune-mediated haemolysis (anaemia, hyperbilirubinaemia, red cell spherocytosis on the blood film, a positive direct antiglobulin test, etc.) in the postoperative period. Those who develop severe anaemia should be transfused with group O red cell concentrates [21].

Donor–recipient matching for Rh (D)

Outside the ABO system, Rh (D) is by far the most immunogenic red cell antigen, and outside the transplant setting anti-D antibody is an important cause of transfusion reactions and haemolytic disease of the newborn. The risk of sensitizing a D-negative patient by a D-positive donor heart and/or lung graft is low, probably in part because of the effects of ciclosporin [24], and there is no requirement to match donors and recipients for Rh (D). However, because the volume of red cells transferred with heart–lung transplants is relatively large, and because there are relatively few data concerning D sensitization in heart–lung transplant recipients, it is policy at our hospital to administer anti-D immunoglobulin to all unsensitized premenopausal

D-negative females who receive a heart–lung transplant from a D-positive donor [24]. (We usually administer 2500 U anti-D within 48 hours of surgery and assess the need for additional anti-D by flow cytometry [25].)

One case has been described in which a D-positive heart–lung transplant patient developed severe haemolysis caused by anti-D of donor origin [26]. Because the frequency of anti-D in the thoracic organ donor population is low, and because haemolysis caused by donor anti-D is rare, it is not practice in the UK to screen thoracic organ transplant donors for anti-D antibody.

Complications of the transplant procedure

Haemorrhage

Bleeding is the most important early complication after lung and heart–lung transplantation, and the blood transfusion requirements of these patients are considerable [6]. Surgical trauma is the most important aetiological factor, particularly in patients with severe chronic inflammatory changes and dense pleural and pericardial adhesions. Other important causes include pre-existing coagulation abnormalities (especially those caused by hepatic venous congestion [9] and deficiency or antagonism of vitamin K), and the adverse haemostatic effects of cardiopulmonary bypass (dilution and activation of clotting factors, thrombin generation, stimulation of fibrinolysis, heparin effects, and most importantly, activation and degranulation of platelets in the bypass circuit) [27].

Important preventative measures include careful patient selection (major liver abnormalities should be regarded as a contraindication to isolated lung transplantation [28]); optimal surgical technique, with adequate access to the pleural space and, with heart–lung and double lung transplants, the posterior mediastinum; reversal of coumarin effect with vitamin K and fresh frozen plasma [29]; and, in patients undergoing cardiopulmonary bypass, use of pharmacological agents such as aprotinin [30,31]. A potent serine protease inhibitor, aprotinin has been shown to reduce perioperative blood loss in a variety of high risk surgical procedures. The precise mechanism of its therapeutic effect remains unknown but probably involves mitigation of the systemic inflammatory response to cardiopulmonary bypass [32].

Most postoperative bleeding has a surgical basis and requires surgical management, though optimization of the patient's haematocrit and clotting status can be achieved through transfusion of red cells, platelets, fresh frozen plasma, and, in selected cases, cryoprecipitate. Such treatment should be guided wherever possible by the re-sults of simple laboratory or bedside tests (prothrombin time, partial thromboplastin time, fibrinogen concentration, activated clotting time, thromboelastography, etc.). In practice, however, the severity of bleeding, and the high frequency with which platelet dysfunction and coagulation abnormalities develop, often require that therapy be administered largely on an empirical basis. The exception is fibrinogen replacement (typically by use of cryoprecipitate), which should be given only to patients whose plasma fibrinogen concentration falls below 0.8 g/L [33]. The thromboelastogram is discussed in Chapter 15.

Heparin-induced thrombocytopenia

The diagnosis of HIT after cardiopulmonary bypass is problematic [11]: first, because thrombocytopenia that develops in this context has a number of causes, many of which are not readily distinguishable from HIT; and, second, because none of the laboratory tests available for detection of HIT antibody has both high sensitivity and high specificity [34]. For this reason we generally reserve HIT antibody testing for patients who develop thrombocytopenia in association with unexplained thrombosis and those in whom a rapidly falling platelet count cannot be satisfactorily attributed to a cause other than heparin [11]. Ultimately, however, the diagnosis of HIT must be based largely on clinical impression [34].

Once HIT has been diagnosed, cessation of all forms of heparin exposure is mandatory. Effective, alternative anticoagulation can be achieved with either danaparoid or lepirudin. Retrospective studies have suggested that the risk of haemorrhage may be greater with lepirudin, though its effects are easier to monitor (by means of the activated partial thromboplastin time) [12]. However, lepirudin is expensive and, because it is renally excreted, needs to be used with caution in patients with impaired renal function. Moreover, there is no simple, readily available antidote for patients who bleed while they are receiving the drug.

Anaemia

Anaemia may develop in lung transplant patients for a number of reasons, the most important of which are perioperative haemorrhage, haemolysis caused by donor ABO antibodies (see above), infections (both viral and bacterial), and myelosuppressive drugs (particularly azathioprine and ganciclovir). There is, in addition, a particular type of anaemia that occurs in lung and heart–lung transplant patients that seems to represent a distinct clinicopathological entity [35–37].

In one study [35] significant anaemia (haemoglobin <10 g/dL) was present in 31% of heart–lung transplant

recipients six months after transplantation, and persisted in 18% of patients beyond two years. The prevalence of anaemia was unrelated to the type of immunosuppressive therapy administered, though affected patients seemed unduly sensitive to the myelosuppressive effects of azathioprine. The disorder shares a number of features with the 'anaemia of chronic disease': the red cell indices are normochromic and normocytic, reticulocyte counts are unremarkable, and reticuloendothelial iron stores are usually plentiful but associated with a low serum iron and low or normal iron-binding capacity [35].

A subsequent study [36] showed that serum erythropoietin levels in both anaemic and nonanaemic lung transplant recipients are decreased compared to controls, a finding that offers a rationale for use of recombinant erythropoietin [37]. However, such therapy is costly and has several side effects (hypertension is perhaps the most important in this clinical context). Erythropoietin should therefore generally be reserved for transplant patients who develop anaemia that cannot be attributed to other causes and which significantly impairs quality of life.

Graft rejection

Acute cellular rejection may be associated with a variety of changes in the peripheral blood but, with the possible exception of the eosinophil count, none of these changes is sufficiently sensitive or specific to be useful as a diagnostic marker. Eosinophilia has been shown to be an early marker of graft rejection in both renal and hepatic allograft recipients, and an increase in the eosinophil count also seems to accompany pulmonary allograft rejection [38]. However, the magnitude of this effect is small (the circulating eosinophil count remains well within normal limits) and its detection requires frequent monitoring by flow cytometry.

Haematological aspects of immunosuppressive therapy

Reversible myelosuppression

The agents used most frequently to prevent graft rejection after heart and lung transplantation are ciclosporin, azathioprine and corticosteroids. Ciclosporin inhibits the release of cytokines, particularly interleukin (IL) 2 and interferon, from T helper cells through inhibition of lymphokine genes at the transcriptional level [39]. The drug may slightly reduce circulating lymphocyte numbers, but otherwise has negligible effects on the peripheral blood count.

Azathioprine, by contrast, causes significant myelosuppression, largely through the action of its metabolites, the 6-thioguanine nucleotides [40]. The white blood cell count must therefore be monitored frequently in patients receiving azathioprine, and the drug must be temporarily discontinued if neutropenia develops. Unfortunately, people vary considerably in their sensitivity to the drug's myelosuppressive effects. Monitoring of red cell 6-thioguanine nucleotide levels has been suggested as one way by which therapy can be tailored to the metabolic capacity of individual patients [40].

The myelosuppressive effects of azathioprine are greatly increased in patients who receive concurrent allopurinol therapy for control of hyperuricaemia [41]. (Hyperuricaemia is common in heart and lung transplant patients, partly because ciclosporin inhibits uric acid excretion by the kidney [42].) It is widely recommended that the dose of azathioprine should be reduced by at least two thirds in patients who receive the combination therapy; failure to follow this recommendation can lead to severe myelosuppression [41] and death [43]. The uricosuric agent benzbromarone has been shown to reduce uric acid levels in renal transplant patients without causing myelosuppression [44]. Generally, however, we discontinue azathioprine in patients who require urate-lowering therapy and substitute mycophenolate mofetil (see below).

Corticosteroids have numerous haematological effects [45], including neutrophilia, monocytosis, thrombocytosis, polycythaemia, lymphocytopenia and eosinopenia. Perhaps the most important of these in the transplant setting is neutrophilia, which occurs commonly in the early post-transplantation period and can mask the bone marrow response to bacterial infection.

Two other immunosuppressive drugs often used in thoracic organ transplant patients are tacrolimus (FK-506) and mycophenolate mofetil. Both agents may have a role in reversing acute rejection that is refractory to standard immunosuppression [46]. The haematological effects of tacrolimus are mild and similar to those of ciclosporin (see above). Mycophenolate, on the other hand, may cause leucopenia, anaemia and thrombocytopenia, which in some cases necessitates the drug's withdrawal [47,48].

Recently, two patients were described who developed striking morphological abnormalities in their circulating neutrophils while receiving mycophenolate mofetil (Figure 24.1) [49]. In both patients the changes heralded the development of neutropenia and were thus a sign of impending haematological toxicity. The mechanism was unclear but probably involved inhibition of guanosine nucleoside synthesis [50]. In both cases the abnormalities resolved after the drug was discontinued.

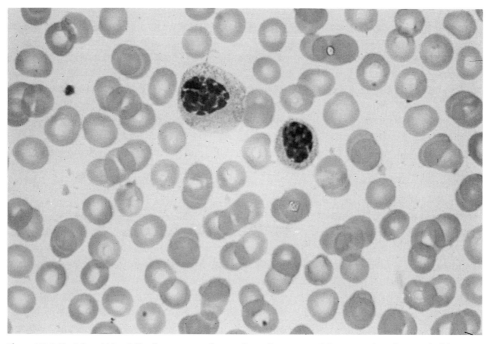

Figure 24.1 Peripheral blood film from a transplant patient who was receiving mycophenolate mofetil because of persistent graft rejection. Two nonlobed neutrophils are present, both of which show coarse chromatin clumping. (May–Grunwald Giemsa stain. 70×.) (Reproduced with permission from ref. 49.)

Red cell alloimmunisation

Despite their huge exposure to foreign red cells [6], heart and lung transplant patients develop red cell alloantibodies infrequently [24]. This phenomenon, which has also been observed in liver transplant patients [51], is probably due to the effects of ciclosporin on the primary immune response [24]. Ciclosporin, however, has no effect on secondary immune responses [52], and lung transplant patients with red cell alloantibodies are at risk of developing severe immune-mediated haemolysis if they are transfused with red cells expressing the corresponding antigen(s) [24].

Graft-versus-host disease

Graft-versus-host disease (GVHD) involves an attack by donor-derived immunocompetent cells on host tissues which express human leukocyte antigen (HLA) class I antigens. The condition is characterized by fever, skin rash, liver abnormalities and bone marrow suppression. In the solid-organ transplant setting, clinical GVHD is rare [53,54], in part because the level of host immunosuppression is seldom severe enough to allow its development. By contrast, histological changes consistent with GVHD ('pseudo-

GVHD') may be relatively common [55], though there is no evidence that such findings are of major clinical importance. For these and other reasons, it is not current practice to administer irradiated blood components to patients undergoing heart and/or lung transplantation in the UK.

Haemolytic-uraemic syndrome/thrombotic thrombocytopenic purpura

Haemolytic-uraemic syndrome (HUS) and the closely related disorder thrombotic thrombocytopenic purpura (TTP) are infrequent but potentially serious complications of solid organ transplantation [56]. Over 90% of reported cases have been in renal transplant patients, with only 1% occurring in lung and heart transplant recipients [56–58]. Affected patients develop fever, drowsiness, microangiopathic haemolysis, thrombocytopenia and renal failure. In approximately 50% of renal transplant patients and in almost all nonrenal solid organ transplant recipients ciclosporin or tacrolimus has been implicated in the pathogenesis [56]. Infective causes, though common outside the transplant setting [59], are rare in solid organ transplant patients [56]. Interestingly, we have seen a heart transplant patient who developed acute TTP in association with disseminated toxoplasmosis [60]. Treatment of HUS/TTP may require discontinuation of ciclosporin/tacrolimus, haemodialysis, plasma exchange, and, in refractory cases, use of defibrotide [60].

Acute leukaemia and myelodysplasia

Both acute lymphoblastic leukaemia and acute myeloblastic leukaemia (AML) have been reported after thoracic organ transplantation. One recently reported case of the former was shown to be of B-cell origin and appeared to represent a form of post-transplantation lymphoproliferative disease (see below): the leukaemic blasts were Epstein–Barr virus (EBV) positive, showed Burkitt-like features, and contained a t(8:14) translocation [61].

In a series of 631 patients who underwent heart transplantation at a single centre, four cases of AML and one case of myelodysplasia were identified [62]. This incidence of myeloid neoplasia is substantially higher than that in the general population and may reflect a number of factors, including chronic immune suppression, the mutagenic effects of azathioprine, and radiation exposure during diagnostic procedures. Leukaemia in this context is invariably fatal [62]. At our hospital we recently treated a patient (Figure 24.2) who developed acute myelomonoblastic leukaemia five years after heart transplantation. He died from overwhelming sepsis during remission induction.

Viral infection

Cytomegalovirus

Cytomegalovirus (CMV) infection is a potentially serious complication of solid organ transplantation, but because of the scarcity of suitable thoracic organs, many transplant centres no longer match transplant donors and patients for CMV antibody status. Most CMV infections that occur in lung transplant recipients represent either a primary infection acquired from the graft or reactivation of latent CMV infection in the host. However, approximately 50–60% of UK blood donors have serological evidence of previous CMV exposure, and CMV is readily transmissable via cellular blood components. The risk of transmitting CMV via (CMV-unscreened) leukodepleted blood components appears to be low [63]. Nevertheless, because transmission of CMV to lung transplant patients can be lethal, many centres are still using only CMV-negative components for CMV-negative recipients of CMV-negative donor grafts.

CMV infection in both immunocompetent and immunosuppressed patients is a well-recognized cause of leukopenia, thrombocytopenia and the appearance of atypical lymphocytes on the blood film [64]. Ganciclovir, an anti-

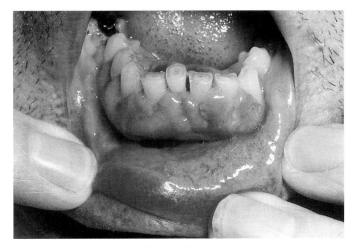

Figure 24.2 Acute myelomonoblastic leukaemia in a thoracic organ transplant recipient. The patient presented with gum hypertrophy due to leukaemic infiltration.

viral agent often used to treat CMV infection, also causes leukopenia [65], largely via bone marrow suppression. CMV-infected patients who develop severe neutropenia may be suitable candidates for treatment with recombinant growth factor granulocyte–macrophage colony stimulating factor or granulocyte colony stimulating factor [66,67].

Hepatitis C

The blood transfusion requirements of patients undergoing heart and lung transplantation are substantial [6] and, prior to the introduction of screening of blood donors in 1991 for antibody to hepatitis C virus (HCV) antibody, these patients were at relatively high risk of becoming infected with HCV. At our hospital, 15 (2.1%) of 724 surviving patients who underwent transplantation between 1980 and 1995 were positive for HCV antibody, and two-thirds of these patients were also positive for HCV RNA [68]. Abnormalities of liver function were relatively common in polymerase chain reaction-positive subjects, and some patients had histopathological evidence of chronic hepatitis. Thus the frequency of persistent HCV infection in our antibody-positive transplant recipients seems to be higher than that reported in antibody-positive immunocompetent subjects, and liver disease in this population may pursue a more aggressive clinical course. The long-term outcome remains to be established.

Parvovirus

Infection with parvovirus B19 has been implicated in a variety of clinical syndromes, including fifth disease, acute monarticular arthropathy, thrombocytopenia, exacerbation of anaemia in patients with chronic haemolysis, and neonatal hydrops fetalis [69]. Parvovirus preferentially infects erythroid progenitors, leading to arrest of red cell production [70]. In immunocompetent subjects this effect is self-limiting and only of clinical importance in patients with a coexistent haemolytic state. In immunosuppressed patients, however, the virus may persist and cause severe transfusion-dependent anaemia [71,72]. The red cell indices in such cases are usually normochromic and normocytic, reticulocytes are absent from peripheral blood, and bone marrow examination reveals profound erythroid hypoplasia, sometimes with presence of giant proerythroblasts.

All lung transplant recipients who develop acute, unexplained anaemia should be tested for presence of parvovirus-specific DNA and IgM anti-parvovirus antibody. High dose intravenous gammaglobulin has been shown to be safe and effective in promoting viral clearance and recovery of erythropoiesis [71,72].

Varicella-zoster virus

Infection with the varicella-zoster virus (VZV) is an important cause of morbidity after solid organ transplantation [73,74]. The greatest risk seems to be in patients who lack immunity to the virus and who receive corticosteroids during the prodrome of the illness. Infection in such circumstances may pursue a fulminant course complicated by pneumonitis, multiorgan failure and disseminated intravascular coagulation (Figure 24.3) [75]. The mortality rate in these cases is high, regardless of treatment.

Transplant-related lymphoproliferative disease

The virology and histopathology of post-transplantation lymphoproliferative disease (PTLD) are covered in chapters 20 and 23. Most cases of PTLD in lung transplant recipients are related to latent infection with EBV [76]. In many cases the disease remains confined to the pulmonary allograft, though extranodal and systemic involvement (Figure 24.4) may occur. Some patients respond, at least initially, to a reduction in pharmacological immunosuppression with or without administration of antiviral therapy. However, refractory cases are common and exhibit clinical and histopathological features that are frequently indistinguishable from those of high grade non-Hodgkin's lymphoma. A wide variety of therapies have been used to treat such patients but, because of the condition's rarity and the absence of controlled studies, assessing the relative efficacy of these therapies is difficult. We have treated several such patients with weekly courses of combination chemotherapy comprising prednisolone, adriamycin, (doxorubicin) cyclophosphamide, bleomycin and vincristine (PACEBO),

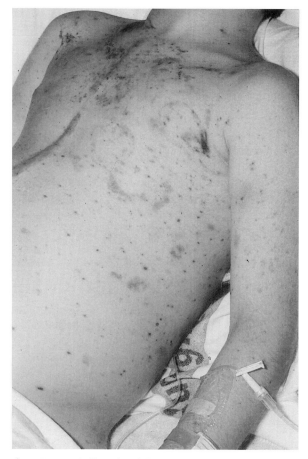

Figure 24.3 Varicella-induced disseminated intravascular coagulation in a heart–lung transplant recipient.

and have observed some gratifying responses. Other therapies that may be effective include interferon alpha [77], anti-CD20 monoclonal antibody [78], and infusions of EBV-specific cytotoxic T cells [79]. Defining the precise role of these treatments will require randomized, multicentre trials.

Conclusions

In attempting to cover the full haematological spectrum of lung transplantation, my coverage of individual subjects has inevitably been somewhat limited. Nevertheless, the interested reader will, I hope, have found the preceding pages a useful starting point from which to explore the subject in depth.

Recent years have seen important developments in this field, particularly in relation to blood transfusion therapy and the haematological effects of immunosuppressive treatment. However, many important challenges remain.

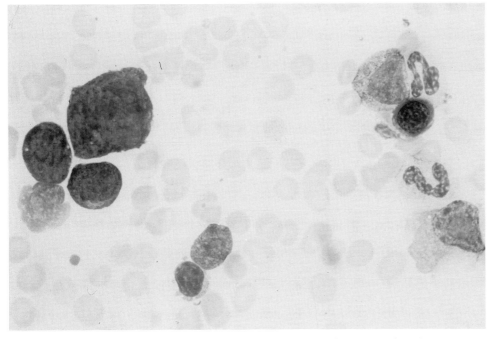

Figure 24.4 Bone marrow aspirate from a heart–lung transplant patient with post–transplantation lymphoproliferative disease. Large, abnormal lymphoid cells are present (May Grunwald Giema stain. 70×.)

There is increasing concern as to what effect the introduction of screening for variant Creuzfeldt–Jakob disease will have on the availability of homologous blood in the UK. Potentially, the impact could be considerable, requiring even greater emphasis to be placed on intraoperative blood conservation strategies, and a reassessment of the role of autologous transfusion. With PTLD, exciting developments in monoclonal antibody therapy and EBV-specific cytotoxic T-cell infusions offer the hope of radically improving the outlook for patients with refractory forms of the disease. Finally, it seems likely that lung transplantation will play an increasingly important role in the management of lung damage caused by primary haematological disorders and their treatment. These are interesting times for the transplant haematologist, and the next few years promise to be more interesting still.

REFERENCES

1 Lindblad A, Glaumann H, Strandvik B. Natural history of liver disease in cystic fibrosis. *Hepatology* 1999; **30**: 1151–1158.

2 Rashid M, Durie P, Andrew M, et al. Prevalence of vitamin K deficiency in cystic fibrosis. *Am J Clin Nutr* 1999; **70**: 378–382.

3 Cornelissen EA, van Lieburg AF, Motohara K, van Osstrom CG. Vitamin K status in cystic fibrosis. *Acta Paediatr* 1992; **81**: 658–661.

4 Klima LD, Kowdley KV, Lewis SL, Wood DE, Aitken ML. Successful lung transplantation in spite of cystic fibrosis-associated liver disease: a case series. *J Heart Lung Transplant* 1997; **16**: 934–938.

5 Dennis CM, McNeil KD, Dunning J, et al. Heart–lung–liver transplantation. *J Heart Lung Transplant* 1996; **15**: 536–538.

6 Hunt BJ, Sack D, Amin S, Yacoub MH. The perioperative use of blood components during heart and heart–lung transplantation. *Transfusion* 1992; **32**: 57–62.

7 Anonymous. Alpha 1-antitrypsin deficiency: memorandum from a WHO meeting. *Bull World Health Organ* 1997; **75**: 397–415.

8 Kramer MR, Marshall SE, Tiroke A, Lewiston NJ, Starnes VA, Theodore J. Clinical significance of hyperbilirubinaemia in patients with pulmonary hypertension undergoing heart–lung transplantation *J Heart Lung Transplant* 1991; **10**: 317–321.

9 Cummins D, Halil O, Amin S, Yacoub MH. Blood transfusion support for patients undergoing heart and lung transplantation: association with preoperative coagulation status. [Abstract.] *Br J Haematol* 1995; **89**(Suppl. 1): 49.

10 Farner B, Eichler P, Kroll H, Greinacher A. A comparison of dana-paroid and lepirudin in heparin-induced thrombocytopenia *Thromb Haemost* 2001; **85**: 950–957.

11 Cummins D, Halil O, Amin S. Which patients undergoing cardiopulmonary bypass should be assessed for development of heparin-induced thrombocytopenia? *Thromb Haemost* 1995; **73**: 890–891.

12 Pamboukian SV, Ignaszewski AP, Ross HJ. Management strategies for heparin-induced thrombocytopenia in heart transplant

candidates: case report and review of the literature. *J Heart Lung Transplant* 2000; **19**: 810–814.

13 Asherson RA, Higenbottam TW, Dinh Xuan AT, Khamashta MA, Hughes GR. Pulmonary hypertension in a lupus clinic: experience with twenty four patients. *J Rheumatol* 1990; **17**: 1292–1298.

14 Simoneau G, Azarian R, Brenot F, Darteville PG, Musset D, Duroux P. Surgical treatment of unresolved pulmonary embolism. A personal series of 72 patients. *Chest* 1995; **107**(1 Suppl): 52S–55S.

15 Putterman C, Polliack A. Late cardiovascular and pulmonary complications of therapy in Hodgkin's disease: report of three unusual cases, with a review of the literature. *Leuk Lymphoma* 1992; **7**: 109–115.

16 Santamauro JT, Stover DE, Jules-Elysee K, Maurer JR. Lung transplantation for chemotherapy-induced pulmonary fibrosis. *Chest* 1994; **105**: 310–312.

17 Rabitsch W, Deviatko E, Keil F, et al. Successful lung transplantation for bronchiolitis obliterans after allogenic bone marrow transplantation. *Transplantation* 2001; **71**: 1341–1343.

18 West LJ, Pollock-Barziv SM, Dipchand AI, et al. ABO-incompatible heart transplantation in infants. *N Engl J Med* 2001; **344**: 843–844.

19 Cooper DK. Clinical survey of heart transplantation between ABO blood group-incompatible recipients and donors. *J Heart Transplant* 1990; **9**: 376–381.

20 Ott GY, Norman D, Ratkovec RR, Hershberger RE, Hosenpud JD, Cobanoglu A. ABO-incompatible heart transplantation: a special case for the A_2 donor. *J Heart Lung Transplant* 1993; **12**: 504–507.

21 Hunt BJ, Yacoub MH, Amin S, Devenish A, Contreras M. Induction of red cell destruction by graft-derived antibodies after minor ABO-mismatched heart and lung transplantation. *Transplantation* 1988; **46**: 246–249.

22 Magrin GT, Street AM, Williams TJ, Esmore DS. Clinically significant anti-A derived from B lymphocytes after single lung transplantation. *Transplantation* 1993; **56**: 466–467.

23 Salerno CT, Burdine J, Perry EH, Kshetty VR, Hertz MI, Bolman RM. Donor-derived antibodies and hemolysis after ABO compatible but nonidentical heart–lung and lung transplantation. *Transplantation* 1998; **65**: 261–264.

24 Cummins D, Contreras M, Amin S, Halil O, Downham B, Yacoub MH. Red cell alloantibody development associated with heart and lung transplantation. *Transplantation* 1996; **59**: 1432–1435.

25 Johnson PRE, Tait RC, Austen EB, Shwe KH, Lee D. The use of flow cytometry in the quantitation and management of feto-maternal haemorrhage. *J Clin Path* 1995; **48**: 1005–1008.

26 Knoop CK, Andrien M, Antoine M, et al. Severe haemolysis due to a donor anti-D antibody after heart–lung transplantation. Association with lung and blood chimerism. *Am Rev Resp Dis* 1993; **148**: 504–506.

27 Webb AR, Shapiro MJ, Singer M, Suter PM, eds. *Oxford textbook of critical care*. Oxford Medical Publications, Oxford, 1998: 973–976.

28 Corris PA. Selection of patients' suitability for lung transplant assessment. In: Schofield PM, Corris PA, eds. *Management of heart and lung transplant patients*. BMJ Books, London, 1998: 15–16.

29 Karck M, Haverich A. Heart transplantation under coumarin therapy: friend or foe? *Eur J Anaesthesiol* 1994; **11**: 475–479.

30 Kesten S, de Hoyas A, Chaparro C, Westney G, Winton T, Maurer JR. Aprotinin reduces blood loss in lung transplant patients. *Ann Thorac Surg* 1995; **59**: 877–879.

31 Spray TL. Use of aprotinin in pediatric organ transplantation. *Ann Thorac Surg* 1998; **65**(6 Suppl): S71–S73.

32 Punjabi PP, Wyse RK, Taylor KM. Role of aprotinin in the management of patients during and after cardiac surgery. *Expert Opin Pharmacotherap* 2000; **1**: 1353–1365.

33 Blood Transfusion Task Force. Transfusion for massive blood loss. *Clin Lab Haematol* 1988; **10**: 265–273.

34 Walenga JM, Jeske WP, Fasanella AR, Wood JJ, Bakhos M. Laboratory tests for heparin-induced thrombocytopenia. *Semin Thromb Hemost* 1999; **25**(Suppl 1): 43–49.

35 Hunt BJ, Amin S, Halil O, Yacoub MH. The prevalence, course and characteristics of chronic anaemia after heart–lung transplantation. *Transplantation* 1992; **53**: 1251–1256.

36 End A, Stift A, Wieselthaler G, et al. Anaemia and erythropoietin levels in lung transplant patients. *Transplantation* 1995; **60**: 1245–1251.

37 End A, Ringl H, Grimm M, et al. Chronic anaemia after lung transplantation: treatment with recombinant erythropoietin. *Transplantation* 1994; **57**: 1142.

38 Trull A, Steel L, Cornelissen J, et al. Association between blood eosinophil counts and acute cardiac and pulmonary allograft rejection. *J Heart Lung Transplant* 1998; **17**: 517–524.

39 Granelli-Piperno A. Cellular mode of action of cyclosporine A. In: Bach JF, ed. *T-cell directed immunointervention*. Blackwell, Oxford, 1993: 3–25.

40 Schutz E, Gummert J, Mohr FW, Armstrong VW, Oellerich M. Should 6-thioguanine nucelotides be monitored in heart transplant recipients given azathioprine? *Ther Drug Monit* 1996; **18**: 228–233.

41 Cummins D, Sekar M, Halil O, Banner N. Myelosuppression associated with azathioprine–allopurinol interaction after heart and lung transplantation. *Transplantation* 1996; **61**: 1661–1662.

42 Burack DA, Griffith BP, Thompson ME, Kahl LE. Hyperuricaemia and gout among heart transplant recipients receiving cyclosporin. *Am J Med* 1992; **92**: 141–146.

43 Adverse Drug Reactions Advisory Committee. Allopurinol and azathioprine. Fatal interaction. *Med J Aust* 1980; **2**: 130.

44 Zurcher RM, Bock HA, Thiel G. Excellent uricosuric effect of benzbromarone in cyclosporin A-treated renal transplant patients: a prospective study. *Nephrol Dial Transplant* 1994; **9**: 548–551.

45 Athens JW. Variations in leukocytes in disease. In: Lee GR, Bithell TC, Foerster J, Athens JW, Lukens JN, eds. *Wintrobe's Clinical*

Haematology, 9th edn. Lea & Febiger, Pennsylvannia, 1993: 1564–1588.

46 Morris RE. Mechanisms of action of new immunosuppressive drugs. *Ther Drug Monitor* 1995; **17**: 564–569.

47 European Mycophenolate Mofetil Cooperative Study Group. Mycophenolate mofetil in renal transplantation: 3-year results from the placebo-controlled trials. *Transplantation* 1999; **68**: 391–396.

48 Kobashigawa J, Miller L, Renlund D, et al. A randomised active controlled trial of mycophenolate mofetil in heart transplant recipients. *Transplantation* 1998; **66**: 507–515.

49 Banerjee R, Halil O, Bain B, Cummins D, Banner N. Neutrophil dysplasia caused by mycophenolate mofetil. *Transplantation* 2000; **70**: 1608–1610.

50 Allison AC, Eugui EM. Purine metabolism and the immunosuppressive effects of mycophenolate mofetil. *Clin Transplant* 1996; **10**: 77–84.

51 Ramsey G, Hahn LF, Cornell FW, et al. Low rate of Rh-immunization from Rh-incompatible blood transfusions during liver and heart transplant surgery. Transplantation 1989; **47**: 993–995.

52 Jones AC. Power DA, Stewart KN, Catto GRD. Cyclosporin A prevents sensitization after blood transfusion in multiparous rats. *Clin Sci* 1988; **74**: 389–392.

53 Chau EM, Lee J, Yew WW, Chiu CS, Wang EP. Mediastinal irradiation for graft-versus-host-disease in a heart–lung transplant recipient. *J Heart Lung Transplant* 1997; **16**: 974–979.

54 Sola MA, España A, Redondo P, et al. Transfusion-associated graft-versus-host-disease in a heart transplant recipient. *Br J Dermatol* 1995; **132**: 626–630.

55 Herman JG, Beschorner WE, Baughman KL, Boitnott JK, Vogelsang GB, Baumgartner WA. Pseudo-graft-versus-host disease in heart and lung transplant recipients. *Transplantation* 1988; **46**: 93–98.

56 Singh N, Gayowski T, Marino IR. Hemolytic uremic syndrome in solid-organ transplant recipients. *Transpl Int* 1996; **9**: 68–75.

57 Mercadal L, Petitclerc T, Assogba U, Beaufils H, Deray G. Hemolytic and uremic syndrome after heart transplantation. *Am J Nephrol* 2000; **20**: 418–420.

58 Walder B, Ricou B, Suter PM. Tacrolimus (FK506)-induced hemolytic syndrome after heart transplantation. *J Heart Lung Transplant* 1998; **17**: 1004–1006.

59 Karmali MA, Petric M, Lim C, Fleming PC, Arbus GS, Lior H. The association between hemolytic uremic syndrome and infection by verotoxin-producing *E. coli. J Infect Dis* 1985; **151**: 775–782.

60 Cummins D, Jenkins G, Hall A, Banner N, Burke M. Thrombotic thrombocytopenic purpura in association with acute toxoplasmosis after cardiac transplantation. [Abstract.] *Br J Haematol* 1999; **67**(Suppl. 1): 40.

61 Tweddle DA, Gennery AR, Reid MM, et al. Posttransplantation B lymphoblastic leukaemia with Burkitt-like features. *Transplantation* 1999; **67**: 1379–1380.

62 Huebner G, Karthaus M, Pethig K, Freund M, Ganser A. Myelodysplastic syndrome and acute myelogenous leukaemia secondary to heart transplantation. *Transplantation* 2000; **70**: 688–690.

63 Pamphilou DH, Rider JR, Barbara JA, Williamson LM. Prevention of transfusion-transmitted cytomegalovirus infection. *Transfus Med* 1999; **9**: 115–123.

64 Elkins CC, Frist WH, Dummer JS, et al. Cytomegalovirus disease after heart transplantation: is acyclovir prophylaxis indicated? *Ann Thorac Surg* 1993; **56**: 1267–1272.

65 Keay S, Petersen E, Icenogle T, et al. Ganciclovir treatment of serious cytomegalovirus infection in heart and heart–lung transplant recipients. *Rev Infect Dis* 1988; **3**(10 Suppl): S563–S572.

66 Gordon MS, O'Donnell JA, Mohler ER III, Cooper MA. The use of granulocyte colony-stimulating factor in the treatment of fever and neutropenia in a heart transplant patient. *J Heart Lung Transplant* 1993; **12**: 706–707.

67 Ippolti G, Negri M, Rovati B, Grossi P, Vigano M. Sequential use of G-CSF and GM-CSF after heart-lung transplantation. *J Heart Lung Transplant* 1997; **16**: 473–475.

68 Cummins D, Banner N, Teo CG, et al. Hepatitis C infection among survivors of thoracic organ transplantation: prevalence, clinical significance and relationship to blood transfusion. [Abstract.] *Transf Med* 1996; **6**(Suppl. 2): 6.

69 Lee GR. The hemolytic disorders: general considerations. In: Lee GR, Bithell TC, Foerster J, Athens JW, Lukens JN, eds. *Wintrobe's Clinical Haematology*, 9th edn. Lea & Febiger, Pennsylvannia, 1993: 948–949.

70 Ozawa K, Kurtzman G, Young N. Productive infection by B19 parvovirus of human erythroid bone marrow cells in vitro. *Blood* 1987; **70**: 384–391.

71 Calvet A, Pujol MO, Bertocchi M, Bastien O, Boissonnat P, Mornex JF. Parvovirus B19 infection in thoracic organ transplant recipients. *J Clin Virol* 1999; **13**: 37–42.

72 Wicki J, Samii K, Cassinotti P, Voegeli J, Rochat T, Beris P. Parvovirus B19-induced red cell aplasia in solid-organ transplant recipients. Two case reports and review of the literature. *Hematol Cell Ther* 1997; **39**: 199–204.

73 McGregor RS, Zitelli BJ, Urbach AH, Malatack JJ, Gartner JC. Varicella in pediatric orthotopic liver transplant recipients. *Pediatrics* 1989; **83**: 256–261.

74 Charkes ND. Purpuric chickenpox: report of a case, review of the literature and classification by clinical features. *Ann Intern Med* 1961; **54**: 745–759.

75 Cummins D. Disseminated intravascular coagulation. In: Webb AR, Shapiro MJ, Singer M, Suter PM, eds. *Oxford textbook of critical care*. Oxford Medical Publications, Oxford, 1998: 668–670.

76 Swerdlow AL, Higgins CD, Hunt BJ, et al. Risk of lymphoid neoplasia after cardiothoracic transplantation: a cohort study of the relationship to Epstein–Barr virus. *Transplantation* 2000; **69**: 897–904.

77 Davis CL, Wood BL, Sabath DE, Joseph JS, Stehman-Breen C, Broudy VC. Interferon-alpha treatment of posttransplant

lymphoproliferative disorder in recipients of solid organ transplants. *Transplantation* 1998; **66**: 1770–1779.

78 Reynaud-Gaubert M, Stoppa AM, Gaubert J, Thomas P, Fuentes P. Anti-CD20 monoclonal antibody therapy in Epstein–Barr virus-associated B-cell lymphoma following lung transplantation. *J Heart Lung Transplant* 2000; **19**: 492–495.

79 Haque T, Amlot P, Helling N, et al. Reconstitution of EBV-specific T-cell immunity in solid organ transplant recipients. *J Immunol* 1998; **160**: 6204–6209.

25

Psychology

Claire N. Hallas and Jo Wray

Harefield Hospital, Harefield, Middlesex, UK

Introduction

The experience of living with chronic respiratory disease is documented in both medical and psychological literature [1,2] however these perspectives are rarely brought together within a medical textbook. Often psychological issues are seen as separate to symptoms, treatment and prognosis; however, this chapter aims to illustrate how the emotional experience of the patient is intrinsically related to their clinical status and management, rehabilitation and prognosis.

To achieve this aim, the chapter is divided into four sections. The first focuses on emotional, cognitive and social issues that are relevant to patients diagnosed with various respiratory conditions, the second discusses the assessment of candidates for lung transplantation, the third focuses on the specific psychological issues that are salient to lung transplant recipients and finally the role of the psychologist within the transplant team is discussed.

Living with respiratory disease: quality of life and psychological adjustment

The measurement of the quality of the outcome of treatment from the patient's perspective is becoming increasingly recognized as an important aspect of decision making in the provision of all aspects of health care. The term 'quality of life' (QoL) is nebulous and its definition and measurement have been a source of controversy and uncertainty in the literature. QoL has been defined in many ways, although for years it was described entirely in physical terms. However, it has become accepted that QoL is a complex concept, its definition comprising various dimensions of function and well-being. A popular definition of QoL that continues to remain relevant to contemporary research was first introduced in 1958 by the World Health Organization as 'a state

of complete physical, mental and social well-being and not merely the absence of disease or infirmity' [3]. This definition of QoL was expanded in 1995 to include 'individuals' perception of their position in life in the context of the culture and value systems in which they live and in relation to their goals, expectations, standards and concerns' [4].

Research investigating the impact of respiratory disease on emotional and physical QoL has focused on the major symptoms of the disease, such as dyspnoea, lung function and limitations in physical activity. Results have shown clear physical differences between the general age-matched population and those diagnosed with respiratory diseases [5]. However, the evidence for the causal effect of pulmonary function on psychological adjustment is unclear, particularly regarding whether differences exist between diagnostic groups. Current evidence suggests that subgroups of patients within respiratory diseases such as chronic obstructive pulmonary disease (COPD) may be more at risk of developing low mood [6], although some studies have contradicted these findings and shown that the prevalence of anxiety and depression does not differ between COPD and non-COPD patients [7]. It is also unclear whether psychological adjustment directly (e.g. via hyperventilation) and/or indirectly (e.g. via behaviour – not using oxygen when needed) affects mortality and morbidity.

It is clear that the most common emotions reported in response to dyspnoea and physical restrictions are mood disturbances, specifically anxiety and depression. Anxiety is particularly related to major restrictions on mobility and energy, difficulties with activities of daily living and dependence on others for care [8]. The main mediator of the relationship between anxiety and poor overall QoL has been identified as lack of sleep and fatigue [9–13]. It is postulated that breathing difficulties are most prevalent at night and significantly disrupt sleeping patterns. A cyclical pattern can develop when poor sleep develops due to worries associated with physical symptoms and psychosocial problems. Lack of sleep and fatigue can subsequently compound anxiety by interacting with any neuropsychological impairments. When a patient has high levels of fatigue and an inability to concentrate and utilize mental flexibility, this combination will significantly impair the patient's ability to employ problem-solving coping strategies to cope with persistent anxieties.

The aetiology of neuropsychological impairments in patients with end-stage respiratory disease can be generated through this synergistic combination of biological, psychological and social factors. Results from the literature indicate, however, that there is not a unique pattern of deficits presented in end-stage disease but instead the affected organs or system are associated with a diffuse cerebral lesion that can manifest itself either as severe and florid disturbances or as subtle but chronic neuropsychological impairments [14,15]. Subtle deficits can include problems with attention and concentration [16], short-term memory loss [17] and poor psychomotor efficiency and coordination [16]. Other areas of impairment have been noted in mental flexibility and abstract thinking, although whether this is pervasive or circumscribed to particular facets of capacity are unknown.

Depending on the respiratory impairment, a proportion of patients who have very limited activity suffer from chronic hypoxaemia, which is a significant predictor of poor prognosis. Long-term oxygen therapy has been shown to significantly improve survival, pulmonary haemodynamics and the frequency and length of hospitalizations; however, there appears to be little impact upon QoL, mood state or neuropsychological function for these patients [6,18].

The evidence for small benefits to QoL were shown by Janssens and colleagues [7]. These authors measured anxiety, depression, severity and frequency of respiratory symptoms, lung function tests, daily distance walked and dyspnoea ratings in a diagnostically heterogeneous group of 79 patients using long-term home-based oxygen therapy.

Results demonstrated that 21% of patients experienced clinical levels of anxiety and 27% clinical levels of depression. There were no differences in mood state between COPD and non-COPD patients and there was no significant change in mood state within 12 months. Anxiety and depression were not associated with dyspnoea scores or pulmonary function tests, but were significantly correlated with number of days spent in hospital over the preceding year. Depression was also significantly related to daily walking distance. Two mechanisms can explain these results; first, being in hospital severely restricts mobility, which increases fatigue through lack of exercise; and, second, many

days spent in hospital also indicate on a perceptual level that the disease may be deteriorating or that treatments are becoming less effective. These two conditions together could determine those individuals who are more susceptible to developing depressive states.

Other evidence suggests that a mediator of the relationship between mobility and depression when patients are at home is dependence on oxygen. Such dependence interferes with mobility due to the embarrassment of wearing oxygen masks, difficulties with managing activities outside of the home and the financial costs involved in acquiring small, mobile cylinders [19].

Studies investigating the psychological adjustment of adult cystic fibrosis (CF) patients have shown more positive outcomes. Anderson et al. [20] recently assessed 34 adults with CF and related their mental health to their objective lung function tests. Results showed that there were very low levels of clinical anxiety and depression in the population and no significant differences were shown in psychological functioning when groups were compared according to disease severity based on forced expiratory volume in 1 s (FEV_1) lung function tests. However, there was a significant main effect of gender that interacted with psychological and physical function; men were at higher risk of depression than women, and depression was significantly associated with more severe lung impairment.

Other studies have reported relatively normal adjustment in older adolescents and adults with CF [21], although some have suggested that there are elevated levels of anxiety (between 12% and 30%), depression and eating disorders [22,23]. Aspin [24] argued that older adolescents or adults with CF adapt well to their lifestyle and employ various coping strategies to deal with admissions to hospital, intravenous medication treatment and recurrent infections. Those CF patients who experience anxiety, depression and denial are those who have more severe symptoms at a younger age, have experienced personal loss (e.g. sibling death, divorce of parents), infertility, are lonely and isolated and have a poor self-esteem and body image.

Does respiratory disease cause panic anxiety to develop?

It has been previously shown that anxiety is one of the most common psychological responses to respiratory disease, with the greatest levels of anxiety associated with more intense dyspnoea and the sensation of impending suffocation. Intense, acute anxiety is associated with physical symptoms such as dyspnoea, palpitations, chest pain and cognitive fears such as a fear of dying or going crazy – this experience is described as a panic attack and is often reported by respiratory disease patients. However, panic anxiety may be uniquely discriminated from other types of anxiety due to the presence of dyspnoea and this in itself is the difficulty with managing panic anxiety in patients with respiratory disease [25]. Evidence currently suggests that the lifetime prevalence of respiratory diseases in patients with clinically diagnosed panic disorder is 47%, compared with 13% in patients with obsessive–compulsive disorder or an eating disorder. In addition the prevalence of panic disorder among respiratory patients appears to be disproportionately high at approximately 11% [26,27].

Therefore the relationship between panic anxiety and respiratory disease is complex, and the nature of this relationship continues to be debated, with evidence being generated from both physiological and psychological models [28–31]. Three models have been proposed to interpret the interrelationships between dyspnoea, panic and hyperventilation; the carbon dioxide hypersensitivity/ suffocation false alarm (HSFA) model, the cognitive–behavioural model and the hyperventilation model (HM) [2]. Evidence suggests that the HSFA model and the HM model may explain how some individuals have a biological susceptibility to developing dyspnoea through the hyperventilation of CO_2 and the triggering of medullary chemoreceptors; however, some conflicting evidence has found inconsistency for these theories, particularly as anxiety attacks can be aborted by some nonoxygen-dependent patients using paper bag re-breathing [32].

The cognitive–behavioural model may be more relevant to explain panic anxiety in respiratory patients, as neither pulmonary function testing nor response to bronchodilators differentiates patients with respiratory disease who panic and those who do not panic. However, those patients who panic have more catastrophic cognitions and fears about bodily sensations – and are more sensitized to interoceptive cues such as dyspnoea, chest tightness and tachycardia [33]. Individuals subsequently misinterpret these sensations as being more dangerous than they actually are, leading to a positive feedback cycle of escalating anxiety and physical symptoms that increases hyperventilation. It has also been shown that catastrophic thoughts tend to develop in response to symptoms or sensations that were unexpected [34]. Therefore it seems that many patients with respiratory disorders experience anxiety due to feelings of suffocation, fear and breathlessness, but that panic anxiety may develop from an unexpected attack of symptoms or sensations that sensitize the individual to misinterpret other regular sensations as catastrophic. In addition, medications used to treat respiratory disorders such as glucocorticoids, beta-adrenergic agonists and anticholinergics can also be anxiogenic – thus pulmonary disease may be a risk factor for the development of panic disorder, although pulmonary impairment is not directly associated with panic anxiety [27,28].

Theoretical rationale for psychological adaptation

As the major psychological responses to the experience of chronic respiratory disease have been highlighted, it seems appropriate to expand on the theoretical rationale for why only a proportion of patients develop negative and maladaptive emotional responses to pulmonary symptoms and function. Various health psychology theories have already been proposed for why certain individuals undertake health-related behaviours [35]. However, the rationale for the development of illness-related perceptions or cognitions that ultimately determine the emotional responses to illness and the motivation for undertaking health-related behaviours have been the centre of some debate. Evidence for the 'Self-Regulatory' theory or the 'Illness Perception' theory as it is also termed is compelling, nevertheless, as it illustrates the cognitive mechanisms that patients employ to adapt to and cope with their illness [36].

Leventhal et al. [36] described the theoretical model as 'the common sense representation of illness danger' and elaborated upon a self-regulatory system for cognitive and emotional activity that was involved in the construction of a representation of illness (Figure 25.1). It was postulated that this representation was conceptualized by five dimensions: causes (ideas that the person has about the cause of the disease), identity (the label placed on the disease and the symptoms associated with it), consequences (the expected outcome and sequelae of the disease), time-line (expectations about the duration and the course of the disease), and controllability/cure (beliefs about the extent to which the disease is amenable to control or cure). Illness perceptions based on these dimensions are developed in response to various individual experiences; however, evidence suggests that lay beliefs and previous experiences of illness and treatment are the primary basis for the development of illness perceptions. In addition, beliefs about medication and treatment are developed in response to these perceptions and these relationships are also illustrated in Figure 25.1.

A detailed account of the evidence for the illness perceptions theory is beyond the scope of this chapter; however, research has shown that cognitive representations of illness are significantly associated with health-related behaviours [37,38], coping strategies [39–41], psychological well-being and greater QoL in a variety of chronic illnesses [42,43].

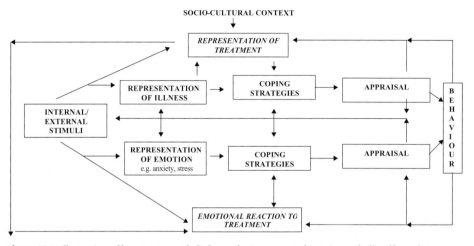

Figure 25.1 Illustration of how treatment beliefs may be incorporated into Leventhal's self-regulatory model and how the continuous feedback of appraisal mediates behaviour change

More recently, illness perceptions have been shown to affect the diagnosis and management of patients with respiratory disorders. In particular, more frequent and debilitating symptoms predict reduced QoL [44,45], lower self-esteem and self-efficacy [46], decreased adherence to self-management programmes and pulmonary rehabilitation [47–49] and social support [50].

One recent study by Scharloo [51] investigated sixty-four patients with COPD and measured the contribution of coping and beliefs about their illness to predict clinical outcome (FEV_1 and forced vital capacity (FVC)). In this longitudinal study, measures of spirometry, coping, functional status and illness perceptions were taken with a 12 month interval between them. Results indicated that perceptions of their illness 'identity' measured at the first assessment, significantly predicted social functioning and health perceptions 12 months later. More 'emotional attributions' (perceptions that others and stress have *caused* the illness) were significantly associated with an increased number of visits to the outpatient clinic over the 12 months.

Coping strategies significantly predicted social functioning, mental health and overall functional status. Passive coping in particular explained 26% of the variance in mental health. Furthermore, FEV_1 function at the first assessment significantly explained 15% of the variance in social functioning, 20% of the variance in perceptions of health and 12% of the variance in overall functional status 12 months later.

These results also confirm previous research [52–54] indicating that the 'identity' with which the person has labelled their disease, and the subsequent symptoms they associate with this label, predict health-related behaviours

(in this case greater attendance at the outpatient clinic and lower levels of sociability).

Therefore, although physical limitations can initiate maladaptive coping strategies, it is also clear that illness perceptions significantly contribute to the development of cognitive sensitivity to symptoms, sensations and treatment efficacy, leading to an overall reduction in emotional state that predicts QoL for patients with respiratory disease. In addition, the psychological profile of patients is of particular importance when their disease becomes end-stage and transplantation is the only treatment option.

End-stage disease: psychosocial assessment for lung transplantation

Clinical criteria for selecting transplant candidates focus on the functional capacity of the patient and his or her prognosis; however, as surgical techniques and medical treatments have improved survival, practitioners have become interested in the mental health of transplant recipients and its impact on postoperative recovery. Psychosocial assessment of transplant candidates has been a widespread practice for many years, with important ethical implications – and this is something of which psychologists and practitioners working within this area must be aware. Methodological and ethical issues relating to the assessment process of lung transplant candidates are important and are discussed below.

The majority of the ethical discussion surrounding psychosocial assessments of transplant candidates has originated from the USA, with position statements being proposed for their value [55] and for the potential discrimination of candidates and lack of validity [56,57]. Within the UK and Europe this debate has been limited, and wide variations exist within centres due to the scarcity of psychological services to transplant programmes. However, it is generally accepted that psychosocial criteria are employed for the following reasons:

1 To determine whether patients are sufficiently educated regarding their role and that of hospital procedures within the transplantation process and to ensure that the patient has adequate understanding in order to give informed consent.

2 To predict how patients will cope with the stress of major surgery.

3 To identify whether patients' perceptions of their illness and their expectations of the surgery are realistic.

4 To establish baseline measures of emotional, cognitive, social and behavioural function in order to be able to monitor postoperative changes.

5 To identify comorbid mental illness or maladaptive behaviours and plan interventions for these conditions.

6 To learn about the psychosocial needs of the patient and his or her family and plan services to assist them during the waiting, recovery and rehabilitation phases of the transplant process.

7 To help the transplant team understand the patient better as a person in order to provide more effective clinical care.

It should be made clear at this point that the psychosocial assessment of patients is *not* a means to rank order them in terms of eligibility for transplantation, or as a 'gatekeeping' function. The assessment should be utilized as a screening process to identify psychosocial factors that may place patients at risk of poor psychological and clinical outcome and to determine whether there is a need to implement an intervention to maximize the QoL benefits of transplantation for this candidate. In fact it is clearly stated within the UK Human Rights Act (2001) [58] and the Americans with Disabilities Act (1990) [56] that it is illegal to discriminate or disadvantage persons in need of healthcare (even when there are limited resources such as organs) on the basis of a mental health or psychosocial disability, provided that all possible services and health care provisions are in place to support their psychosocial needs.

Assessment tools

Assessments of transplant candidates are based upon individual need; however, a standard battery of tests should be implemented to measure various aspects of QoL and to facilitate a method of comparing and evaluating psychological outcomes. Various psychometric measures can be employed depending on the limitations of the patient and his or her current emotional and cognitive function, although it is also necessary to conduct a thorough interview with the patient. The literature indicates that previous psychiatric history and current mood state, neuropsychological function, QoL, illness perceptions and health-related behaviours (e.g. adherence), coping strategies, social networks and support should be assessed during the interview [55]. Brief screening measures encompassing the domains of attention, visuospatial capacity and psychomotor capacity can be administered to establish whether a full cognitive assessment is needed. Commonly used measures include the Trailmaking Test [59], Symbol Digit Modalities Test [60] and the Grooved Pegboard Test [61].

Although the literature has focused on a range of modality-specific psychometric measures, both as individual outcomes and summary assessments, no assessments have been specifically designed for lung transplant candidates. Two scaled formats that have been used to a limited degree to summarize the results of psychosocial assessments of various types of transplant candidates will be discussed here in conjunction with more respiratory specific measures.

The Psychosocial Assessment of Candidates for Transplant (PACT) has eight items that are rated on a five-point scale. Higher scores on the PACT indicate fewer psychological risk factors for transplantation [62]. The Transplant Evaluation Rating Scale (TERS) consists of 10 items rated on a three-point scale [63]. A prior psychiatric history (mood disorders) weights the highest on the TERS. Preliminary evidence indicates that the PACT and the TERS have reasonable internal consistency and that they correlate fairly highly with each other.

The PACT final rating and psychopathology subscale has been shown to predict mortality and referral for psychological treatment in liver, heart and bone marrow transplant recipients but its predictive qualities have not been tested for lung transplant recipients [62]. The TERS is a reliable instrument that utilizes a weighting system to predict clinical outcome from psychosocial characteristics. Adherence to medication and health care, overall success of the transplant and positive health-related behaviours have been significantly related to the overall TERS score. QoL was not, however, associated with the overall TERS score [63].

Prospective studies to document the predictive value of the TERS and PACT in addition to its relationship to patient reports of QoL have not been conducted. This is necessary, however, as evidence has previously shown that professional and patient reports of QoL do not correlate highly together [64]. Communication difficulties between the medical team and the patient and dissatisfaction with the health care process by the patient are often cited as the underlying factors for this nonsignificant relationship, which ultimately results in poor adherence to the treatment regime and misunderstanding and dissatisfaction from the medical team.

Various measures of health-related QoL specifically designed for assessing the impact of respiratory disease have been designed, although few studies have compared measures and outcomes. Lanuza et al. [65] recently reviewed the research literature investigating the QoL of single, double and bilateral-sequential lung transplant candidates. The authors examined the conceptual and operational definitions of QoL, identified measures used to assess QoL and determined relevant methodological issues. A number of recommendations were made as a result of the review: first, that the purpose of the assessment, the theoretical framework and the conceptual definition of QoL should guide any decisions regarding the selection of the QoL measurement tool. This tool should consider the generic and disease-specific dimensions of QoL, give consideration to the number and type of QoL dimensions to be measured and identify whether the individual's subjective evaluation or judgement of the value of the outcomes is important.

One study by Hajiro et al. [66] that compared the discriminant properties among three measures, the Breathing Problems Questionnaire (BPQ) [67], St George's Respiratory Questionnaire (SGRQ) [68] and the Chronic Respiratory Disease Questionnaire (CRQ) [69], indicated that there were no substantial differences between the measures in discriminating physiological parameters. It was shown, however, that the BPQ was less discriminatory than the SGRQ and the CRQ in evaluating QoL cross-sectionally. The CRQ was shown to be more influenced by psychological status than physiological function. These measures focus on the patient's experience of dyspnoea, fatigue, emotional function, mastery of their condition, symptoms, activity levels and the impact of the disease – and are typical of health-related QoL measures for respiratory diseases.

It is also important to note that a comprehensive assessment is conducted with ethical and professional principles in mind and that it is applied with the following guidelines (adapted from Orentlicher [56]):

1 The psychosocial assessment must find meaningful differences among candidates in the extent to which they will benefit from transplantation.
2 There must be a reliable process for undertaking psychosocial assessments.
3 Psychosocial assessments should be individualized and must reflect specific issues related to the patient, not generalizations.

4 Reasonable psychological and social services must be provided to assist patients to overcome the emotional, cognitive and/or social issues that may hinder them from maximizing any potential benefit from a transplant.

Psychosocial issues relating to live-lobe donors

Although this chapter focuses on the psychological issues relating to respiratory diseases and the psychosocial assessments of lung transplant candidates it is also worth mentioning that individuals who wish to donate a lung lobe to their relative with end-stage pulmonary disease also require rigorous psychosocial assessment. This assessment should include domains of function that have been previously mentioned but must also determine the donor's motivation to donate the lobe, the decision making process and coping strategies to undergo surgery themselves and to cope with the outcome of the recipient's surgery. Little information exists on the cognitive processes and decisions that live-lobe donors make, although this is an area of clinical progression, particularly as the supply of available donor lungs is insufficient to meet the demand of those individuals who are currently on the lung transplant waiting list.

Psychological issues after transplantation

Although it is now more than two decades since the first successful heart–lung transplant was carried out, most of the psychosocial literature on lung transplantation focuses only on global or physical-functional QoL [70]. In common with the findings for other transplant populations, marked improvement in overall function after lung transplantation has been widely demonstrated [71], although the literature on lung transplant recipients is rather less extensive and comprehensive than that for most other transplant groups. Physical function has received detailed attention and dominates the post-transplantation literature. In contrast, mental health outcomes in lung recipients have received far less consideration and have tended to be measured as part of broad quality of life evaluations or with brief situational mood measures [70]. To clarify the key psychological issues for lung recipients, a review of each area of functioning will be addressed individually.

Quality of life

Most of the literature looking at aspects of psychological functioning post-transplantation is concerned with an evaluation of 'quality of life'. Several prospective longitudinal [72–76] and cross-sectional [77,78] studies have described the QoL of lung and heart–lung candidates and recipients. Such studies have indicated that lung transplantation has a significant impact on, and affects a wide range of, QoL domains [79]. Prospective studies demonstrate significant improvements across many domains of health after transplantation (in one case the improvement was such that the patient was able to complete a marathon [80]). In particular, energy, physical functioning and mobility improve and symptoms such as breathlessness and anxiety reduce [8]. There are improvements in self-esteem and body image after transplantation [81], although functioning is at a lower level than that of a normative sample. However, there may be an increase in overall symptomatology that is probably attributable to adverse effects of immunosuppressive drugs (although it is not immunosuppression per se that does this) [82]. Whilst scores on health-related QoL indices have been found to be lower than for normative samples [82], Littlefield et al. [83] found that not only did lung recipients report better functioning than heart or liver transplant patients in physical, psychological and social domains but their level of functioning was equivalent to, or better than, those of a normative sample. Recipients' perceptions of satisfaction with life and health are also significantly more positive after transplantation than before [75].

There is little information on differences in QoL between different diagnostic groups. CF has been the exclusive focus of attention in some studies [73,76,84,85] and a further study looked at differences between heart–lung and single lung patients who had emphysema [86], but small sample sizes have tended to preclude meaningful comparisons. A further limitation of many studies is their cross-sectional nature – comparing candidates with recipients, with the additional factor of small sample sizes, makes interpretation difficult at best. Changes in QoL at different time points after transplantation have also been assessed cross-sectionally [74,87] and longitudinally [8,72,77,86]. In those studies assessing the same patient cohort at different time intervals, no significant changes in QoL scores were found.

Three studies have addressed patients' satisfaction with their decision to undergo transplantation [75,77,88] and found that almost 90% were very satisfied with their decision and 91% would encourage others to undergo transplantation. However, no attempts were made to offer any theoretical understanding of the decision making process to undergo transplantation or to assess potential response bias.

One further finding addressed in a number of studies is that, although recipients report improved QoL, functioning and satisfaction as compared with before transplantation,

relatively few return to work [77,83,88]. Working prior to transplantation, an underlying diagnosis of emphysema, cystic fibrosis or primary pulmonary hypertension and a belief in being physically able to work distinguished recipients who were employed from those who were not, but type of lung transplantation procedure did not determine employment [89]. In contrast, one study of 31 lung transplant recipients five years after transplantation found that 23 (74%) were working full-time and had no limitations in daily living [90].

Postoperative organic mental syndromes

In a study of 30 patients, 22 (73%) demonstrated one or more organic mental syndromes during the first 14 days after lung transplantation [91], 16 of whom had delirium with severe agitation, hallucinations and/or delusions. Undergoing cardiopulmonary bypass, having higher ciclosporin levels and moving house from a distant location to await surgery were associated with an increased risk of postoperative delirium. Anxiety, agitation, disorientation, nightmares and psychosis associated with the use of ciclosporin have been reported in liver transplant recipients [92]. With the lung transplant recipients, the presence of agitation and delirium complicated their medical management and also resulted in some instances in nonadherence with required procedures. Such difficulties led the Toronto Group to introduce the routine administration of intravenous haloperidol for the first 10 postoperative days, which was effective in minimizing anxiety and agitation and improving patient alertness and cooperation [91].

Depression

Few studies specifically address depression, despite the anecdotal evidence for the significance of depression in lung recipients. A prospective evaluation of 24 patients found significant improvements in depression scores from preoperative levels, which were higher than reported norms [8]. In contrast, Limbos et al. [93] found no differences in depression scores in female patients who were waiting for ($n = 7$) or had undergone ($n = 84$) lung transplantation, although the disparate group sizes and cross-sectional nature of the comparison makes meaningful interpretation of such results difficult. Use of mean depression scores can also give a misleading picture, as Stilley et al. [70] found with their post-transplantation sample. Whilst the mean level of depression was not significantly higher than in the normative sample, the proportion of recipients with clinically meaningful depression was relatively large.

Anxiety

In contrast to depression, elevated mean levels of anxiety have been more widely reported in lung recipients [70, 81], with clinically significant anxiety present in a sizeable proportion [70,93]. Such findings are consistent with the documented high prevalence of anxiety symptoms in patients with chronic lung disease [11] and also indicate that anxiety remains relatively common after transplant. In contrast, Caine et al. [74] found that mean anxiety scores and prevalence of clinically significant anxiety dropped significantly from pretransplant levels and did not differ from normative levels after transplantation. However, these were all heart–lung recipients, an unspecified number of whom had a previous diagnosis of Eisenmenger's syndrome rather than of a primary lung condition.

Attitudes to the donor

Adequate incorporation of the transplanted organs into the body image is considered as a prerequisite for the long-term success of organ transplantation [94]. In a study assessing patients' attitudes to different allografts, Schlitt et al. [94] found that optimal identification with the graft was better in lung recipients (75%) than in any other organ group, with female gender, higher educational level and better graft function being associated with optimal integration of the graft. Lung recipients also expressed greater interest in their donors.

Attitudes of recipients to donors in living donor lung transplant programmes suggest that when the recipient does well, there are psychosocial benefits for both recipient and donor, but that when the recipient experiences rejection of the donor's lobe, or other related complications, there are significant difficulties for the donor [95]. However, Cohen et al. [96] reported that, for donors, 'quality of life and satisfaction with having participated are uniformly high' – even in instances where the recipient died.

Recipient attitudes to the living donor have not been extensively studied. Adolescent recipients express multiple concerns about such donors from moral, social and pragmatic perspectives and indicate clear preferences for acceptability of lobes from given donors [95].

Complications

Chronic transplant dysfunction is the major complication after lung transplantation. Despite bronchiolitis obliterans syndrome (BOS) affecting nearly half of the long-term survivors of heart–lung and lung transplantation and being the major cause of mortality after the first postoperative year, the psychological implications have received scant attention. Comparison of patients with and without BOS indicated poorer health-related QoL in those with BOS [77,97], with pain in particular worsening with BOS [77]. Other complications, such as acute rejection episodes and cytomegalovirus pneumonitis, may be risk factors for the development of obliterative bronchiolitis but the indications are that these complications do not influence health-related QoL, with a reduction in health-related QoL becoming apparent only after a diagnosis of BOS [97]. This may also suggest that it is being given a diagnosis of BOS and its likely prognosis, with its concomitant cognitions, that affects a patient's perceptions of their functioning and levels of pain rather than BOS per se causing the changes, at least in the early stages after BOS is diagnosed.

With a lack of effective treatment for BOS, retransplantation offers the only chance of improved well-being. Despite the numerous psychological and ethical issues involved and the increasing numbers of single and double lung retransplantations now being performed, no systematic evaluation of patients' decision making processes to consent to, or refuse, a second transplant has been undertaken, nor has there been any attempt to assess psychological functioning in this group of patients.

Adherence to treatment and follow-up

With the increasing numbers of successful organ transplants has come an increase in the number of patients displaying nonadherence in medication and follow-up care resulting in graft loss [98]. Nonadherence has been reported in heart [99] and kidney [100,101] recipients and has been found to worsen over time [99]. Pretransplant adherence has been identified as a significant predictor of survival after transplantation in heart [102,103] and renal [104] patients.

Complex cognitive processes underlie adherence, which may result in unintentional nonadherence (e.g. memory loss resulting in forgetting to take medication) as well as the more commonly recognized intentional nonadherence. Understanding such differences is crucial in the management of these patients. Studies on adherence in lung transplant recipients are limited, but a recent study elucidated this complex nature in this patient group [105]. The authors found that, although the patients rated themselves as being compliant with aspects of their self-care, such as taking medication daily, on more subtle measures of adherence – such as the time between onset of fever and contacting the hospital – 'considerable noncompliance' was evident. In addition, patients receiving a transplant more recently were more compliant and those with CF used their spirometer more often than patients with other lung diseases. Family support was also found to be significantly correlated with self-reported adherence.

These findings highlight the difficulty in defining and measuring adherence. In particular it is important to determine not only the degree of adherence but also the underlying reasons and mechanisms in order to facilitate 'adherence-promoting strategies', such as maintaining more frequent contact with patients, providing positive feedback and empowering patients to take responsibility for their health care. These strategies have been found to increase adherence in recipients participating in an electronic home spirometry programme [106].

Sexual dysfunction

Few studies have included a measure of sexual functioning, despite the documentation of impotence in men following heart transplantation [107,108], which has been postulated to be attributable to the immunosuppressive drug therapy. Heart transplant recipients reported impaired sexual confidence and performance due to altered roles and responsibilities between spouses, concerns about sexual attractiveness, loss of autonomy, physiological effects of medication, performance anxiety, depressed mood and fear of coital death [109]. A further fear of this patient group was of assuming the sexual behaviour of the anonymous donor.

Two studies of lung transplant recipients used a specific, comprehensive measure of sexual functioning [81,93]. The earlier study focused exclusively on female lung transplant patients and found no overall difference in overall sexual functioning before and after transplant, but patients prior to transplantation reported a higher sex drive. Furthermore, 12% of the recipients identified sexual functioning (particularly lack of interest in sexual activity) as a significant problem. In their later study, Limbos et al. [81] found no difference in mean scores on any of the sexual functioning subscales between pre- and post-transplantation ratings, with scores in the average range in terms of satisfaction with sexual functioning, overall sexual satisfaction and affectivity in comparison with a clinical sample of healthy adults. Percentile scores for the 'drive' subtest were below average before and after transplantation for women only.

Rehabilitation

As recipients experience the reality of life post-transplantation, they are challenged to find ways to cope

with feelings of vulnerability and to relinquish unrealistic and 'magical' expectations concerning the outcome of the surgery [110]. The hope for complete independence from the health care system can be strong, in response to feelings of helplessness and lack of control prior to transplantation. Having to continue in the patient role, whilst at the same time being encouraged to abandon the sick role, can cause confusion and concern. Whilst increased autonomy and independence are highly desirable goals following transplantation, some recipients experience difficulty in separating themselves from the transplant environment [111] and forging their post-transplantation identity. Returning home and leaving the protective environment of the hospital, together with the security of relationships formed with other patients and staff, may result in considerable apprehension. Unacknowledged anxiety regarding separation from the perceived security of the transplant environment led to somatic complaints, overinvolvement in hospital issues and transplant-based activities and problems in assuming independence [110]. Within their home environment, recipients may experience problems reintegrating due to the difficulty others have in comprehending the transplant experience and empathizing with the patient. Re-establishing their niche within their family and in society and fulfilling their own and others' expectations regarding day-to-day living can be overwhelming and cause significant problems with maintaining a sense of personal control. Such factors combined with the need for regular hospital checkups and continuing drug regimens and self-monitoring for signs of rejection and infection may precipitate episodes of depression and/or nonadherence. The additional psychological concomitants if a patient develops bronchiolitis obliterans syndrome – anger, disappointment, vulnerability – indicate the need for realistic and appropriate psychosocial interventions, targeted early on in the transplantation process. The importance of education as an essential component of rehabilitation is now recognized and introduced when patients are accepted for transplant [112].

The special case of adolescence

For the adolescent, the challenge is to achieve the desired independence and autonomy whilst also maintaining close and supportive links with the nuclear family [113]. A sense of identity and self-understanding are created through social relationships with peers, self-reflection and future expectations [114]. Illness at this time exaggerates the challenge. Chronically ill adolescents may be particularly vulnerable to social isolation and delayed development of peer-support networks [115,116] and issues such as body image and self-perception are particularly important at this time.

The need to undergo transplantation during adolescence makes increased dependence unavoidable, thereby curtailing the move towards autonomy. The development of a sense of self is threatened by the downward trajectory of the chronic illness and the need for a lung transplant to survive [117], thus making adolescence a particularly vulnerable time for considering life-altering treatment. Adolescents frequently have a belief in their own immortality which can result in nonadherence to aspects of the drug and treatment regimen [118]. They may exhibit risk-taking behaviours, common among adolescents, by choosing to delay transplantation or not take medication, which functions to fulfil developmental needs for independence, autonomy and self-competence [119]. Facilitating the adolescent's active participation in the transplant decision allows them to gain control over their life and creating hope provides a way to integrate the present with the future.

Research has shown that adherence to a specific treatment regimen is poorer for adolescents when it interferes with developmental needs and daily activities with peers [120]. There is also a strong association between adherence decisions and QoL [121], with QoL for adolescents being characterized largely by the extent to which physical symptoms limit their participation in age-appropriate activities and affect psychological and social functioning [122]. Patients undergoing lung transplantation in adolescence more frequently have an illness with which they have had to cope all their lives, such as congenital heart disease or CF, than an acquired illness and may view lung transplantation as a 'magical cure' – the one therapeutic alternative that offers them real hope to live a normal life. The conflict between expectations and the realities of lung transplantation can increase the likelihood of nonadherence post-transplantation, and there is significant concern about the prevalence of medical nonadherence in the adolescent lung transplant population [123]. A study of 19 CF adolescent lung recipients found that the need to control as many aspects of their lives as possible whilst dealing with parental overprotection was one of the major themes identified [124] and issues such as education and the difficulties of reintegration after transplantation experienced by some patients have also been highlighted [125].

The challenges of undergoing lung transplantation in adolescence are very different from those of the adult population and it is essential that this is recognized if the benefits afforded to the patient by successful lung transplantation are to be maximized.

Family roles

There is a paucity of literature concerning family members at any stage of lung transplantation, but a study of support groups for families of heart transplant recipients found that change in role and responsibility was among the most frequently mentioned topics [126]. Prior to transplantation, family members may have to assume roles previously held by the patients, and recipients' spouses have commented on increased responsibilities in a number of domains, including running the home and becoming the major wage earner [127]. Family members also have to share responsibility for the care of the patient – which can be particularly disruptive to social functioning – and the burden of waiting for a transplant can put enormous strains on relationships between family members.

A study of 12 spouses of lung recipients found that, after transplantation, the core theme explaining their experiences was a 'roller coaster ride' [128]. Sleep difficulties [129,130] and distress levels above normal [131] have been reported for spouses of heart transplant recipients in the early postoperative phase, although distress levels did decline after the first postoperative year [131]. In the early postoperative stage, family members have to relinquish the control of the patient's life that they had during the waiting period and hand over responsibility to the medical and nursing teams [132]. In a further study of heart transplant recipients and their spouses, Grundbock et al. [133] found that role performance was rated as poorer after transplantation than before, which was related to recipients' spouses' unwillingness to relinquish their new roles adopted during the illness. However, role changes may, in the longer term, be beneficial for family members and result in increased self-esteem as a result of acquiring new skills and lower levels of psychological distress post-transplantation [129,131]. Research with renal patients has shown that the adjustment of a spouse is associated with the patient's adjustment and recovery [134]. The importance of the spouse reinvesting emotionally in the patient, whose life has now been extended by transplantation, has been highlighted for spouses of heart transplant recipients [135]. Such findings may well be applicable to lung transplant recipients as it is the couple, rather than just the patient, who have to adapt to the problems of life after transplantation [128].

In situations where the recipient has had a long history of ill health and required significant input from a family member, overprotection may be a problem. Conversely, if the family member feels that the recipient's progress is too slow and their continuing dependency becomes a source of frustration, too little support may be provided to the recipient and the anger and subsequent guilt experienced by the family member may result in depression.

Information on family members other than spouses is scant, but in terms of role changes adolescents in families of heart transplant recipients became depressed, resentful and angry over the focus on the transplant patient [126], and with the corresponding shift in responsibility and the need for them to assume new roles, which in turn caused disruption to their daily lives.

The management of respiratory disease: the role of the psychologist

The role of the psychologist is varied when working with patients and families living with respiratory disease and following lung transplantation. Psychological assessments and therapeutic intervention are necessary at various stages of the disease and treatment process, although a generic basis can be adapted to the individual needs of the patient. However, the systematic evaluation of interventions is also required to evaluate their effectiveness and to promote scientific understanding of the psychology of respiratory disease.

Psychological intervention

The previous sections have demonstrated that emotional status, not lung function, is the greatest predictor of QoL. In addition, the prevalence of panic, anxiety and depression in pre- and postoperative patients is significantly higher that in the general population. Studies have indicated the benefits of psychotropic medical therapy for these patients [136]; however, medication side effects such as orthostatic hypotension are common. Furthermore, although medication helps to reduce negative mood states it does not change the cognitions that initiate these negative emotions and so a psychological alternative is also needed.

Cognitive–behavioural therapy (CBT) for adult patients awaiting lung transplantation has enhanced coping abilities, reduced anxiety, dyspnoea and sleep disturbance, promoted health and exercise adherence and improved their QoL [137–141], and has been used effectively with adolescents with CF [142].

However, other studies utilizing relaxation alone or combined interventions have shown little impact on anxiety [143]. Evidence suggests that the more severe the psychological symptoms, the more significant the impact of an intervention on improving pulmonary function tests and QoL. The longevity of any gain and the psychological mech-anism that mediates this change is still unclear from current studies; however, it has been suggested that an increase in self-efficacy to control symptoms and an increase in knowledge can reduce anxiety and increase adherence to oxygen and medical therapy, subsequently improving the perception of physical function [144]. Pretransplant stress management training has been suggested as a means of lowering pretransplant stress and anxiety and increasing post-transplantation psychological status, QoL and adher-ence [145]. Following transplantation interventions should be targeted at key times such as the diagnosis of the first acute rejection episode or obliterative bronchiolitis, an area that has been neglected in the literature.

Summary

It is clear that lung transplantation generally results in significant improvements in physical and psychological health, even though transplant recipients are a heterogeneous group with different pretransplant respiratory conditions. However, limitations in study design, such as small sample sizes and cross-sectional assessment have precluded comparison of changes within different diagnostic groups. Investigators are now beginning to look at the prognostic implications of emotional health, with preoperative QoL scores predicting survival post-transplantation [6]. It seems that there is a complex pathway for the development of psychiatric symptomatology in respiratory diseases. Evidence clearly indicates that anxiety and depression are the most common psychological consequences, but these symptoms are not closely related to lung function. Therefore it seems that other variables mediate the relationship between mood, panic and symptomatology; these have been postulated as illness perceptions and beliefs, fatigue and dependence on oxygen therapy and others for care. However, the failure to identify a theoretical framework needs to be addressed by future research. Evidence from health psychology literature indicates that the Self-Regulatory Theory provides a basis for understanding the development of cognitive representations of respiratory illness that is integral to the manifestation of emotions, QoL and clinical outcome. However, the model lacks definition relating cognition and behaviour, particularly how emotional responses mediate this relationship and the global outcome of QoL.

Evidence suggests that, although recipients with a psychiatric disorder may be more able to identify and deal with psychological difficulties and are thus better able to cope with the significant stressors which occur post-transplantation [146], a proportion of individuals and their families experience negative emotions and poor physical and psychological QoL both before and after lung transplantation. Even the presence of significant psychological symptomatology pretransplantation does not preclude successful adaptation to transplantation and should not be seen as a contraindication. To facilitate optimal psychological adaptation post-transplantation a flexible approach to their care should be negotiated.

The clinical role of the health psychologist as an integral part of the transplant team is crucial for the emotional, social and behavioural management of patients and their families. Results clearly indicate the importance of targeting appropriate psychosocial interventions at the earliest possible time and for isolating psychological risk factors for adaptation to transplantation. Future research needs to focus on developing prospective, longitudinal studies utilizing an appropriate theoretical framework with larger sample sizes, and administering multivariate approaches in order to assess the efficacy of such interventions.

REFERENCES

1 Scharloo M, Kaptein AA, Weinman J, et al. Illness perceptions, coping and functioning in patients with rheumatoid arthritis, chronic obstructive pulmonary disease and psoriasis. *J Psychosom Res* 1998; **44**: 573–585.

2 Smoller JW, Pollack MH, Otto MW, Rosenbaum JF, Kradin RL. Panic anxiety, dyspnea and respiratory disease. *Am J Respir Crit Care Med* 1996; **154**: 6–17.

3 World Health Organization. *The First Ten Years. The Health Organization.* WHO, Geneva, 1958.

4 WHOQoL Group. The World Health Organization Quality of Life Assessment (WHOQOL): position paper from the World Health Organization. *Soc Sci Med* 1995; **41**: 1403–1409.

5 McSweeny J, Labuhn KT. *Chronic obstructive pulmonary disease.* In: Spilker B, ed. *Quality of life assessments in clinical trials.* Raven Press, Ltd. New York, 1990: 391–417.

6 Squier HC, Reis AL, Kaplan RM, et al. Quality of well-being predicts survival in lung transplantation candidates. *Am J Respir Crit Care Med* 1995; **152**: 2032–2036.

7 Janssens J-P, Rochat T, Frey J-G, Dousse N, Pichard C, Tschopp J-M. Health-related quality of life in patients under long-term oxygen therapy: a home based descriptive study. *Respir Med* 1997; **91**: 592–602.

8 TenVergert EM, Essink-Bot ML, Geertsma A, van Enckevort PJ, de Boer WI, van der Bij W. The effect of lung transplantation on health-related quality of life. *Chest* 1998; **113**: 358–364.

9 Cohen L, Littlefield C, Kelly P, Maurer I, Abbey S. Predictors of quality of life and psychological adjustment after lung transplantation. *Chest* 1998; **113**: 633–644.

10 Porzelius J, Vest M, Nochmovitz M. Respiratory anticipation, cognitions, and panic in chronic obstructive pulmonary disease. *Behav Res Ther* 1992; **30**: 75–77.

11 Karajgi BA, Rifkin S, Doddi S, Kolli R. The prevalence of anxiety disorders in patients with chronic obstructive pulmonary disease. *Am J Psychiatry* 1990; **147**: 200–201.

12 Heaton RK, Grant I, McSweeny J, Adams KM, Petty TL. Psychological effects of continuous oxygen therapy in hypoxaemic chronic obstructive pulmonary disease. *Arch Intern Med* 1982; **143**: 1941–1947.

13 McSweeny J, Grant J, Heaton RK, Adams KM, Timms RM. Life quality of patients with chronic obstructive pulmonary disease. *Arch Intern Med* 1982; **142**: 473–478.

14 Tarter RE, Switala J. Cognitive assessment in organ transplantation. In: Trzepacz P, Dimartini A, eds. *The transplant patient. Biological, psychiatric and ethical issues in organ transplantation.* Cambridge University Press, Cambridge, 2000: 164–186.

15 Incalzi R, Gemma A, Marra C, Muzzulon R, Capparella O, Carbonin P. Chronic obstructive pulmonary disease. An original model of cognitive decline. *Am Rev Respir Dis* 1993; **148**: 412–424.

16 Farmer M. Cognitive deficits related to major organ failure. The potential role of neuropsychological testing. *Neuropsychol Rev* 1994; **4**: 117–160.

17 Etnier J, Johnston R, Dagenbach D, Pollard RJ, Rejeski WJ, Berry M. The relationships among pulmonary function, aerobic fitness, and cognitive functioning in older COPD patients. *Chest* 1999; **116**: 953–960.

18 Weitzenblum E, Apprill M, Oswald M. Benefit from long-term O_2 therapy in chronic obstructive pulmonary disease patients. *Respiration* 1992; **59**: 14–17.

19 Strom K. Long-term oxygen therapy in parenchymal lung diseases: an analysis of survival. *Eur Respir J* 1993; **6**: 1264–1270.

20 Anderson DL, Flume PA, Hardy KK. Psychological functioning of adults with cystic fibrosis. *Chest* 2001; **119**: 1079–1084.

21 Blair C, Cull A, Freeman C. Psychosocial functioning of young adults with cystic fibrosis and their families. *Thorax* 1994; **49**: 798–802.

22 Pearson D, Pumariega A, Seilheimer D. The development of psychiatric symptomatology in patients with cystic fibrosis. *J Am Acad Child Adolesc Psychiatry* 1991; **30**: 290–295.

23 Cowen L, Coney M, Simmons R, Keenan N, Robertson J. Levenson H. Growing older with cystic fibrosis: psychosocial adjustment. *Arch Disabil Child* 1984; **56**: 538–543.

24 Aspin AJ. Psychological consequences of cystic fibrosis in adults. *Br J Hosp Med* 1991; **45**: 368–371.

25 Perna G, Bertani A, Diaferia G, Arancio C, Bellodi L. Prevalence of respiratory diseases in patients with panic and obsessive compulsive disorders. *Anxiety* 1994; **1**: 100–101.

26 Pollack MH, Kradin R, Otto MW, et al. Prevalence of panic in patients referred for pulmonary function testing at a major medical center. *Am J Psychiatr* 1996; **153**: 110–113.

27 Verberg K, Griez E, Meijer J, Pols I. Respiratory disorders as a possible predisposing factor for panic disorder. *J Affect Disord* 1995; **33**: 129–134.

28 Spinhoven P, Sterk PJ, van der Kamp L, Onstein EJ. The complex association of pulmonary function with panic disorder:

a rejoinder to Ley (1998). *J Behav Ther Exp Psychiatry* 1999; **30**: 341–356.

29 Ley R. Pulmonary function and dyspnea/suffocation theory of panic. *J Behav Ther Exp Psychiatry* 1998; **29**: 1–11.

30 Spinhoeven P, Onstein EJ, Sterk PJ. Pulmonary function in panic disorder. Evidence against the dyspnea–fear theory. *Behav Res Ther* 1995; **33**: 457–460.

31 Asmundson GJG, Stein MB. A preliminary analysis of pulmonary function in panic disorder: implications for the dyspnea–fear theory. *J Anxiety Disord* 1994; **8**: 63–70.

32 Papp LA, Klein DF, Gorman JM. CO_2 hypersensitivity, hyperventilation and panic disorder. *Arch Gen Psychiatry* 1993; **150**: 1149–1157.

33 Otto MW, Wittal ML. Cognitive–behaviour therapy and the longitudinal course of panic disorder. *Psychiatry Clin North Am* 1995; **18**: 803–820.

34 Nutt D, Lawson C. Panic attacks: a neurochemical overview of models and mechanisms. *Br J Psychiatry* 1992; **160**: 165–178.

35 Bennett P, Murphy S. *Psychology and health promotion.* Open University Press, Milton Keynes, 1997.

36 Leventhal H, Meyer D, Nerenz DR. The common sense representations of illness danger. In: Rachman S, ed. *Contributions to medical psychology*, Vol. 2. Pergamon, New York, 1980: 17–30.

37 Moss-Morris R. Measuring cognitive representations of illness: a revision of the Illness Perceptions Questionnaire. Paper presented at the International Congress of Behavioral Medicine, Brisbane, Australia.

38 Petrie K, Weinman JA, Sharpe N, Buckley J. Role of patients' view of their illness in predicting return to work and functioning after myocardial infarction: longitudinal study. *Br Med J* 1996; **312**: 1191–1194.

39 Maes S, Leventhal H, De Ridder DTD. Coping with chronic diseases. In: Zeider M, Endler NS, eds. *Handbook of coping.* Wiley, New York, 1996: 221–251.

40 Reesor KA, Craig KD. Medically incongruent chronic back pain: physical limitations, suffering and ineffective coping. *Pain* 1988; **32**: 35–45.

41 Leventhal H, Nerenz DR, Steele DJ. Illness representations and coping with health threats. In: Baum A, Taylor SE, Singer JE, eds. *Handbook of psychology and health*, Vol. 4. Erlbaum, Hillsdale, N J, 1984: 219–252.

42 Scharloo M, Kaptein AA. Measurement of illness perceptions in patients with chronic somatic illness: a review. In: Petrie KJ, Weinman JA, eds. *Perceptions of health and illness: current research and applications.* Harwood, London, 1997: 103–154.

43 Dalal AK, Singh AK. Role of causal and recovery beliefs in the psychological adjustment to a chronic disease. *Psychol Health* 1992; **6**: 193–203.

44 Maille AR, Koning CJM, Zwinderman AH, Willems LNA, Dijkman JH, Kaptein AA. The development of the 'Quality of Life for Respiratory Illness Questionnaire (QOL-RIQ)': a disease-specific quality of life questionnaire for patients with mild to moderate chronic non-specific lung disease. *Respir Med* 1997; **91**: 297–309.

45 Kaptein AA, Brand, PLP, Dekker FW, Kerstjens HAM, Postma DS, Sluiter HJ, the Dutch CNSLD Study Group. Quality of life in a long-term multicentre trial in chronic nonspecific lung disease: assessment at baseline. *Eur Respir J* 1993; **6**: 1479–1484.

46 Kaplan RM, Ries AL, Prewitt LM, Eakin E. Self-efficacy expectations predict survival for patients with chronic obstructive pulmonary disease. *Health Psychol* 1994; **13**: 366–368.

47 Eakin EG, Russsell E. The patients' perspective on the self-management of chronic obstructive pulmonary disease. *J Health Psychol* 1997; **2**: 245.

48 Scherer Y, Schmeider LE. The effect of a pulmonary rehabilitation program on self-efficacy, perception of dyspnea and physical endurance. *Heart Lung* 1997; **26**: 15–22.

49 Zimmerman BW, Brown ST, Bowman JM. A self-management program for chronic obstructive pulmonary disease: relationship to dyspnea and self-efficacy. *Rehabil Nurs* 1996; **21**: 253–257.

50 Graydon JE, Ross E. Influence of symptoms, lung function, mood and social support on level of functioning of patients with COPD. *Res Nurs Health* 1995; **18**: 525–533.

51 Scharloo M, Kaptein AA, Weinman JA, Willems NA, Rooijmans HGM. Physical and psychological correlates of functioning in patients with chronic obstructive pulmonary disease. *J Asthma* 2000; **37**: 17–29.

52 LaCroix JM, Martin B, Avendano M, Goldstein R. Symptom schemata in chronic respiratory patients. *Health Psychol* 1991; **10**: 268–273.

53 Millard RW, Wells N, Thebarge RW. A comparison of models describing reports of disability associated with chronic pain. *Clin J Pain* 1991; **7**: 283–291.

54 Gil KM, Abrama MR, Philips G, Keefe FJ. Sickle cell disease pain: relation of coping strategies to adjustment. *J Consult Clin Psychol* 1989; **57**: 725.

55 Levenson JL, Olbrisch ME. Psychosocial screening and selection of candidates for organ transplantation. In: Trzepacz P, Dimartini A, eds. *The transplant patient. Biological, psychiatric and ethical issues in organ transplantation.* Cambridge University Press, Cambridge, 2000: 21–41.

56 Orentlicher D. Psychosocial assessment of organ transplant candidates and the Americans with Disabilities Act. *Gen Hosp Psychiatry* 1996; **18**: 5S-12S.

57 Levenson JL, Olbrisch ME. Psychosocial evaluation of organ transplant candidates: a comparative survey of process, criteria and outcomes in heart, liver and kidney transplantation. *Psychosomatics* 1993; **34**: 324–325.

58 *Human Rights Act.* HMSO, London, 1998.

59 Reitan R. Validity of the trailmaking test as an indicator of organic brain damage. *Percept Motor Skills* 1958; **8**: 271–276.

60 Smith A. *Symbol digit modalities test.* Western Psychological Services: Los Angeles, CA, 1973.

61 Costa L, Vaughn H, Levita E, Farber N. Purdue pegboard as a predictor of the presence and laterality of cerebral lesions. *J Consult Psychol* 1963; **27**: 133–137.

62 Levenson JL, Best A, Presberg B, et al. Psychosocial assessment of candidates for transplantation (PACT) as a predictor of transplant outcome. In *Proceedings of the 41st Annual Meeting of the Academy of Psychosomatic Medicine* 1994: 39.

63 Twillman RK, Manetto C, Wellisch DK, Wolcott DL. The Transplant Evaluation Rating Scale. A revision of the psychosocial levels system for evaluating organ transplant candidates. *Psychosomatics* 1993; **34**: 144–153.

64 Barry CA, Stevenson FA, Britten N, Barber N, Bradley CP. Giving voice to the lifeworld. More humane, more effective medical care? A qualitative study of doctor-patient communication in general practice. *Soc Sci Med* 2001; **53**: 487–505.

65 Lanuza DM, Lefaiver CA, Farca GA. Research on the quality of life of lung transplant candidates and recipients: an integrative review. *Heart Lung* 2001; **29**: 180–195.

66 Hajiro T, Nishimura K, Tsukino M, Ikeda A, Koyama H, Izumi T. Comparison of discriminative properties among disease-specific questionnaires for measuring health-related quality of life in patients with chronic obstructive pulmonary disease. *Am J Crit Care Med* 1998; **157**: 785–790.

67 Reichenspurner HRE, Girgis RC, Robbins KL, et al. Stanford experience with obliterative bronchiolitis after lung and heart–lung transplantation. *Ann Thorac Surg* 1996; **62**: 1467–1472.

68 Burke CM, Theodore J, Dawkins KD, et al. Post-transplant obliterative bronchiolitis and other late lung sequelae in human heart–lung transplantation. *Chest* 1984; **86**: 824–829.

69 Valentine VG, Robbins RC, Berry GJ, et al. Actuarial survival of heart–lung and bilateral sequential lung recipients with obliterative bronchiolitis. *J Heart Lung Transplant* 1996; **15**: 371–383.

70 Stilley CS, Dew MA, Stukas AA, et al. Psychological symptom levels and their correlates in lung and heart–lung recipients. *Psychosomatics* 1999; **40**: 503–509.

71 Dew MA, Switzer GE, Goycoolea JM, et al. Does transplantation produce quality-of-life benefits: a quantitative review of the literature. *Transplantation* 1997; **64**: 1261–1273.

72 O'Brien BJ, Banner NR, Gibson S, Yacoub MH. The Nottingham Health Profile as a measure of quality of life following combined heart and lung transplantation. *J Epidemiol Commun Health* 1988; **42**: 232–234.

73 Dennis C, Caine N, Sharples L, et al. Heart–lung transplantation for end-stage respiratory disease in patients with cystic fibrosis at Papworth Hospital. *J Heart Lung Transplant* 1993; **12**: 893–902.

74 Caine N, Sharples LD, Dennis C, Higenbottam TW, Wallwork J. Measurement of health-related quality of life before and after heart–lung transplantation. *J Heart Lung Transplant* 1996; **15**: 1047–1058.

75 Lanuza DM, Lefaiver C, McCabe M, Farcas GA, Garrity E. Prospective study of functional status and quality of life before and after lung transplantation. *Chest* 2000; **118**: 115–122.

76 Caine N, Sharples LD, Smyth R, et al. Survival and quality of life of cystic fibrosis patients before and after heart–lung transplantation. *Transplant Proc* 1991; **23**: 1203–1204.

77 Gross CR, Savik K, Bolman RM, Hertz MI. Long-term health status and quality of life outcomes of lung transplant recipients. *Chest* 1995; **108**: 1587–1593.

78 Ramsey SD, Patrick DL, Lewis S, Albert RK, Raghu G. Improvement in quality of life after lung transplantation. *J Heart Lung Transplant* 1995; **14**: 870–877.

79 Gross CR, Raghu G. The cost of lung transplantation and the quality of life post-transplant. *Clin Chest Med* 1997; **18**: 391–403.

80 Stanghelle JK, Koss JO, Bjortuft O, Geiran O. Case report: marathon with cystic fibrosis and bilateral lung transplant. *Scand J Med Sci Sports* 2000; **10**: 42–46.

81 Limbos MM, Joyce DP, Chan CKN, Kesten S. Psychological functioning and quality of life in lung transplant candidates and recipients. *Chest* 2000; **118**: 408–416.

82 MacNaughton KL, Rodrigue JR, Cicale M, Staples EM. Health related quality of life and symptom frequency before and after lung transplantation. *Clin Transpl* 1998; **12**: 320–323.

83 Littlefield C, Abbey S, Fiducia D, et al. Quality of life following transplantation of the heart, liver and lungs. *Gen Hosp Psychiatry* 1996; **18**: 36S–47S.

84 Busschbach JJV, Horikx PE, van den Bosch JMM, de la Rivière AB, de Charro FT. Measuring the quality of life before and after bilateral lung transplantation in patients with cystic fibrosis. *Chest* 1994; **105**: 911–917.

85 Lama R, Alvarez A, Santos J, et al. Long-term results of lung transplantation for cystic fibrosis. *Transplant Proc* 2001; **33**: 1624–1625.

86 Al-Kattan K, Tadjkarimi S, Cox A, Banner N, Khaghani A, Yacoub M. Evaluation of the long-term results of single lung versus heart–lung transplantation for emphysema. *J Heart Lung Transplant* 1995; **14**: 824–831.

87 Stavem K, Bjortuft O, Lund MB, Kongsshaug K, Geiran O, Boe J. Health-related quality of life in lung-transplant candidates and recipients. *Respiration* 2000; **67**: 159–165.

88 Lanuza DM, Norton N, McCabe M, Garrity JE. Lung transplant patients' quality of life and symptom experiences. *Circulation* 1997; **96** (Suppl 1): 440.

89 Paris W, Diercks M, Bright J et al. Return to work after lung transplantation. *J Heart Lung Transplant* 1998; **17**: 430–436.

90 Chaparro C, Scavuzzo M, Winton T, Keshavjee S, Kesten S. Status of lung transplant recipients surviving beyond five years. *J Heart Lung Transplant* 1997; **16**: 511–516.

91 Craven JL, the Toronto Lung Transplant Group. Postoperative organic mental syndromes in lung transplant recipients. *J Heart Lung Transplant* 1990; **9**: 129–132.

92 De Groen PC, Aksamit AJ, Rakela J, Forbes GS, Krom RAF. Central nervous system toxicity after liver transplantation: the role of cyclosporine and cholesterol. *New Engl J Med* 1987; **317**: 861–866.

93 Limbos MM, Chan CK, Kesten S. Quality of life in female lung transplant candidates and recipients. *Chest* 1997; **112**: 1165–1174.

94 Schlitt HJ, Brunkhorst R, Schmidt HHJ, Nashan B, Haverich A, Raab R. Attitudes of patients before and after transplantation towards various allografts. *Transplantation* 1999; **68**: 510–514.

95 Markovitz MS, Doyle A, Shaner MA, Schuller D, Sweet SC. Pediatric living donor lung transplantation: psychosocial considerations. *J Heart Lung Transplant* 2001; **20**: 245.

96 Cohen RG, Starnes VA. Living donor lung transplantation. *World J Surg* 2001; **25**: 244–250.

97 Van den Berg JWK, Geertsma A, van den Bijw, et al. Bronchiolitis obliterans syndrome after lung transplantation and health-related quality of life. *Am J Respir Crit Care Med* 2000; **161**: 1937–1941.

98 Schweizer RT, Rovelli M, Palmeri D, Vossler E, Hull D, Bartus S. Noncompliance in organ transplant recipients. *Transplantation* 1990; **49**: 374–377.

99 Dew MA, Roth L, Thompson M, Kormos R, Griffith B. Medical compliance and its predictors in the first year after heart transplantation. *J Heart Lung Transplant* 1996; **15**: 631–645.

100 Didlake RH, Dreyfus K, Kerman RH, van Buren CT, Kahan BD. Patient noncompliance: a major cause of late graft failure in cyclosporine-treated renal patients. *Transplant Proc* 1988; **10**: 63–69.

101 Dunn J, Golden D, van Buren CT, Lewis RM, Lawen J, Kahan, BD. Causes of graft loss beyond two years in the cyclosporine era. *Transplantation* 1990; **49**: 349–353.

102 Chacko R, Harper R, Grotto J, Young J. Psychiatric interview and psychometric predictors of cardiac transplant survival. *Am J Psychiatry* 1996; **153**: 1607–1612.

103 Dew MA, Kormos R, Roth L, Murali S, DiMartini A, Griffith B. Early post-transplant medical compliance and mental health predict morbidity and mortality one to three years after heart transplantation. *J Heart Lung Transplant* 1999; **18**: 549–562.

104 Douglas S, Blixen C, Bartucci R. Relationship between pre-transplant noncompliance and posttransplant outcomes in renal transplant recipients. *J Transplant Coord* 1996; **6**: 53–58.

105 Teichman BJ, Burker EJ, Weiner M, Egan TM. Factors associated with adherence to treatment regimens after lung transplantation. *Progr Transplant* 2000; **10**: 113–121.

106 Chlan L, Snyder M, Finkelsteins, et al. Promoting adherence to an electronic home spirometry research program after lung transplantation. *Appl Nurs Res* 1998; **11**: 36–40.

107 Lough ME, Lindsay AM, Shinn JA, et al. Impact of symptom frequency and symptom distress on self-reported quality of life in heart transplant recipients. *Heart Lung* 1987; **16**: 193–200.

108 Mai F, McKenzie FN, Kostuk WJ. Psychosocial adjustment and quality of life following heart transplantation. *Can J Psychiatry* 1990; **35**: 223–227.

109 Tabler JB, Frierson RL. Sexual concerns after heart transplantation. *J Heart Transplant* 1990; **9**: 397–403.

110 Kelly P, Bart C, Craven J. Lung transplantation. In: Craven J, Rodin GM, eds. *Psychiatric aspects of organ transplantation.* Oxford Medical Publications, Oxford, 1992: 205–223.

111 Craven JL, Bright J, Dear CL. Psychiatric, psychosocial and rehabilitative aspects of lung transplantation. *Clin Chest Med* 1990; **11**: 247–257.

112 Palmer SM, Tapson VF. Pulmonary rehabilitation in the surgical patient. *Respir Care Clin North Am* 1998; **4**: 71–83.

113 Eiser C. *Growing up with a chronic disease: the impact on children and their families.* Jessica Kingsley Publishers Ltd, London, 1993: 70–92.

114 Sroufe LA, Cooper RG, DeHart GB. *Child development.* McGraw-Hill, New York, 1996.

115 Melzer SM, Leadbeater B, Reisman L, Jaffe LR, Lieberman KV. Characteristics of social networks in adolescents with end stage renal disease treated with renal transplantation. *J Adolesc Health Care* 1989; **10**: 308–312.

116 Noll RB, Bukowski WM, Davies WH, Koontz K, Kulkarni R. Adjustment in the peer system of adolescents with cancer: a two-year study. *J Pediatr Psychol* 1993; **18**: 351–364.

117 Christian BJ, D'Auria JP, Moore CB. Playing for time: adolescent perspectives of lung transplantation for cystic fibrosis. *J Pediatr Health Care* 1999; **13**: 120–125.

118 Suddaby EC. No simple answers: ethical conflicts in pediatric heart transplantation. *J Transpl Coord* 1999; **9**: 266–270.

119 Millstein SG, Igra V. Theoretical models of adolescent risk-taking behavior. In: Wallander JL, Siegel LJ, eds. *Adolescent health problems.* Guilford, New York, 1995: 52–71.

120 LaGreca LM. Issues in adherence with pediatric regimens. *J Pediatr Psychol* 1990; **15**: 423–436.

121 Thompson RJ, Gustafson KE. *Adaptation to childhood chronic illness.* American Psychological Association, Washington, DC, 1996.

122 Spieth LE, Harris CV. Assessment of health-related quality of life in children and adolescents: an integrative review. *J Pediatr Psychol* 1996; **21**: 175–193.

123 Serrano-Ikkos E, Lask B, Whitehead B, Eisler I. Incomplete adherence after pediatric heart and heart–lung transplantation. *J Heart Lung Transplant* 1998; **17**: 1177–1183.

124 Durst CL, Horn MV, MacLaughlin EF, Bowman CM, Starnes VA, Woo MS. Psychosocial responses of adolescent cystic fibrosis patients to lung transplantation. *Pediatr Transplant* 2001; **5**: 27–31.

125 Wray J, Long T, Radley-Smith R, Yacoub M. Returning to school after heart or heart–lung transplantation: how well do children adjust? *Transplantation* 2001; **72**: 100–106.

126 Hyler BJ, Corley MC, McMahon D. The role of nursing in a support group for heart transplant recipients and their families. *Heart Transplant* 1985; **4**: 453–456.

127 Baumann LJ, Young CJ, Egan JJ. Living with a heart transplant: long-term adjustment. *Transpl Int* 1992; **5**: 1–8.

128 Kurz JM. Experiences of well spouses after lung transplantation. *J Advan Nurs* 2001; **34**: 493–500.

129 Buse SM, Pieper B. Impact of cardiac transplantation on the spouse's life. *Heart Lung* 1990; **19**: 641–648.

130 Erdman RAM, Horstman L, van Domburg RT, Meeter K, Balk AHHM. Compliance with the medical regimen and partner's quality of life after heart transplantation. *Qual Life Res* 1993; **2**: 205–212.

131 Canning RD, Dew MA, Davidson S. Psychological distress among caregivers to heart transplant recipients. *Soc Sci Med* 1996; **42**: 599–608.

132 Smolin TL, Aguiar LJ. Psychosocial and financial aspects of lung transplantation. *Crit Care Nurs Clin North Am* 1996; **8**: 293–303.

133 Grundbock A, Bunzel B, Schubert MT. Changes in partnership after cardiac transplantation. In: Walter PJ, ed. *Quality*

of life after open heart surgery, Kluwer Academic Publishers, Dordrecht, 1992: 483–490.

134 White Y, Grenyer B. The biopsychosocial impact of end-stage renal disease: the experience of dialysis patients and their partner. *J Advan Nurs* 1999; **30**: 1312–1320.

135 Frierson R, Tabler J, Spears R. Heart transplantation. In: Craven J, Rodin GM, eds. *Psychiatric aspects of organ transplantation.* Oxford Medical Publications, Oxford, 1992: 164–176.

136 Smoller JW, Otto MW. Panic dyspnea, and asthma. *Curr Opin Pulmon Med* 1998; **9**: 90–95.

137 Kunick ME, Braun U, Stanley MA, et al. One session cognitive behavioural therapy for elderly patients with chronic obstructive pulmonary disease. *Psychol Med* 2001; **31**: 717–723.

138 Littlefield C. Psychological treatment of patients with end-stage pulmonary disease. *Monaldi Arch Chest Dis* 1995; **50**: 58–61.

139 Sachs G, Harber P, Spiess K, Moser G. Effectiveness of relaxation groups in patients with chronic respiratory tract diseases. *Wien Klin Wochenschr* 1993; **105**: 603–610.

140 Gift AG, McCrone SH. Depression in patients with COPD. *Heart Lung* 1993; **22**: 289–297

141 Atkins CJ, Kaplan RM, Timms RM, Reinsch S, Lofback K. Behavioural exercise programmes in the management of chronic obstructive pulmonary disease. *J Consult Clin Psychol* 1984; **52**: 591–603.

142 Hains AA, Davies WH, Behrens D, Biller JA. Cognitive behavioral interventions for adolescents with cystic fibrosis. *J Pediatr Psychol* 1997; **22**: 669–687.

143 Eiser N, West C, Evans S, Jeffers A, Quirk F. Effects of psychotherapy in moderately sever COPD: a pilot study. *Eur Respir J* 1997; **10**: 1581–1584.

144 Peters ML. The effects of follow-up treatment following multidisciplinary pulmonary rehabilitation program on dyspnea, functional status, psychological symptoms and adherence to discharge recommendations for patients with COPD. *Dissert Abstr Int Sect B* 2000; **60**: 5787.

145 Cohen L, Littlefield C, Kelly P, Maurer J, Abbey S. Predictors of quality of life and adjustment after lung transplantation. *Chest* 1998; **113**: 633–644.

146 Woodman CL, Geist LJ, Vance S, Laxson C, Jones K, Kline JN. Psychiatric disorders and survival after lung transplantation. *Psychosomatics* 1999; **40**: 293–297.

26

The current status of lung transplantation

Allan R. Glanville

St Vincent's Hospital, Sydney, Australia

Introduction

Three critical factors led to the birth of heart–lung transplantation (HLT) in 1981; the visionary approach of Norman Shumway [1], the application of Bruce Reitz [2] and the availability of the novel immunosuppressive agent ciclosporin [2,3]. The new discipline had a difficult birth and a tumultuous childhood. The world's first heart–lung transplant recipient spent four months in hospital due in part to bilateral phrenic nerve paresis. Despite restrictive physiology [4] and early concerns regarding the relevance of the Hering–Breuer reflex in mammalian species [5] the outcome was eminently successful, at least for five years. Her ultimate demise from complications of acute renal failure occurred after a fall at home in which she transected her short gastric artery. At postmortem the transplanted organs were pristine. This abbreviated case history of the first HLT recipient emphasizes the multiorgan complexity of lung transplantation and the potential risks associated with a simple fall in the immunosuppressed host.

The ensuing 21 years have been just as exciting for those privileged to be involved in this new dimension of care of patients for whom no other therapy offered the chance of ongoing survival and quality of life. The science of lung transplantation has evolved from an experimental procedure, through an investigative procedure, to be accepted as a legitimate mainstream therapy for patients with life-threatening pulmonary diseases. Similarly, living lobar pulmonary transplantation was first performed in 1993 and has now achieved a position as accepted therapy, with survival rates equivalent to lung transplantation using a cadaveric donor [6].

The development of an international guidelines document [7] for the referral of patients for consideration of lung transplantation sets a benchmark for international collaboration in the field of organ transplantation. Importantly, it signifies the willingness of the lung transplant community to identify and solve key problem areas in this continually developing field. As a result of this type of collaboration, adequately powered multicentre trials of new immunosuppressive agents are building on earlier single centre studies [8] to identify superior drug combinations for the prevention of rejection and the development of obliterative bronchiolitis [9]. Similar trials using everolimus (Novartis Pharmaceuticals East Hanover, New Jersey, USA) are investigating effective therapies for established bronchiolitis obliterans syndrome (BOS) and a new position paper has been developed to assist in the diagnosis of BOS [10].

The growth of a burgeoning industry in lung transplantation has enabled new insights into other orphan diseases such as primary pulmonary hypertension (PPH) [11–14], alpha-1-antitrypsin deficiency (AATD) [15] and pulmonary lymphangioleiomyomatosis [16]. Viable alternatives to lung transplantation have been developed for selected patients, including for PPH [17], post-thromboembolic pulmonary hypertension [18] and, most importantly, for emphysema, where the role of lung volume reduction surgery is under review [19].

Diagnostic bronchoscopic techniques such as transbronchial lung biopsy [20] and interventional techniques such as laser therapy [21], balloon dilatation and stent placement have undergone major advances as a direct result of the need to examine the allograft for rejection and infection [22], and to manage the sequelae of bronchial anastomotic strictures [23–26]. These techniques have been transferred to the management of patients with diverse conditions including lung cancer, post-tuberculosis stricture and tracheo-oesophageal fistula [27].

The development of isolated lung transplantation, coupled with the early high perioperative mortality rates reported for HLT has led to a reduction in the yearly rate of HLT from a plateau of about 220 procedures per annum in the years 1988–1995 to only 104 procedures in the year 2000 [28]. For the 2550 HLT patients in the International Society for Heart and Lung Transplant (ISHLT) Registry 2001 database the one year survival is 60% and the five year survival 40%. However, while the overall half-life $t_{1/2}$ is only 2.8 years, the conditional $t_{1/2}$ (for one year survivors) is 8.2 years. By contrast, our one year survival for HLT at St Vincent's (Sydney, Australia) is 81% overall and 93% during the last decade ($n = 42$). For experienced units, this is still an excellent operation, with a substantial number of patients now in the 10–20 year survival group. Predominant indications remain congenital heart disease (32.4%), PPH (25.4%), cystic fibrosis (CF) (16.3%), chronic obstructive pulmonary disease (COPD) (4.4%), AATD (3.1%), and idiopathic pulmonary fibrosis (IPF) (2.8%). The majority of units now routinely service all conditions other than congenital heart disease with lung-only procedures where possible. HLT seems to confer no additional benefit [29]. Arguments still exist regarding the equity of performing this triple organ transplant where separation of the donor block might service two or even three individuals. In truth, few surgeons have achieved experience with the nuances of HLT of latter years and this alone biases towards the performance of separate heart- and lung-only procedures [30]. Moreover where the heart transplant team dominates the discussion regarding organ allocation, there are often patients who seem to have a more pressing need than the potential HLT recipient.

For lung-only transplants an activity plateau of about 1350 procedures per annum was reached between the years 1996 and 2000. The numbers of bilateral sequential single lung transplants (BSSLT) have risen slowly during that time to occupy just over half the procedures performed per annum. It is of note that while the one year ISHLT international survival figures for single lung transplant (SLT) and BSSLT are superior to HLT at 69% and 70%, with $t_{1/2}$ of 3.6 years and 4.5 years, respectively, the five year survival for SLT is inferior at 40% while BSSLT is equivalent at 48%. The conditional $t_{1/2}$ values are 5.7 years and 7.9 years, respectively. St Vincent's has an 89% survival at one year for BSSLT ($n = 171$) and 80% for SLT ($n = 129$) with five year survivals of 60% and 53%, respectively.

The ISHLT Registry reports that the indications for SLT remain the non-suppurative parenchymal diseases such as COPD (47%), IPF (21%), and AATD (11%). By comparison, CF (33.3%) comprises the largest group for BSSLT, followed by COPD (20.1%), AATD (9.8%), PPH (9%) and IPF (7.8%). IPF followed by CF has the highest mortality rates on the waiting list [31]. Differences in organ allocation systems throughout the world are associated with regional differences in mortality rates on the waiting list. The equity of duration of time waiting versus medical urgency as a criterion for priority of transplantation remains questionable. Late referral compounds this problem particularly for patients with IPF [32].

Some 44% of all lung transplant recipients are in the age range 50–64 years and the mean donor age has risen from 24 to 34 years between 1990 and 2000. Paediatric recipients (aged less than 10 years) have been static at 20 per annum during this time, emphasizing that no paediatric lung transplantation programme can have the benefits that accrue from the experiences gained from a high volume transplant unit turnover. Registry data confirm lower survival rates for units performing fewer than nine lung transplantations per annum [28]. Coupling adult and paediatric units in adjacent facilities may allow sharing of expertise, better outcomes and increasing rates of paediatric transplantations if a cooperative approach is utilized.

Long-term outcomes

Survival

The causes of death after lung transplantation vary with the time post-transplantation, and to provide ease of grouping of like causes it is useful to divide the time after lung transplantation into operative, perioperative (within 30 days of transplantation), early (defined as within the first post-operative year), medium term (one to three years), and late (beyond three years). To add some complexity to this analysis it is important to acknowledge that causes of death are still evolving, representing the dynamic nature of developments in the field over the past 10 years. While some units have reached maturation, many have become defunct. Only a few have taken up the challenge anew in this most difficult area. In fact only 44 of 126 centres that have performed HLT are still active compared with 91 of 161 single lung transplant centres and 91 of 148 bilateral lung transplant centres [28].

Thirty-day mortality is predominantly dependent on surgical factors, factors related to donors, organ harvesting, ex vivo preservation and early high dose immunosuppression. In order of prevalence, causes of death include non-specific graft failure (NSGF) (38%), noncytomegalovirus (non-CMV) infection (33%), technical factors (12%), cardiac causes (11%), acute rejection (5%), and lastly obliterative bronchiolitis (OB) (1%).

Early deaths are largely due to non-CMV infections (52%), and NSGF (20%), with an increasing prevalence of

OB (9%), post-transplantation lymphoproliferative disease (PTLD) (4%), CMV (4%) and malignancy (2%). Deaths related to cardiac causes (4%), technical factors (3%), and acute rejection (2%) are less frequent.

Medium term, the pendulum has begun to swing towards OB, which now accounts for 35% of deaths, other major causes being non-CMV infection (30%), and NSGF (18%). Less frequent causes include malignancy (4%), cardiac (4%), PTLD (3%), acute rejection (3%), CMV (2%), and technical factors (1%).

OB (40%), non-CMV infection (28%) and NSGF (14%) dominate late deaths. Malignancy now accounts for 8%, with the incidence of less frequent causes including cardiac (4%), PTLD (2%), acute rejection (2%), CMV (1%) and technical factors (1%) remaining fairly static.

It is perhaps disappointing that NSGF accounts for so many deaths as it suggests that an in-depth analysis of aetiology has not been made nor has postmortem information been available [33]. While acute rejection does not account for a significant proportion of deaths, these data do not include an assessment of the relationship between therapy for rejection and resulting infection. This potential relationship is perhaps even more important in the nexus between OB and infectious death. The major trend, however, is the dominance of OB as the sole cause and the increasing frequency of malignancy as a late cause. Risk factor analysis from the ISHLT Registry identifies the major risks for one year survival as: transplantation from a ventilator (odds ratio (OR) 3.48), diagnosis of congenital heart disease (OR 2.04), diagnosis primary pulmonary hypertension (OR 1.50), CMV mismatch of donor and recipient (OR 1.44), transplantation year 1988–1991 (OR 1.37) and retransplantation (OR 1.35). Both linear and quadratic analyses of survival identify risk of increasing age (age 65 OR 1.86), increasing body mass index (BMI) (BMI 32: OR 1.32), reducing donor height (height 140 cm: OR 1.41), decreasing centre volume ($p < 0.0001$), and increasing donor age ($p < 0.002$), as well as a combination of increasing donor age with increasing ischaemic time ($p = 0.03$). For the active unit the challenge is to provide maximal utilization of available donors. While the results of a position paper from the ISHLT are awaited it is clear that rational donor use may be expanded outside traditional arbitrary guidelines [34–36]. The cost to the individual patient of not using a particular donor needs to be considered in the risk–benefit equation.

Recipient age and BMI remain important risk factors for five year survival as do transplantation from a ventilator (OR 3.01), CMV mismatch (OR 1.42), and transplant year 1988–1991 (OR 1.21). By comparison, protective factors include female sex of recipient (OR 0.85), diagnosis AATD (OR 0.83), diagnosis COPD (OR 0.56), age 20 (OR 0.82), low BMI (BMI 17, OR 0.83), and tall donor (height 200 cm, OR 0.76). All but donor height remain relevant for five year survival, where bilateral lung transplant assumes a survival advantage (OR 0.84) perhaps indicative of superior pulmonary functional reserve inherent in this procedure [28]. Evaluating data for AATD/COPD patients who receive bilateral lung transplants might now provide evidence of a survival benefit [37].

Morbidity

Overview

The most prevalent serious complications are hypertension, renal dysfunction, hyperlipidaemia and diabetes mellitus. All are related to immunosuppressive therapy with calcineurin inhibitors [38] and corticosteroids. Preventative strategies now exist for the majority of these predictable sequelae.

Surgical complications

Despite recent improvements in perioperative mortality rates, morbidity related to wound dehiscence remains an important cause of prolonged inpatient stay. Usual causes include wound infection with common bacterial pathogens, particularly methicillin-resistant *Staphylococcus aureus* (MRSA) [39]. Fastidious organisms such as *Mycoplasma hominis* also cause wound breakdown and should be considered where wound swabs show pus cells but no organisms on Gram stain [40]. Culture for this particular organism takes five to eight days, so plates should not be discarded early. Preliminary evidence also implicates *Chlamydia pneumoniae* as a potential contributor to early postoperative mortality from airway dehiscence and inflammatory airway disease [41] but confirmation of diagnosis requires more sophisticated tools such as polymerase chain reaction (PCR) of bronchoalveolar lavage fluid. The majority of laboratories are not able to culture wild-type strains. Fungal anastomotic infection may present with exsanguinating haemoptysis due to erosion into the pulmonary artery. Preventative strategies include the use of prophylactic inhaled amphotericin in the perioperative period [42].

An inevitable consequence of bilateral thoracosternotomy performed for bilateral lung transplantation is cutaneous paraesthesia and commonly dysaesthesia related to surgical section of cutaneous nerves. Return of sensation is variable and it is prudent to warn patients of the likely alterations in chest wall and nipple sensation at the time of acquiring informed consent.

Phrenic nerve palsy, whether by inadvertent intraoperative section, thermal trauma or traction may delay weaning from assisted ventilation and pose ongoing problems with breathing whilst recumbent, particularly at the time of bronchoscopy.

Postoperative arrhythmias are predominantly atrial in origin and probably no more frequent than after other forms of thoracic surgery [43]. Most patients cope well with the rate disturbance but the risk of embolic phenomena makes it worth considering prophylaxis and/or early electroconversion. Pharmacological therapy with amiodarone is often effective but the potential risks of acute and chronic pulmonary toxicity should be borne in mind, particularly if pulmonary infiltrates develop [44]. Inherent in the risk profile of thoracic surgery is the risk of operative ischaemic events, perhaps related to inadvertent hypotension and hypoperfusion secondary to uncontrolled bleeding. Pulmonary vein thrombosis has been reported with an increased frequency in lung transplantation [45]. The use of cardiopulmonary bypass, however, does not necessarily protect from these events and adds a significant risk of cognitive dysfunction, which may persist in the long term [46]. Atrial anastomotic thrombus, which may be detected by transoesophageal echocardiography, adds another potential embolic risk for neurological deficit.

One surgical complication, which may respond to medical therapy, is the development of significant gastroparesis with secondary gastro-oesophageal reflux (GOR) due either to section, traction or thermal trauma to vagal efferents. Therapy with dietary advice, elevation of the head of the bed, prokinetic agents, acid suppression and newer antireflux therapies such as proton pump inhibitors may ameliorate symptoms. It is often the passage of time, however, that affords resolution of simple traction or thermal injuries. Abdominal weight loss is important in this group to further reduce the risk of aspiration. Silent nocturnal aspiration of gastric contents is recognized as a potential risk factor for the development of BOS [47]. The mechanism may be complex, involving the interaction of a competent immune response to epithelial injury followed by the development of an autonomous propagation of the response to alloepithelial antigens [48]. If there are to be surgical attempts at cure using fundoplication, they should be undertaken before permanent airway damage ensues.

Iatrogenic complications

Bronchoscopy, with transbronchial biopsy (TBBx), carries an appreciable iatrogenic risk for patients undergoing lung transplantation. In services where a policy of allograft surveillance with TBBx is followed, the majority of patients will undergo at least six procedures in the first postoperative year. The total risk for an individual patient therefore is the unit risk per procedure multiplied by the number of procedures. Complications of TBBx in lung transplant recipients include pneumothorax (1–3%), pulmonary haemorrhage (10–15%), postprocedure fever (5–7%), need for assisted ventilation (0.1–0.5%), arrhythmia (2%), upper airway obstruction requiring intervention (10%) and cardiorespiratory arrest and death ($\sim 0.01\%$) [49]. The risk to the patient of not performing an interventional diagnostic procedure must be balanced against these known risks. Early therapeutic intervention resulting from the diagnostic procedure may well prevent development of permanent allograft dysfunction.

Interventional bronchoscopy for the management of airway anastomotic breakdown or stricture, by its very nature, has a much higher risk profile. Torrential bleeding from granulation tissue, airway rupture, creation of a false passage, misplacement of a stent, migration of a stent and late stent occlusion from granulation tissue or inspissated secretions are all recognized complications. Nevertheless, excellent results can be obtained with long-term good-quality survival, but results are inferior to those seen in patients who do not need airway intervention [25].

Other common but potentially risky procedures include insertion of central venous access devices, particularly Swan–Ganz catheters [50–52] and vascaths for dialysis, pleural drainage tubes and urinary catheters. Death from perforation of the jugular vein leading to haemothorax and hypotension, air embolism [53], undiagnosed tension pneumothorax, lacerations of intercostal arteries, splenic puncture and direct myocardial transfixion have all been recorded [54,55].

In addition to morbidity related to immunosuppressive agents there are three relatively common idiosyncratic adverse drug reactions that seem to have a predilection for transplant patients. Ciprofloxacin-associated Achilles tendon disease is characterized by pain, gait disturbance, swelling and occasionally rupture, and is reported to occur frequently in lung transplant recipients [56]. It does not appear to be a dose-related phenomenon. Nor is it related to postoperative steroid dose, age or underlying disease process. Aminoglycoside ototoxicity is mentioned to remind readers that this potential complication is worth considering in addition to renal toxicity and may occur even with inhaled therapy. Risks are even more difficult to assess in the ventilated patient. Formal audiological testing at the time of transplant assessment is particularly useful in patients with CF to identify patients at high risk. Statin-related acute and chronic rhabdomyolysis may be a devastating complication with profound global weakness, myoglobinuria and renal failure or present simply with subtle fatiguability [57]. Triazole antifungal agents alter calcineurin metabolism so that catastrophic levels of muscle breakdown may ensue in patients taking statins. Pravastatin is reported to have the lowest rate of this effect at low and intermediate dosages.

Generic complications of immunosuppression

Opportunistic infections are perhaps the most frequent cause of morbidity and direct mortality after lung transplantation. Common agents include CMV [58,59], MRSA, other herpes group viruses including Epstein–Barr virus (EBV) and varicella-zoster and potentially human herpesvirus 8 [60], typical and atypical mycobacteria [61], *Pneumocystis carinii*, *Aspergillus fumigatus*, *Nocardia asteroides*, *Burkholderia cepacia* [62] and *Pseudomonas aeruginosa* (see Chapters 20 and 21). Multiresistant agents such as vancomycin-resistant *Enterococcus* (VRE) pose a constant threat to all transplant units.

PTLD is found more commonly after lung transplantation than other forms of solid organ transplantation, which may reflect the bulk of lymphoid tissue transplanted with the pulmonary allograft, the tendency for young lung transplant recipients to be EBV naive or simply the use of a higher level of immunosuppression after lung transplantation [63,64]. EBV mismatch, where an EBV-naive recipient receives an EBV-positive graft is reported to carry such a high incidence (30–50%) [65] of PTLD that serious questions have been raised regarding the utility of transplant for EBV-naive recipients, as PTLD is often fatal. A recent report outlines a strategy to reduce the incidence of PTLD to an acceptable, almost negligible level, by using lifelong specific antiviral therapy in the high risk group of EBV-mismatched recipients [66]. PTLD represents 53% of post-transplantation malignancy occurring in the first postoperative year but only 17% by the fifth year post-transplantation. Conversely, cutaneous malignancy assumes a more important role as time passes after transplantation. At one year it causes 15% of malignancy but by five years 56% of cases [28]. In particular, cutaneous squamous cell carcinoma (SCC) in the immunosuppressed lung transplant recipient has a predilection for metastatic spread, thereby causing significant morbidity and mortality in this group. While exhortations to practise sun-safe behaviour are frequently made to this group, it is more likely that the rate of SCC reflects solar damage that occurred 10–20 years previously. Regular and frequent dermatological review is nevertheless important to detect early SCCs at a stage where interventional management may be efficacious to avoid disfiguring surgery.

The issues of female genital health and especially the risk of accelerated genital tract neoplasm related to human papillomavirus infection have received scant attention in the literature to date. Our recent review records a higher rate of cervical intraepithelial neoplasia (CIN grades 1–3) after lung transplantation [67]. Frequent surveillance Papanicolaou (PAP) smears are needed to detect early recurrence after therapeutic endeavours. Extensive surgery may be required for vulval intraepithelial neoplasia. Routine surveillance mammography for the early detection of breast carcinoma after lung transplantation has not been proved to have an advantageous cost–benefit ratio; however, logic dictates that benefits might accrue to individual patients who have higher risk profiles.

Lung cancer may occur in the transplanted lung, but more reports have dealt with the problem of cancer in either the explanted lung or the remaining native lung [68]. Depending on the underlying disease process it may be very difficult to detect a small primary neoplasm and, where patients spend a protracted time on the waiting list, it is wise to perform review thoracic CT scans on a six monthly basis to detect early lesions. The cost efficiency of this strategy is such that only 1 case per 100 lung transplants needs to be detected to provide a favourable cost–utility ratio. No prospective data on the potential role or cost–efficiency ratio exist for the use of positron emission tomography (PET) scans in this group. Careful review of chest radiography performed on the night of transplantation is of course invaluable to detect larger lesions (>1 cm) but chest X-ray is neither sensitive nor specific and the decision to defer lung transplantation is difficult in this situation. The risk of proceeding needs to be weighed against the likelihood that a particular lesion is malignant.

Multifactorial complications

Coronary artery disease (CAD) rarely causes death after lung transplantation but transplant-related CAD after HLT occurs frequently in conjunction with OB, suggesting that both may be forms of chronic allograft rejection. Transplantation CAD is often difficult to appreciate on standard coronary angiography, which underestimates the severity and extent of the pathology owing to the diffuse and concentric nature of the intimal changes [69]. Hypertension is the most frequent complication after lung transplantation. Therapy with calcineurin inhibitors, corticosteroids, renal dysfunction, obesity and underlying disease states all combine to produce an incidence of hypertension of 48% at one year and 62.5% at five years. Hypertension is often refractory to therapy with conventional agents but may respond to angiotensin converting enzyme (ACE) receptor antagonists, which fortunately have a lower rate of troublesome cough and angioedema than ACE inhibitors per se.

Oral health is not always appreciated as a *sine qua non* of optimum success after lung transplantation, but recent studies have demonstrated improvements in quality of life and outcome measures with attention to oral health issues. Severe gingival hyperplasia related to ciclosporin therapy may require conversion to alternative agents.

Changes in libido may occur in both directions after lung transplantation. Alterations in body image, postoperative chest pain, side effects of medications especially corticosteroids, and changes in the dynamics of longstanding relationships related to shifts in the need for care/caregiving may all impact negatively on the desire to maintain a sexual relationship. Conversely, the freedoms that accrue with the liberation from the shackles of oxygen therapy, improvements in exercise tolerance and a general feeling of health all conspire in the opposite direction. It may be commented that the desire to procreate often transcends common sense in healthy young transplant recipients. A considered, individualized approach is advised as the preferred method of discussing these issues, after which optimum perinatal care is required for both mother and child [70].

Corticosteroids

Whilst the ramifications of corticosteroid therapy are legion and well known, it is puzzling that more attempts to individualize therapy based on solid pharmacokinetic data are not made. It is as if the oldest and most frequently prescribed immunosuppressive in the pharmacopoeia is somehow blighted by the curse of familiarity and hence our patients pay a heavy penalty of unwanted and largely preventable side effects. A move towards routine performance of area under the curve (AUC) monitoring for prednisolone therapy may assist in the rational utilization of this most dangerous medication [71].

Subtle alterations in bone mineral density occur promptly after lung transplantation and it is the first six months in which the greatest damage is done [72,73]. Steroids combine with calcineurin inhibitors to promote rapid bone loss during this time and pre-emptive strategies to prevent this trend should be part of routine management [74,75]. The risk of osteoporosis after lung transplantation should not be underestimated. Osteoporosis is a mortality risk factor in some series, and the reduction of quality of life and rehabilitation potential associated with pathological fracture due to osteoporosis is well recognized [75].

Proximal myopathy related to steroid therapy seriously hinders rehabilitation as well and may be so severe as to prevent independent walking and resumption of activities of daily living. Relative inactivity due to proximal myopathy forms part of a vicious cycle leading to further deconditioning and loss of function [77,78]. In addition to the direct effects of steroid therapy, post-transplantation myopathy is a complex end result of pretransplantation deconditioning [79], the pre-existing disease state [80] and ciclosporin effects [81,82]. The success or failure of lung transplantation as a discipline depends ultimately on the functionality of the survivors, so it behoves all working in the area to act aggressively in the interests of optimum patient care to minimize the incidence of these catastrophic complications. In one sense, lung transplantation is perhaps the key for true pulmonary rehabilitation for selected patients [83].

Cutaneous fragility remains problematical even on low dose steroid therapy and is a great source of concern to many older patients. Seemingly minor trauma often results in significant skin tears requiring surgery, with or without skin grafting, to repair the defect. The risk of secondary infection further compounds the impact of this all too frequent complication. In the younger age group, by comparison, acne is the usual problem and, while it may be controlled by topical therapies, it is the passage of time that more often provides resolution. Again the distress of what we see as a relatively minor complication cannot be overestimated. Quality of life may be significantly impaired due to alterations in personal image. Acne may therefore require more aggressive systemic therapy in selected patients.

Diabetes mellitus occurs de novo after transplantation in 15–20% of patients. Patients with CF and patients on tacrolimus are at the highest risk but onset is often related to augmented immunosuppression with high dose corticosteroids given for rejection. In addition to the usual risks of ketoacidosis and therapy-related hypoglycaemia, diabetes mellitus may be associated with accelerated microvascular disease and thereby contribute to overall vasculopathy in the transplant recipient. Dietary management is important to help maintain optimal BMI and a balanced nutritional intake [84–86]. Many transplant recipients blame their overeating on their steroid therapy and, for this reason alone, attempts to minimize steroid dosage are justifiable. Hyperlipidaemia is of course, exacerbated by dietary indiscretion, poor diabetic control, and excessive alcohol intake. Calcineurin inhibitors and sirolimus, in particular, all contribute to the difficulty of normalizing lipids after transplantation.

Posterior subcapsular cataract formation is the ocular hallmark of steroid therapy after lung transplantation and is so frequent that it is good policy to incorporate yearly eye examination into the transplant patient's preventative maintenance schedule [87]. Thankfully, lens extraction is now performed as a minor procedure and thus the burden of diminished visual acuity in this group may be reduced. The accelerated nature of cataract formation in this group mandates expediting ophthalmic surgery to maximize quality of life.

Avascular necrosis of the femoral head presents with pain and a limp. Bone scan findings are typical and treatment of choice is total hip replacement for severe cases. Perhaps 5% of patients are so afflicted but age and previous treatment are relevant cofactors in assessing relative risk.

Obstructive sleep apnoea syndrome (OSAS) is an important but little appreciated cause of morbidity after lung transplantation [88]. Whereas lung transplantation cures OSAS in the immediate postoperative period, a proportion of subjects develop OSAS rapidly thereafter, as if lung transplantation were an accelerated model for the development of OSAS. Pulmonary denervation per se does not cause sleep disturbance [89,90]. Mechanisms postulated include localized fat deposition in and around the upper airway and steroid-induced myopathy of the genioglossus. Weight gain is both a cause and consequence of OSAS in this group. Other sequelae include sleep fragmentation, hypertension, cardiac dysfunction, and a tendency to desaturate during fibreoptic bronchoscopy. The latter may be managed by therapeutic, or indeed prophylactic, insertion of a nasopharyngeal tube [91].

Calcineurin inhibitors

The relative roles of the principal calcineurin inhibitors, ciclosporin and tacrolimus in the generation of hypertension, hyperlipidaemia, diabetes mellitus and oral health issues have already been discussed. It is hypertension, particularly in the younger patient that is implicated in the potentially fatal complication of cerebral neurotoxicity manifest by major motor epilepsy and, on occasion, status epilepticus [92]. Blood pressure control is essential for satisfactory short-term management. Other forms of neurotoxicity include tremor, an exaggerated physiological tremor that may be ameliorated by the use of a small dose of beta-blocker, and peripheral neuropathy, which may respond to dose reduction if detected early. Delirium may be seen as an idiosyncratic response in new transplant recipients with initial drug exposure. Hypomagnesaemia and hypokalaemia are thought to be contributory factors [92]. High dose steroids alone may cause a similar response.

Hirsuitism may seem a small price to pay for adequate immunosuppression, but in so far as it may impact negatively on self-esteem and thereby limit social interaction it can defeat the aim of lung transplantation to return functional patients to real world situations [93]. Therefore, a proactive strategy is needed to enable patients so afflicted access to optimal therapies to manage this problem.

Nephrotoxicity was and is the major complication that requires on-going consideration [94]. Some 36% of lung transplant recipients have significant renal dysfunction by five years post-transplantation [28]. This rate alone calls for an urgent reappraisal of current immunosuppressive strategies. The technology and pharmacological knowledge already exist to allow more sophisticated use of current drugs and for the sake of renal preservation we must forego outmoded approaches and embrace a new strategy [95]. Every nephron is important and the minor inconvenience of performing AUC monitoring or a limited sampling strategy is eminently worth the investment of time and cost if superior outcomes can be achieved.

Bronchiolitis obliterans syndrome

Other authors in earlier chapters have covered the issues regarding BOS but it would be remiss in this summary of the status of lung transplantation not to provide some further commentary. It is important when discussing BOS to clearly differentiate it from the diagnosis of obliterative bronchiolitis (OB), which is a pathological description [96–98]. The two conditions are not mutually exclusive, however, and the majority, but not all patients with OB will have BOS and vice versa. A distinct proportion with BOS will have other diagnoses such as undetected invasive fungal infection, necrotizing bronchiolitis, chondromalacia, native lung volume hyperinflation syndrome, mycobacterial infection, chlamydial infection or PTLD. The value of postmortem studies as a teaching tool in this regard should not be discounted. The logical corollaries are: first, that all attempts to achieve a firm tissue diagnosis should reasonably be made within a suitable risk–benefit framework; and, second, that empiric augmented immunosuppression carries a mortality risk for a percentage of patients with BOS [99].

Several studies have linked the finding of acute pulmonary allograft rejection with the subsequent development of BOS but none has then analysed the positive predictive value of the diagnosis of BOS for the confirmation of OB at postmortem in sufficient numbers to allow meaningful analysis [100–104]. The possibility that treatment of BOS confounds the natural history should not be excluded from any proper discussion in this area. The nexus between the finding of perivascular and parenchymal lymphocytic infiltrates and the subsequent development of OB is not clear in a pathogenic sense. Perhaps the more useful signal for the development of (possibly) BOS or (certainly) OB will be the severity and persistence of lymphocytic bronchiolitis on TBBx. It seems strange that the focus for so long in this area has been on the parenchyma rather than the airway.

Approaches to the management of BOS have been described in this volume and elsewhere [105,106]. Early recognition signals [107] are needed to allow institution of therapies at a stage where maximum preservation of lung function can be achieved. Every terminal bronchiole is important and, once lost to fibrosis, will never be recovered. A suitable metaphor for the concept of the effect of OB is to consider the total cross-sectional area of the 30 000 terminal bronchioles summed together as the area of a clockface. As the area of a single terminal bronchiole is lost to fibrosis, just over a second passes. Initially, there is no clinical evidence of disease because the lung has such great functional reserve. By 6 o'clock the loss of 50% of the cross-sectional area is now appreciable, physiologically and symptomatically. Much irreversible damage has already been done and it is here that the majority of interventional studies have usually commenced management! It is no wonder that the rate of effectiveness of any therapeutic agent is so small. Proven effective treatments can be established only by properly powered multicentre trials that are not biased to a negative result by time of entry to the study. We need the best evidence as soon as it can be collected to guide management in this area that is most critical to the long-term viability of individual patients and to lung transplantation per se. Similarly, in the scientific domain, research should focus on vascular and epithelial injury patterns [108] and the fibroproliferative response of the human lung fibroblast [109,110]. This information will then allow a rational choice of therapies for individual patients. Ultimately, the goal remains prevention, which we hope will make early detection and therapy redundant.

Future trends

The future of lung transplantation remains as much of an enigma now as it ever was. However, there are some positive trends to guide forward planning and development. Consensus documents from the international community are available to guide listing of candidates, to diagnose and grade acute and chronic pulmonary allograft rejection and to describe and grade BOS. The latter document has recently been revised and now includes a more sensitive descriptor of small airway dysfunction, with the aim of identifying BOS at an earlier stage when it may be more amenable to reversal with interventional therapy, or at least to stabilization with maximal preservation of pulmonary functional reserve [10]. The results of trials designed to prevent and manage BOS are awaited with great interest. Whether positive or not, the proper template now exists to examine these questions in a scientifically rigorous manner. The recognition of the precious nature of donor resources has led rightly to the re-evaluation of evidence describing the acceptable criteria for pulmonary organ utilization. A position paper is in preparation and it is to be expected that analysis of the recommendations contained therein will be tested in the crucible of clinical practice. Knowledge gained from the study of patients with orphan diseases referred for transplantation has led to the development of therapeutic alternatives for pulmonary hypertension and emphysema, with further refinements of listing criteria ensuing. It is likely that organ allocation strategies will continue to reflect the dynamics of the local transplant community, with major differences existing between countries and indeed within some larger countries. It is to be hoped that inequities of organ allocation thus accruing can be solved ultimately by a system that takes cognisance of differing rates of urgency between disease states. Only thus can we, as a global community, hope to minimize the phenomenon of death on the waiting list.

Summary and conclusions

The attention on advanced respiratory failure that has been generated by clinical lung transplantation has contributed to new therapies for specific conditions and to alternative approaches to transplantation. However, transplantation remains the optimal therapy for appropriately selected patients with advanced respiratory failure or severe pulmonary vascular disease refractory to other therapies.

Traditional conservative concepts of the optimal donor are being superseded by a reasoned, outcome-based approach with acceptable clinical results (taking into account the 'opportunity cost' of not using a suboptimal donor for a potential individual recipient). With regard to recipient selection, the concept of whom to exclude from transplantation has been superseded by the approach of whom to include within an acceptable risk–benefit ratio for the specific patient.

Monitoring and individualizing drug regimens have become more widespread. High rates of post-transplantation renal dysfunction mandate the use of more sophisticated techniques such as 'area under the curve' monitoring and limited sampling strategies to control therapy with calcineurin inhibitors. The availability of techniques to examine the response to immunosuppressive agents 'in vitro' may be able to provide an insight into the likely response of an individual patient 'in vivo'. We must be vigilant to the long-term non-immunological side effects of immunosuppressive agents and careful management of risk factors for coronary, and other, vascular disease is essential for optimal long-term outcomes.

We are now in a position where multicentre clinical trials can be used to help to answer important questions about the optimum treatment both before and after lung transplantation and such studies are now under way.

Obliterative bronchiolitis remains the main factor limiting the long-term benefit of lung transplantation; its conquest remains the 'Holy Grail' for all those involved in the field.

Acknowledgment

The author acknowledges with much gratitude the privilege of being involved with the lung transplant community over the last 17 years and in particular the experiences and lessons learned from exposure to this remarkable patient group.

REFERENCES

1 Shumway, NE. Thoracic transplantation. *World J Surg* 2000; **24**: 811–814.
2 Reitz BA, Wallwork JL, Hunt SA, et al. Heart–lung transplantation: successful therapy for patients with pulmonary vascular disease. *N Engl J Med* 1982; **306**: 557–564.
3 Modry DL, Oyer PE, Jamieson SW, et al. Cyclosporine in heart and heart–lung transplantation. *Can J Surg* 1985; **28**: 274–280, 282.
4 Glanville AR, Theodore J, Harvey J, Robin ED. Elastic behavior of the transplanted lung. Exponential analysis of static pressure–volume relationships. *Am Rev Respir Dis* 1988; **137**: 308–312.
5 Nakae S, Webb WR, Theodorides T, Sugg WL. Respiratory function following cardiopulmonary denervation in dog, cat, and monkey. *Surg Gynecol Obstet* 1967; **125**: 1285–1292.
6 Cohen RG, Starnes SV. Living donor lung transplantation. *World J Surg* 2001; **25**: 244–250.
7 Maurer JR, Frost AE, Estenne M, Higenbottam T, Glanville AR. International guidelines for the selection of lung transplant candidates. The International Society for Heart and Lung Transplantation, the American Thoracic Society, the American Society of Transplant Physicians, the European Respiratory Society. *J Heart Lung Transplant* 1998; **17**: 703–709.
8 Griffith B, Bando K, Hardesty R, et al. A prospective randomized trial of FK506 versus cyclosporine after human pulmonary transplantation. *Transplantation* 1994 **57**: 848–851.
9 Corris P, Glanville A, McNeil K, et al. One year ananysis of an ongong international randomised study of mycophenolate

10 mofetil (MMF) vs azathioprine (AZA) in lung transplantation. *J Heart Lung Transplant* 2001; **20**: 208.
10 Estenne M, Maurer JR, Boehler A, et al. Bronchiolitis obliterans syndrome 2001: an update of the diagnostic criteria. *J Heart Lung Transplant* 2001; **21**: 297–310.
11 Rubin, LJ. Primary pulmonary hypertension. *N Engl J Med* 1997; **336**: 111–117.
12 Fouty B, Rodman DM. Pulmonary vascular gene transfer: prospects for successful therapy of pulmonary hypertension. *Am J Respir Cell Mol Biol* 1999; **21**: 555–557.
13 D'Alonzo, GE, Barst RJ, Ayres SM, et al. Survival in patients with primary pulmonary hypertension. Results from a national prospective registry. *Ann Intern Med* 1991; **115**: 343–349.
14 Glanville AR, Burke CM, Theodore J, Robin ED. Primary pulmonary hypertension. Length of survival in patients referred for heart–lung transplantation. *Chest* 1987; **91**: 675–681.
15 Janus EBJ. Alpha-1-antitrypsin deficiency and emphysema: new horizons in treatment. *Aust NZ J Med* 1990; **20**: 755–757.
16 Taylor J, Ryu J, Colby T, Raffin T. Lymphangioleiomatosis. *N Engl J Med* 1990; **323**: 1254–1260.
17 Conte JV, Gaine SP, Orens JB, Harris T, Rubin LJ. The influence of continuous intravenous prostacyclin therapy for primary pulmonary hypertension on the timing and outcome of transplantation. *J Heart Lung Transplant* 1998; **17**: 679–685.
18 Archibald CJ, Auger WR, Fedullo PF, et al. Long-term outcome after pulmonary thromboendarterectomy. *Am J Respir Crit Care Med* 1990; **160**: 523–528.
19 Meyers BF, Patterson GA. Lung transplantation versus lung volume reduction as surgical therapy for emphysema. *World J Surg* 2001; **25**: 238–243.
20 Higenbottam T, Stewart S, Penketh A, Wallwork J. Transbronchial lung biopsy for the diagnosis of rejection in heart–lung transplant patients. *Transplantation* 1988; **46**: 532–539.
21 Hertz MI, Harmon KR, Knighton DR, et al. Combined laser phototherapy and growth factor treatment of bronchial obstruction after lung transplantation. *Chest* 1991; **100**: 1717–1719.
22 Sibley RK, Berry GJ, Tazelaar HD, et al. The role of transbronchial biopsies in the management of lung transplant recipients. *J Heart Lung Transplant* 1993; **12**: 308–324.
23 Chhajed PN, Malouf M, Tamm M, Spratt P, Glanville AR. Interventional bronchoscopy for the management of airway complications following lung transplantation. *Chest* 2001; **120**: 1894–1899.
24 Chhajed PN, Malouf M, Tamm M, Glanville AR. Early experience with nitinol (ultraflex) stents for the management of benign airway lesions. *Am J Respir Crit Care Med* 2001; **163**: A700.
25 Aboyoun CL, Tamm M, Chhajed PN, et al. Diagnostic value of follow-up transbronchial lung biopsy after lung rejection. *Am J Respir Crit Care Med* 2001; **164**: 460–463.
26 Schafers H-J, Haydock DA, Cooper JD. The prevalence and management of bronchial anastomotic complications in lung transplantation. *J Thorac Cardiovasc Surg* 1991; **101**: 1044–1052.

27 Chhajed PN, Malouf M, Glanville AR. Bronchoscopic dilatation in the algorithmic management of benign (non-transplant) tracheobronchial stenosis. *Intern Med J* 2001; **31**: 512–516.

28 Hosenpud JD, Bennett LE, Keck BM, Boucek MM, Novick RJ. The Registry of the International Society for Heart and Lung Transplantation: 18th official report–2001. *J Heart Lung Transplant* 2001; **20**: 805–815.

29 Barlow CW, Robbins RC, Moon MR, Akindipe O, Theodore J, Reitz BA. Heart–lung versus double-lung transplantation for suppurative lung disease. *J Thorac Cardiovasc Surg* 2000; **119**: 466–476.

30 Glanville AR, Marshman D, Keogh A, et al. Outcome in paired recipients of single lung transplants from the same donor. *J Heart Lung Transplant* 1995; **14**: 878–882.

31 De Meester J, Smits JM, Persijn GG, Haverich A. Listing for lung transplantation: life expectancy and transplant effect, stratified by type of end-stage lung disease, the Eurotransplant Experience. *J Heart Lung Transplant* 2001; **20**: 518–524.

32 Lok S. Interstitial lung disease clinics for the management of idiopathic pulmonary fibrosis: a potential advantage to patients. *J Heart Lung Transplant* 1999; **18**: 884–890.

33 Christie JD, Bavaria JE, Palevsky HI, et al. Primary graft failure following lung transplantation. *Chest* 1998; **114**: 51–60.

34 Gabbay E, Williams TJ, Griffiths AP, et al. Maximizing the utilization of donor organs offered for lung transplantation. *Am J Respir Crit Care Med* 1999; **160**: 265–271.

35 Bhorade SM, Vigneswaran W, McCabe MA, Garrity ER. Liberalization of donor criteria may expand the donor pool without adverse consequence in lung transplantation. *J Heart Lung Transplant* 2000; **19**: 1199–1204.

36 Novick RJ, Bennett LE, Meyer DM, Hosenpud JD. Influence of graft ischemic time and donor age on survival after lung transplantation. *J Heart Lung Transplant* 1999; **18**: 425–431.

37 Hosenpud JD, Bennett LE, Keck BM, Edwards EB, Novick RJ. Effect of diagnosis on survival benefit of lung transplantation for end-stage lung disease. *Lancet* 1998; **351**: 24–27.

38 Henry M. Cyclosporine and tacrolimus (FK506): a comparison of efficacy and safety profiles. *Clin Transplant* 1999; **13**: 209–220.

39 Lowy FD. *Staphylococcus aureus* infections. *N Engl J Med* 1998; **339**: 520–532.

40 Hopkins, P. A cluster of *Mycoplasma hominis* infection in heart–lung transplantation. *J Heart Lung Transplant* 2001; **20**: 223–224.

41 Glanville AR. *Chlamydia pneumonia* is associated with graft dysfunction after lung transplantation. *J Heart Lung Transplant* 2001; **20**: 171.

42 Reichenspurner H, Gamberg P, Nitschke M, et al. Significant reduction in the number of fungal infections after lung, heart–lung, and heart transplantation using aerosolized amphotericin B prophylaxis. *Transplant Proc* 1997; **29**: 627–628.

43 Hoffman TM, Rhodes LA, Wieand TS, Spray TL, Bridges ND. Arrhythmias after pediatric lung transplantation. *Pediatr Transplant* 2001; **5**: 349–352.

44 Ashrafian H, Davey P. Is amiodarone an underrecognized cause of acute respiratory failure in the ICU? *Chest* 2001; **120**: 275–282.

45 Leibowitz, DW, Smith CR, Michler RE, et al. Incidence of pulmonary vein complications after lung transplantation: a prospective transesophageal echocardiographic study. *J Am Coll Cardiol* 1994; **24**: 671–675.

46 van Dijk D, Keizer AM, Diephuis JC, Durand C, Vos LJ, Hijman R. Neurocognitive dysfunction after coronary artery bypass surgery: a systematic review. [see comments]. *J Thorac Cardiovasc Surg* 2000; **120**: 632–639.

47 Reid KR, McKenzie FN, Menkis AH, et al. Importance of chronic aspiration in recipients of heart–lung transplants. *Lancet* 1990; **336**: 206–208.

48 Burke CM, Glanville AR, Theodore J, Robin ED. Lung immunogenicity, rejection, and obliterative bronchiolitis. *Chest* 1987; **92**: 547–549.

49 Chhajed PN, Aboyoun CL, Malouf MA, Hopkins PM, Plit ML, Glanville AR. Risk factors and management of bleeding associated with transbronchial biopsy in lung transplant recipients. *J Heart Lung Transplant*: in press.

50 Robin ED. The cult of the Swan–Ganz catheter. Overuse and abuse of pulmonary flow catheters. *Ann Intern Med* 1985; **103**: 445–449.

51 Robin ED. Death by pulmonary artery flow-directed catheter. Time for a moratorium? *Chest* 1987; **92**: 727–731.

52 Robin ED. Defenders of the pulmonary artery catheter. *Chest* 1988; **93**: 1059–1066.

53 Muth CS, ES. Gas embolism. *N Engl J Med* 2000; **342**: 476–482.

54 Kleinfeld G. Iatrogenic splenic trauma. *JAMA* 1980; **244**: 1784.

55 Hesselink DA, Van Der Klooster JM, Bac EH, Scheffer MG, Brouwers JW. Cardiac tamponade secondary to chest tube placement. *Eur J Emerg Med* 2001; **8**: 237–239.

56 Chhajed PN, Plit M, Hopkins P, Malouf M, Glanville AR. Achilles tendon disease in lung transplant recipients and its association with ciprofloxacin. *Eur Respir J* 2002; **21**: 547–554.

57 Malouf MA, Bicknell M, Glanville AR. Rhabdomyolysis after lung transplantation. *Aust NZ J Med* 1997; **27**: 186.

58 Duncan AJ, Dummer JS, Paradis I, et al. Cytomegalovirus infection and survival in lung transplant recipients. *J Heart Lung Transplant* 1991; **10**: 638–646.

59 Burke CM, Glanville AR, Macoviak JA, et al. The spectrum of cytomegalovirus infection following human heart–lung transplantation. *J Heart Transplant* 1986; **5**: 267–272.

60 Ho, M. Human herpesvirus 8 – let the transplantation physician beware. *N Engl J Med* 1998; **339**: 1391–1392.

61 Malouf MA, Glanville AR. The spectrum of mycobacterial infection after lung transplantation. *Am J Respir Crit Care Med* 1999; **160**: 1611–1616.

62 Aris RM, Gilligan PH, Neuringer IP, Gott KK, Rea J, Yankaskas JR. The effects of panresistant bacteria in cystic fibrosis patients on lung transplant outcome. *Am J Respir Crit Care Med* 1997; **155**: 1699–1704.

63 Yousem SA, Randhawa P, Locker J, et al. Posttransplant lymphoproliferative disorders in heart–lung transplant recipients. *Hum Pathol* 1989; **20**: 361–369.

64 Swerdlow AJ, Higgins CD, Hunt BJ, et al. Risk of lymphoid neoplasia after cardiothoracic transplantation. *Transplantation* 2000; **69**: 897–904.

65 Aris RM, Maia DM, Neuringer IP, et al. Post-transplantation lymphoproliferative disorder in the Epstein–Barr virus-naive lung transplant recipient. *Am J Respir Crit Care Med* 1996; **154**: 1712–1717.

66 Malouf MA, Chhajed PN, Hopkins P, Plit M, Turner J, Glanville AR. Antiviral prophylaxis reduces the incidence of lymphoproliferative disease in lung transplant recipients. *J Heart Lung Transplant* 2002; **19**: 469–471.

67 Malouf MA, Hopkins PM, Singleton L, Chhajed PN, Plit ML, Glanville AR. Female sexual health issues after lung transplantation: the importance of screening. *Am J Res Crit Care Med* 2002; **165**: A391.

68 Stagner LD, Allenspach LL, Hogan KK, Willcock LC, Higgins RS, Chan KM. Bronchogenic carcinoma in lung transplant recipients. *J Heart Lung Transplant* 2001; **20**: 908–911.

69 Glanville AR, Baldwin JC, Hunt SA, Theodore J. Long-term cardiopulmonary function after human heart–lung transplantation. *Aust NZ J Med* 1990; **20**: 208–214.

70 Armenti VT, Radmski JS, Mortiz MJ, Philips LZ, McGrory CH, Coscia LA. Report from the National Transplantation Pregnancy Registry (NTPR): outcomes of pregnancy after transplantation. *Clin Transpl* 2000: 123–34.

71 Morton JM, Mcwhinney B, Hickman PE, Potter JM. Therapeutic drug monitoring (TDM) of prednisolone in lung transplantation. *J Heart Lung Transplant* 2001; **20**: 192.

72 Henderson K, Eisman J, Keogh A, et al. Protective effect of short-tem calcitriol or cyclical etidronate on bone loss after cardiac or lung transplantation. *J Bone Miner Res* 2001; **16**: 565–571.

73 Sambrook P, Henderson NK, Keogh A, et al. Effect of calcitriol on bone loss after cardiac or lung transplantation. *J Bone Miner Res* 2000; **15**: 1818–1824.

74 Aris RM, Lester GE, Renner JB, et al. Efficacy of pamidronate for osteoporosis in patients with cystic fibrosis following lung transplantation. *Am J Respir Crit Care Med* 2000; **162**: 941–946.

75 Spira A, Gutiérrez C, Chaparro C, Hutcheon MA, Chan CK. Osteoporosis and lung transplantation: a prospective study. *Chest* 2000; **117**: 476–481.

76 Shane E, Papadopoulos A, Staron R, et al. Bone loss and fracture after lung transplantation. *Transplantation* 1999; **68**: 220–227.

77 Epstein FH. Exercise limitation in health and disease. *N Engl J Med* 2000; **343**: 632–641.

78 Morrison WL, Gibson JN, Scrimgeour C, Rennie MJ. Muscle wasting in emphysema. *Clin Sci* (Colch) 1988; **75**: 415–420.

79 Williams TJ, Patterson GA, McClean PA, Zamel N, Maurer JR, Maximal exercise testing in single and double lung transplant recipients. *Am Rev Respir Dis* 1992; **145**: 101–105.

80 Otulana B, Hifenbottam T, Wallwork J, Causes of exercise limitation after heart–lung transplantation. *J Heart Lung Transplant* 1992; **11**: S244–S251.

81 Evans AB, Al-Himyary AJ, Hrovat MI, et al. Abnormal skeletal muscle oxidative capacity after lung transplantation by ^{31}P-MRS. *Am J Res Crit Care Med* 1997; **155**: 615–621.

82 Wang XN, Williams TJ, McKenna MJ, et al. Skeletal muscle oxidative capacity, fiber type, and metabolites after lung transplantation. *Am J Respir Crit Care Med* 1999; **160**: 57–63.

83 Resnikoff PM, Ries AL. Pulmonary rehabilitation for chronic lung disease. *J Heart Lung Transplant* 1998; **17**: 643–650.

84 Schwebel C, Pin I, Barnoud D, et al. Prevalence and consequences of nutritional depletion in lung transplant candidates. *Eur Respir J* 2000; **16**: 1050–1055.

85 Snell GI, Bennetts K, Bartolo J, et al. Body mass index as a predictor of survival in adults with cystic fibrosis referred for lung transplantation. *J Heart Lung Transplant* 1998; **17**: 1097–1103.

86 Madill J, Maurer JR, de Hoyos A. A comparison of preoperative and postoperative nutritional states of lung transplant recipients. *Transplantation* 1993; **56**: 347–350.

87 Ng P, McCluskey P, McCaughan G, Glanville A, MacDonald P, Keogh A. Ocular complications of heart, lung, and liver transplantation. *Br J Ophthalmol* 1998; **82**: 423–428.

88 Malouf MA, Chhajed PN, Jankelson D, Aboyoun C, Grunstein R, Glanville AR. Prevalence of sleep disordered breathing after lung transplantation. *J Heart Lung Transplant* 2001; **20**: 225.

89 Shea SA, Horner RL, Banner NR, et al. The effect of human heart–lung transplantation upon breathing at rest and during sleep. *Respir Physiol* 1988; **72**: 131–149.

90 Sanders MH, Costantino GP, Owens GR, et al. Breathing during wakefulness and sleep after human heart–lung transplantation. *Am Rev Respir Dis* 1989; **140**: 45–51.

91 Chhajed PN, Aboyoun C, Malouf M, et al. Management of acute hypoxaemia during flexible bronchoscopy with insertion of a nasopharyngeal tube in lung transplant recipients. *Chest* 2002; **121**: 1350–1354.

92 Goldstein LS, Haug MT III, Perl J II, et al. Central nervous system complications after lung transplantation. *J Heart Lung Transplant* 1998; **17**: 185–191.

93 Cohen L, Littlefield C, Kelly P, Maurer J, Abbey S. Predictors of quality of life and adjustment after lung transplantation. *Chest* 1998; **113**: 633–644.

94 Imoto EM, Glanville AR, Baldwin JC, Theodore J. Kidney function in heart–lung transplant recipients: the effect of low-dosage cyclosporine therapy. *J Heart Transplant* 1987; **6**: 204–213.

95 Dumont RJ, Partovi N, Levy RD, Fradet G, Ensom MH. A limited sampling strategy for cyclosporine area under the curve monitoring in lung transplant recipients. *J Heart Lung Transplant* 2001; **20**: 897–900.

96 Burke CM, Theodore J, Dawkins KD, et al. Post-transplant obliterative bronchiolitis and other late lung sequelae in human heart-lung transplantation. *Chest* 1984; **86**: 824–829.

97 Berry GJ, Brunt EM, Chamberlain D, et al. A working formulation for the standardization of nomenclature in the diagnosis of heart and lung rejection: Lung Rejection Study Group. The International Society for Heart Transplantation. *J Heart Transplant* 1990; **9**: 593–601.

98 Yousem SA, Berry GJ, Cagle PT, et al. Revision of the 1990 working formulation for the classification of pulmonary allograft rejection: Lung Rejection Study Group. *J Heart Lung Transplant* 1996; **15**: 1–15.

99 Glanville AR, Baldwin JC, Burke CM, Theodore J, Robin ED. Obliterative bronchiolitis after heart–lung transplantation: apparent arrest by augmented immunosuppression. *Ann Intern Med* 1987; **107**: 300–304.

100 Keller CA, Cagle PT, Brown RW, Noon G, Frost AE. Bronchiolitis obliterans in recipients of single, double, and heart–lung transplantation. *Chest* 1995; **107**: 973–980.

101 Girgis RE, Tu I, Berry GJ, et al. Risk factors for the development of obliterative bronchiolitis after lung transplantation. *J Heart Lung Transplant* 1996; **15**: 1200–1208.

102 Heng D, Sharples LD, McNeil K, Stewart S, Wreghitt T, Wallwork J. Bronchiolitis obliterans syndrome: incidence, natural history, prognosis, and risk factors. *J Heart Lung Transplant* 1998; **17**: 1255–1263.

103 Sharples LD, Tamm M, McNeil K, Higenbottam TW, Stewart S, Wallwork J. Development of bronchiolitis obliterans syndrome in recipients of heart–lung transplantation – early risk factors. *Transplantation* 1996; **61**: 560–566.

104 Husain AN, Siddiqui MT, Holmes EW, et al. Analysis of risk factors for the development of bronchiolitis obliterans syndrome. *Am J Respir Crit Care Med* 1999; **159**: 829–833.

105 Trulock EP. Lung transplantation. *Am J Respir Crit Care Med* 1997; **155**: 789–818.

106 Glanville AR. Current and prospective treatments of obliterative bronchiolitis. *Curr Opin Organ Transpl* 2000; **5**: 396–401.

107 Reynaud-Gaubert M, Thomas P, Badier M, Cau P, Giudicelli R, Fuentes P. Early detection of airway involvement in obliterative bronchiolitis after lung transplantation. Functional and bronchoalveolar lavage cell findings. *Am J Respir Crit Care Med* 2000; **161**: 1924–1929.

108 Zheng L, Orsida BE, Ward C, et al. Airway vascular changes in lung allograft recipients. *J Heart Lung Transplant* 1999; **18**: 231–238.

109 Jonosono M, Fang K, Keith F, et al. Measurement of fibroblast proliferative activity in bronchoalveolar lavage fluid in the analysis of obliterative bronchiolitis among lung transplant recipients. *J Heart Lung Transplant* 1999; **18**: 972–985.

110 Tamm M, Roth M, Malouf M, et al. Primary fibroblast cell cultures from transbronchial biopsies of lung transplant recipients. *Transplantation* 2001; **71**: 337–339.

Part 3

Future directions

27

Tissue engineering

Larry L. Hench[1], Julian R. Jones[1], Rubia F. S. Lenza[2] and Wander L. V. Vasconcelos[2]

[1]Imperial College London, UK
[2]Federal University of Minas Gerais Belo Horizonte, MG, Brazil

Objective

Growing three-dimensional tissue-engineered constructs is one of the few alternatives to the use of heart–lung transplants for critically ill patients. Creating a large, complex viable construct that is capable of supporting human life is a formidable challenge. Ten years ago such an enterprise would have been technically impossible. However, recent results from two fields of materials science indicate that in vitro formation of three-dimensional functional organs may be feasible within the next decade. The developments are: (1) bioactive materials that activate the regenerative potential of tissues and release proteins needed for organogenesis, and (2) sol-gel processing of hierarchical porous materials that can direct growth of three-dimensional (3-D) interconnected structures that mimic the natural architecture of tissues.

The objective of this chapter is to review the concepts of these two fields and indicate how they can be directed towards the goal of engineering biomolecularly tailored 3-D constructs for growth of tissues and organs. The function of the bioactive composition will be to stimulate and control the rate and sequence of differentiation and proliferation of the tissues, whereas the role of the hierarchical bioactive matrix will be to direct formation of the 3-D architecture of the engineered tissue.

Introduction

Tissue engineering combines biology, materials science and biomedical engineering to achieve long-term repair and replacement of failing human tissues and organs [1–3]. Three strategies can be employed: (1) in vitro construction of bioartificial tissues from cells harvested from the patient or from cell lines, (2) in vivo alteration of cell growth and function, and (3) a combination of (1) and (2) [1].

The aims of the first approach are to seed cells onto the appropriate 3-D scaffolds, and then stimulate the cells to proliferate and differentiate to form specific tissues that mimic the complex structure and physiological behaviour of natural tissues. After a critical period of growth, the engineered tissue or organ can be implanted in a patient [1].

The interactions between cells and surfaces play a major biological role in cellular behaviour. Cellular interactions and artificial surfaces are mediated through adsorbed proteins [4–5]. If cells can recognize the proteins adsorbed onto the surface of a biomaterial they can attach to it and start to differentiate, inducing tissue formation or regeneration. However, if cells do not recognize the proteins as part of natural tissues, they will initiate a chronic inflammation that can result in encapsulation of the material or cell death [4,6].

A common strategy in tissue engineering is to modify the biomaterial surface to selectively interact with a cell through biomolecular recognition events. Adsorbed bioactive peptides can allow cell attachment onto biomaterials, and allow 3-D structures modified with these peptides to preferentially induce tissue formation consistent with the cell type seeded, either on or within the device [7].

Besides promoting cell surface recognition, bioactive peptides can be used to control or promote many aspects of cell physiology, such as adhesion, spreading, activation, migration, proliferation and differentiation [8].

Bioactive glasses are special compositions of CaO-SiO_2-based materials that can bond to both hard and soft tissue [9] owing to carbonate hydroxyapatite (HCA) layer formation on the surface of the material on contact with physiological fluids. The HCA layer is similar in structure and composition to the natural apatite found in bone, and hence a strong bond can form between bioactive glasses and bone.

For soft tissues, the bond occurs by tissue incorporation around HCA nodules. In order to enhance the properties of these materials or adapt them to soft tissue engineering, researchers have tried to incorporate growth factors and proteins that promote cell recognition and adhesion, and can be released in a controlled manner, having a beneficial effect on tissue formation [3,10,11].

Polymeric systems for drug and protein delivery are numerous. However, there are presently no biomaterials that exhibit simultaneously controlled biomolecule release and bioactive behaviour [7]. A goal of our research is to synthesize materials that release proteins in a controlled way while at the same time serving as a support for tissue ingrowth and direct organogenesis.

Incorporation of bioactive peptides in 3-D scaffolds as an approach to tissue engineering is challenging because of the fragile nature, chemical complexity and geometric complexity of these macromolecules [6,12]. Several prerequisites must be satisfied in order to successfully graft bioactive molecules to produce materials that demonstrate cell surface recognition and promote cell adhesion, proliferation and differentiation [4,6]. The way that proteins or other bioactive peptides interact with the surfaces can alter their biological functionality. In order to achieve full functionality, peptides have to adsorb specifically. They also must maintain conformation in order to remain functional biologically. Chemical groups, such as amine and mercaptan groups are known to control the ability of surfaces to interact with proteins [4,7–8]. In addition, these chemical groups can allow protein–surface interactions to occur such that the active domains of the protein can be oriented outwards where they can be maximally effective in triggering biospecific processes [7].

Webb et al. [13] related that the adsorption of some proteins, such as bovine serum albumin, fibronectin and laminin, led to differential cell adhesion depending on whether the protein was adsorbed on different chemically functional groups. This finding indicates that proteins can have differential effects on cell behaviour depending on substrate surface chemistry. Healy [7] cited various successful peptide attachments on inorganic and organic matrices utilizing chemical functional groups and demonstrated that the cell behaviour at surfaces could be controlled in vitro by selective immobilization of peptides.

Matrices utilized for simultaneous tissue support and delivery of angiogenic factors must exhibit an appropriate pore structure, bioactive properties, peptide release kinetics and controlled resorbtion rates. We have recently developed a method to incorporate proteins in bioactive sol-gel matrices modified with amine and mercaptan groups [14]. This process avoids the use of high temper-

ature and organic solvents that can denature proteins. We also developed a novel protocol to modify the surface of bioactive foams (58S and 70S30C) [14], using organosilane reagents. These approaches may be ideal to incorporate and deliver angiogenic factors at controlled rates of release owing to the gentle processing conditions utilized.

This chapter describes the protein release profiles for surface modified foams used as carriers for albumin and laminin proteins, respectively. These proteins are selected as molecular models for the eventual tailoring of scaffold chemistry to engineer growth of various tissues and organs. We also studied the influence of chemical groups and adsorbed protein on the in vitro bioactive behaviour of the foams. The 3-D architecture of the foams mimics the scale and interconnectivity of structures needed to grow many complex tissues in vitro. The next phase of research will be an attempt to impregnate the 3-D bioactive foam with various cells that can proliferate and differentiate into a functioning lung lobe.

Synthesis of bioactive foams surface modified with laminin

The binary 70%SiO$_2$–30%CaO (70S30C) and the ternary 60%SiO$_2$–36%CaO–4%P$_2$O$_5$ (58S) foams modified with amine and mercaptan groups were prepared by the sol-gel foam method as described [14]. Processing, structural characterization and specifics of the protein release kinetics have been given [15]. A scanning electron micrograph of both compositions of bioactive foam scaffolds is given in Figure 27.1.

Protein adsorption was carried out by soaking 0.10 g of foams in a phosphate-buffered saline (PBS) solution containing 20 μg of laminin (from human placenta, Sigma) at 37 °C for five hours under constant agitation. The efficiency of the process, in terms of protein loading, was higher than 99%, as was demonstrated by the amount of laminin release from the foams after the PBS wash procedure.

Protein release experiments

Protein release studies were performed by immersing the samples (silica-based glasses and foams modified with adsorbed proteins) in 1 mL PBS and placing them in an orbital shake rotating at 175 rpm at 37 °C. The protein concentration in the solutions was measured based on UV-VIS spectroscopy with a Unicam UV-500 Spectrophotometer using the Peterson method [15]. Absorbance values were

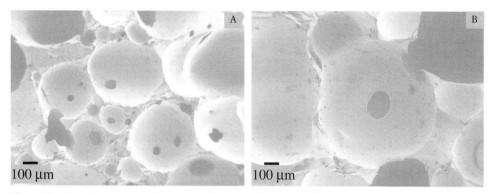

Figure 27.1 Scanning electron micrographs of (A) 58S and (B) 70S30C bioactive foam scaffolds.

taken at a wavelength of 750 nm, at which the protein solutions showed an absorbance maximum.

The UV-VIS spectroscopy was also used to characterize the conformational change/denaturation of the proteins in the release solution after four weeks of immersion in PBS. Interaction between the proteins and the material surface may lead to a conformational change in the ternary structure, which can be revealed by the change in its absorption spectrum [12].

In vitro bioactivity assessment

The in vitro bioactivity assessment was carried out by immersing 0.05 g of each foam (with and without laminin) in 20 mL simulated body fluid (SBF) at pH 7.2 in polyethylene vials. The vials were placed in an orbital shaker rotating at 175 rpm at 37 °C. After various reaction times (up to seven days), the samples were removed and dried with acetone to terminate the reactions. The concentrations of silicon (Si), calcium (Ca) and phosphorus (P) in solution were determined for different time periods using inductively coupled plasma atomic emission spectroscopy (ICP-AES). The foam surfaces were characterized by Fourier transform infrared spectroscopy (FTIR).

The cumulative protein release profiles for the 70S30C foams are shown in Figure 27.2.

A rapid release of laminin was observed during the first 24 hours after immersion in PBS, reaching laminin release values of 5–8% of total protein incorporated for 70S30C foams and 11–15% for 58S foams. From this point, the process becomes slower, obtaining values of 32–40% for 70S30C foams and 33–39% of total protein incorporated for the 58S foams. For the binary and ternary foams, the amount of laminin release at the end of the experiment was larger for the nonmodified foam. The amount of laminin released from the 70S30C foam modified with mercaptan was

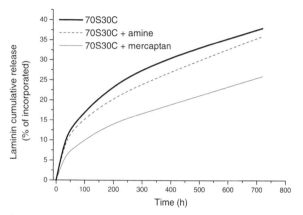

Figure 27.2 Cumulative laminin release trends, as a function of immersion time, from 70S30C foams with no surface modification, modification with amine groups and modification with mercaptan groups.

much lower than that released from the other binary foams. For the ternary (58S) system, the amount of laminin released from the foam modified with amine was a little lower than the amount of protein released from the other foams.

Figure 27.3 shows the changes produced in the SBF during the immersion of the laminin-soaked 70S30C foams. A continuous Ca^{2+} and Si^{4+} release from the foams with and without modification with chemical groups and adsorption of laminin was observed. Two distinct regions with different kinetics were observed in the ion release profiles: a fast release of Ca^{2+} and Si^{4+} occurred for the first 24 hours, after which the rate of ion release decreased. This agrees with previous studies on 58S powders [16]. For the 70S30C foam modified with amine and laminin, Ca^{2+} concentration increased from around 110 ppm (initial value) to approximately 375 ppm after 24 hours, whereas for the foam modified with mercaptan group and laminin, the Ca^{2+}

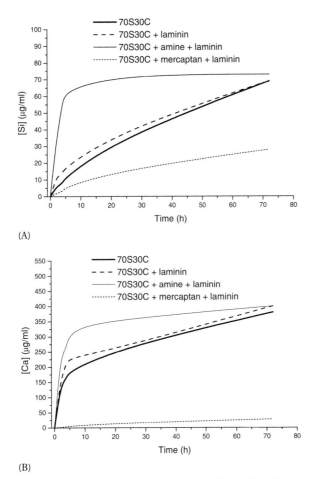

(A)

(B)

Figure 27.3 Dissolution profile trends of (A) Si^{4+} and (B) Ca^{2+} concentrations in SBF for 70S30C foams, as a function of immersion time up to 72 hours.

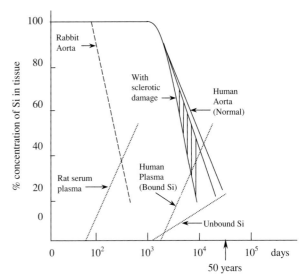

Figure 27.4 Schematic graph showing the effect of ageing on the concentration of biogenic silicon in rabbit and human aorta.

concentration remained approximately constant. The calcium and silica ionic concentration increased with time without reaching a clear saturation point during the three day immersion experiment, except for the 70S30C foam modified with amine and laminin, for which the the Si^{4+} concentration increased rapidly, reaching saturation of 75 ppm within the first 24 hours of immersion in SBF.

For the binary system the presence of amine groups together with laminin increased the dissolution rate of the material, whereas the presence of mercaptan groups significantly decreased the rate of ion exchange from the material surface and solution. For the ternary system the original foam had the highest dissolution rate, and the foams modified with mercaptan and amine groups and coated with laminin exhibited a similar dissolution profile.

Control of dissolution profiles is an important characteristic of the bioactive scaffold for several reasons. All

connective tissues contain critical amounts of bound silicon [17]. One of the roles of biogenic silicon appears to be related to stabilization of the extracellular components of the connective tissue matrix [17,18]. This is especially the case for the arterial wall and the wall of blood vessels. Studies indicate that silicon forms complexes not only with the components of the connective tissue matrix, such as glycosaminoglycans, but also with proteins, collagen and elastin [18], all critical constituents of a tissue-engineered pulmonary artery and lung construct. The presence of biogenic silicon is indicated to have an antiatheromatous function as well [19].

Figure 27.4 shows the effect of ageing on the concentration of biogenic silicon in rabbit and human aorta. There is a continuing decrease in the biologically fixed silicon, with a concomitant increase of unbound, free silicon in plasma. Patients that exhibit sclerotic damage have lost biologically bound silicon from the aorta at a rate that is two to three times as fast as that of normal humans. This effect is attributed to the biologically cross-liked silicon inhibiting permeability of blood lipids to conjunctive tissues [19].

These findings indicate that it may be necessary to deliver to various connective tissue constructs growing in vitro critical amounts of silicon to enhance stable cross-linking of proteoglycans during formation of the extracellular matrix and 3-D structures. Bioactive glasses are an ideal delivery vehicle for controlled release of biogenic silicon because their rate of reaction is a function of the percentage of network-forming silicon in their composition [20–22]. The rate of release of silicon can be controlled to match the rate of cell growth and organogenesis. The bioactive foams described herein with amine or mercaptan groups provide a means to deliver the optimal concentrations of soluble silicon as the extracellular matrix is formed in vitro.

Discussion

The proteins used in this work, laminin and bovine serum albumin (BSA), are of special biomedical significance. Laminin (about 850 kDa) is a component of the extra-cellular matrix. Laminin consists of various combinations of a long chain (α chain) and two shorter chains (β and γ) linked together to form an elongated cruciform shape [23–25]. Laminin has binding sites for type IV collagen, heparin and integrins on cell surfaces. The collagen in-teracts with laminin, which in turns interacts with inte-grins or other laminin receptor proteins, thus anchoring the basal lamina to the cells. Basal laminae are special-ized areas of the extracellular matrix that surround epithe-lial cells amongst others. Glycoproteins containing an RGD amino acid sequence bind to laminin and are major cell at-tachment factors [23]. Laminin is known to promote cell adhesion, proliferation and differentiation [26–29].

Albumin (69 kDa) is the major protein of human plasma. BSA is homologous to human serum albumin, and it is well studied and characterized. Albumin consists of one polypeptide chain of 585 amino acid residues and con-tains 17 disulfide bonds, conforming in a ellipsoidal shape. Albumin is known to enhance the biocompatibility of implants. The most outstanding property of albumin is its ability to bind reversibly a large variety of ligands. Many drugs and other peptides bind to albumin and this feature has important pharmacological and biomedical implications [5,23].

The use of organosilanes with post-deposition process-ing or in the initial mixture of sol-gel systems allows the creation of patterned surfaces with chemically functional groups. Amine and mercaptan groups are known to control protein adsorption in a way that the molecule can freely in-teract with the cell surface receptors [7].

The sol-gel-derived monoliths incorporated with BSA were found to be a highly porous material, with a specific surface area exceeding $800 \, m^2/g$ and average pore diam-eters between 2.0 and 2.8 nm. These textural properties can provide numerous sites for cell–material interactions. Incorporation of a large protein such as albumin, which is a good model protein for growth factors [11], apprecia-bly affects the surface area and the pore structure of the silica-based glasses. The pores containing the protein seem to behave differently from the protein-free pores. The lat-ter exhibit pore collapse when the pore liquid evaporates, whereas the BSA-containing pores conform to the size of the protein. As the protein was added to the sol, protein–sol interactions occurred as the protein became encap-sulated in the growing network. This has been reviewed elsewhere [21].

The binary and ternary foams exhibit a hierarchical 3-D structure consisting of a highly interconnected macro-porous network, with a mesoporous texture (Figure 28.1). The macroporous network has the potential to allow tissue ingrowth, vascularization and nutrient delivery throughout the scaffold, which is essential for cell survival and organo-genesis [29]. The patterned surfaces of the foams allow the interaction between laminin and the surface of the mate-rials without promoting denaturation of the protein. The chemically functional groups on the surface of the foams act as ligands, to which the specific binding sites of the protein bond covalently.

The in vitro release experiment showed that the bioactive foams release proteins in a controlled and continuous way over a long period of time. Other protein carriers cited in the literature, such as calcium phosphate coatings, release the majority of proteins within the first 48 hours of immer-sion [11]. In contrast, our new bioactive scaffolds released less than 10% protein in the first 24 hours of immersion and maintain a sustained release for a period as long as one month. This form of protein release is advantageous for applications that require release of bioactive molecules throughout a long period for the full biological effect to be realized, such as for tissue formation or regeneration.

The protein release process for the bioactive foams shows kinetics very similar to those of the dissolution of the foams in SBFs. These data seem to demonstrate that laminin re-lease from the bioactive foams is driven by the dissolution rate of the material network. A high surface area material with interconnected pore structure increases rates of ion exchange and especially network dissolution [30]. As re-lated in prior work [14], foams modified with mercaptan groups exhibit a mesoporous texture with a surface area of $80–84 \, m^2/g$ and a pore volume of $0.03–0.12 \, cm^3/g$, while the original foams and amine modified foams have a sur-face area of $155–176 \, m^2/g$, and a pore volume of $0.89–0.63$ cm^3/g. Since the ionic exchange between the material and SBF are influenced by the biomaterial texture, we can con-clude that this feature is the major parameter in the release kinetics of this type of material.

Implications for tissue engineering of a pulmonary artery and lung lobe

This work has demonstrated the viability of using a low temperature sol-gel method to incorporate proteins in bioactive gel–glass scaffolds that have a 3-D hierarchical interconnected pore network needed to grow 3-D tissue-engineered constructs. The change in the pore structure of silica-based glasses with incorporation of BSA suggests that protein–matrix interactions facilitate the formation of size-specific pores for the protein molecules. The patterned surface of the binary (70S30C) and ternary (58S) foams allowed interaction between laminin and the surface of the material without promoting significant conformational changes in the protein chain. The protein release from the scaffolds takes place over several weeks in a sustained and time-dependent manner. The BSA release from the silica-based glasses is controlled by the diffusion of the protein through the porous structure. The presence of amine groups decreases the diffusion rate of the protein, whereas the protein release rate increases with increasing mercaptan group concentration. The laminin release from the foams seems to be controlled by the dissolution rate of the material under the conditions used.

The foams with and without modification are bioactive in vitro and form a nanometre scale hydroxycarbonate apatite (HCA) layer on the foams' surface on exposure to SBF. The foams resorb in vitro at a controlled rate and release critical concentrations of silicon and calcium ions needed for cross-linking extracellular matrix proteins. The results indicate that the chemically modified materials have a high potential as a carrier for angiogenic factors and can provide the complex architecture and chemical stimuli needed for the engineering of soft tissues such as a pulmonary artery and lung lobe.

Recent research, as yet unpublished, by Dr Anne Bishop and Professor Julia Polak shows that type II pneumocytes survive and organize into 3-D structures on these bioactive scaffolds. The importance of these findings from the standpoint of tissue engineering is that it shows the potential to design a matrix or scaffold that satisfies several critical functions simultaneously: (1) an optimal composition that releases constituents to enhance growth, proliferation and differentiation of cells in vitro, (2) a composition that enables formation of a stable extracellular matrix similar to that present in vivo, (3) a geometry that directs cellular formation of the correct 3-D architecture of the tissue construct, (4) nanometre scale porosity that enables gases to permeate to the cells and maintain vitality, (5) channels that can direct formation of a blood supply and innervation of the construct, (6) progressive resorbtion of the matrix or scaffold as the constituents are consumed during growth so that the final product mimics a natural organ, (7) controlled release of proteins that enhance cell proliferation and differentiation, and (8) controlled release of ions (Si^{4+} and Ca^{2+}) needed for cross-linking of the extracellular

matrix. None of the presently used polymeric materials provide these complex functions in vitro. Future developments based upon molecular design and sol-gel processing of hierarchical bioactive inorganic matrices offer the potential to achieve all eight functions within a single material system.

Acknowledgement

Two of the authors (L.L.H. and J.R.J.) acknowledge support of the EPSRC and the MRC and two authors (R.F.S.L. and W.V.) thank CAPES (Brazil) for financial support of this work.

REFERENCES

1 Berthiaume F, Yarmush ML. Tissue engineering. In: Bronzino JD, ed. *The biomedical engineering handbook*. CRC Press LLC, Boca Raton, 2000: 1556–1566.
2 Senuma Y, Franceschin S, Hilborn JG. Bioresorbable microspheres by spinning disk atomisation as injectable cell carrier from preparation to *in vitro* evaluation. *Biomaterials* 2000; **21**: 1135–1144.
3 Sheridan MH, Shea LD, Peters MC, Mooney DJ. Bioabsorbable polymer scaffolds for tissue engineering capable of sustained growth factor delivery. *J Controll Release* 2000; **64**: 91–102.
4 Mansur HS, Vasconcelos WL, Lenza RFS, Oréfice RL, Reis EF, Lobato ZP. Sol-gel silica based networks with controlled chemical properties. *J Non-Crystal Solids* 2000; **273**: 109–115.
5 Chin JA, Slack SM. Biomaterials: protein–surface interactions. In: Bronzino JD, ed. *The biomedical engineering handbook*. CRC Press LLC, Boca Raton, 2000: 1597–1608.
6 Ratner BD, Shi H. Recognition templates for biomaterials with engineered bioreactivity. *Curr Opin Solid Mater Sci* 1999; **4**: 395–402.
7 Healy KE. Molecular engineering of materials for bioreactivity. *Curr Opin Solid Mater Sci* 1999; **4**: 381–387.
8 Drumheller PD, Hubbell JA. Surface immobilisation of adhesion ligands for investigations of cell-substrate interactions. In: Bronzino JD, ed. *The biomedical engineering handbook*. CRC Press LLC, Boca Raton, 2000: 1583–1592.
9 Hench LL. Bioceramics: from concept to clinic. *J Am Ceram Soc* 1991; **74**: 1487–1510.
10 Ducheyne P, Qiu Q. Bioactive ceramics: the effect of surface reactivity on bone formation and bone cell function. *Biomaterials* 1999; **20**: 2287–2303.
11 Nicoll SB, Radin S, Santos EM, Tuan RS, Ducheyne P. *In vitro* release kinetics of biologically active transforming growth factor β1 from a novel xerogel carrier. *Biomaterials* 1997; **18**: 853–859.
12 Liu DM, Chen IW. Encapsulation of protein molecules in transparent porous silica matrices via an aqueous colloidal sol-gel process. *Acta Mater* 1999; **18**: 4535–4544.
13 Webb K, Hlady V, Tresco PA. Relative importance of surface wettability and charged functional groups on NIH 3T3 fibroblast

attachment, spreading, and cytoskeletal organisation. *J Biomed Mater Res* 1998; **41**: 422–430.

14 Lenza RFS, Jones JR, Vasconcelos WL, Hench LL. Surface-modified 3D scaffolds for tissue engineering. *J Mater Sci Mater Med* 2002; in press.

15 Peterson GL. A simplification of the protein assay method of Lowry *et al.* which is more generally applicable. *Analyt Biochem* 1977; **83**: 346–356.

16 Sepulveda P, Jones JR, Hench LL. *In vitro* dissolution of melt-derived 45S5 and sol-gel derived 58S bioactive glasses. *J Biomed Mater Res* 2002; **61**: 301–311.

17 Hench LL, West JK. Biological applications of bioactive glasses *Life Chem Rep* 1996; **13**: 187–241.

18 Carlisle E. Biological silicon. In: Evered D, ed. *Silicon biochemistry*, Ciba Foundation. Symposium no. 121. J. Wiley and Sons, Chichester, 1986: 123–136.

19 Najda J, Gminski J, Drozdz M, Flak A. The effect of silicon (Si) on lipid parameters in blood serum and arterial wall. *Biol Trace Element* Res 1991; **31**: 235–247.

20 Hench LL. *Ultrastructure processing of sol-gel silica.* Noyes Publications, New York, 1998.

21 Hench LL. Sol-gel materials for bioceramic applications. *Curr Opin Solid State Mater Sci* 1997; **2**: 604–610.

22 Wheeler DL, Stokes KE. *In vivo* evaluation of sol-gel Bioglass®. Part 1: histological findings. Transactions of the 23rd Annual Meeting of the Society for Biomaterials, New Orleans, 1997.

23 Murray RK, Granner DK, Mayes PM, Rodwell VW. *Harper's biochemistry.* Appleton & Lange, Hartford, CT, 1996: 868.

24 Tian M, Hagg T, Denisova N, Knusel B, Engvall E, Jucker M. Laminin-α2 chain-like antigens in CNS dendritic spines. *Brain Res* 1997; **764**: 28–38.

25 de Arcangelis A, Neuvil A, Boukamel R, Lefebvre O, Kedinger M, Simon-Assmann P. Inhibition of laminin α1-chain expression leads to alteration of basement membrane assembly and cell differentiation. *J Cell Biol* 1996; **133**: 417–430.

26 Lekmine F, Lausson S, Pidoux E, et al. Influence of laminin substratum on cell proliferation and CALC 1 gene expression in medullary thyroid carcinoma C cell lines. *Mol Cell Endocrinol* 1999; **157**: 181–189.

27 Nomizu M, Weeks BS, Weston CA, Kim WH, Kleinman HK, Yamada Y. Structure-activity study of a laminin α1 chain active peptide segment Ile-Lys-Val-Ala-Val(IKVAV). *FEBS Lett* 1995; **365**: 217–231.

28 Nomizu M, Kim WH, Yamamura K, et al. Identification of cell binding sites in the laminin α1 chain carboxyl-terminal globular domain by systematic screening of synthetic peptides. *J Biol Chem* 1995; **270**: 20583–20590.

29 Sepulveda P, Jones JR, Hench LL. Bioactive sol-gel foams for tissue repair. *J Biomed Mater* Res 2002; **59**: 340–348.

30 Pereira MM, Hench LL. Mechanism of hydroxyapatite formation on porous gel-silica substrates. *J Sol-Gel Sci Technol* 1996; **7**: 59–68.

28

Xenotransplantation

Agnes Azimzadeh, Carsten Schroeder and Richard N. Pierson III

Vanderbilt University Medical Center, Nashville, Tennessee, USA

Overview

The impetus to develop the clinical application of xenografts is provided by the shortage of available human donor organs. For the example of end-stage lung disease, despite increasingly flexible donor acceptance criteria, about 20% of lung transplant candidates die while waiting [1] owing to lack of timely availability of suitable donor organs. Meanwhile arbitrary age restrictions are commonly used to exclude from consideration many other patients with end-stage lung and heart disease, primarily to minimize the imbalance between the waiting list and the supply of suitable donors. Xenotransplantation – in this instance of animal organs to humans – represents one potential solution to this problem. Ethical, logistic and infectious disease considerations have focused preclinical xenotransplant efforts on development of the pig as a potential donor species [2,3].

The primary immunological barrier to pig-to-human xenotransplantation is hyperacute rejection (HAR) (Figure 28.1); this phenomenon of immediate (within minutes or hours) capillary leak and parenchymal necrosis defines a 'discordant' xenograft [4]. Pig-to-human grafts are known to be discordant on the basis of several clinical attempts [5–8] and multiple other experiences with ex vivo perfusion of lungs, kidneys, livers, and hearts [5,6,9–15]. Additional possible barriers, including risk of introducing infection ('xenozoonosis') or fundamental biochemical incompatibilities, seem likely to prove manageable once the immune barriers are breached [16].

Scientific background: the role of antibody and complement in hyperacute rejection

The principal cause of HAR is activation of the 'classical pathway' of complement activation, which occurs subsequent to interaction of innate 'natural' antibody circulating in the blood of the recipient with target antigens in the graft [17]. For hearts or kidneys, many different approaches have been shown to prevent HAR during ex vivo perfusion with fresh whole blood [18–23], including in primates [24–29]. HAR of pig hearts and kidneys can be inhibited by removing preformed antidonor antibody [11,30,31], indicating that the classical pathway is central, and that the antibody-independent 'alternative' pathway of complement activation contributes secondarily [32,33] or not at all [34]. Supporting a central role for complement in HAR, pharmacological complement inhibitors such as soluble complement receptor type 1 (sCR1, sCD35: TP10) [26,35–40], compstatin [18,41], and C1 esterase inhibitor (C1-Inh) [19,42–44] are each sufficient as monotherapy to prevent HAR in various in vitro or in vivo models. Similarly, organs from pigs transgenic for human complement regulatory proteins such as decay accelerating factor (hDAF, CD55), membrane cofactor protein (hMCP, CD46), and C8 binding protein (hCD59) are usually protected from HAR in ex vivo perfusion models [27] and when transplanted into primates [20,28,29,45]. On the basis of these experimental findings, HAR of pig organs is mediated primarily through binding of pre-existing 'natural' antibody and activation of the complement cascade.

In primate models where HAR is successfully prevented, grafts often fail within days, even in the context of intense immune suppression. The relatively acellular histological picture associated with this phenomenon is described as 'acute vascular rejection (AVR)' or 'delayed xenograft rejection'. Endothelial activation, intraparenchymal haemorrhage, and intravascular thrombosis are typical, and quite different from the lymphocytic cellular infiltrate seen with acute rejection of allografts. AVR is usually associated with high or rising titres of induced antibody, typically of the immunoglobulin (Ig) G isotype (often in addition to 'natural'

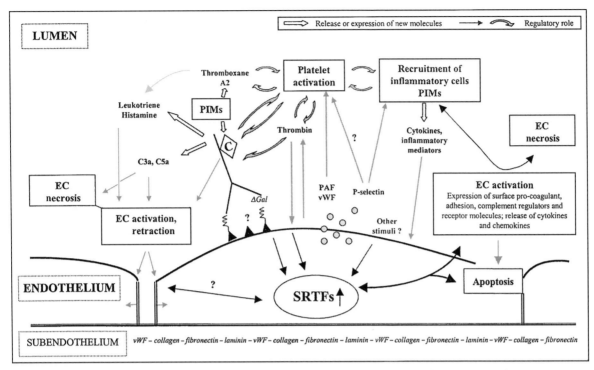

Figure 28.1 Model of lung xenograft hyperacute rejection. Whereas complement inhibition is sufficient to prevent hyperacute rejection (HAR) of pig heart and kidney xenografts beyond several days without further treatment, survival of lung xenografts is limited to a few hours. Possible mechanisms of rejection involved in late HAR (4–24 hours) are presented. In the current dogma of HAR, recipient natural antibodies and complement (c) induce porcine endothelial cell (EC) changes with resultant retraction of ECs from one another, leading to vascular permeability, exposure or release of von Willebrand factor (vWF), platelet activating factor (PAF), expression of P-selectin and other procoagulant and proinflammatory molecules. This results in recruitment and activation of platelets, leading to promotion of coagulation and release of inflammatory mediators (leukotriene, histamine, thrombin). The graft is ultimately rejected (loss of function) in the context of interstitial haemorrhage and intravascular thrombosis. Complement inhibition is usually sufficient to prevent these events for organs other than lung.

Lung xenografts are more sensitive to complement activation, or to injury independent of complement. Incompletely characterized amplification loops of activation are triggered by inflammatory mediators such as platelets [86], thrombin [90], thromboxane, and neutrophils [87]. Natural antibodies, inflammatory mediators, cytokines, adherent blood cells and perhaps other stimuli may ultimately activate stress-responsive transcription factors (SRTFs) in ECs, perhaps even in the absence of complement pathway byproducts [100–102]. EC activation triggers shape change, expression of proinflammatory and procoagulant surface molecules such as tissue factor, and cytokine production, and in certain conditions, may trigger apoptosis. Similar effects may be triggered on other lung cell types such as pulmonary intravascular macrophages (PIMs) [87], thereby amplifying the proinflammatory response. SRTFs may include, but not be limited to nuclear factor κB, activator protein 1, and signal transducer and activator of transcription. DAF, decay accelerating factor; TF, tissue factor; IL, interleukin.

IgM), but its pathogenesis remains controversial. Consistently preventing AVR using a regimen with acceptable toxicity is currently the principal hurdle to clinical application of cardiac and renal xenografts.

Hyperacute lung rejection: a special case?

The initial reports describing transplantation of pig lungs into baboons and monkeys suggested that the lung was relatively resistant to hyperacute rejection [46]. Kaplon

et al. described remarkably preserved lung histology for up to nine hours after transplantation, and were unable to demonstrate deposition of antidonor antibody or activation of complement in the grafts at the conclusion of the experiment. They concluded that the lung was deficient in antigenic targets recognized by anti-pig antibody, and therefore resistant to injury via the classical complement pathway.

However, we and others have since clearly demonstrated the central importance of anti-species antibody and complement to hyperacute lung rejection (HALR). We believe that Kaplon et al.'s observations were probably a consequence of using a model where function of the lung was not directly assessed in a life-supporting mode, and of the difficulties inherent in performing immunohistochemistry on the lung. Pig lungs exposed to human blood develop profound elevation in pulmonary vascular resistance (PVR) within seconds, and rapidly develop pulmonary oedema. Antibody and complement pathway components are demonstrable on the endothelium in pig lungs exposed to human blood [12,47,48] or transplanted into primates [49]. Specifically, immunoglobulin, C3b and C5b-9 are rapidly deposited on pulmonary endothelium [33,48]. C3a is elaborated when unmodified pig lungs are perfused with human blood [33,50,51]. This parameter of complement activation is diminished in association with expression of various human complement regulatory proteins in the organs of genetically modified 'transgenic' pigs. Thus histological and biochemical evidence supports the preponderance of physiological data, and directly implicates anti-pig antibody and complement in HALR.

Anti-species antibody in hyperacute lung rejection

For other organs, efficient antibody absorption or carbohydrate-blocking strategies reliably prevent HAR. For the lung, however, results using analogous approaches have been disappointing [12,52–54]. Although Gal-specific antibody columns remove the majority of anti-species antibody, HALR is not reliably prevented [33,47,53]. Similarly, conventional plasmapheresis, removing all immunoglobulins as well as other plasma proteins, or columns that remove all immunoglobulins, showed no significant advantages for the lung [55], in contrast to findings in other organs [30]. As first shown by Macchiarini et al., lung preperfusion yielded better results for short-term protection, as we and others have confirmed [53,56]. These experiments admit several possible interpretations: antigenic targets exist in the lung that are more efficient in activating injury pathways; lung-specific antigens are of particular importance for HALR; the lungs defences against injury are lower than those of other organs; the lung used for preperfusion removes cellular or other bloodborne elements (platelets) that are important to the kinetics and character of HAR. These nonexclusive possibilities are explored below.

We have focused our experimental efforts on approaches to prevent HALR without completely removing anti-pig antibody for four reasons. First, we have found that completely removing all anti-pig antibody is difficult in vivo. In addition, preventing antibody rebound without substantial

host toxicity is even more challenging. Understanding mechanisms of lung injury that are driven by antibody, and learning to control them, are therefore likely to be critical to both short- and long-term success. Second, presence of antidonor antibody under appropriate circumstances is not inconsistent with graft survival, and may actually facilitate long-term 'accommodation' of the graft [57]. Third, even when antidonor antibodies are efficiently depleted, important physiological perturbations are common [47,53], and lung xenograft function is usually inadequate to permit recipient survival without intensive support [56,58]. Finally, in the setting of effective regulation of complement activation, for pig hearts and kidneys depletion of antidonor antibody is unnecessary to achieve prolonged, life-supporting function in primates [35,36]. In light of these considerations, and since regulation of complement activation is the cornerstone of efforts to modify pigs for xenotransplantation, it seems sensible, if possible, to identify an approach which is successful even without directly modulating host antigraft antibody.

Complement in hyperacute lung rejection

There is compelling evidence that the lung is particularly sensitive to complement-mediated injury, and that the pig lung exposed to human blood is injured by complement. Systemic complement activation, either directly, by administration of cobra venom factor (CVF) or zymosan-activated plasma, or indirectly, in association with endotoxin or sepsis, causes acute lung injury; which in each instance is attenuated by anticomplement strategies [59,60]. In addition, the lung has a particular sensitivy to ischaemia and reperfusion, which is mediated in part through activation of the complement cascade [61–63]. Since the lung is particularly susceptible to complement injury, and antibody-driven activation of the classical pathway is the principal mediator of HAR of other organs [34], we reasoned that effective regulation of complement activation should be particularly effective for preventing HALR.

Paradoxically we and others have found that even potent strategies to regulate complement activation are inadequate to prevent lung injury, at least in the setting of anti-pig antibody. Using human plasma to perfuse lungs from pigs transgenic for hDAF and CD59, two groups have seen improved function with the transgene [22,23]. With these same transgenic constructs, improved graft function is also seen using whole fresh human blood [63] or baboon blood [50] in ex vivo perfusion. However, although graft appearance and function were improved, and despite impressive reduction in complement activation across the lung (measured as C3a elaboration), these grafts accumulated significant oedema fluid, as gauged by significant increase in weight over the three to four hour interval studied in these experiments. When lungs from one of these transgenic lines were transplanted into baboons in a life supporting setting, a previous lung-immunoadsorption showed the best results [56]. The transpulmonary blood flow was stable up to 11 hours, with a nearly normal cardiac output in the recipient. Mild inotropic support was required to overcome rising pulmonary vascular resistance and support systemic perfusion pressure. Although gross and microscopic appearance was improved relative to recipients treated in other ways, gross pulmonary oedema was observed in at least some grafts, and PVR was significantly increased.

In a recent study, we evaluated the role of common complement pathway activation in HALR. Pig lungs transgenic for hDAF were perfused with and without the addition of a soluble inhibitor (sCR1) of the C3/C5 convertase [65] (Figure 28.2). Expression of hDAF alone was associated with

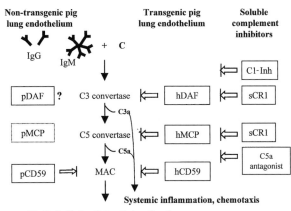

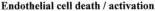

Endothelial cell death / activation

Figure 28.2 Regulation of complement activation in porcine lungs. Binding of complement fixing natural antibody (pentavalent IgM or bivalent IgG) to the porcine endothelium triggers complement (C) activation. In a nontransgenic lung endothelium, the endogenous porcine CD59 (pCD59) may inhibit C activation, but is overwhelmed by the intensity of activation, leading to endothelial cell destruction. Decay accelerating factor (DAF) is expressed in a wide range of pig tissues, but its regulatory role on endothelium is still controversial [103].

Although pMCP is expressed on pig endothelium elsewhere, it is absent from porcine lung endothelium. In the transgenic endothelium, complement inhibition may be reinforced by expression of one or more human C regulators (hDAF, hMCP, hCD59). Finally, the addition of soluble inhibitors (C1-Inh, sCR1, C5a antagonist) may act synergistically to block specific activation steps in the lung or elsewhere in the graft recipient. MAC, membrane attack complex.

reduced deposition of complement C3b and C5b-9 fragments on pulmonary vascular endothelium, and survival of hDAF (+) lungs was significantly prolonged relative to farm-bred controls. However, soluble phase complement activation was not effectively regulated by hDAF expression, as evidenced by production of C3a and sC5b-9. The proportion of lungs surviving, mean survival duration and complement inhibition were further improved by additional use of sCR1. We conclude that complement activation plays an important role in HALR, and that porcine lung is particularly vulnerable to injury by complement. The synergistic effect of hDAF and sCR1 suggests that the cofactor I activity (which is provided by the regulatory molecule sCR1, in addition to its decay accelerating activity similar to DAF) plays an important role in HALR. This idea is in line with the recent finding that MCP (which also provides cofactor I activity), is not expressed on porcine lungs. Assuming that other pig regulatory proteins (such as CD59) may inhibit human complement, as recently suggested, limited protection of the hDAF lung may in part reflect an insufficient 'dose' of regulators of complement activation (RCA). This has been reviewed elsewhere [65]. In this case selection of pig lines that exhibit high constitutive levels of pig RCA protein or higher levels of human RCA protein on the lung endothelium may confer an important advantage to hDAF (+) lungs, particularly if they operate synergistically or at different steps in the complement cascade.

Thus, while results with transgenic lungs are significantly better than those with control lungs, they are substantially worse than have been reported for other transgenic organs. Further, baboons with profound systemic depletion of complement after CVF pretreatment exhibited poor function of pig lungs despite documented reduction in CH50 to very low levels. These observations show that, although complement plays an important role in lung HAR, the lung may be more sensitive to injury by complement. Because CVF generates anaphylatoxins, this experiment leaves open the critical question: are complement-independent pathways particularly important to HALR?

Adhesive interactions and the coagulation pathway

Adhesion molecules play a critical role in ischaemia–reperfusion injury, and mediate the lung injury seen with systemic complement activation [66,67]. Where they have been examined, the interaction between most pig and human integrin and selectin ligands appears to occur under circumstances analogous to those described within either species, and may thus be considered to occur in an appropriate 'physiological' manner. P-selectin and inter-cellular adhesion molecule 1 (ICAM-1) are examples of adhesion molecules whose function has been well char-acterized in this species combination, and found to func-tion physiologically [68,69]. In the xenogeneic situation, other 'nonphysiological' molecular interactions may also trigger pathogenic adhesive interactions between porcine endothelium and primate platelets and neutrophils.

Like complement activation, activation of the coagula-tion cascade occurs most efficiently on activated cell sur-faces. Interestingly, coagulation pathway dysregulation was recently shown to play a central role in clinical acute lung injury, in that administration of activated protein C was associated with decreased morbidity and mortality in the acute respiratory distress syndrome/systemic inflamma-tory response syndrome [70–73].

In the coagulation pathway several 'nonphysiological' interactions between porcine endothelium and human platelets and coagulation factors have been identified that are potentially important to HAR [74–78]. Whereas quies-cent human platelets do not bind to human von Wille-brand factor (vWF), porcine vWF binds to human platelets through a nonphysiological interaction via GP1b and the $\alpha 1$ domain of vWF [79]. Human thrombin activation is actively inhibited by regulatory proteins on human en-dothelium, but constitutive activation of human throm-bin occurs when human plasma is exposed to quiescent porcine endothelium [80]. Thrombomodulin and ecto-ADPase, potent anticoagulant molecules expressed by nor-mal endothelium, are rapidly downregulated or lost after exposure of porcine endothelium to human blood con-stituents, leading to a procoagulant endothelial phenotype [81,82]. Porcine vWF appears to bind human complement even in the absence of anti-pig antibody [83], suggesting that pig vWF itself may serve as a primary nidus for inflam-mation. In addition, high shear stress, which occurs at sites of vasoconstriction, causes platelet aggregation to vWF, and shedding of procoagulant microparticles [84]. Finally, ag-gregated platelets coated with vWF, or vWF multimers re-leased from the surface of injured or activated endothelial cells, may thus activate complement in soluble phase, trig-gering productions of anaphylatoxins in the blood as well as where they are expressed in the organ [49]. Thus, even if pig endothelium is not activated by other interactions, platelet adhesion and binding of complement are likely to occur, and to trigger prothrombotic and proinflammatory events in the graft and elsewhere in the organ recipient.

Physiological characteristics of pulmonary blood flow may predispose the lung to injury mediated through dys-regulated adhesive interactions. Adhesive interactions for platelets and neutrophils to endothelium are mediated by

P-selectin, E-selectin, and vascular cell adhesion molecule 1 (VCAM-1) (but not L-selectin). Adhesion of platelets and neutrophils occurs more efficiently in conditions of low shear stress, and is inefficient under conditions of high shear stress [85]. In the absence of P-selectin or other inte-grins (or nonphysiological ligands) leukocytes do not nor-mally adhere, become activated, or translocate. Each of several adhesion mechanisms depends critically on shear stress at the interface between blood and endothelium, which is governed by the relationship between pressure, flow and vessel size as follows: $\tau = 4\eta Q/\rho r^3$ (τ is shear stress, Q is flow, ρ is fluid density, η is viscosity). Vascular resistance may be presumed to be equal in vessels of a specified length and lumen radius, and the pressure in the pulmonary circulation is roughly one third of that in the sys-temic circulation. Thus flow through – and therefore shear stress in – the resistance vessels of the lung is normally low, about one third of that in the kidney. This environment should favour rolling of formed blood elements, and thus their subsequent adhesion, translocation, and activation in response to proinflammatory influences.

In our estimation, the nonphysiological interaction be-tween porcine vWF and human platelet glycoprotein 1b (GP1b), is likely to occur with greater efficiency under the low shear stress conditions found in the lung, but this ques-tion has not been addressed. If so, the lung's particular propensity to sequester platelets in the early moments of perfusion with human blood may in part account for the rapid induction of high vascular resistance in the lung and subsequent inflammatory events characteristic of HALR. Alternatively, increased shear stress conditions occurring as a consequence of high vascular resistance may augment vWF-driven platelet adhesion and the release of vWF into the blood, and thus more efficiently trigger soluble phase complement activation. In support of this paradigm, we have identified a particularly important role for platelets [86] and neutrophils [87] in HALR, while Holzknecht et al. [49] have found evidence for circulating multimers of vWF in baboons undergoing HALR, a phenomenon that has not been reported for other organs. Two independent reports suggested that endothelial cells from the lung contain 5 to 50 times higher concentrations of vWF (protein and mRNA) than endothelial cells of similar-sized vessels from other or-gans such as liver or kidney [88,89], which may account for the high avidity of the lung for platelets and for its apparent propensity to shed vWF in large amounts during injury.

To evaluate the influence of platelet vWF/GPIb-V-IX and thrombin–fibrinogen/GPIIbIIIa receptor interactions in HALR, an inhibitor of platelet–GPIb interactions with vWF (aurintricarboxylic acid, ATA), a synthetic GPIIbIIIa inhibiting molecule (SC51202) or both agents were added to heparinized whole human blood prior to perfusion of isolated piglet lungs [86]. Addition of ATA or SC alone prior to lung perfusion significantly reduced the rise in PVR, diminished histamine release, and extended mean survival to 31 min from 8 min for untreated control lungs. When the agents were combined, mean survival reached 156 min, a significant increase over either monotherapy. To our surprise, complement activation was delayed by platelet receptor blockade, and only when the drugs were used together. This basic observation raises the possiblity that platelet aggregation is fundamental to efficient complement cascade in vivo.

Since the production of thrombin was significantly decreased during platelet receptor blockade, we asked whether similar results could be reproduced by specific inhibition of thrombin, which we achieved using bivalirudin, a semi-synthetic analogue of hirudin. Bivalirudin controlled thrombin production, limited the rise in PVR, attenuated histamine release and significantly improved mean lung survival, from 8 to 77 minutes [90]. Importantly, because results with bivalirudin also consistently delayed complement activation, similar to combined platelet receptor blockade, we infer that endothelial thrombin formation may be a crucial primary stimulus for the initiation of platelet aggregation and activation, and thus for complement cascade amplification during HALR.

Our knowledge regarding mechanisms by which thrombin can affect inflammation and coagulation processes has been growing rapidly [91–95]. In our estimation, improved mechanistic definition of the interaction between these various triggers – antibody, complement, adhesion molecules, platelets, and other coagulation pathway constituents – will be necessary to devise efficient strategies for aborting the various pathogenic positive feedback loops outlined here, and thus to develop clinically suitable approaches for lung xenografting (Figure 28.1).

Preclinical studies of lung xenotransplantation

We believe that a life-supporting model is necessary to acquire meaningful information regarding potential clinical efficacy of various strategies. As illustrated by Kaplon et al. [46] indirect assessments and histology can be very misleading. We have found very high PO_2 in the pulmonary vein effluent of lungs with trivial transpulmonary blood flow, showing that the blood is oxygenated during its slow transit through the lung, and limiting the utility of this parameter as a measure of function unless the recipient is fully dependent on the graft. PVR can not exceed the capacity of a normal (or perhaps conditioned) right heart under

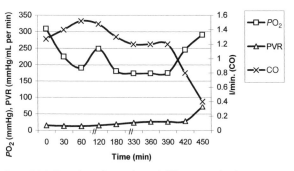

Figure 28.3 Function of an orthotopic life-supporting lung xenotransplanta. Physiological measurements during seven hours of life-supporting lung xenotransplant after cross-clamping of the right pulmonary artery. Left-sided single lung transplantation was performed using an hDAF (decay accelerating factor) transgenic donor pig. The baboon recipient was treated with C1-Inh (complement inhibitor), 1-benzylimidazole (thromboxane inhibitor), diphenhydramine (antihistamine), steroids, and inhaled nitric oxide. Lung function was assessed by serial measurement of partial oxygen pressure (PO_2) and pulmonary vascular resistance (PVR) and was stable until 390 min. Similarly, the flow through the graft, assessed by cardiac output (CO), was normal (>1.2 L/min) for a baboon of this size without inotropic support. Progressive lung oedema and increasing PVR lead to elective termination of the experiment.

physiological flow conditions and using inotropic support at clinically applicable levels.

Our preclinical results have been generally disappointing, as have been those of other investigators [50,51,56,64,96], even using lungs that express complement regulatory proteins. We have transplanted three hDAF transgenic lungs in cynomolgus monkeys and three more in baboons. Even with additional interventions to block thromboxane, histamine and complement, we rarely obtained life-supporting xenogenic lung function for more than a few minutes. In one instance, additional use of αGal-column immunoadsorption daily for three days prior to transplant yielded seven hour life-supporting survival in a baboon lung transplant recipient. Additional therapies used in this case included an hDAF(+) lung, C1 esterase inhibitor (Berinert P®), thromboxane and histamine inhibition, methylprednisolone, and inhaled nitric oxide. Gas exchange, cardiac output and pulmonary artery pressure remained stable for seven hours without any inotropic requirement (Figure 28.3). After 6.5 hours the major histological abnormality was marked perivascular oedema and lymphatic dilation in the lobular septa, without intravascular thrombi. The small arteries show morphological evidence of endothelial activation, including nuclear enlargement and 'plumping up' of the individual endothelial cells (Figure 28.4). This approach was not successful

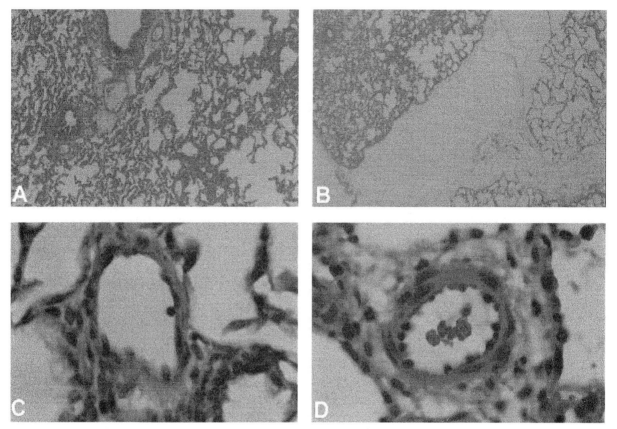

Figure 28.4 Histology of an orthotopic life-supporting lung xenotransplant. (A) After 6.5 hours, the alveolar parenchyma is free from intravascular thrombi and without significant pathological change (haematoxylin and eosin (H&E) 25x). (B) The major histological abnormality is oedema of the perivascular compartment, with marked dilatation of intraseptal lymphatic channel (H&E, 12.5x). (C) An artery from the contralateral (nonperfused) right lung shows unobstructive flat endothelial cells and normally spindled endothelial nuclei (H&E, 250x). (D) In contrast, a close view of a small artery from the grafted lung (H&E, 250x) shows morphological evidence of mononuclear cells and endothelial activation, including nuclear enlargement and 'plumping up' of the individual endothelial cells, and perivascular interstitial oedema extending to the alveolar septi.

when applied in two additional animals that had previously been sensitized during rejection of a previous pig heart graft. The only other report of life-supporting pig lung function in a primate was also accomplished with highly efficient antibody adsorption, in that instance using preperfusion through a pig lung [56]. In summary, this experience suggests that preperfusion through a lung will provide the most reliable protection of a subsequent graft, particularly in the context of high anti-pig antibody titres against non-Gal antigens.

Clinical lung xenotransplantation: general considerations

Xenotransplantation potentially offers the opportunity to avoid lung injury associated with brain death. While some ischaemia–reperfusion is unavoidable, the mechanisms contributing to this lung injury are well understood, and, when anticipated, can be addressed specifically. However, because we do not yet know how to reliably protect the pig lung from acute injury in a human blood environment, these theoretical advantages have not yet been fully investigated in the preclinical work performed to date.

Lung xenotransplantation might advance to the clinic under one of two circumstances. If the basic science and preclinical primate models demonstrate consistent results suggesting that lung xenotransplantation is likely to succeed in the clinic, then a clinical trial could be justified and performed in patients who would otherwise die. Alternatively, if the initial hurdles (HAR) are overcome, pig organs might be tested as an alternative to long-term mechanical gas exchange devices such as ECMO (extracorporeal membrane oxygenation (heart and lung machine)), as a bridging strategy to lung recovery or lung allotransplant.

As summarized in the recent ISHLT report on thoracic organ xenotransplantation, lung xenotransplantation should be offered initially to patients who (1) have an extremely limited life expectancy without transplantation, (2) have no realistic chance of a human cadaveric or living lung transplant in their estimated survival time, and (3) have no severe contraindications or risk factors for transplantation [97]. Those requiring prolonged mechanical ventilation or ECMO support and with poor prognosis for lung recovery constitute an appropriate initial study population.

The initial trial will probably be undertaken as a bridge to a lung allograft. The bridging procedure could consist of a single or bilateral pig lung transplant, or ex vivo perfusion in a paracorporeal 'ECMO'-type circuit. It would seem sensible that a bridging procedure should be as simple as possible in keeping with adequate respiratory support, and that a fallback strategy (exchange of the pig lung or ECMO) be available in case a human lung is not available and in case the first pig lung fails. Unless organ allocation policy is adjusted, initial lung xenotransplantation recipients might have to be supported by the pig lung for an extended period of time. The likelihood of successful allotransplantation in such a 'bridged' patient is probably lower than in patients awaiting a cardiac allograft on mechanical support, particularly since multiple invasive procedures and administration of immunosuppressive or nephrotoxic agents will probably be necessary to protect the pig lung from injury. In our judgement, this type of application should not be undertaken until successful long-term support seems likely.

Once the feasibility of prolonged support with a lung xenograft has been demonstrated in preclinical models and in initial clinical trials, its application might be extended to other high risk patient groups who are not so critically ill, and in whom the lung xenograft would be performed as 'destination therapy' rather than as a 'bridge' to an allograft. Patients with end-stage idiopathic pulmonary fibrosis and primary pulmonary hypertension have the shortest life expectancy on the lung transplant waiting list. For example, in Europe the mortality for idiopathic pulmonary fibrosis is 1.55 times higher than for patients with cystic fibrosis. While selection criteria to identify appropriate patients will depend on prospective studies using objective markers of disease severity, and will vary by underlying lung pathology, validated criteria would be an appropriate tool to identify potential candidates for a careful high risk clinical trial. When considered for 'definitive' rather than 'bridge' therapy, the choice of operation (single versus double) would presumably be dictated primarily by

recipient diagnosis and other considerations, as currently for allotransplantation.

When will we be ready for clinical lung xenotransplantation?

Clinical trials of porcine cell and tissue xenotransplantation are already being undertaken, in both the USA and Europe [98]. These trials are associated with little immediate risk to the patient, and valuable information will hopefully be gleaned from them, particularly with regard to the risk of xenozoonoses. Trials of ex vivo pig liver perfusion in patients with fulminant liver failure are also ongoing, and again may be a source of data that proves valuable when trials of whole organ xenotransplantation are initiated.

The considerations that should govern initial trials of clinical lung xenotransplantation were recently reviewed in detail by an advisory committee to the International Society for Heart and Lung Transplantation [97].

Three main questions have to be answered before a clinical trial in lung xenotransplantation is initiated. (1) Will the transplanted organ adequately support the patient? With regard to the lung, there is as yet no evidence that porcine lung survival can be prolonged beyond a few hours. (2) Is the regimen necessary to protect the graft also safe for use in appropriate patients with end-stage lung disease? It is likely that candidate immunomodulatory regimens will first be evaluated for other organs. Risk of infection would be of particular concern for the lung because of its obligate exposure to airborne pathogens. (3) Is the risk low of transmitting an infectious agent into the human recipient? Porcine endogenous retrovirus, for example, might or might not cause disease in this nonphysiological incidental host. Secondary transmission to intimate acquaintances is very unlikely, but the acquired immune deficiency syndrome epidemic provides a sobering example of the consequence of latent infection crossing from a primate species to humans. While it might be acceptable to a dying patient to risk being infected with a porcine microorganism with no known pathogenicity for humans, other members of the community may feel differently. Broad public education, rational public health guidelines, and careful monitoring of xenograft recipients will all be necessary for safe clinical application.

Differing ethical standards could lead to what some members of society may consider an unacceptably risky or unethical procedure. However, we maintain that if the new procedure is likely to be both safe and effective based on sound scientific principles and objective data, and if it is motivated primarily by an otherwise unmet medical need, then assent of an informed majority and informed consent by the subject are sufficient to proceed. A secondary benefit to society may be anticipated, in new knowledge and improved care of future patients. Safeguards must be in place to assure that the procedure itself is not harmful to the subject or other members of society, and the patient must not be misled or given false hope about the outcome [99].

In view of the considerations outlined above, we believe that a clinical trial of lung xenotransplantation must await substantial scientific progress.

Summary

While it remains possible that more efficient complement control will yield clinically useful lung protection, the weight of evidence supports the conclusion that the lung is not fully protected from HAR by anticomplement strategies alone. Events triggered by antibody binding and coagulation system activation, and mediated by activation of lung macrophages and endothelial cells, are probably in part complement independent, and particularly important to the pathogenesis of HALR. Defining the lung's vulnerability to HAR at a mechanistic level is important in devising effective protection strategies, and thus to progress towards eventual clinical application of lung xenografts. Meanwhile, the lung may offer a valuable window into the importance of dysregulated coagulation and other adhesive interactions to the immediate events occurring in HAR, and clues to subsequent vascular events associated with acute vascular rejection/delayed xenograft rejection. In our estimation, understanding these interactions and developing approaches to control them are likely to prove crucial to xenografting of the lung and other organs. Xenotransplantation will advance to the clinic only when preclinical models consistently demonstrate that success is possible.

Acknowledgements

Many former members of our laboratory contributed to the work summarized in this essay, as did numerous collaborators and colleagues. The authors wish particularly to thank Joyce Johnson, George Zorn and Steffen Pfeiffer for their outstanding technical contributions, and Jacek Hawiger and Tim Blackwell for helpful discussions. The authors' research has been supported by Vanderbilt University, the VUMC Clinical Research Center, and the Nashville VAMC, and by grants from the American Association of Thoracic Surgeons (R.N.P.), the Thoracic Surgery Foundation for Research and Education (S.P.), American Lung Association (R.N.P., A.A.), NIH (R.N.P.), VA Merit Review (R.N.P.), and Imutran-Novartis Pharma (R.N.P.). C.S. is the recipient of a fellowship from the German Research Foundation.

REFERENCES

1 Hosenpud JD, Bennett LE, Keck BM, Boucek MM, Novick RJ. The Registry of the International Society for Heart and Lung Transplantation: 18th Official Report - 2001. *J Heart Lung Transplant* 2000; **20**: 805–815.
2 Buhler L, Friedman T, Iacomini J, Cooper DK. Xenotransplantation – state of the art – update 1999. *Front Biosci* 1999; **4**: 416–432.
3 Lambrigts D, Sachs DH, Cooper DK. Discordant organ xenotransplantation in primates: world experience and current status. *Transplantation* 1998; **66**: 547–561.
4 Calne RY. Organ transplantation between widely disparate species. *Trans Proc* 1970; **3**: 21–26.
5 Markman, JF, Barker CF. Basic and clinical considerations in the use of xenografts. *Curr Prob Surg* 1994; **31**: 385–468.
6 Auchincloss H Jr. Xenogeneic transplantation: a review. *Transplantation* 1986; **46**: 1–20.
7 Makowka L, Wu GD, Hoffman A, et al. Immunohistopathologic lesions associated with the rejection of a pig-to-human liver xenograft. In *Proceedings of the Second International Congress on Xenotransplantation*, Cambridge, UK, 1993: Abstract no.32.
8 Czaplicki J, Blonska B, Religa Z. The lack of hyperacute xenograft heart transplant rejection in a human. *J Heart Lung Transplant* 1992; **11**: 393–397.
9 Bryant LR, Eiseman B, Avery M. Studies of the porcine lung as an oxygenator for human blood. *J Thorac Cardiovasc Surg* 1968; **55**: 255–261.
10 Pierson RN III, Tew DN, Konig WK, Dunning JJ, White DJG, Wallwork J. Pig lungs are susceptible to hyperacute rejection by human blood in a working ex vivo heart–lung model. *Transplant Proc* 1994; **26**: 1318–1319.
11 Pierson RN III, Dunning JJ, Konig WK, Tew DF, White DJG, Wallwork J. Mechanisms governing the pace and character of pig heart and lung rejection by human blood. *Transplant Proc* 1994; **26**: 2337–2338.
12 Pierson RN III, Kaspar-Konig W, Tew DN, et al. Hyperacute rejection in a pig-to-human lung transplant model. (1) The role of anti-species antibody and complement. *Transplantation* 1997; **63**: 594–603.
13 Dunning JJ, Pierson RN III, Braidley PC, White DJG, Wallwork J. A comparison of the performance of pig hearts perfused with pig or human blood using an ex-vivo working heart model. *Eur J Cardiothorac Surg* 1994; **8**: 204–206.
14 Kirk AD, Heinle JS, Mault JR, Sanfilippo F. Ex vivo characterization of human anti-porcine hyperacute cardiac rejection. *Transplantation* 1993; **56**: 785–793.
15 Shah AS, O'Hair DP, Kaplon RJ, et al. Absence of hyperacute rejection in pig-to-primate double lung xenografts. *J Heart Lung Transplant* 1995; **14**(2): S83.

16 Cooper DKC, Kemp E, Platt JL, White DJG, eds. *Xenotransplantation: the transplantation of organs and tissues between species*, 2nd edn. Springer-Verlag, Heidelberg, 1997.

17 Platt JL, Lindman BJ, Geller RL, et al. The role of natural antibodies in the activation of xenogenic endothelial cells. *Transplantation* 1991; **52**: 1037–1043.

18 Fiane AE, Mollnes TE, Videm V, et al. Compstatin, a peptide inhibitor of C3, prolongs survival of ex vivo perfused pig xenografts. *Xenotransplantation* 1999; **6**: 52–65.

19 Fiane AE, Videm V, Johansen HT, Mellbye OJ, Nielsen EW, Mollnes TE. C1-inhibitor attenuates hyperacute rejection and inhibits complement, leukocyte and platelet activation in an ex vivo pig-to-human perfusion model. *Immunopharmacology* 1999; **42**: 231–243.

20 McCurry KR, Kooyman D, Diamond L, Byrne GW, Logan JS, Platt JL. Human complement regulatory proteins in transgenic animals regulate complement activation in xenoperfused organs. *Proceedings of the XVth International Congress of the Transplantation Society*, Kyoto, Japan, 1998, Abstract no.288.

21 Dunning JJ, Pierson RN III, Braidley PC, White DJ, Wallwork JA. Comparison of the performance of pig hearts perfused with pig or human blood using an ex-vivo working heart model. *Eur J Cardiothorac Surg* 1994; **8**: 204–206.

22 Daggett CW, Yeatman M, Lodge AJ, et al. Swine lungs expressing human complement-regulatory proteins are protected against acute pulmonary dysfunction in a human plasma perfusion model. *J Thorac Cardiovasc Surg* 1997; **113**: 390–398.

23 Kroshus TJ, Bolman RM III, Dalmasso AP, et al. Expression of human CD59 in transgenic pig organs enhances organ survival in an ex vivo xenogeneic perfusion model. *Transplantation* 1996; **61**: 1513–1521.

24 Leventhal JR, Sakiyalak P, Witson J, et al. The synergistic effect of combined antibody and complement depletion on discordant cardiac xenograft survival in nonhuman primates. *Transplantation* 1994; **57**: 974–978.

25 Kobayashi T, Taniguchi S, Neethling FA, et al. Delayed xenograft rejection of pig-to-baboon cardiac transplants after cobra venom factor therapy. *Transplantation* 1997; **64**: 1255–1261.

26 Pruitt SK, Bollinger RR, Collins BH, et al. Effect of continuous complement inhibition using soluble complement receptor type 1 on survival of pig-to-primate cardiac xenografts. *Transplantation* 1997; **63**: 900–902.

27 Young VK, Pierson RN III, Kaspar-Konig W, et al. Pig hearts transgenic for human decay accelerating factor are protected from hyperacute rejection. *J Heart Lung Transplant* 1995; **14**: S82.

28 Zaidi A, Schmoeckel M, Bhatti F, et al. Life-supporting pig-to-primate renal xenotransplantation using genetically modified donors. *Transplantation* 1998; **65**: 1584–1590.

29 Vial CM, Ostlie DJ, Bhatti FN, et al. Life supporting function for over one month of a transgenic porcine heart in a baboon. *J Heart Lung Transplant* 2000; **19**: 224–229.

30 Kroshus TJ, Bolman RM III, Dalmasso AP. Selective IgM depletion prolongs organ survival in an ex vivo model of pig-to-human. *Transplantation* 1996; **62**: 5–12.

31 Simon PM, Neethling FA, Taniguchi S, et al. Intravenous infusion of Galα1–3Gal oligosaccharides in baboons delays hyperacute rejection of porcine heart xenografts. *Transplantation* 1998; **65**: 346–353.

32 Blum MG, Collins BJ, Chang AC, et al. Complement inhibition by FUT-175 and K76-COOH in a pig-to-human lung xenotransplant model. *Xenotransplantation* 1998; **5**: 35–43.

33 Zhang JP, Blum MG, Chang AC, et al. Immunohistologic evaluation of mechanisms mediating hyperacute lung rejection, and the effect of treatment with K76-COOH, FUT-175, and anti-Gal column immunoadsorption. *Xenotransplantation* 1999; **6**: 249–261.

34 Dalmasso AP, Vercellotti GM, Fischel RJ, Bolman RM, Bach FH, Platt JL. Mechanism of complement activation in the hyperacute rejection of porcine organs transplanted into primate recipients. *Am J Pathol* 1992; **140**: 1157–1166.

35 Zaidi A, Masroor S, Vial CM, Soin B, et al. A short course of perioperative TP10 (sCR1) therapy improves early graft function following life-supporting xenotransplantation of hDAF transgenic pig kidneys, exposed to prolonged cold ischemia, into cynomolgous monkeys. Oral Abstract no.181A, *Fifth Congress of the International Xenotransplantation Association*, Nagoya, Japan, 27 October 1999; Abstract book p. 63.

36 Soin B, Vial CM, Masroor S, et al. Extended survival of hDAF transgenic pig kidneys after prolonged cold ischemia in pig-to-primate xenotransplantation using cyclophosphamide, cyclosporin A and TP10 (sCR1) at induction and RAD and corticosteroids as a maintenance therapy. Oral abstract no.182, *Fifth Congress of the International Xenotransplantation Association*, Nagoya, Japan, 27 October 1999; Abstract book p. 63.

37 Bennet W, Sundberg B, Elgue G, Larsson R, Korsgren O, Nilsson B. A new in vitro model for the study of pig-to-human vascular hyperacute rejection. *Xenotransplantation* 2001; **8**: 176–184.

38 Chrupcala M, Pomer S, Staehler G, Waldherr R, Kirschfink C. Prolongation of discordant renal xenograft survival by depletion of complement. Comparative effects of systemically administered cobra venom factor and soluble complement receptor type 1 in a guinea-pig to rat model. *Transpl Int* 1994; **7**: 650–653.

39 Davis EA, Pruitt SK, Greene PS, et al. Inhibition of complement, evoked antibody, and cellular response prevents rejection of pig-to-primate cardiac xenografts. *Transplantation* 1996; **62**: 1018–1023.

40 Candinas D, Lesnikoski BA, Robson SC, et al. Effect of repetitive high-dose treatment with soluble complement receptor type 1 and cobra venom factor on discordant xenograft survival. *Transplantation* 1996; **62**: 336–342.

41 Morikis D, Assa-Munt N, Sahu A, Lambris JD. Solution structure of compstatin, a potent complement inhibitor. *Protein Sci* 1998; **7**: 619–627.

42 Matsunami K, Miyagawa S, Yamada M, Yoshitatsu M, Shirakura R. A surface-bound form of human C1 esterase inhibitor improves xenograft rejection. *Transplantation* 2000; **69**: 749–755.

43 Heckl-Ostreicher B, Wosnik A, Kirschfink M. Protection of porcine endothelial cells from complement-mediated cytotoxicity by the human complement regulators CD59, C1 inhibitor, and soluble complement receptor type 1. Analysis in a pig-to-human in vitro model relevant to hyperacute xenograft rejection. *Transplantation* 1996; **62**: 1693–1696.

44 Dalmasso AP, Platt JL. Prevention of complement-mediated activation of xenogeneic endothelial cells in an in vitro model of xenograft hyperacute rejection by C1 inhibitor. *Transplantation* 1993; **56**: 1171–1176.

45 White DJG. HDAF transgenic pig organs: are they concordant for human transplantation? *Xenotransplantation* 1996; **4**: 50–54.

46 Kaplon RJ, Platt JL, Kwiatkowski PA, et al. Absence of hyperacute rejection in pig-to-primate orthotopic pulmonary xenografts. *Transplantation* 1995; **59**: 410–416.

47 Pfeiffer S, Zorn GL III, Kelishadi S, et al. Role of anti-Galα1,3Gal and anti-platelet antibodies in hyperacute rejection of pig lung by human blood. *Ann Thorac Surg* 2001; **72**: 1681–1689; discussion 1690.

48 Macchiarini P, Mazmanian GM, Oriol R, et al. Ex vivo lung model of pig-to-human hyperacute xenograft rejection. *J Thorac Cardiovasc Surg* 1997; **114**: 315–325.

49 Holzknecht ZE, Coombes S, Blocher BA, et al. Immune complex formation after xenotransplantation: evidence of type III as well as type II immune reactions provides clues to pathophysiology. *Am J Pathol* 2001; **158**: 627–637.

50 Yeatman M, Daggett CW, Lau CL, et al. Human complement regulatory proteins protect swine lungs from xenogeneic injury. *Ann Thorac Surg* 1999; **67**: 769–775.

51 Yeatman M, Daggett CW, Parker W, et al. Complement-mediated pulmonary xenograft injury: studies in swine-to-primate orthotopic single lung transplant models. *Transplantation* 1998; **65**: 1084–1093.

52 Lin SS, Kooyman DL, Daniels LJ, et al. The role of natural anti-Galα1–3Gal antibodies in hyperacute rejection of pig-to-baboon cardiac xenotransplants. *Transpl Immunol* 1997; **5**: 212–218.

53 Macchiarini P, Oriol R, Azimzadeh A, et al. Evidence of human non-alpha-galactosyl antibodies involved in the hyperacute rejection of pig lungs and their removal by pig organ perfusion. *J Thorac Cardiovasc Surg* 1998; **116**: 831–843.

54 Lau CL, Daggett WC, Yeatman MF, et al. The role of antibodies in dysfunction of pig-to-baboon pulmonary transplants. *J Thorac Cardiovasc Surg* 2000; **120**: 29–38.

55 Leventhal JR, John R, Fryer JP, et al. Removal of baboon and human antiporcine IgG and IgM natural antibodies by immunoadsorption. *Transplantation* 1995; **59**: 294–300.

56 Daggett CW, Yeatman M, Logge AJ, et al. Total respiratory support from swine lungs in primate recipients. *J Thorac Cardiovasc Surg* 1998; **115**: 19–27.

57 Platt JL. A perspective on xenograft rejection and accommodation. *Immunol Rev* 1994; **141**: 127–149.

58 Blum M, Chang AC, Collins BJ, Knaus SA, Christman BW, Pierson RN III. The effect of nitric oxide and thromboxane blockade on pulmonary vascular resistance in a pig-to-primate lung transplant model. *Fourth International Congress for Xenotransplantation*, Nantes, France, September 1997.

59 Mulligan MS, Lentsch AB, Ward PA. In vivo recruitment of neutrophils: consistent requirements for L-arginine and variable requirements for complement and adhesion molecules. *Inflammation* 1998; **22**: 327–339.

60 Mulligan MS, Warner RL, Rittershaus CW, et al. Endothelial targeting and enhanced antiinflammatory effects of complement inhibitors possessing sialyl Lewis X moieties. *J Immunol* 1999; **162**: 4952–4959.

61 Stammberger U, Hamacher J, Hillinger S, Schmid RA. sCR1sLe ameliorates ischemia/reperfusion injury in experimental lung transplantation. *J Thorac Cardiovasc Surg* 2000; **120**: 1078–1084.

62 Zamora MR, Davis RD, Keshavjee SH, et al. Complement inhibition attenuates human lung transplant reperfusion injury: a multicenter trial. *Chest* 1999; **116**(Suppl 1): 46S.

63 Heller T, Hennecke M, Baumann U, et al. Selection of a C5a receptor antagonist from phage libraries attenuating the inflammatory response in immune complex disease and ischemia/reperfusion injury. *J Immunol* 1999; **163**: 985–994.

64 Kulick DM, Salerno CT, Dalmasso AP, et al. Transgenic swine lungs expressing human CD59 are protected from injury in a pig-to-human model of xenotransplantation. *J Thorac Cardiovasc Surg* 2000; **119**: 690–699.

65 Azimzadeh A, Zorn GL III, Blair KSA, et al. Synergistic effect of soluble and membrane complement inhibition to attenuate porcine pulmonary hyperacute rejection. *Xenotransplantation* 2002; in press.

66 Mulligan MS, Warner RL, Rittershaus CW, et al. Endothelial targeting and enhanced antiinflammatory effects of complement inhibitors possessing sialyl Lewis^x moieties. *J Immunol* 1999; **162**: 4952–4959.

67 Mulligan MS, Schmid E, Till GO, et al. C5a-dependent upregulation in vivo of lung vascular P-selectin. *J Immunol* 1997; **158**: 1857–1861.

68 Simon AR, Warrens AN, Sykes M. Efficacy of adhesive interactions in pig-to-human xenotransplantation. *Immunol Today* 1999; **20**: 323–330.

69 Warrens AN, Simon AR, Theodore PR, Sykes M. Human–porcine receptor–ligand compatibility within the immune system: relevance for xenotransplantation. *Xenotransplantation* 1999; **6**: 75–78.

70 Bernard GR, Vincent JL, Laterre PF, et al. Recombinant human protein C Worldwide Evaluation in Severe Sepsis (PROWESS) Study Group. Efficacy and safety of recombinant human activated protein C for severe sepsis. *N Engl J Med* 2001; **344**: 699–709.

71 Grey ST, Tsuchida A, Hau H, Orthner CL, Salem HH, Hancock WW. Selective inhibitory effects of the anticoagulant activated

protein C on the responses of human mononuclear phago-cytes to LPS, IFN-gamma, or phorbol ester. *J Immunol* 1994; **153**: 3664–3672.

72 Hirose K, Okajima K, Taoka Y, et al. Activated protein C reduces the ischemia/reperfusion-induced spinal cord injury in rats by inhibiting neutrophil activation. *Ann Surg* 2000; **232**: 272–280.

73 Grinnell BW, Hermann RB, Yan SB. Human protein C inhibits selectin-mediated cell adhesion: role of unique fucosylated oligosaccharide. *Glycobiology* 1994; **4**: 221–225.

74 Robson SC, Young VK, Cook NS, et al. Thrombin inhibition in an ex vivo model of porcine heart xenograft hyperacute rejection. *Transplantation* 1996; **61**: 862–868.

75 Robson SC, Kaczmarek E, Seigel JB, et al. Loss of ATP diphos-phohydrolase activity with endothelial activation. *J Exp Med* 1997; **185**: 153–163.

76 Nagayasu T, Saadi S, Holzknecht RA, Plummer TB, Platt JL. Ex-pression of tissue factor mRNA in cardiac xenografts: clues to the pathogenesis of acute vascular rejection. *Transplantation* 2000; **69**: 475–482.

77 Alwayn IP, Appel JZ, Goepfert C, Buhler L, Cooper DK Robson SC. Inhibition of platelet aggregation in baboons: therapeu-tic implications for xenotransplantation. *Xenotransplantation* 2000; **7**: 247–257.

78 Bustos M, Saadi S, Platt JL. Platelet-mediated activation of en-dothelial cells: implications for the pathogenesis of transplant rejection. *Transplantation* 2001; **72**: 509–515.

79 Schulte am Esch J II, Cruz MA, Siegel JB, Anrather J, Robson SC. Activation of human platelets by the membrane-expressed A1 domain of von Willebrand factor. *Blood* 1997; **90**: 4425–4437.

80 Siegel JB, Grey ST, Lesnikoski BA et al. Xenogeneic endothelial cells activate human prothrombin. *Transplantation* 1997; **64**: 888–896.

81 Kalady MF, Lawson JH, Sorrell RD, Platt JL. Decreased fibri-nolytic activity in porcine-to-primate cardiac xenotransplan-tation. *Mol Med* 1998; **4**: 629–637.

82 Saadi S, Holzknecht RA, Patte CP, Stern DM, Platt JL. Complement-mediated regulation of tissue factor activity in endothelium. *J Exp Med* 1995; **182**: 1807–1814.

83 Holzknecht ZE, Coombes S, Blocher BA, Lau CL, Davis RD, Platt JL. Identification of antigens on porcine pulmonary mi-crovascular endothelial cells recognized by human xenoreac-tive natural antibodies. *Lab Invest* 1999; **79**: 763–773.

84 Miyazake Y, Momura S, Miyake T, et al. High shear stress can initiate both platelet aggregation and shedding of procoagu-lant containing microparticles. *Blood*; **88**: 3456–3464.

85 Finger EB, Puri KD, Alon R, Lawrence MB, Andrian UH, Springer TA. Adhesion through L-selectin requires a thresh-old hydrodynamic shear. *Nature* 1996; **379**: 266–269.

86 Pfeiffer S, Zorn GL III, Zhang JP, et al. Hyperacute lung rejec-tion in the pig-to-human model. 3. Platelet receptor inhibitors synergistically modulate complement activation and lung in-jury. *Transplantation* 2003, in press.

87 Collins BJ, Blum MG, Parker RE, et al. Thromboxane medi-ates pulmonary hypertension and lung inflammation during hyperacute lung rejection. *J Appl Physiol* 2001; **90**: 2257–2268.

88 Bahnak BR, Wu QY, Coulombel L, et al. Expression of von Willebrand factor in porcine vessels: heterogeneity at the level of von Willebrand factor mRNA. *J Cell Physiol* 1989; **138**: 305–310.

89 Yamamoto K, de Waard V, Fearns C, Loskutoff DJ. Tissue distri-bution and regulation of murine von Willebrand factor gene expression in vivo. *Blood* 1998; **92**: 2791–2801.

90 Zorn GL, Pfeiffer S, Azimzadeh A, Pierson RN III. Thrombin inhibition protects the pulmonary xenograft from hyperacute rejection. *Surgical Forum* 2000; **XLXI**: 338–340.

91 Esmon CT. Role of coagulation inhibitors in inflammation. *Thromb Haemost* 2001; **86**: 51–56.

92 Cocks TM, Moffatt JD. Protease-activated receptor-2 (PAR2) in the airways. *Pulm Pharmacol Ther* 2001; **14**: 183–191.

93 Yokasaki Y, Sheppard D. Mapping of the cryptic integrin-binding site in osteopontin suggests a new mechanism by which thrombin can regulate inflammation and tissue repair. *Trends Cardiovasc Med* 2000; **10**: 155–159.

94 Murphy JT, Duffy SL, Hybki DL, Kamm K. Thrombin-mediated permeability of human microvascular pulmonary endothelial cells is calcium dependent. *J Trauma* 2001; **50**: 213–222.

95 Chi L, Li Y, Stehno-Bittel L, et al. Interleukin-6 production by endothelial cells via stimulation of protease-activated re-ceptors is amplified by endotoxin and tumor necrosis factor-alpha. *J Interferon Cytokine Res* 2001; **21**: 231–240.

96 Kamholz SL, Brewer RJ, Grijalva G, et al. Laboratory studies in cross-species lung transplantation. *World J Surg* 1997; **21**: 951–955.

97 Cooper DKC, Keogh AM, Brink J, et al. Report of the Xeno-transplantation Advisory Committee of the International So-ciety for Heart and Lung Transplantation: the present status of xenotransplantation and its potential role in the treatment of end-stage cardiac and pulmonary diseases. *J Heart Lung Transplant* 2000; **19**: 1125–1165.

98 Cooper DKC, Lanza RP *Xeno – the promise of transplanting an-imal organs into humans*. Oxford University Press, New York, 2000.

99 Hammer C. Comments on ethics in human transplantation. In: Cooper DKC, Kemp E, Platt JL, White DJG, eds. *Xenotrans-plantation: The Transplantation of Organs and Tissues between species*, 2nd edn. Springer-Verlag, Heidelberg, 1997: 766–775.

100 Maruyama S, Cantu E III, Pernis B, et al. Alpha-galactosyl anti-body redistributes alpha-galactosyl at the surface of pig blood and endothelial cells. *Transpl Immunol* 1999; **7**: 101–106.

101 Di Carlo A, Tector AJ, Tan M, et al. Complement inactivation does not attenuate endothelial cell activation in pig-to-human liver xenotransplantation. *Surg Forum* 2001; **52**: 299–300.

102 Grehan JF, Benson BA, Bolman RM, Dalmasso AP. Porcine interleukin-4 protects porcine aortic endothelial cells from human complement-mediated injury. *Surg Forum* 2001; **52**: 301–302.

103 Perez de la Lastra JM, Harris CL, Hinchliffe SJ, Holt DS, Rush-mere NK, Morgan BP. Pigs express multiple forms of decay-accelerating factor (CD55), all of which contain only three short consensus repeats. *J Immunol* 2000; **165**: 2563–2573.

29

The artificial lung

Brack G. Hattler[1,2] and William J. Federspiel[2]

[1]University of Pittsburgh Medical Center, Pittsburgh, Pennsylvania, USA
[2]University of Pittsburgh, Pennsylvania, USA

Introduction

Over the last 50 years, we have seen remarkable progress in the area of cardiac support as it pertains to artificial organs. Artificial hearts and ventricular assist devices have changed the way we think about end-stage chronic heart failure. Yet the area of the artificial lung has lingered behind many of these accomplishments, not because the need was not recognized but because a full understanding of the engineering problems and the unique material requirements had not reached a level of development to be fully evident. This has changed, and at the centre of this progress has been a close collaboration between the clinician-scientist and the engineer. Here, the underlying concepts that are fundamental to gas exchange in blood have been instrumental in guiding research and in defining the haemodynamic impact on the host as it pertains to both extra- and intracorporeal artificial lung devices [1]. An overview of how this change has occurred and where it appears to be leading us is the subject of this chapter.

Background

Artificial lung technology can be broadly classified into current and next generation (Figure 29.1). What is presently available to clinicians derives from the pioneering work of John Gibbon and his contemporaries who, in the 1950s, developed the early prototypes of the heart–lung machine [2–5]. The goal of these pioneers was to support the heart and the lungs during heart surgery, and the objectives in the design of their oxygenators predicted many of the parameters for artificial lungs under current development. As Galletti and Brecher enumerated, the 'ideal' oxygenator must achieve the following [6]:

1 Oxygenation of venous by blood safely and efficiently bringing blood into close proximity to the oxygen source. The barrier posed by large diffusion distances must be overcome while providing oxygenation over a wide range of venous inlet conditions.

2 Carbon dioxide must be safely and efficiently eliminated to avoid both arterial hyper- and hypocapnia.

3 The oxygenator must avoid high shear stress, turbulence, and incompatible surfaces so as to minimize damage to blood cells, platelets and proteins.

4 The oxygenator must be able to perform its functions with a small priming volume.

5 The oxygenator must be easy and safe to operate, minimizing especially the possibility of air embolism.

These design objectives and early work evolved over the ensuing 40 years to the cardiopulmonary bypass circuits that we use today, with an excessive area of external, synthetic material exposed to the blood through tubes and cannulas, heat exchangers, and several square metres of membrane surface area in the oxygenator – overall a very bioactive environment conducive to the activation of the complement and coagulation cascades along with a host of inflammatory mediators. A goal, therefore, to improving any support systems in the future includes a means of reducing synthetic material interactions by reducing the bulk of material to which the blood is exposed. Next generation technology takes into consideration this fact and attempts to reduce the synthetic material exposed to blood whether in a paracorporeal or intracorporeal configuration.

ECMO

Although support of the lungs was integral to cardiopulmonary bypass during heart surgery, the emphasis was not on the lungs or on any form of targeted lung disease.

Artificial Lung Technology

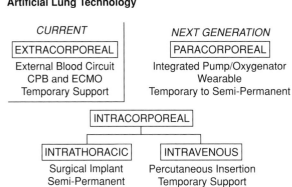

Figure 29.1 Artificial lung technology: current and next generation. CPB, cardiopulmonary bypass; ECMO, extracorporeal membrane oxygenation.

ECMO For Respiratory Failure
(U. of Michigan Experience)

	Numbers	Mortality
Neonates	586	12%
Children	132	30%
Adults	146	44%

Figure 29.2 Recent results from the University of Michigan experience with extracorporeal membrane oxygenation.

Therefore, as attention turned to the lungs, a natural extension of cardiopulmonary bypass for heart surgery was extracorporeal membrane oxygenation (ECMO), which used the same approach and equipment but concentrated on support of the lungs. In spite of the fact that early trials with ECMO in the 1970s were not encouraging and had mortality rates as high as 80–90% in adult patients with the acute respiratory distress syndrome (ARDS), interest in extracorporeal lung support has continued [7,8]. More recent trials by experienced clinicians such as the Michigan group have lowered this mortality in the adult to 40–50% (Figure 29.2) [9]. This is still a challenge to be further improved upon but clearly a great deal has been learned since the early trials of ECMO that could be applied to the concept of an artificial lung.

Artificial lungs

Artificial lung development can be categorized broadly into devices that are intended as implantable or paracorporeal for prolonged and total support, and intravenous devices

The Artificial Lung

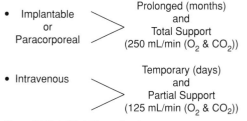

Figure 29.3 Artificial lung development.

The Artificial Lung

- Chronic Lung Disease (Months of support) ⟶ Bridge to Transplant
- Acute Respiratory Failure (Days to weeks of support) ⟶ Bridge to Recovery

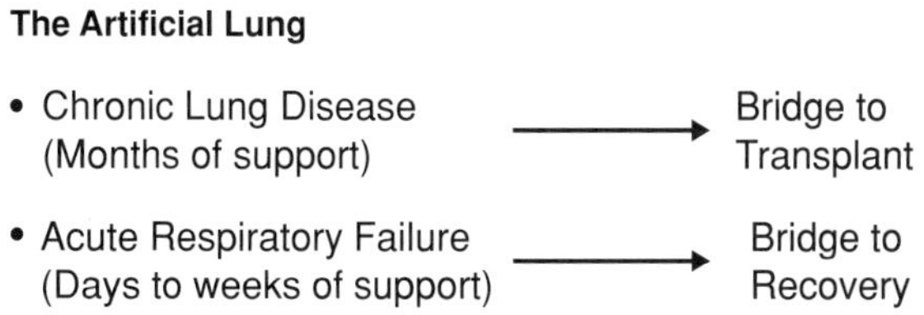

Figure 29.4 The artificial lung as a bridge to transplant or to recovery.

that will provide only temporary and partial support for the lung (Figure 29.3). At present, both implantable and paracorporeal devices would function as a bridge to transplant, whereas intravenous devices that provide only partial support can be used only in the setting where the natural lungs should recover either from a reversible disease or from an acute exacerbation of a chronic lung condition.

Whether one is considering total or partial support, the metabolic requirements for basal gas exchange are different. Total and prolonged support is usually conceptualized in the setting of chronic irreversible lung disease and the invasiveness involved with its implementation makes it less attractive as a temporary support measure (Figure 29.4). Partial support as a bridge to recovery, however, depends on the fact that, even with severe acute respiratory failure, there are areas of the lung that retain relatively normal architecture and compliance [10]. These areas can be accessed for their contribution to gas exchange along with what would in addition be provided by a partial support device. The extent to which partial support assists in gas exchange would enhance the ability to proportionally reduce tidal volumes and peak inspiratory pressures while managing the ventilator in the patient with acute respiratory failure. A 22% reduction in mortality was recently reported in ARDS patients treated with low tidal volume ventilation (6 mL/kg) when compared with the increased death rate with higher tidal volumes (12 mL/kg) [11]. The gas exchange goal of partial support of the lungs is also different from that of total support. Partial support attempts only to

Oxygen Provided By Respiratory Assist Catheter as a Function of Percentage of Lung Functioning

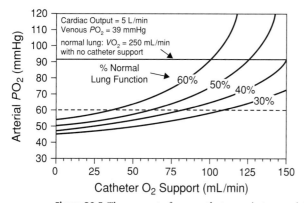

Figure 29.5 The amount of oxygen that a respiratory assist catheter positioned in the venous system would have to add to an adult patient with a normal hematocrit, cardiac output, and venous PCO_2 39 mmHg (1 mmHg $\approx$ 133.3 Pa) as determined by the amount of residual lung still functional.

supplement, in the case of oxygen, by adding enough O_2 to the patient's blood to raise the pressure of oxygen (PO_2) to 60 mmHg (8 kPa) or a saturation of 90% or greater. Adding 100–125 mL O_2/min to the patient represented graphically in Figure 29.5 would be life sustaining, even though only 30% of the patient's lung is functional.

Basic principles for artificial lungs

Before considering examples of artificial lungs that are at various stages of development, it is important to remember several principles of gas exchange, for both O_2 and CO_2, as they would apply to any artificial lung. An in-depth review of these concepts and the theoretical basis behind them can be found in a recent review [1]. The more important of these principles are summarized here:

1 Positioned within the bloodstream, microporous hollow fibre membranes, the working component for gas exchange of any artificial lung, function by diffusion gradients determined by the partial pressures of O_2 and CO_2 on either side of the hollow fibre membrane wall. The gas flow in the lumen of these hydrophobic hollow fibres is 100% oxygen, here represented as 760 mmHg (101 kPa) at sea level (Figure 29.6), which allows oxygen to enter the blood. The concentration of carbon dioxide within the blood promotes entry into the fibres and removal with the exhaust gas. These hollow fibres are usually coated with a micrometre thick or thinner layer of a silicon polymer that prevents plasma from leaking into the fibre

How Microporous Hollow Fibre Membranes Work

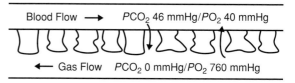

Figure 29.6 Diffusion gradients for O_2 and CO_2 as established by blood flow on one side of the wall of a hollow fibre membrane and gas flow on the opposite side. Oxygen diffuses into the blood and CO_2 into the hollow fibre membrane lumen.

after prolonged use. In addition, heparin is bonded to the fibre lumen surface to enhance thrombo-resistance and in general promote a reduced reactive response engendered by any artificial surface.

2 Gas transfer for oxygen and carbon dioxide from the hollow fibre lumen of an artificial lung to the blood and vice versa is determined at both the membrane level and the blood level by permeability coefficients (K) for each gas, which take into account how the gas diffuses initially in its gaseous (K_g) environment, when it encounters the membrane (K_m) and finally when it reaches the liquid–blood barrier (K_l). The mass transfer for oxygen (KO_2) can therefore be expressed as: $KO_2 = K_g + K_m + K_l$. Diffusion of a gas in a gaseous environment is essentially unimpeded, and therefore the only two components of the equation that are of practical importance would be diffusion through the hollow fibre membrane wall (K_m) and diffusion on the liquid side (blood side) of the fibres (K_l). Thus liquid-side and membrane gas permeabilities dictate overall gas exchange and represent serial transport processes with the micrometre thin liquid boundary layer (K_l) adjacent to the fibre wall representing the predominant resistance to gas diffusion.

3 Agitated blood flow as provided by a pulsating balloon leads to improved gas exchange when compared to unagitated flow because it enhances the permeability coefficient (K) for oxygen and carbon dioxide, especially as it relates to its effect in improving permeability at the liquid boundary layer (K_l).

4 Fibres woven into constrained fibre mats (as compared to free fibres) enforce a precise spacing between fibres, increasing the uniformity and reproducibility of balloon-generated blood flow through the hollow fibre membrane fabrics and eliminating the potential for fibres to clump together once exposed to blood.

5 Finally, the gas exchange can be improved if the blood flows at right angles to the hollow fibres, a condition known as cross-flow, which is significantly more efficient

Design Specifications for an Implantable Artificial Lung

- Capable of transferring > 200 mL/min of O_2 and CO_2
- Minimal shunting
- Blood-side pressure loss < 15 mmHg at blood flow rates of 4–6 L/min
- Low gas-side pressures to avoid gas embolism
- Compliant housing chamber
- Size and configuration to fit in hemithorax
- Thromboresistant and otherwise biocompatible
- Reliability and durability to function at least 2–3 months

Figure 29.7 Specifications for an implantable artificial lung designed for total support.

at O_2–CO_2 transfer than parallel flow, where the blood flow is parallel to the fibres.

Keeping these principles in mind, design specifications for an implantable total artificial lung are listed in Figure 29.7 [12]. Most of these specifications are obvious, such as biocompatibility, gas transfer requirements, size, and function for two to three months. Other specifications require comment such as blood-side pressure loss, which must be as low as possible to avoid failure of the right ventricle as it provides inflow to the oxygenator. Also, the need for a compliant chamber as part of the oxygenator is important when one remembers that the natural lungs work under conditions of low resistance and high compliance. Both of these conditions are favourable to the right ventricle, and compliance allows red cells to be distributed to the pulmonary capillaries both in the systolic and diastolic phases of the cardiac cycle.

Next-generation artificial lungs

Artificial lung technology for the next generation has proponents for both paracorporeal and intracorporeal implementation (Figure 29.8). The paracorporeal approach involves invasively sewing grafts onto the right atrium and pulmonary artery or the right atrium and aorta, bringing these grafts through the chest wall and attaching them to an integrated pump oxygenator (Figure 29.9). Paracorporeal devices are intended to be tethered by very short grafts to the patient and to be wearable. In reality, they are simplified forms of ECMO or ECCO$_2$R (extracorporeal carbon dioxide removal). The oxygenator, however, is smaller and more efficient, and there is less synthetic material exposed to the blood. A paracorporeal device that is being developed at the University of Pittsburgh has a rotating disk of hollow fibres that spins and propels the blood while oxygenating and removing CO_2 (Figure 29.10). The ability

Artificial Lung Technology

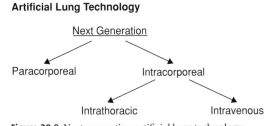

Next Generation

Paracorporeal   Intracorporeal

Intrathoracic   Intravenous

Figure 29.8 Next generation artificial lung technology.

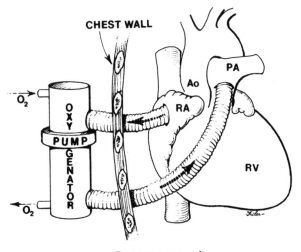

CHEST WALL

O_2

OXYGENATOR

PUMP

O_2

PA

Ao

RA

RV

Paracorporeal

Figure 29.9 Paracorporeal configuration for total pulmonary support. The integrated pump-oxygenator is tethered to the chest wall. PA, pulmonary artery; RV, right ventricle; RA, right atrium; AO, aorta.

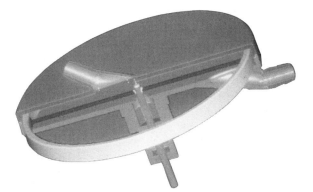

Figure 29.10 A spinning disk oxygenator that both oxygenates and propels blood, being developed as a paracorporeal device.

to have access to the oxygenator should it fail is attractive. Also, it becomes clear that, with a paracorporeal approach, one is following down the same path that cardiac ventricular assist devices did years ago. A paracorporeal device that is being developed by Tatsumi and colleagues in Japan has been able to provide total gas exchange requirements in goats for five to seven days with the animals ambulatory [13]. The benefits of a paracorporeal device include, therefore, its compact size and its integrated functions.

With intracorporeal or implantable devices, there are two choices – intrathoracic or intravenous (Figure 29.8). The intrathoracic requires a surgical implant, the oxygenator is intended to be internally positioned with oxygen lines exiting the left chest. It is a semi-permanent support as a bridge to transplant, less suitable for temporary support in its present configuration because of the invasiveness involved. Although intended for intracorporeal use, these devices are tested in the research laboratory, with the oxygenator positioned paracorporeally, although connected to the native vasculature as if the device were intrathoracic. Intrathoracic insertion involves placing the device either in series (Figure 29.11) where the right ventricle drives the blood through the oxygenator and then returns it to the distal pulmonary artery with no communication between the proximal and distal pulmonary artery, or the oxygenator can be placed in parallel where blood is returned to the left atrium (Figure 29.12). A third possibility not represented is that blood would be returned from the oxygenator to both the pulmonary artery and the left atrium in a so-called hybrid configuration. A distinct advantage of the hybrid configuration is that, in providing some pulmonary

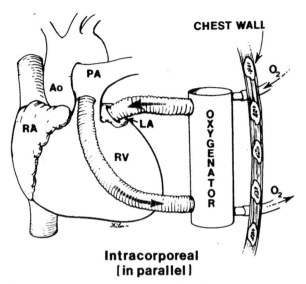

Intracorporeal [in parallel]

Figure 29.12 Intracorporeal, in parallel, artificial lung. Partial banding of the distal pulmonary artery (not shown) controls the volume of blood diverted to the oxygenator. For abbreviations, see Figure 30.9.

artery flow, it helps to maintain nongas exchange properties of the lung as they pertain to metabolic and hormonal functions.

Two groups have devoted a considerable effort in the development of an intrathoracic lung, the group at the University of Michigan under the leadership of Drs Bartlett, Montoya and Lynch, and the group at Northwestern University under the leadership of Drs Mockros and Vaslef (present address, Duke University Medical Center). An example of the Michigan lung is seen in Figure 29.13, with its contained attachment grafts and, in its most recent configuration, a compliant external housing made of an elastomir, which allows for improved haemodynamics as far as the right ventricle is concerned as it ejects into a compliant chamber before the blood is distributed to the oxygenator [14–18]. Sheep have been totally supported for up to seven days with the Michigan lung with no pump except the right ventricle to drive the blood. These devices are frequently called 'pumpless devices' because there is no artificial blood pump. Mockros et al. have also developed an intracorporeal-intrathoracic lung also with a compliant casing [14, 19–22]. This pumpless artificial lung (Figure 29.14) has been tested mainly in a parallel configuration with a proximal graft sewn to the pulmonary artery that receives the output of the right ventricle and the distal graft sewn to the left atrium. By banding the distal pulmonary artery, the amount of blood directed through the oxygenator can be controlled. Total gas exchange in

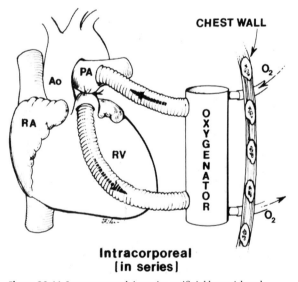

Intracorporeal [in series]

Figure 29.11 Intracorporeal, in series artificial lung. A band between the proximal and distal pulmonary artery assures that all right ventricular output is diverted to the oxygenator. For abbreviations, see Figure 29.9.

Michigan Lung

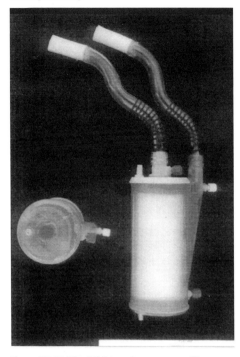

Figure 29.13 The Michigan intracorporeal lung. A compliant external housing can be seen receiving the graft connected to the proximal pulmonary artery (not shown). The tubing and graft exiting the centre of the oxygenator connects to the distal pulmonary artery.

A Thoracic Artificial Lung

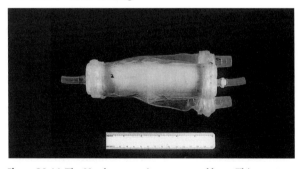

Figure 29.14 The Northwestern intracorporeal lung. This most recent prototype shows very clearly the compliant external layer surrounding the fibre bundle that receives the output of the right ventricle.

The Artificial Lung (Areas of Concern)

	Intracorporeal (Intrathoracic Artificial Lung)	Paracorporeal (Artificial Lung)
Invasiveness	+	+
RV Strain	+	–
Need for Blood Pump	–	+
Blood Trauma	–	+
Blood side Pressure Loss (oxygenator flow)	+	–
Potential for Mechanical failure	–	+
Potential for Oxygenator failure	+	+

Figure 29.15 A comparison of intracorporeal and paracorporeal devices. Intracorporeal devices, although tested in the research laboratory outside the chest, are intended for intrathoracic placement. RV, right ventricular.

pigs has been provided for over 24 hours with the artificial lung providing complete support. So, comparing intrathoracic (implantable) lungs with paracorporeal lungs that are intended as a wearable device outside the body, the following points can be made (Figure 29.15):

1 They are both significantly invasive.
2 Right ventricular strain is not a concern with a paracorporeal device driven by an external pump.
3 Blood trauma over a prolonged period of time is of greater concern with paracorporeal devices because of the higher shear stresses potentially involved with the pump function.
4 Blood-side pressure losses are a concern if the right ventricle is the driving force for propelling blood through the oxygenator.

Both paracorporeal and intracorporeal (implantable) devices are being readied for clinical trials in the next three to five years.

Artificial lungs can best be thought of as those that are being developed as bridge to transplant and those that are intended as a bridge to recovery for short-term use in the treatment of reversible, acute respiratory failure. Short-term support with the intracorporeal artificial lung is the only technology that has been tested in humans and occurred when the intravascular oxygenator (IVOX) developed by J. D. Mortensen underwent clinical trials, following its insertion into the human vena cava, in the early 1990s [23] (Figure 29.16). The device consisted of a bundle of microporous hollow fibre membranes through which oxygen was extracted under vacuum. Devices tested clinically ranged in membrane surface area from 0.21 to 0.51 m². The hollow fibre membranes of the IVOX were crimped

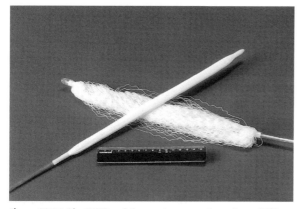

Figure 29.16 The IVOX and the respiratory assist catheter (HC) juxtaposed. The IVOX as seen here was used in clinical trials [23].

along their length in an effort to produce secondary fluid currents around the fibres. Otherwise, the device resided in the central venous system and was dependent upon passive parallel flow past the fibres to promote gas exchange. The fibres were free-floating and, lacking constraint, randomly assumed their position, including the propensity for some fibres to clump together once placed in the venous system. The polypropylene microporous hollow fibre membranes of the IVOX had an ultrathin siloxane coating, permeable to O_2 and CO_2, but impermeable to water, thus preventing the membrane pores from being subject to plasma leakage. A second coating applied to all components of the IVOX was a covalently bonded heparin derivative intended to increase the thrombo-resistance of the device. The IVOX is the only intracorporeal device to have undergone phase I and phase II human clinical trials in the early 1990s. The phase I trials established the safety for introducing an intravascular oxygenator in humans, and the phase II trial examined the clinical efficacy and gas exchange performance for this device. A total of 160 patients from the USA and Europe was studied. Once entry criteria for acute lung failure were met, patients underwent a right internal jugular or femoral vein cutdown for device implantation. The largest size IVOX (0.21–0.51 m^2 membrane surface area) was chosen for implantation according to the vena cava size determined by ultrasound and the suitability of the access vein. The IVOX was furled during insertion and guided over a wire into position in the inferior vena cava, right atrium, and superior vena cava, where unfurling occurred to fully expose the hollow fibre membranes to the returning venous blood. Heparinization (activated clotting time 180–200 s) was maintained during use of the device. After activation of the IVOX, attempts were made to reduce the fraction of oxygen in inspired gas (F_IO_2) and minute ventilation as long as blood gases could

be maintained, with oxygen saturations over 90%. The IVOX trials confirmed earlier animal experiments and proved the feasibility of extended intravenous respiratory gas exchange in severe acute respiratory failure patients [23]. In some patients, peak O_2 and CO_2 transfer rates varying between 40 and 70 mL/min were noted. During IVOX utilization, some clinical trial patients showed improvement in blood gas partial pressures and the ability to reduce the intensity of mechanical ventilation. The IVOX functioned in some patients for weeks without adverse effects. In these severely ill patients with acute respiratory failure, 60% survived to have the device removed, but only 30% improved to a point where mechanical ventilation could be discontinued. These same patients were hospital survivors and were discharged for an average 30% survival rate. Further trials of the IVOX were not pursued because of failure to show improvement in survival compared with historical controls. Food and Drug Administration consideration was not in question because of the lack of concurrent controls and randomization in the clinical trials. Nevertheless, as the first and only trial of a short-term intravenous oxygenator designed for support of the patient while the lungs recover, the IVOX provided valuable evidence that gas exchange (O_2 and CO_2) occurs in humans, but at a level that at the very best met only 30% of patients' needs and was frequently not reproducible. Very significantly, the trial demonstrated that hollow fibre membranes could reside in the human vena cava for prolonged periods without haemodynamic compromise or thrombus formation. Those involved in the clinical trial of the IVOX felt that, in order to be clinically useful, an intravenous respiratory assist device would have to supply 50% of basal metabolic needs (Figure 29.5), be relatively easily insertible, and demonstrate consistent and reproducible gas exchange in patients with acute respiratory failure. These recommendations for improvements have been instrumental in our approach to designing devices dedicated to gas exchange in the venous system.

Gas exchange within the venous system

Our interest in the development of an intravenous hollow fibre membrane lung-assist device, the Hattler Respiratory Support Catheter, or Hattler Catheter (HC)* began

---

* Also reported in previous publications as the Intravenous Membrane Oxygenator (IMO) for use in intracorporeal membrane oxygenation. The catheter-based device, however, exchanges both oxygen and carbon dioxide. Simply describing it as a membrane oxygenator is not sufficient. It is intended for temporary respiratory support in cases of acute respiratory failure.

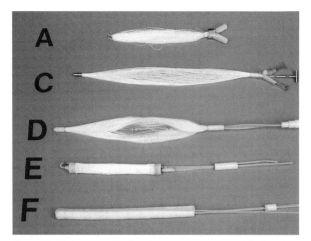

Figure 29.17 An example of various prototypes tested during the development of the respiratory assist catheter (HC). Prototype 'A' was the earliest prototype, tested in 1984.

with early prototype design and animal testing in 1984 [1]. These initial efforts were primitive compared to devices now being tested and involved bulky bundles of hollow fibres through which 100% oxygen would flow (Figure 29.17). Both ends of each hollow fibre were potted into a single proximal manifold so that O_2 and CO_2 exchange would occur as the oxygen traversed the full length of the fibre (Figure 29.17, example A). To avoid gas emboli, oxygen was extracted by vacuum through the fibres. In vivo testing of these devices following surgical placement in the vena cava of dogs revealed that O_2 and CO_2 exchange occurred, but at levels that were not considered of clinical value [1]. It became apparent during these early experiments that passive and undisturbed flow of blood in the vena cava, flow that was largely parallel to the hollow fibres, did not provide adequate gas exchange. Our efforts have evolved, therefore, over the ensuing years in defining conditions that allow for better mixing of the blood with the hollow fibre membrane bundle and in providing cross-flow to the fibres that are represented within the hollow fibre membrane mats [1, 24–40]. The devices on which we have concentrated our efforts have always been intended to be catheter based, and introduced and removed through either the jugular or the femoral vein. Once in the venous system, the goal has been to provide up to 50% of the basal oxygen and carbon dioxide exchange requirements in the adult patient over a 7–10 day interval of support (Figure 29.5). In reality, shorter intervals of support may be of benefit. A recent National Institutes of Health trial has provided evidence that, as early as 48 hours following the institution of a lung protective strategy, an improvement in the pulmonary status of ARDS patients can be seen [11]. Zwishenberger et al.

have confirmed these clinical findings in an ovine smoke inhalation model of acute lung injury [41]. Our goals, therefore, in developing a respiratory assist catheter have been as follows:

1 Provision of active mixing of blood at right angles and across the hollow fibre membranes.
2 Provision of O_2 and CO_2 exchange at approximately 125 mL/min for both (50% of basal requirements) with the ability of CO_2 exchange to progressively increase with permissive hypercapnea, as is seen with reduced tidal volume ventilation as a lung protective strategy in the therapy of acute respiratory failure.
3 The device must maintain its gas exchange functions for 5–10 days in the therapy of patients with reversible acute lung injury.
4 The device must be relatively thrombo-resistant and resistant to plasma leakage into the hollow fibres by incorporating a thin polymer coating (less than 1 μm) to which a heparin molecule is attached. Under these conditions, and with a device that actively moves blood through the fibres, the need for full anticoagulation is decreased.
5 The device must be made of constrained hollow fibre mats, thus preventing fibre clumping. Fibres are thus maintained in a consistent configuration regardless of their contained vessel, which enhances reproducible gas exchange for devices of identical membrane surface area.
6 The device, although initially requiring a cut-down to directly expose the vein for insertion, should eventually be designed for percutaneous insertion.

The catheter-based device that has been designed to meet these requirements is shown in Figure 29.18. For comparison, the IVOX that was used in the clinical trials in the early 1990s and the respiratory assist catheter (HC) are

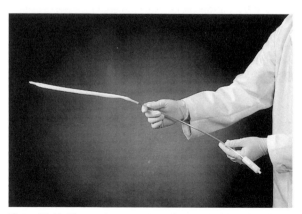

Figure 29.18 The respiratory assist catheter (HC) being held by a technician.

Operational Features of the IMO

- Pulsating balloon within device captures normal vena cava blood flow and drives it across hollow fibre membranes.

- This 'active' mixing leads to more gas transfer (O_2 and CO_2), less required fibre area. Better artificial respiration.

- Constrained fibre bundles are designed not to occupy the entire cross-section of the vena cava.

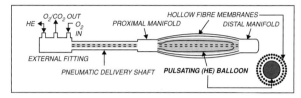

Figure 29.19 The respiratory assist catheter (HC) in position.

Description of IMO

- Insert through femoral or jugular vein

- Resides in superior and inferior vena cava, incorporating right atrium

- Oxygenates venous blood and removes carbon dioxide before blood reaches the lungs

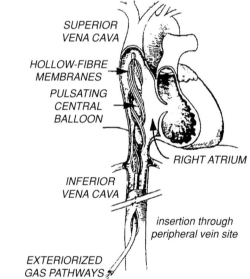

Figure 29.20 Operational features of the respiratory assist catheter (HC or IMO) (see text).

superimposed on each other as seen in Figure 29.16. A schematic of the respiratory assist catheter (HC) that is being readied for clinical trials in Europe in 2004 is shown in Figure 29.19 and how it would sit in a patient in Figure 29.20. Hollow fibre membrane mats surround a central balloon in concentric layers. These hollow fibres are potted into proximal and distal manifolds at each end of the device. The gas exchange component therefore sits at the end of a catheter through which 100% oxygen flows to the proximal manifold and is extracted by vacuum from the distal manifold after traversing down the length of each hollow fibre. A separate port provides helium to the balloon

and is driven by a console capable of completely inflating and deflating the balloon at 300 beats/min or greater. The device is inserted at present through a cut-down on the common femoral or internal jugular vein where it then occupies the inferior vena cava, right atrium, and superior vena cava positions. Biocompatibility of the HC is dependent on reducing sheer stress and the potential for blood clotting and fibrin and cellular deposition on the surface of the hollow fibre membranes. A heparin bond linked to a <1 μm thick siloxane coating covering the pores of the hollow fibre membrane has been used to enhance biocompatibility at the blood–membrane interphase. In addition, we have demonstrated that nitric oxide as part of the sweep-gas within the hollow fibres markedly diminishes cellular and platelet deposition on the membrane surface [30]. Other than the use of specialized coatings and controlling the composition of the oxygen mixture being vacuumed through the hollow fibres, a general principle applied to the design of the HC has been to minimize sheer stress as a means of promoting biocompatibility. Flow in the vena cava is largely laminar where sheer stresses occur because adjacent fluid layers travel at different speeds. Fluid in the centre of the stream moves more quickly than fluid near the vessel wall. Therefore sheer rate is highest at the wall and lowest at the centre, where friction is minimal. Flow velocity profiles visualized in the laboratory have shown that balloon pulsation not only improves gas exchange but also disrupts the layer of fluid next to the vessel wall (area of high sheer stress), therefore reducing overall sheer and potential damage to the formed elements of blood (Figure 29.21). Since the HC depends on blood flowing freely around the device where blood is captured and directed towards the fibres by balloon pulsation, very low blood-side pressure drops across the device (2–3 mmHg) have been noted in large animal implants. By reducing the pressure drop, a reduction in sheer stress at the same flow rate is noted, which promotes overall biocompatibility.

Once inserted in the venous system, the respiratory assist catheter (HC) occupies the superior and inferior vena cava, spanning the right atrium. Studies in calves have shown that, while carbon dioxide exchange was studied, the average carbon dioxide flux was 305 ± 25 mL/min per m^2 with the device in the right atrium whereas in the inferior vena cava position it was approximately 265 ± 18 mL/min per m^2. This is not unanticipated, since under these latter

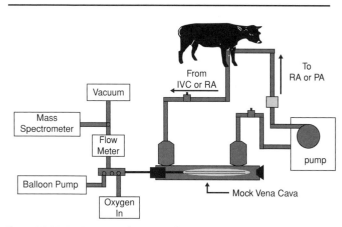

Ex-Vivo Vena Cava Circuit

Figure 29.22 Ex vivo circuit for testing the respiratory assist catheter (HC). Blood from the cow's right atrium (RA) fills a mock vena cava where the HC is positioned. Oxygenated blood is then returned to the pulmonary artery (PA). IVC, intravenous catheter.

conditions, blood entering the right atrium from the upper body would not be exposed to the gas exchange fibres, creating a significant shunt fraction with reduced overall gas exchange. With the HC in the desired position, the total hollow fibre membrane surface area that the blood is exposed to is no more than 0.43 m^2 of membrane surface area. This decreases the magnitude of blood–synthetic material interactions.

In addition to extensive bench-testing, the respiratory assist catheter (HC) has been tested in ex vivo circuits using calves 90–100 kg in weight (Figure 29.22). The HC is positioned in a mock vena cava, which receives blood from the right atrium. The blood, once oxygenated, is pumped back to the pulmonary artery. Continuous gas exchange is measured with a mass spectrometer. Since the IVOX implanted in humans was tested under similar protocols a comparison can be made to the respiratory assist catheter (HC). As seen in Figure 29.23, with no pulsation, the IVOX and respiratory assist catheter (IMO) perform similarly in an ex vivo circuit. However, with balloon pulsation, the respiratory assist catheter significantly increases its gas exchange capability both ex vivo and in vivo following implantation into the calf.

For in vivo testing of the HC over one to five days, we have used calves extensively monitored for haemodynamic and gas exchange parameters. Here the catheter is inserted through the jugular vein. In vivo carbon dioxide removal progressively increases with balloon pulsations up to 300 beats/min (Figure 29.24). Results of short-term implants in cows are seen in Figure 29.25 comparing devices

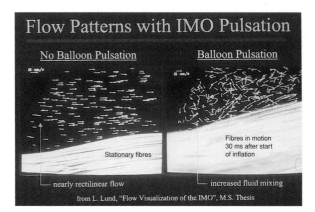

Figure 29.21 The effect of balloon pulsation with a respiratory assist catheter positioned in a flow visualization chamber seeded with fluorescent particles. The computer assigns vectors to each particle's motion.

IMO Gas Exchange Performance

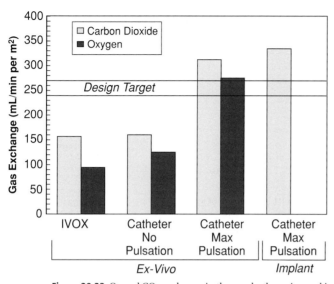

Figure 29.23 O_2 and CO_2 exchange in the cow both ex vivo and in vivo (implant). With no balloon pulsation, the IVOX and the IMO (HC) perform equally. With balloon pulsation (300 beats/min), the HC significantly increases its gas exchange performance both ex vivo and in vivo.

In Vivo CO$_2$ Removal vs. Beat Rate

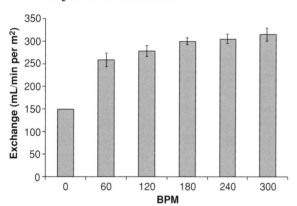

Figure 29.24 In vivo CO_2 gas exchange in the cow as determined by balloon pulsation rate (BPM, beats per minute).

constructed from constrained fibre fabric mats with devices made from free-floating, nonconstrained fibres. Free fibre devices have diminished gas exchange capabilities largely because groups of free floating fibres tend to clump together once in the bloodstream, creating fibres at the centre of the clump that are not exposed to blood.

In chronic experiments carried out over four to five days, gas exchange is maintained constant in the awake and standing animal over this entire time interval [42]. Here,

Acute In Vivo Implantation of IMO

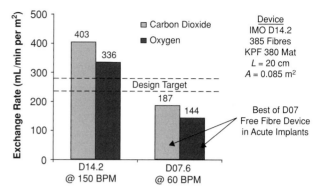

Figure 29.25 In vivo gas exchange performance for two respiratory assist catheters tested in cows. Devices made of fibre mats uniformly perform significantly better than devices made of free floating, non-constrained fibres. L, length; A, area. BPM, beats/min.

haemodynamics, including cardiac output, mean arterial pressure, pulmonary artery pressure, and venous pressures do not change with positioning of the device in the venous system. This is because the device is chosen purposely not to occupy the entire diameter of its containing vessel (i.e. vena cavae and right atrium). Unimpeded flow around the device is essential in order to allow the pulsating balloon to capture and direct blood towards the fibre mat in a cross-flow configuration. Plasma-free haemoglobin rises early in these chronic experiments but returns to levels of 2–4 mg/dL. Autopsies of these animals showed no distal emboli or end-organ failure.

If permissive hypercapnoea is allowed to occur in the calves, the device will increase its CO_2 output as the PCO_2 rises and the minute ventilation drops, raising the possibility that the device could function effectively in patients as tidal volumes are reduced in the therapy of acute respiratory failure (Figure 29.26). Diseases where temporary support may be beneficial are listed in Table 29.1.

Permissive Hypercapnea in the Calf and CO$_2$ Exchange Rate With the Hattler Catheter

PCO_2 (mmHg)	VCO_2 (mL/min per m2)	Minute Ventilation (L/min)
50	320–28	20
60	426–32	–
70	480–45	11

Figure 29.26 The respiratory assist catheter (HC) increases its CO_2 output as the PCO_2 rises with decreased minute ventilation.

Table 29.1. Disease states where temporary support of the lungs may be beneficial

Severe acute respiratory failure

Hypercapnic respiratory failure

Medically resistant status asmaticus

Toxic (chemical) damage to the lungs

In the perioperative lung transplant interval

Persistent pulmonary air leaks

Any setting where reduced ventilation would be beneficial, including patients difficult to wean from the ventilator

Severe reactive pulmonary hypertension with right ventricular failure

Summary

Technology to implement temporary and partial support of the lungs is available today but awaits clinical trials. Technology for chronic (months) and total support of the lungs is being actively investigated with a goal of clinical trials in the next three to five years. Beyond where we are now, the future of artificial lungs will be part of the exciting new field of hybrid organs with genetically engineered stem cells mounted to altered biomaterials (Figure 29.27). This area is with us today in the laboratory and will be part of our future in the care of patients with acute and chronic lung diseases.

Acknowledgements

The work described in this chapter from our group was supported by the US Army Medical Research, Development, Acquisition and Logistics Command, under prior Contract no. DAMDA 17-94-C-4052 and current grant no. DAMD 17-98-1-8638. The views, opinions and findings contained in this chapter are those of the authors and should not be construed as an official Department of the Army position.

REFERENCES

1 Hattler BG, Federspiel WJ. Gas exchange in the venous system: support for the failing lung. In: Vaslef SN, Anderson RW, eds. *The artificial lung.* Landes Bioscience, Austin, TX, 2002.

2 Gibbon JH, Kraul CW. An efficient oxygenator for blood. *J Lab Clin Med* 1941; **26**: 1803–1809.

3 Gibbon JH. Application of a mechanical heart–lung apparatus to cardiac surgery. *Minn Med* 1954; **37**: 171–180.

4 DeWall, Warden HE, Read RC, et al. A simple expendable artificial oxygenator for open heart surgery. *Surg Clin North Am* 1956; **36**: 1025–1034.

5 McCaughan JS, Weeder RR, Schuder JC, et al. Evaluation of new non-wetable microporous membranes with high permeability coefficients for possible use in a membrane oxygenator. *J Thorac Cardiovasc Surg* 1969; **40**: 574–581.

6 Galletti PM, Brecher GA. Bubble oxygenation and membrane oxygenation. In: Heart–lung bypass: principles and techniques of extracorporeal circulation. Grune and Streatton, New York, 1962: 61–78, 108–120.

7 Zapol WM, Snider MT, Hill JD, et al. Extracorporeal membrane oxygenation in severe acute respiratory failure: a randomized prospective study. *JAMA* 1979; **242**: 2193–2196.

8 Gattinoni L, Pesenti A, Masheroni D, et al. Low-frequency positive pressure ventilation with extracorporeal CO_2 removal in severe acute respiratory failure. *JAMA* 1986; **256**: 881–886.

9 Bartlett RH, Roloff DW, Custer JR, et al. Extracorporeal life support: the University of Michigan experience. *JAMA* 2000; **283**: 904–908.

10 Ware LB, Matthay MA. The acute respiratory distress syndrome. *N Engl J Med* 2000; **342**: 1334–1349.

11 The Acute Respiratory Distress Syndrome Network. Ventilation with lower tidal volumes as compared with traditional tidal volumes for acute lung injury and the acute respiratory distress syndrome. *N Engl J Med* 2000; **342**: 1301–1308.

12 Vaslef SN. Implantable artificial lungs: fantasy or feasibility. *New Surg* 2001; **1**: 116–126.

13 Tatsumi E, Takewa Y, Akagi H, et al. Development of an integrated artificial heart–lung device for long-term cardiopulmonary support. *ASAIO J* 1996; **42**: M827–M832.

14 Vaslef SN, Anderson RW. Development of an implantable artificial lung. In: Vaslef SN, Anderson RW, eds. *The artificial lung.* Landes Bioscience, Austin, TX, 2001.

15 Fazzalari RL, Montoya JP, Bonnell MR, et al. The development of an implantable artificial lung. *ASAIO J* 1994; **40**: M728–M731.

16 Fazzalari FL, Bartlett RH, Bonnell MR, et al. An intrapleural lung prosthesis: rationale, design, and testing. *Artif Organs* 1994; **18**: 801–805.

The Future of Artificial Lungs

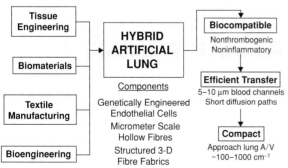

Figure 29.27 The future of artificial lungs will evolve from a close interaction between the life sciences and engineers. 3-D, three dimensional; A/V, area/volume.

17 Lynch WR, Montoya JP, Brant DO, et al. Hemodynamic effect of a low-resistance artificial lung in series with the native lungs of sheep. *Ann Thorac Surg* 2000; **69**: 351–356.

18 Lynch WR, Hatt JW, Montoya JP, et al. Partial respiratory support with an artificial lung perfused by the right ventricle: chronic studies in an active animal model. *ASAIO J* 2000; **46**: 202.

19 Vasleff SN, Mockros LF, Cook KE, et al. Computer-assisted design of an implantable intrathoracic artificial lung. *Artif Org* 1994; **18**: 813–817.

20 Boschetti F, Perlman CE, Cook KE, et al. Hemodynamic effects of attachment modes and device design of a thoracic artificial lung. *ASAIO J* 2000; **46**: 42–48.

21 Vaslef SN, Cook KE, Leonard RJ, et al. Design and evaluation of a new, low pressure loss, implantable artificial lung. *ASAIO J* 1994; **40**: M522–M526.

22 Cook KE, Makarewicz AJ, Backer CL, et al. Testing of an intrathoracic artificial lung in a pig model. *ASAIO J* 1996; **42**: M604–M609.

23 Conrad SA, Bagley A, Bagley B, et al. Major findings from the clinical trials of the intravascular oxygenator. *Artif Organs* 1994; **18**: 846–863.

24 Hattler BG, Johnson PC, Sawzik PJ, et al. Respiratory dialysis: a new concept in pulmonary support. *ASAIO J* 1992; **38**: M322–M325.

25 Reeder GD, Hattler BG, Rawleigh J, et al. Current progress in the development of an intravenous membrane oxygenator. *ASAIO J* 1993; **39**: M461–M465.

26 Hattler BG, Reeder GD, Sawzik PJ, et al. Development of an intravenous membrane oxygenator (IMO): enhanced intravenous gas exchange through convective mixing of blood around hollow fibre membranes. *Artif Organs* 1994; **18**: 806–812.

27 Hattler BG, Reeder GD, Sawzik PJ, et al. Development of an intravenous membrane oxygenator: a new concept in mechanical support for the failing lung. *J Heart Lung Transplant* 1995; **13**: 1003–1007.

28 Federspiel WJ, Hewitt T, Hout MS, et al. Recent progress in engineering the Pittsburgh intravenous membrane oxygenator. *ASAIO J* 1996; **42**: M435–M442.

29 Macha M, Federspiel WJ, Lund LW, et al. Acute in vivo studies of the Pittsburgh intravenous membrane oxygenator. *ASAIO J* 1996; **42**: M609–M615.

30 Konishi R, Shimizer R, Firestone L, et al. Nitric oxide prevents human platelet adhesion to fiber membranes in whole blood. *ASAIO J* 1996; **42**: M850–M853.

31 Lund LW, Federspiel WJ, Hattler BG. Gas permeability of hollow fiber membranes in a gas–liquid system. *J Membr Sci* 1996; **117**: 207–219.

32 Lund LW, Hattler BG, Federspiel WJ. Is condensation the cause of plasma leakage in microporous hollow fiber membrane oxygenators? *J Membr Sci* 1998; **147**: 87–93.

33 Federspiel WJ, Hattler BG. Sweep gas flowrate and CO_2 exchange in artificial lungs. *Artif Org* 1996; **20**: 1050–1056.

34 Hout MS, Hattler BG, Federspiel WJ. Validation of a model for flow-dependent carbon dioxide exchange in artificial lungs. *Artif Organs* 2000; **24**: 114–119.

35 Federspiel WJ, Williams JL, Hattler BG. Gas flow dynamics in hollow fiber membranes. *Ann Inst Chem Eng J* 1996; **42**: 2094–2099.

36 Hewitt TJ, Hattler BG, Federspiel WJ. A mathematical model of gas exchange in an intravenous membrane oxygenator. *Ann Biomed Eng* 1998; **26**: 166–178.

37 Federspiel WJ, Hewitt TJ, Hattler BG. Experimental evaluation of a model for oxygenation exchange in a pulsating intravascular artificial lung. *Ann Biomed Eng* 2000; **28**: 160–167.

38 Federspiel WJ, Hout MS, Hewitt TJ, et al. Development of a low flow resistance intravenous oxygenator. *ASAIO J* 1997; **45**: M725–M730.

39 Federspiel WJ, Golob JF, Merrill TL, et al. Ex-vivo testing of the intravenous membrane oxygenator (IMO). *ASAIO J* 2000; **46**: 261–267.

40 Golob JF, Federspiel WJ, Merrill TL, et al. Acute in-vivo testing of an intravascular respiratory support catheter. *ASAIO J* 2001; **47**: 432–437.

41 Jayroe JB, Alpard SK, Donfang W, et al. Hemodynamic stability during arteriovenous carbon dioxide removal for adult respiratory distress syndrome: a prospective randomized outcomes study in adult sheep. *ASAIO J* 2001; **47**: 211–214.

42 Hattler BG, Lund LW, Golob J, et al. A respiratory gas exchange catheter: in-vitro and in-vivo tests in large animals. *J Thorac Cardiovasc Surg* 2002; **124**: 520–530.

Index